Role Play in
MRCP-PACES

Role Play in MRCP-PACES

Mohammad Ali FCPS MCPS D-Card

Clinical Professor of Medicine and Head
Dhaka Central International Medical College and Hospital
Shyamoli, Dhaka, Bangladesh

Foreword

Quazi Deen Mohammad

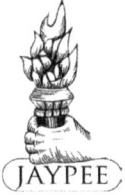

JAYPEE BROTHERS MEDICAL PUBLISHERS
The Health Sciences Publisher

New Delhi | London

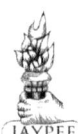

Jaypee Brothers Medical Publishers (P) Ltd

Headquarters
EMCA House
23/23-B, Ansari Road, Daryaganj
New Delhi 110 002, India
Landline: +91-11-23272143, +91-11-23272703
+91-11-23282021, +91-11-23245672
E-mail: jaypee@jaypeebrothers.com

Corporate Office
Jaypee Brothers Medical Publishers (P) Ltd.
4838/24, Ansari Road, Daryaganj
New Delhi 110 002, India
Phone: +91-11-43574357
Fax: +91-11-43574314
E-mail: jaypee@jaypeebrothers.com

Overseas Office
JP Medical Ltd.
83, Victoria Street, London
SW1H 0HW (UK)
Phone: +44-20 3170 8910
Fax: +44(0)20 3008 6180
E-mail: info@jpmedpub.com

Website: www.jaypeebrothers.com
Website: www.jaypeedigital.com

© 2023, Jaypee Brothers Medical Publishers

The views and opinions expressed in this book are solely those of the original contributor(s)/author(s) and do not necessarily represent those of editor(s) or publisher of the book.

All rights reserved. No part of this publication may be reproduced, stored or transmitted in any form or by any means, electronic, mechanical, photocopying, recording or otherwise, without the prior permission in writing of the publishers.

All brand names and product names used in this book are trade names, service marks, trademarks or registered trademarks of their respective owners. The publisher is not associated with any product or vendor mentioned in this book.

Medical knowledge and practice change constantly. This book is designed to provide accurate, authoritative information about the subject matter in question. However, readers are advised to check the most current information available on procedures included and check information from the manufacturer of each product to be administered, to verify the recommended dose, formula, method and duration of administration, adverse effects and contraindications. It is the responsibility of the practitioner to take all appropriate safety precautions. Neither the publisher nor the author(s)/editor(s) assume any liability for any injury and/or damage to persons or property arising from or related to use of material in this book.

This book is sold on the understanding that the publisher is not engaged in providing professional medical services. If such advice or services are required, the services of a competent medical professional should be sought.

Every effort has been made where necessary to contact holders of copyright to obtain permission to reproduce copyright material. If any have been inadvertently overlooked, the publisher will be pleased to make the necessary arrangements at the first opportunity.

Inquiries for bulk sales may be solicited at: jaypee@jaypeebrothers.com

Role Play in MRCP-PACES / Mohammad Ali

First Edition: 2023

ISBN: 978-93-5696-117-3

Dedicated to

My Beloved Son

Maher Ali Rusho

(Ideal Google Boy, Self-learner, Researcher – Future Scientist)

— My inspiration

"The physician must be able to tell the antecedents, know the present, and foretell the future—must mediate these things, and have two special objects in view with regard to disease, namely, to do good or to do no harm."

— **Hippocrates** (460 BC–370 BC)
Father of Medicine

Foreword

I am delighted to write the foreword to this book, written by my student, Professor Mohammad Ali.

The role-play format is the most attractive and unique point of this book. It shows realistic pictures of how a doctor should approach his patient. From welcoming a patient to the doctor, talking to him, listening to him, taking his full history, examining him properly, finding out an appropriate diagnosis and treatment for him, fulfilling the patient's concerns and queries as well as saying goodbye to him, all these are shown through the role-play manner in every topic of this book. I believe candidates will enjoy the journey of their PACES exam with the role-play manner of this book, the postgraduation exam is to prove oneself professionally efficient by applying one's clinical knowledge within the stipulated time, a complete mirror image of which is given in this book. I believe the student will find the difference between this book from the other.

In this book, the author has tried to keep the most important topics that the previous candidates faced at the PACES exam. This book has four main chapters: In physical examination—candidates will learn how to present a case in a confident, fluent, systematic and well-structured manner; appropriate and professional techniques of physical examination and how to identify physical signs correctly. In clinical communication—how to explain clinical information, apply clinical knowledge including knowledge of ethics, manage a case or situation, patient's concerns and maintain patient's welfare respectfully and sensitively, ensuring their comfort, safety, and dignity. In clinical consultation—the candidate will learn focused history taking and focused clinical examination, acknowledge and address the patient's concerns with multiple realistic cases as a role-play station between a patient and a candidate. In history taking—the candidate will learn about detailed history taking and management plans of a patient on the basis of history.

This will be a helping handbook for the MRCP-PACES exam and all the other postgraduate examinations particularly MD, FCPS and other allied. I congratulate the author and editors for their collaborative effort to bring together their experience and expertise to make this book need-based and useful.

Quazi Deen Mohammad
FCPS MD Fellow in Neurology (USA)
President of Bangladesh College of
Physicians and Surgeons (BCPS)
Founding Director of the
National Institute of Neuroscience
Dhaka, Bangladesh

Preface

Practice assessment of clinical examination skills (PACES) is designed to assess a physician's clinical, diagnostic, medicolegal, and communication skills in close to real-life scenarios with a real patient.

Truly, this book is primarily intended to help candidates prepare for MRCP-PACES. Many undergraduate medical students and other postgraduate examinations (such as FCPS and MD in my country) have adopted a similar assessment model. Therefore, candidates who are preparing for these examinations may also find this book beneficial.

This is one volume text giving candidates complete preparation for the PACES examination within one portable volume. Here around 200 cases are organized into the five stations of the PACES exam involving respiratory, cardiovascular, abdominal, neurology examination, communication and ethics, history taking as well as clinical consultation. Engaging question and answer approach between candidate and surrogate/patient and candidate and examiner—Just as a role play in our real-life practice to pass the exam. The format lends itself to individual study and group role play, which will stimulate dialogue around the theme introduced. Exploring the themes and topics presented in each of the cases in accordance with the framework will equip candidates with the necessary skills to negotiate the PACES process.

Expose yourself to clinical signs and scenarios. Then practice, practice, and practice. Examine the patient who is ill, examine the patient who is well, examine your friends, your relatives, your partner, your siblings, or your parents. Remember, you always have the best chance to succeed if you practice wholeheartedly.

I hope the candidate will both enjoy and benefit from this book and their PACES preparation.

Best of luck!

Mohammad Ali
Clinical Professor of Medicine and Head

Few Words

I am glad and proud to write a few words about the *"Role Play in MRCP-PACES"* book by Dr Mohammad Ali. This book sheds light on the important aspects of different diseases covering all the important sections for MRCP-PACES. While going through the manuscript of this book, I keenly observed that all the chapters in this book are arranged in an excellent way, of awesome quality and reader-friendly. This book is the first of its kind in the country as well as overseas enlightening the crucial facts of history taking, clinical examination, communication skills, eliciting patient's concerns and their solution, cross-questions, and spot diagnosis of different diseases, which will primarily help MRCP students and also undergraduate (MBBS) and postgraduate (FCPS/MD) students of different specialties. Even intern doctors, trainees, and general practitioners will be greatly benefitted from this book. Dr Mohammad Ali has written this book in such an arithmetical and magical way that I firmly believe it will become a powerful tool for gathering knowledge for doctors of all specialties which will positively impact to make a real physician.

Dr Mohammad Ali graduated from Dhaka Medical College in 2003. He self-retired from government job and joined the Department of Medicine in the Dhaka Central International Medical College. We are working together in the same department.

I am very much proud of being his colleague. He is a truly inspiring, student-loving well-read teacher, and has such fundamental knowledge. I always feel that he could teach anything about medicine.

He is an excellent clinician, compassionate and good listener to patients, and an expert in making accurate diagnoses and management. All his qualities and hardship make this book real. Being his colleague and as a principal of this Institute, I wish the success for his book. Finally, I would like to express my special thanks to Professor Dr Mohammad Ali for his hardship and devotion.

Bidhu Bhushan Das MBBS MD (Med)
Principal
Dhaka Central International Medical College

"Role Play in MRCP-PACES" is a well-structured, problem-oriented book of medicine. I have gone through the book partially and found all aspects need to cover with proper history taking, skillful clinical examination, and evaluation and ethical management, counseling, and appropriate referral of a patient. I strongly believe that all practicing physicians, postgraduate students as well as undergraduate examinees should exercise the problems in the book to become more methodical and well-organized in their daily patient management. Definitely, patients will be more favored by such types of physicians.

Md Shoeb Nomany FCPS MD
Associate Professor of Nephrology

It is nice to know the publication of such a book which can give a virtual guide for practicing cases relevant for MRCP (UK) PACES examination preparation. Role play is the latest ad-on in clinical learning method which is utilized in this book. This book is mostly intended for MRCP (UK) PACES examinees. MRCP (UK) examination is the most reliable examination in the field of clinical medicine in the world. I believe this book can be a model for any other clinical exam preparation. The author was much more serious about choosing words in the text of the book, which made the book a unique one. Readers can find required information for different stations of PACES very easily in a palatable way. MRCP (UK) examination process is regularly under evaluation and modification in its structure, but the core materials of the exam are unchanged. I agree, the author of the book was quite alert to this and tried his best to keep the book useful for learners forever. Wishing the best to the author of such a useful book.

M Osman Gani MBBS MRCGP MRCP
Associate Professor of Medicine

I am really delighted to write forward for this wonderful book *"Role Play in MRCP-PACES"* by Professor Mohammad Ali, whom I know for more than three decades. He is very famous as a teacher among his students. I had an opportunity to observe his sound and deep knowledge of medicine. I was surprised to see his dedication to writing this book. He has not tried to make this book comprehensive by including all topics but has tried to focus on important and common cases. It is easier to understand. I hope this book will have wide acceptance among MRCP examinees as well as FCPS, and MD examinees of our country.

Kazi Abdullah Al Mamun FCPS MD
Associate Professor of Neurology

Contents

CHAPTER 1 **Clinical Consultation** 1
- Approach to a Scenario in Clinical Consultation Station 2
- Spot Diagnosis 4
- Hypothyroidism 32
- Graves' Disease 38
- Cushing Syndrome 43
- Acromegaly 47
- Addison's Disease 52
- Diabetic Foot 56
- Ankylosing Spondylitis 60
- Back Pain 65
- Systemic Lupus Erythematosus 69
- Systemic Sclerosis 75
- Rheumatoid Arthritis 79
- Gout 86
- Optic Atrophy 90
- Diplopia 94
- Retinitis Pigmentosa 98
- Vitreous Hemorrhage 102
- Pyoderma Gangrenosum 106
- Psoriasis 110
- Pleural Effusion 114
- Chronic Obstructive Pulmonary Disease 118
- Pulmonary Embolism 122
- Atrial Fibrillation 127
- Congestive Cardiac Failure 131
- Lambert–Eaton Myasthenic Syndrome 136
- Transient Ischemic Attack 140
- Transient Ischemic Attack in Young Female 144
- Marfan Syndrome 148
- Osteogenesis Imperfecta 152
- Post-transplant Lymphoproliferative Disorder 155
- Sexually Transmitted Infection 159
- Crohn's Disease 163

CHAPTER 2	**History Taking**	**167**

- Hemoptysis 168
- Headache 173
- Joint Pain 178
- Abdominal Bloating 183
- Night Sweats 187

CHAPTER 3	**Clinical Examination: Cardiovascular System**	**193**

- Cardiovascular System Examination 194
- Aortic Stenosis 198
- Aortic Regurgitation 200
- Mixed Aortic Valve Disease 202
- Mitral Stenosis 204
- Mitral Regurgitation 207
- Mitral Valve Prolapse 210
- Mixed Mitral Valve Disease 212
- Pulmonary Stenosis 214
- Prosthetic Aortic Valve 216
- Prosthetic Mitral Valve 218
- Atrial Septal Defect 220
- Ventricular Septal Defect 222
- Patent Ductus Arteriosus 224
- Intracardiac Device 226

CHAPTER 4	**Clinical Examination: Respiratory System**	**229**

- Respiratory System Examination 230
- Interstitial Lung Disease 235
- Rheumatoid Lung 237
- Bronchiectasis 239
- Cystic Fibrosis 242
- Pneumonia 244
- Chronic Obstructive Pulmonary Disease 246
- Cor-pulmonale 249
- Bronchial Asthma 251
- Lung Cancer 253
- Lobectomy 256
- Pneumonectomy 258
- Lung Transplant 260

CHAPTER 5 Clinical Examination: Gastrointestinal System   263

- Gastrointestinal Tract Examination   264
- Chronic Liver Disease   269
- Cirrhosis with Portal Hypertension   273
- Hepatomegaly with No Stigmata of Chronic Liver Disease   276
- Hereditary Hemochromatosis   278
- Primary Biliary Cholangitis/Cirrhosis   280
- Ascites   283
- Hepatosplenomegaly   286
- Isolated Splenomegaly   288
- Hemolytic Anemia (Hereditary Spherocytosis)   290
- Autosomal Dominant Polycystic Kidney Disease   292
- Renal Transplant   295
- Liver Transplantation   298
- Renal-pancreas Transplant   301
- Chronic Pancreatitis   303
- Crohn's Disease   305
- Percutaneous Endoscopic Gastrostomy   307

CHAPTER 6 Clinical Examination: Nervous System   309

- Examination of Upper Limb   310
- Examination of Lower Limb   314
- Examination of Cranial Nerves   317
- Examination for Disequilibrium   321
- Examination of Eye   323
- Peripheral Neuropathy   327
- Peripheral Neuropathy: Atypical Features   330
- Chronic Inflammatory Demyelinating Polyneuropathy   332
- Sensory Ataxia   334
- Charcot–Marie–Tooth Disease   336
- Claw Hand   338
- Spastic Paraparesis   340
- Cord Compression   342
- Cervical Myelopathy   344
- Stroke/Cerebrovascular Disease   346
- Cerebellar Disorder (Upper Limb)   349
- Cerebellar Ataxia   350
- Multiple Sclerosis   352
- Motor Neuron Disease (Kennedy's Disease)   354
- Bulbar Palsy (Motor Neuron Disease)   356
- Myotonic Dystrophy   358

- Myasthenia Gravis (Ocular) 361
- Parkinson's Disease 364
- Tardive Dyskinesia 367
- Involuntary Movement (Chorea) 368

CHAPTER 7 Clinical Communication Skills and Ethics 371

- Brief Discussion on Communication and Ethics 372
- Lifestyle Modification of a Rheumatoid Arthritis Patient 376
- Rheumatoid Arthritis 381
- Transient Ischemic Attack 384
- Addison's Disease 387
- Ulcerative Colitis with the Refusal to Admit Hospital 390
- Celiac Disease 393
- Patient with the First Fit 396
- Emphysema with Smoking Cessation 399
- Counseling of an Alcohol Drinker 403
- Discussion on Breaking Bad News 406
- Pancreatic Carcinoma 407
- Multiple Sclerosis 410
- Delayed Diagnosis of Cancer 414
- Dementia 417
- Renal Biopsy 420
- Percutaneous Endoscopic Gastrostomy Tube Insertion 424
- Intercostal Chest Drain 427
- Hickman Line 430
- Lumbar Puncture 432
- Oesophago-gastro-duodenoscopy Procedure 435
- Offer a Blood Transfusion 438
- Needle Stick Injury 440
- Newly Diagnosed Human Immunodeficiency Virus 443
- Hospital Superbug-1 447
- Hospital Superbug-2 450
- Genetic Counseling 453
- Counseling for Anticoagulation 456
- Patient with Poor Compliance 458
- Nonorganic Disease 461
- Medical Error-1 464
- Medical Error-2 467
- Medical Trial 469
- Cancer Withhold 471

- Live Organ Donation   474
- Advance Care Decision   477
- Decision about Do-not-resuscitate   480
- End of Life Decision   483
- Brainstem Death Testing   486
- Brainstem Death and Organ Donation   489
- Hospital Postmortem   492
- Coroner's Postmortem   495

Index   *499*

Introduction

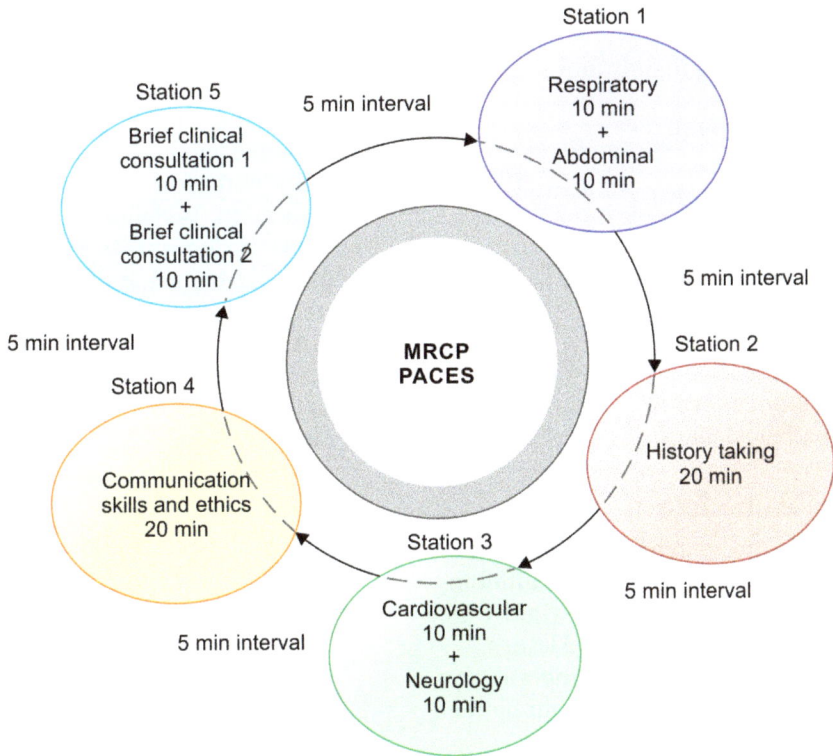

7—Clinical Skills are Assessed during the PACES Exam

1. *Clinical communication skills*: Try to elicit history relevant to the complaint and explain information to the patient in a focused, fluent, and professional manner.
2. *Physical examination*: In a correct, appropriate, well-practiced, and professional manner.
3. Identifies correct physical signs.
4. *Differential diagnosis*: Constructs a sensible differential diagnosis, including the correct diagnosis.
5. *Clinical judgement*: Selects sensible and appropriate investigations and treatment.
6. *Managing patients' concerns*: Detects, acknowledges, and attempts to address patient's concerns in an empathetic way.
7. *Maintaining patient's welfare*: Treat patients respectfully and sensitively and ensure comfort, safety, and dignity.

In the clinical consultation station (station 5) all seven things are assessed by the examiner.

But in respiratory, abdominal, CVS, and neurological station examination—five things are mainly assessed that including:
1. Physical examination
2. Identifying physical signs
3. Differential diagnosis
4. Clinical judgment
5. Managing patient welfare

In clinical communication, mainly four things are assessed:
1. Clinical communication
2. Clinical judgment
3. Managing patient concern
4. Managing patient welfare

In history taking, mainly five things are assessed:
1. Clinical communication
2. Differential diagnosis
3. Clinical judgment
4. Managing patient concern
5. Managing patient welfare

Top Tips for PACES Exam

- Give yourself time to read the instruction carefully and think about diagnosis, differential diagnosis, relevant investigations, management plans and any ethical issues.
- During PACES examination, examiners always tell you the patient's name. Greet your patient in their family name.
- The candidate should always have sleeves rolled above the elbow.
- *During clinical consultation*:
  - At first, take a full history, presenting complaint, systems review, past medical history, drugs and allergies, social history, and family history. Be systematic—you will be marked down for being unsystemic and presenting in an unstructured way. Whenever you need to ask about sexual history, do it sensitively with an introduction such as "do you mind if I ask you a very personal question."
  - Try to make your differential diagnoses for each symptom initially in broad categories, not individual diseases, e.g., causes of chest pain may be cardiac, respiratory, thromboembolic, musculoskeletal, gastro-esophageal reflux disease, etc.
  - Always remember that you are an SHO/registrar in the clinic with a consultant next door. You should inform the patient that you will discuss your plan with your consultant. Any investigations and follow-up should be best practiced and, within reason, not limited by resources.
- You must wash your hands before and after touching the patient. The antiseptic liquid is provided to you in the station.
- See the patient as a whole, do not rush to examination. Bedside clues and other clues are very important during the examination and clinical consultation.
- Be gentle to your patient and examiner. Do not hurt the patient. Always ask, "do you have any pain or discomfort?" Then take permission from the patient to talk or examine always, do not miss it.
- Respect the patient's dignity during exposure and maintain the patient's welfare.
- Never argue with the examiner. Maintain eye contact with both examiners. Remember, most examiners try to pass you if possible. If any examiner offers help and gives you hints to diagnosis, you must be very vigilant to accept the offer.
- The clinical examination needs to be smooth and spontaneous and answering questions in MRCP-PACES needs cortical reflex where your brain cells to answer.
- Hold your hands together behind your back, do not point to your body, do not turn your head to the patient. Always hold your stethoscope in your hand, do not put it over your shoulder.
- Examiners like an easy life, if they ask you a question, try to answer them and give them your reason.
- When presenting the case—comment on signs observed or bedside clues first before commenting on the system examined.

In the end, say I would like to complete my examination by (important other bedside examination like doing bedside urine dipstick for proteinuria in a diabetic patient).

Formulate your comment and diagnosis that include—important positive and negative findings, the diagnosis—bronchiectasis, possible cause—cystic fibrosis, possible complications due to disease (cor-pulmonale) or treatment (cushingoid appearance due to steroid use).

Common diseases are common. Never try to impress your examiner with something uncommon unless they force you to do so. When you say something uncommon diagnosis get ready to answer the questions pertaining to that illness.

Try to avoid "verbal constipation" try to say something when the examiner asks you. If you are lucky, they might guide you to answer and help to come to a diagnosis. Never say something obviously wrong and stupid.

You must have the ability to say simple management when talking about management and any disease—four important things need to be covered:

1. First, outline the investigations that we want to do—try to say the expected findings of the investigations for your diagnosis (such as in case of pneumonia—I would like to do a chest X-ray, which will show consolidation) to exclude the differential diagnosis, to identify complications as well as investigations for etiology.
2. Secondly, counseling and explanation—you must tell the patient his/her diagnosis and explain to them easily (without jargon) if the disease is a chronic one.
3. Regarding management of the patient, first talk about the nonpharmacological approach as it is an important part of a holistic approach to a patient, especially in chronic one.
4. The final part of your management is, of course, your pharmacological approach and a surgical approach if required.

Always Remember This

- In clinical communication station, the most important part is for successful communications:
  - To identify the patient agenda.
  - To explore the patient's ideas, concerns, and expectations (ICE).
  - To show empathy and sympathy to the patient in an appropriate manner.

CHAPTER 1

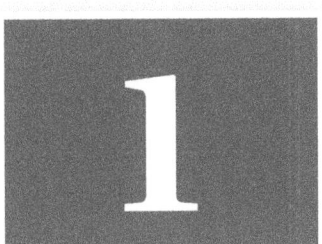

Clinical Consultation

- Approach to a Scenario in Clinical Consultation Station
- Spot Diagnosis
- Hypothyroidism
- Graves' Disease
- Cushing Syndrome
- Acromegaly
- Addison's Disease
- Diabetic Foot
- Ankylosing Spondylitis
- Back Pain
- Systemic Lupus Erythematosus
- Systemic Sclerosis
- Rheumatoid Arthritis
- Gout
- Optic Atrophy
- Diplopia
- Retinitis Pigmentosa
- Vitreous Hemorrhage
- Pyoderma Gangrenosum
- Psoriasis
- Pleural Effusion
- Chronic Obstructive Pulmonary Disease
- Pulmonary Embolism
- Atrial Fibrillation
- Congestive Cardiac Failure
- Lambert–Eaton Myasthenic Syndrome
- Transient Ischemic Attack
- Transient Ischemic Attack in Young Female
- Marfan Syndrome
- Osteogenesis Imperfecta
- Post-transplant Lymphoproliferative Disorder
- Sexually Transmitted Infection
- Crohn's Disease

Approach to a Scenario in Clinical Consultation Station

Two sorts of cases are typical during the Practical Assessment of Clinical Examination Skills (PACES) exam in clinical consultation stations:

The patient presenting with a common discrete medical presentation in the medical outpatient clinic, ward, or emergency department such as "the patient complains of sharp pain in the chest" and the patient with a spot diagnosis; most often with dermatological, rheumatological, endocrinological or (probably less likely), ophthalmological diagnoses.

Candidates will be given written instructions for each of the stations, usually in the form of short notes or referral letters during 5-minutes interval before each station. The instructions to the candidate will give definite direction, and these must be followed; there is simply no time for going "off-track." Once you get this clinical scenario, start to think about your diagnosis and differential diagnoses and plan for taking focused history as well as focused examination.

Each station, as you know, will be 20 minutes which includes history taking, clinical examination, and explanation to the patient. Here, history taking is an essential component of their assessment and it is absolutely important that as a candidate you use the most scientific and modern way of collecting important information from the patient while keeping the patient the center of this exercise. So traditionally we have had things such as the presenting complaint followed by a history of present illness, followed by past medical history (PMH), followed by drug history, allergies, family history (FH), travel history, personal history, social history, and systems review while all of these are still very relevant and very important.

It is important to take history and do the examination in a patient-centered approach. We should consider the **Calgary Cambridge framework** during clinical consultation under five headlines that include:

1. **Initiating the session:** Introduce yourself to the patient; shake the hand; establish their identity by getting the name, date of birth, and address; take the patient's consent for speaking to them; then move on to establishing the agenda for the consultation and start with open questions. All of these can be considered under the headline initiating the session.
2. **Gathering the information:** Move from open questions to closed questions to analyze the presenting symptoms. At the same time an initial careful inspection for few seconds may provide essential clues, which may, for example guide further questioning and examination. Keeping a suspected diagnosis in your mind from the obvious clinical appearance as well as initial focused history, go for short-targeted history to establish your diagnosis, exclude the differential diagnosis, complications, causes, identify risk factors, and associated conditions. Then go for quick systemic review, PMH, FH, treatment and social history according to your provisional and differentials. It is very important to **explore the patient's ideas, concerns, expectations (ICE).** To explore the patient's ideas, e.g., if the patient does come in with chest pain, what are their ideas about what

could be causing this? And, what are their concerns? What are they worried about? The patient could be worried about this being a heart attack and then expectations, what are they expecting from your consultation? What would they like to be? In the end, maybe the patient would like to have been investigated and treated. So, this is under gathering information.

3. **Physical examination:** Take permission and do the focused examination based on the patient's history and spot diagnosis, e.g., if a patient complains of breathlessness, his focused systemic examination will be the respiratory and or cardiovascular system. Note the bedside clues and examine the patient in appropriate and professional manners to identify physical signs correctly. You can examine the patient after taking the complete history, or you can take history for the first few minutes, then start examination and continue taking the history at the same time.

4. **Explanation and planning:** You have gathered the information, explore the physical signs and address the patient's ICE, now move on to the explanation and planning. Here, you need to give the patient an explanation of what you have found from the history and examination, your idea about the patient's problem, your next plan, check the understanding, and acknowledge the patient's concerns. Since you are giving chunks of information to the patient, give a pause so that the patient can take it in and then check the patient's understanding—did you follow that? Did you follow what I have just said to you? Am I clear so far? Not only here, but you should also **take pauses throughout the station** to giving time to the patient to interrupt you so that patient can ask you things. All above, you should **avoid medical jargon, do not use complex medical terms** that the patient will not understand or will have difficulty understanding. If you use a complex medical term, please explain what does it mean, e.g., in a patient with autoimmune disease, you should explain the autoimmune disease by saying "It is a disease due to disturbance in our defensive system which is supposed to attack bugs and germs. Sometimes, our immune system instead of attacking germs and bugs, go crazy for an unknown reason, and it starts attacking our own tissues."

5. **Closing the session:** Now move to close the interview, there are certain fundamental landmarks of this part of clinical consultation. At this point, you need to summarize what you have obtained from this conversation. Then again, ask if the patient has **any further concern or anything to mention** that you have not asked already. Then, negotiate a mutual plan of action and remember this, you are going to negotiate, this is not a one-way street, so the doctor is not to dictate their plan to the patient. So, suggest the patient about the investigation, treatment, admission, referral, or follow-up and ask is that okay with them or not? Moreover, finally, we can call it as a final safety net— **"Have I missed anything, or do you want to add anything more?"**

Spot Diagnosis

Many of the patients seen in station 5 will have spot dermatological, rheumatological, endocrinological, or ophthalmological diagnosis.

Vitiligo (Fig. 1)

Well-demarcated depigmented macules and patches surrounded by normal skin with a hyperpigmented border without loss of sensation (which exclude differential diagnosis of leprosy).

Look for distributions such as the face, dorsal hands, axilla, nipple, umbilicus, sacrum, and anogenital region.

It may be associated with other autoimmune disorders, so ask about the suggestive history of other autoimmune disorders such as hypo or hyperthyroidism, pernicious anemia, Addison's disease, diabetes mellitus (DM), and alopecia areata.

Look for signs of associated autoimmune disorders including thyroidectomy scar, needle marks for DM, and evidence of peripheral neuropathy for pernicious anemia.

Alopecia Areata (Figs. 2A and B)

Loss of hair with no signs of scarring or inflammation with some small, tiny hairs at the periphery. It may be associated with nail pitting and other autoimmune disorders. So, proceed as a case of vitiligo described earlier. Usually, this is treated with topical steroids and minoxidil.

Lichen Planus (Fig. 3)

Itchy, flat-topped, pink, or purple papules in the arms, legs, or buccal mucosa with white Wickham striae on the surface. This may be associated with longitudinal nail ridge. Certain infections such as

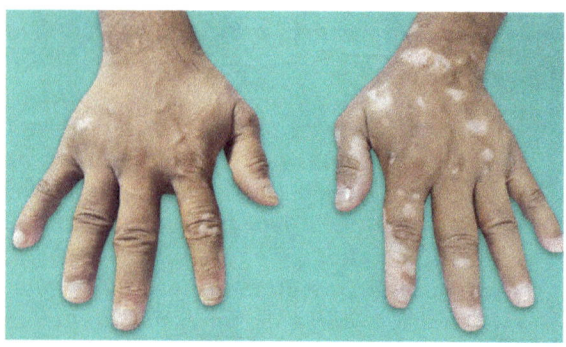

FIG. 1: Vitiligo.

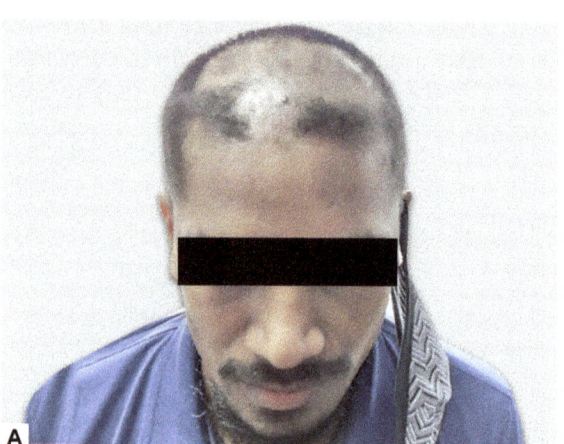

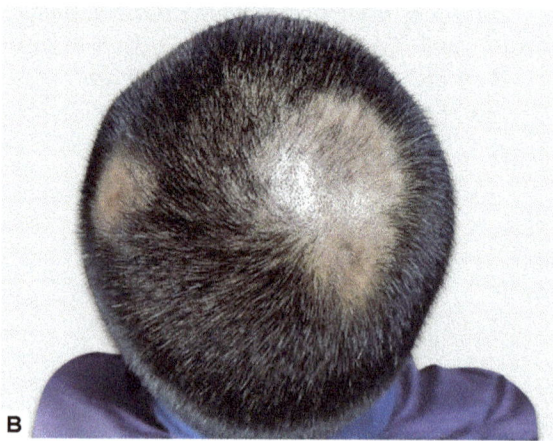

FIGS. 2A AND B: Alopecia areata.

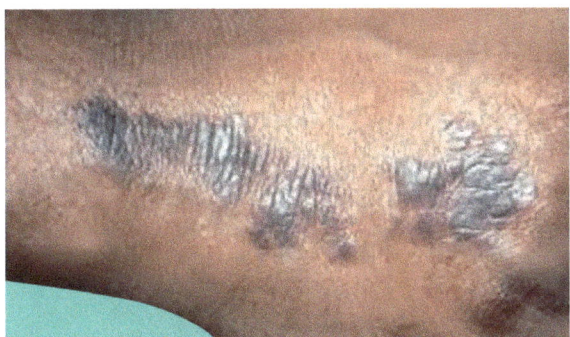

FIG. 3: Lichen planus.

hepatitis C virus (HCV) infection and medications such as beta-blockers, thiazide diuretics, metformin, and antimalarials may trigger lichen planus.

It can affect different organs, so ask about:
- Change of voice or shortness of breath (? larynx)
- Difficulty or painful swallowing [?gastrointestinal tract (GIT)]
- Dysuria (? renal)
- Redness in the eye (? conjunctiva)

Diagnosis is confirmed by biopsy and usually treated with local steroid, but systemic steroid may be required in severe and widespread disease.

Necrobiosis Lipoidica (Fig. 4)

Sharply defined, a thin, shiny, atrophic area with yellowish waxy center (feels like candle wax) with overlying dilated blood vessels (telangiectasia) in the skin.

It is a rare and chronic skin condition that may be associated with DM. So, ask about the suggestive history of DM and its complications; look for BM testing pricks and insulin injections sites which indicate associated DM. Potent topical steroids/tacrolimus/intralesional steroids are the treatment of choice. However, oral steroid and/or cyclosporine may be required in a refractory case.

Sturge–Weber Syndrome (Fig. 5)

Flat, pink, red, or purple colored patch (port-wine stain) in one side of the face (caused by the

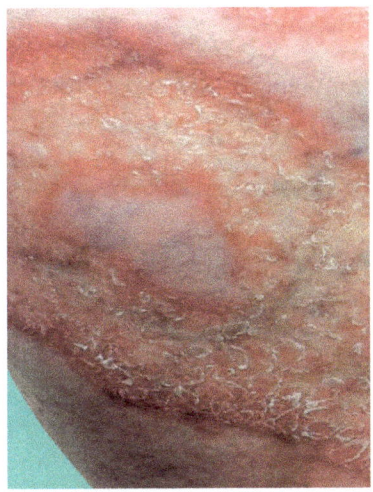

FIG. 4: Necrobiosis lipoidica.

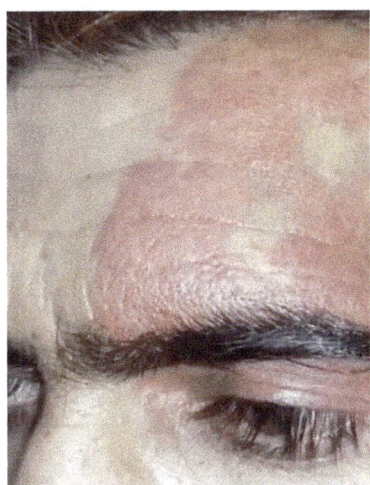

FIG. 5: Sturge–Weber syndrome.

concentration of dilated tiny blood vessels called capillaries-hemangioma).

Ask about fits or weakness (brain hemangioma) if present, then think it is a case of Sturge–Weber syndrome (caused by *GNAQ* gene mutation).

Then ask about pain in the eye or decrease vision (it can be associated with glaucoma).

Now examine the lower limbs neurologically for weakness and fundus for glaucoma or choroidal hemangioma.

It is congenital (presents from birth). Brain imaging [computed tomography (CT)/magnetic resonance imaging (MRI)] and a genetic test is the investigation of choice.

Neurofibromatosis Type-1 (Figs. 6A and B)

Multiple soft and firm, sessile, mobile nodules along the course of peripheral nerves (neurofibroma).

Now examine for:
- Light brown, evenly pigmented macules (Café-au-lait spots).
- Gold-tan to brown in color—dome-shaped gelatinous masses, developed on the surface of the iris [Lisch nodule characteristics of neurofibromatosis (NF)-1].
- Small circular spots on the axillary skin that are darker than the surrounding skin due to deposit of melanin (axillary freckling).
- Large nodules containing multiple neurofibromas "bag of worms" (plexiform neuroma).
- Any scar from previous surgery.

Now ask about:
- Tinnitus, hearing loss or balance problem (unilateral or bilateral acoustic neuroma for NF-2).
- Take suggestive histories and examine for cranial nerves involvement.
- Any weakness in the limbs for spinal involvement.

It is an autosomal dominant inheritance (chromosome 17—NF-1, and chromosome 22—NF-2). Genetic screening and MRI are the investigations of choice. Surgical removal and antiepileptics are treatment options.

Hereditary Hemorrhagic Telangiectasia (Fig. 7)

Multiple telangiectasias (visible small linear red blood vessels) on the tongue, but look for distribution in the face, especially around the mouth, nailbed, and palate.

Now ask about:
- Do you bleed from any part of the body such as mouth or nose? Do you have any hematemesis or melena (recurrent bleeding)?
- Any shortness of breath, racing of the heart, or do you look pallor (? anemia)?
- Do you have any bleeding with your bowel motion [? bowel arteriovenous (AV)]?
- Do you have any blood with your waterworks [? Kidney AV]?
- Do you have any weakness or clumsiness (? Brain AV)?
- Do you have coughed up blood (? Lung AV)?
- Family history [autosomal dominant disorder; mutation in Endoglin on chromosome 9 or ACVRL1 gene on chromosome 12; characterized

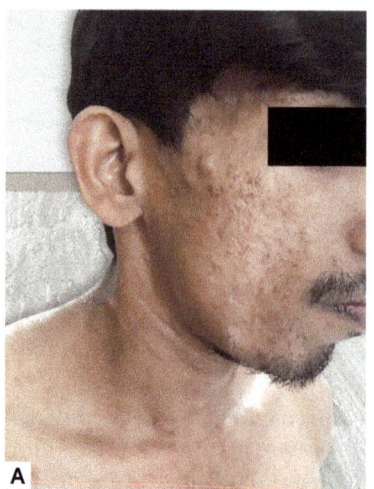 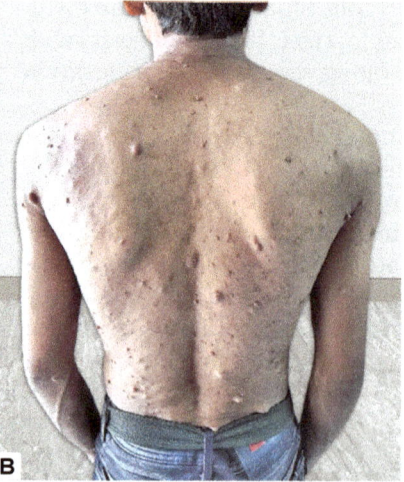

FIGS. 6A AND B: Neurofibromatosis type-1.

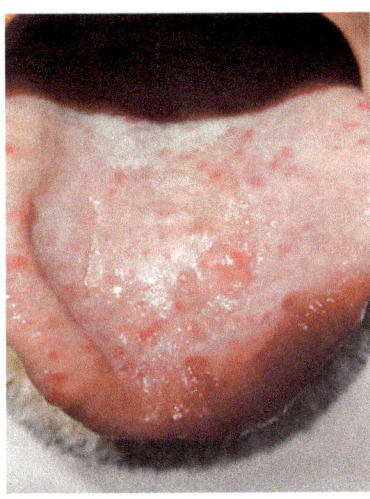

FIG. 7: Hereditary hemorrhagic telangiectasia.

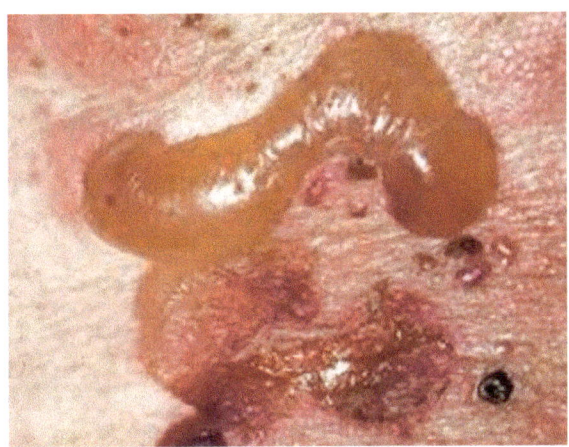

FIG. 9: Bullous pemphigoid.

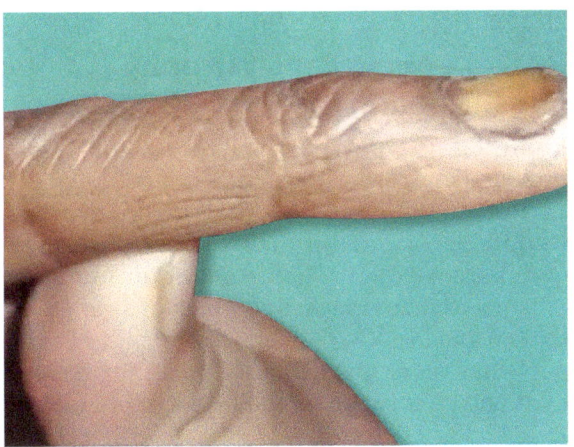

FIG. 8: Look for anemia and signs of Iron deficiency anemia (koilonychia) for evidence of chronic blood loss.

by epistaxis, cutaneous telangiectasia, and visceral arteriovenous malformations (AVMs)]

Examine the liver for enlargement and bruit (? AVM).

Neurological examination if weakness is present.

Examine the lung for pulmonary bruits especially in the lower lobe (? pulmonary AVM)

Look for anemia and signs of iron deficiency anemia (IDA) (koilonychia) for evidence of chronic blood loss **(Fig. 8)**.

Bullous Pemphigoid (Fig. 9)

Multiple bullae are arising from normal skin or red skin filled with clear or yellow or hemorrhagic fluid, which is large, tense, and involving inner thigh, upper arms, and trunk.

Ask about:
- Itching (It is intensely itchy lesion).
- Any weight loss, anorexia, nausea, vomiting, hematemesis, and lumps (underlying malignancy).
- Any joint pain, butterfly rash [underlying systemic lupus erythematosus (SLE)].
- Any precipitating drug history [captopril, gliptins, antibiotics, nonsteroidal anti-inflammatory drugs (NSAIDs), furosemide].
- Any history of radiation (precipitating events).

Now examine the lymph nodes and abdomen for underlying malignancy.

Diagnosis is confirmed by biopsy for histopathology and immunofluorescence shows deposition of immunoglobulin G (IgG) and C3 in dermoepidermal junction. Treatment includes steroid and azathioprine.

Porphyria Cutanea Tarda (Fig. 10)

Multiple bullae (fluid-filled sacs), milia (small, dome-shaped white, or yellow bumps) and scarring over the sun-exposed area particularly on the dorsal hands, forearms, face, and ears.

Ask about predisposing factors such as alcohol intake, history of hepatitis or liver disease (hemochromatosis), or estrogen-containing drugs.

Family history (commonly sporadic but sometimes AD)

Diagnosis is confirmed by 24-hour urine for uroporphyrin; if it is confirmed, then consider hepatitis screen, iron, or ferritin level (to exclude hemochromatosis) and alpha-fetoprotein (to exclude hepatocellular carcinoma).

Treatment options include:
- Removal of offending agents
- Sun avoidance
- Phlebotomy, and
- Antimalarial (chloroquine)

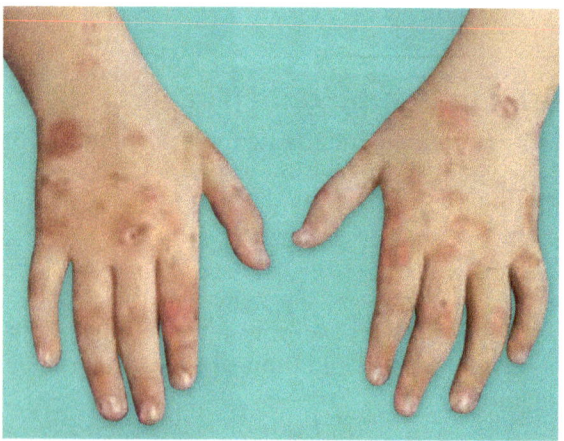

FIG. 10: Porphyria cutanea tarda.

Rheumatoid Hand and Foot (Figs. 11 and 12)

Picture illustrates Z-deformity of the thumb and swan neck deformity of the other fingers and gross wasting of the small muscle of the hand.

Look for ulnar subluxation of the metacarpophalangeal (MCP) joints and ulna at the carpal joint, Boutonniere deformity, nail infarct, palmar erythema, carpal tunnel syndrome, and scars of previous surgery.

Look for rheumatoid nodule and disease activity (joint swelling and tenderness).

Assess the functional status of the joint and joint movement (active and passive).

Look for evidence of extra-articular manifestations—pulmonary [diffuse parenchymal lung disease (DPLD)], eye (uveitis, scleritis), and Felty's syndrome (anemia and splenomegaly).

Becker's Muscular Dystrophy (Figs. 13A and B)

Enlarged calves (pseudohypertrophy) and proximal muscle wasting.

Presented with proximal myopathy and waddle gait (walk on their toes or push their abdomen forward when walking to maintain balance and compensate for lack of strength in the hip and legs).

Other signs particularly check for dilated cardiomyopathy can be the first sign of Becker's

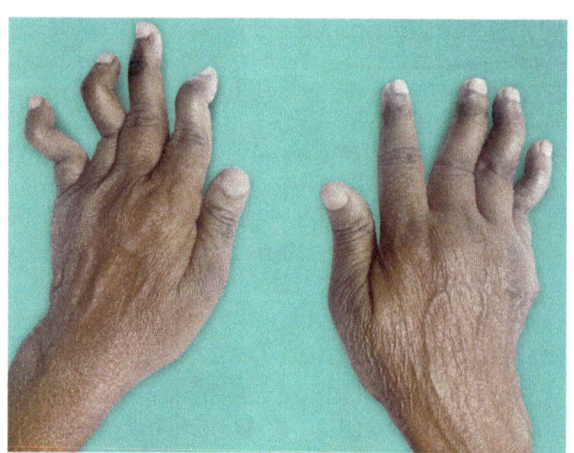

FIG. 11: Rheumatoid hand.

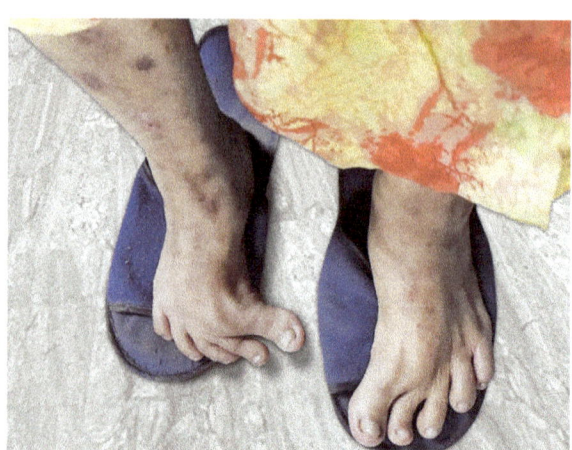

FIG. 12: Rheumatoid feet.

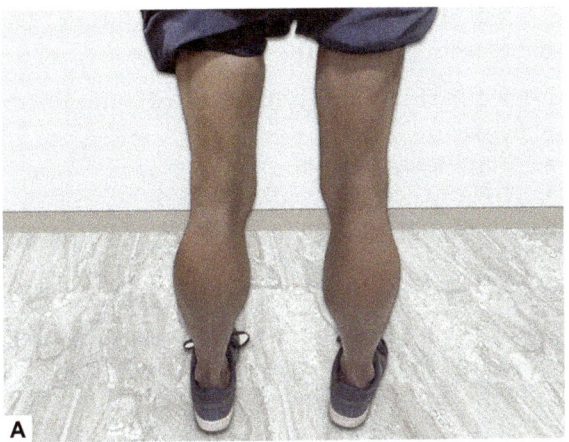 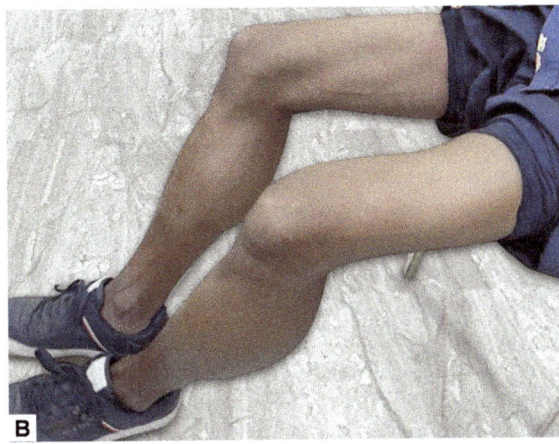

FIGS. 13A AND B: Becker's muscular dystrophy.

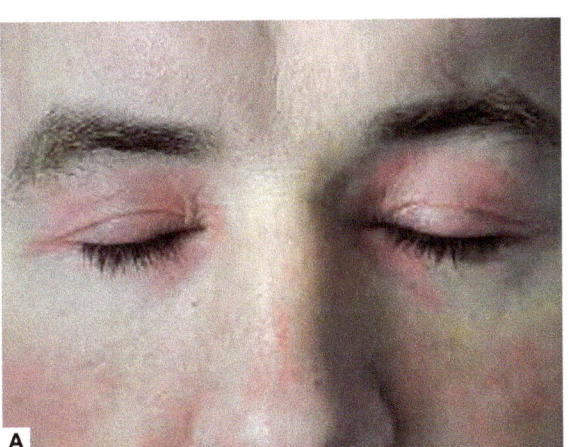 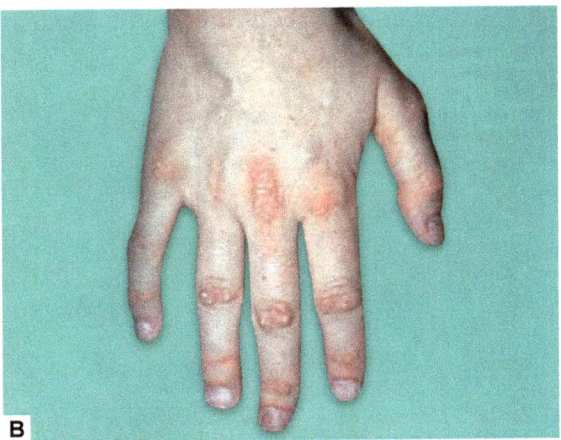

FIGS. 14A AND B: Dermatomyositis.

muscular dystrophy (BMD). On neurological exam—reduced muscle power with preserved reflex and sensation.

Becker muscular dystrophy is an X-linked recessive inherited disorder caused by mutations in the dystrophin gene. Slowly progressing muscle weakness of the legs and pelvis. Symptoms usually appear in teenage or early adult years.

Diagnosis based on history, examination, and investigations include elevated serum creatinine kinase, dystrophin gene deletion analysis, electromyography (EMG), and muscle biopsy with dystrophin antibody staining. Electrocardiogram (ECG) and echocardiography for cardiomyopathy.

There is no cure for BMD. Only treatment option is symptomatic care under multidisciplinary team (MDT).

Dermatomyositis (Figs. 14A and B)

Purple or red colored erythematous rash around eyes (heliotrope rash), over the knuckles (gottron's papule).

Look for rash in other parts of the body around the neck (shawl rash), chest, and back—above the breast (V-sign).

Ask about:
- Weakness in climbing stairs, combing hair (? proximal myopathy).
- Shortness of breath, cough (? lung fibrosis).

- Painful hand joints, butterfly rash with photosensitivity [? mixed connective tissue disease (MCTD)].
- Fever, weight loss, anorexia, difficulty in swallowing, hematemesis (? underlying malignancy).

Examine for proximal myopathy, chest for signs of DPLD or any evidence of malignancy (lymph node, abdomen).

Investigations include a blood test [creatine phosphokinase (CPK), anti-Jo Ab, complete blood count (CBC), C-reactive protein (CRP)], EMG and screening for malignancy depending on the symptoms (CT, endoscopy, or colonoscopy).

Amiodarone Facies (Fig. 15)

Deep, bluish gray discoloration around malar area, nose, and cheeks.

Ask about drug history (? amiodarone) and the reason for taking the drug.

Look for signs and symptoms of amiodarone toxicity:
- Pulmonary fibrosis
- Thyrotoxicosis/hypothyroidism
- Liver impairment

Pretibial Myxedema (Fig. 16)

Waxy discolored induration of the skin- given the characteristic appearance of Peau-d-orange on the anterior aspect of the lower leg spreading to the dorsum of the foot (pretibial myxedema) **(Fig. 16)**.

Now look for the *myxedematous face* **(Figs. 17A and B)** (expressionless face with apathetic look, periorbital swelling, puffiness of the face with baggy eyelids, loss of outer one-third of the eyebrows, xanthelasma).

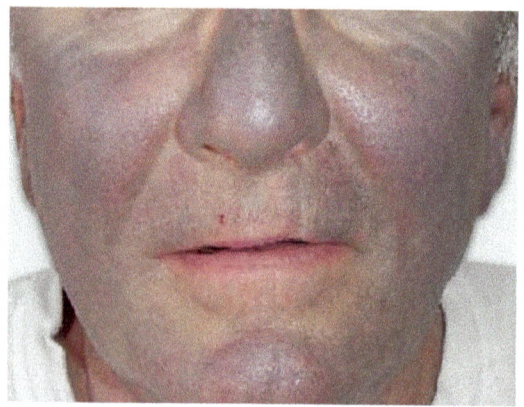

FIG. 15: Amiodarone facies.

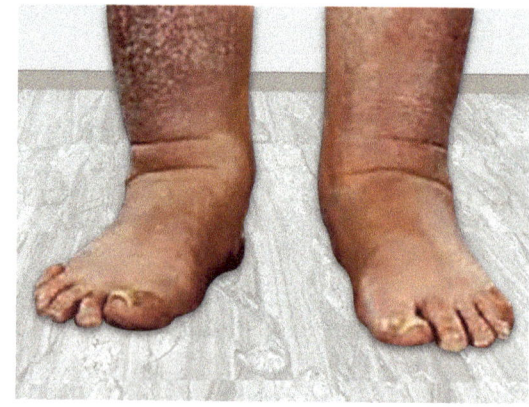

FIG. 16: Pretibial myxedema.

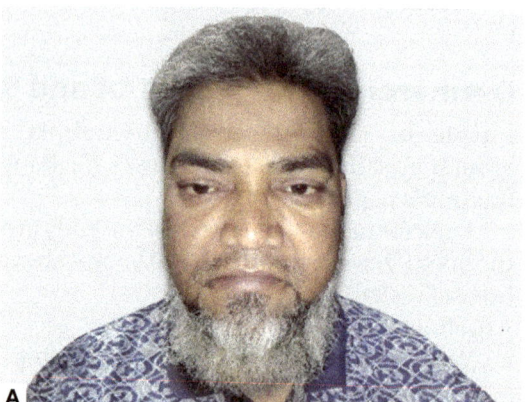

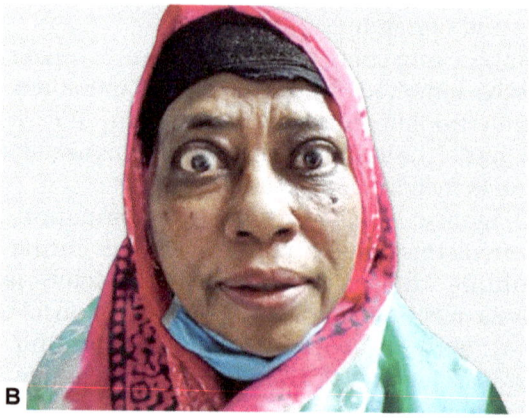

FIGS. 17A AND B: Myxedematous face.

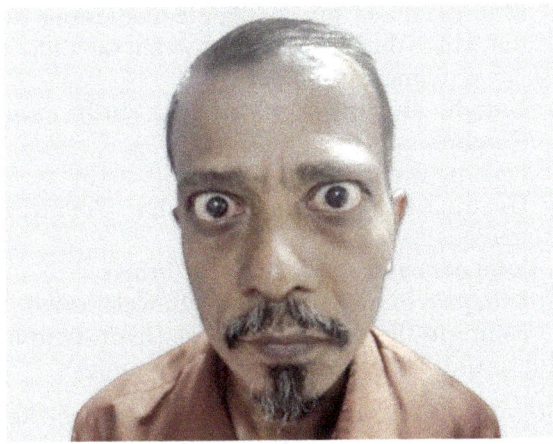

FIG. 18: Thyrotoxic face.

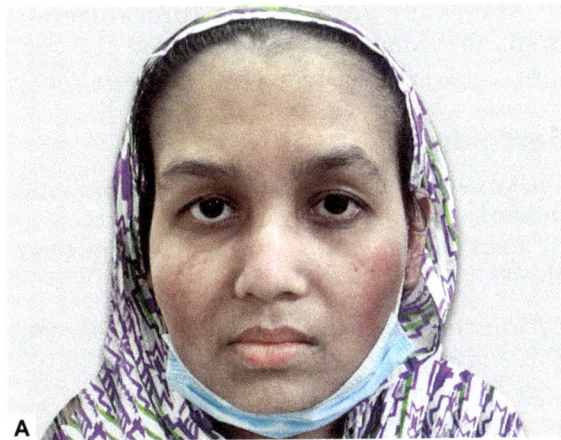

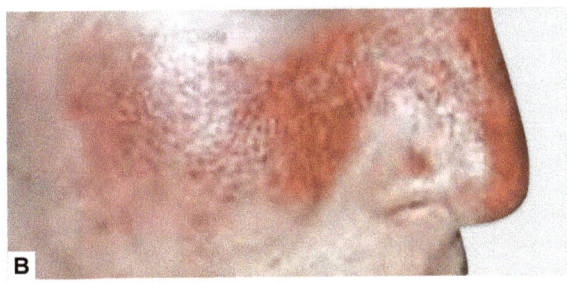

FIGS. 20A AND B: Photosensitive rash.

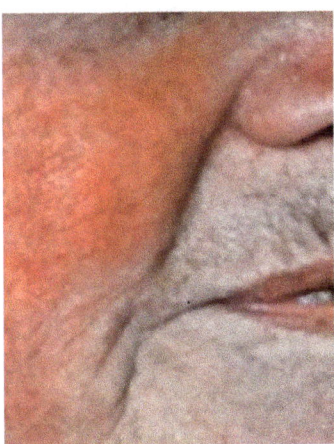

FIG. 19: Mitral facies.

Or, *thyrotoxic face* (**Fig. 18**) (patient appears anxious, restless, and fidgety with unilateral or bilateral proptosis).

Now examine for thyroid status and thyroid gland.

Mitral Facies (Fig. 19)

Malar flush—rosy, flushed cheeks, and dilated capillaries. The rash correlates with the severity of mitral stenosis due to reduced cardiac output.
- Look for signs of mitral stenosis, evidence of pulmonary hypertension or right ventricular hypertrophy, heart failure, and infective endocarditis.
- Listen for a hoarse voice (left vocal cord paralysis secondary to left atrial enlargement in mitral stenosis).
- Ask about rheumatic heart disease.
Exclude SLE; facial telangiectasia occurs in outdoor workers.

Photosensitive Rash (Figs. 20A and B)

Rash over both cheeks and bridge of the nose with sparing of the nasolabial fold—butterfly rash of SLE.

Differential diagnosis: MCTD, dermatomyositis, leprosy, erysipelas, post kala-azar dermal leishmaniasis (PKDL), and rosacea.

Look for other signs: Discoid rash (typically sun-exposed area), oral ulcer, periungual erythema, nail fold telangiectasia, livedo reticularis, alopecia, hyperpigmentation, purpura, and urticaria.

Ask about drug history (procainamide, isoniazid, hydralazine—drug induced SLE), and thrombosis [antiphospholipid (APLA) syndrome].

Sarcoidosis (Figs. 21A to D)

Dusky blue or purple plaque on the nose (lupus pernio).

Look for other sites of involvement (ears, cheeks, lips, and forehead).

Differential diagnosis: Rhinophyma (Rosacea), SLE, and leprosy.
Look for other signs:
- Erythematous tender bumps on the lower leg—erythema nodosum.
- Multiple dusky purple plaque like lesions in the skin of the different parts—skin sarcoid.

Ask for systemic symptoms:
- Cough, shortness of breath, chest pain (? pulmonary)
- Red and watery eye (? uveitis)
- Headache, confusion, malaise [?central nervous system (CNS)]
- Joint pain and or swelling (? arthritis)
- Loin pain or hematuria (? nephrocalcinosis)

Examine the heart, lung, eye, liver, lymph nodes, and CNS according to the symptoms.

Targeted investigations: CBC with erythrocyte sedimentation rate (ESR), CRP, chest X-ray

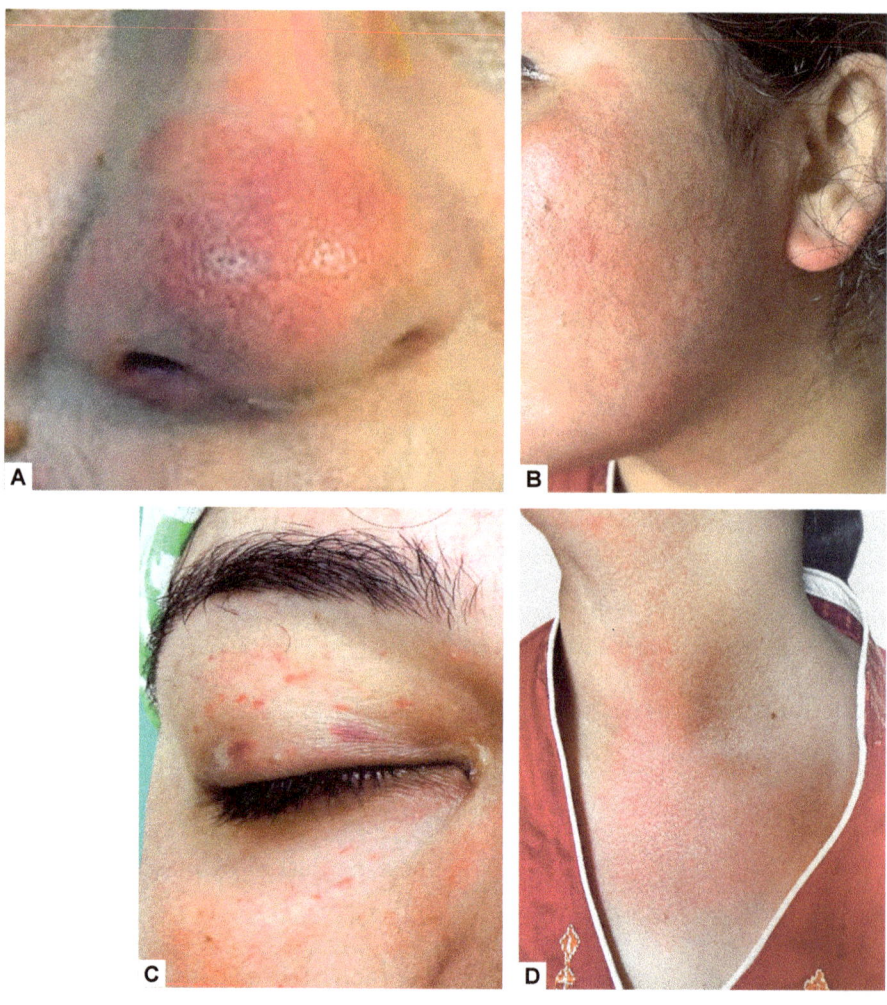

FIGS. 21A TO D: Sarcoidosis.

(CXR), serum calcium, serum angiotensin converting enzyme (ACE) level, skin biopsy, and lung function test, if required, high-resolution CT (HRCT) chest.

Ask about drug history (procainamide, isoniazid, hydralazine—drug induced SLE), and thrombosis (APLA syndrome).

Plethoric Face (Fig. 22)

Differential diagnosis: Cushing syndrome, mitral facies, SLE, dermatomyositis, and polycythemia rubra vera.

Oral Ulcer (Fig. 23)

Hard palate ulcer likely to have SLE.

Psoriasis (Figs. 24A and B)

Symmetrical multiple scattered well-demarcated raised erythematous plaques with silvery white scale on the extensor surface of the knee, elbows, and hand.

Look for other sites of involvement such as scalp, umbilicus, groin, and natal cleft.

Ask about FH of psoriasis and inflammatory back pain or arthritis.

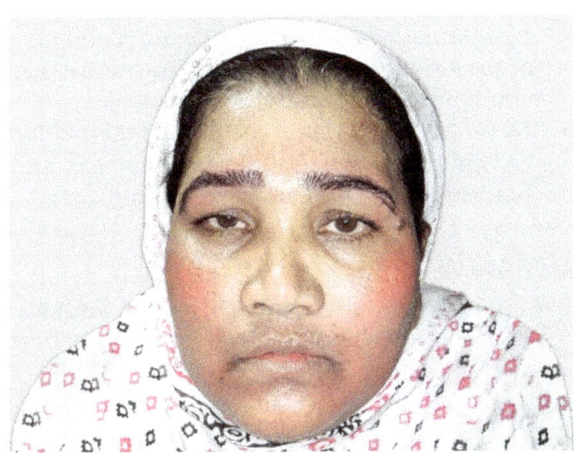

FIG. 22: Plethoric face.

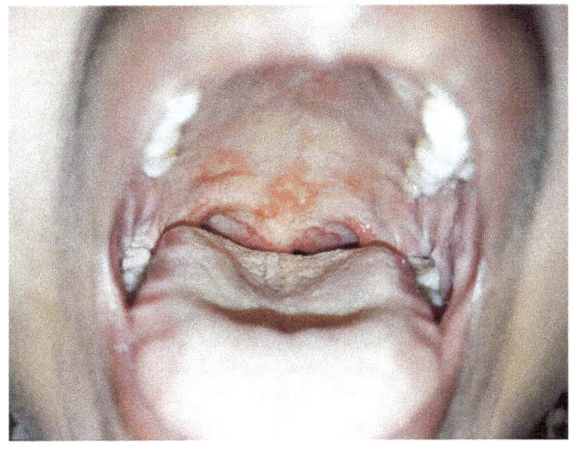

FIG. 23: Oral ulcer.

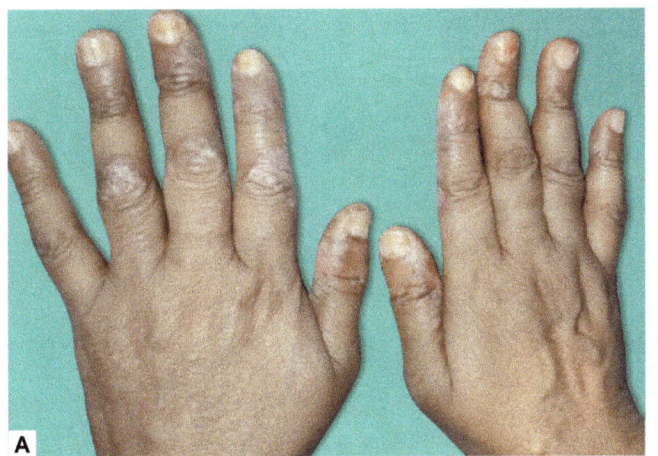

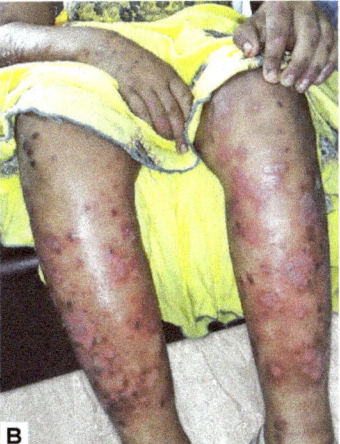

FIGS. 24A AND B: Psoriasis.

Ask about joint pain, swelling or back pain, red eye, or blurring of vision (uveitis).

Look for any nail changes (pitting, onycholysis, subungual hyperkeratosis).

Angioedema (Fig. 25)

Localized, nonpitting swelling of the face, involving periorbital areas, nose, and lips.

Ask and examine for involvement in tongue, larynx, hand, feet, and genitalia.

Ask about:
- Family history (hereditary angioedema—bradykinin-mediated)
- Prior history or episode
- Medication history (? ACE inhibitor—bradykinin-mediated)
- Urticaria (suggests histamine mediated but absent in hereditary and ACE-inhibitor induced angioedema)
- Features of anaphylaxis (histamine-mediated)
- Trigger factors—foods, drugs (NSAIDs, opioids, radiocontrast), infections, and hypothyroidism (histamine-mediated).
- Life-threatening respiratory symptoms (breathlessness, cough, cyanosis)
- Gastrointestinal tract (GIT) symptoms; abdominal pain.

Treatment:
- *Histamine-mediated angioedema*: Avoidance of precipitating foods, drugs (intramuscular epinephrine, antihistamine, steroids).
- *Hereditary/bradykinin-mediated angioedema*: C-1 inhibitor concentrate replacement and bradykinin receptor antagonist (icatibant).

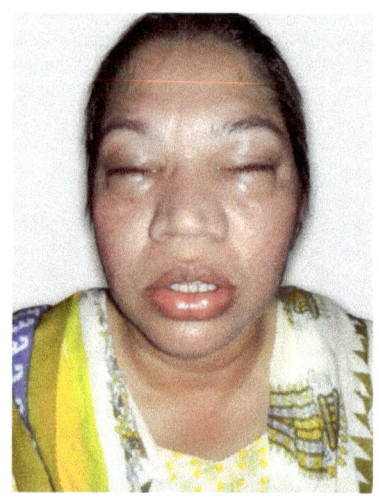

FIG. 25: Angioedema.

Urticaria (Figs. 26A and B)

Raised, itchy, circular skin rash, spread throughout the body particularly upper arm and chest with variable sizes.

Cushing Syndrome (Figs. 27A and B)

Rounded, plethoric face giving rise to moon face appearance, and acne.

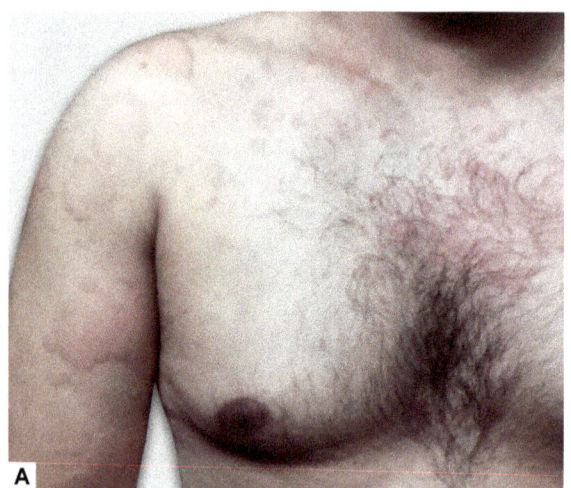
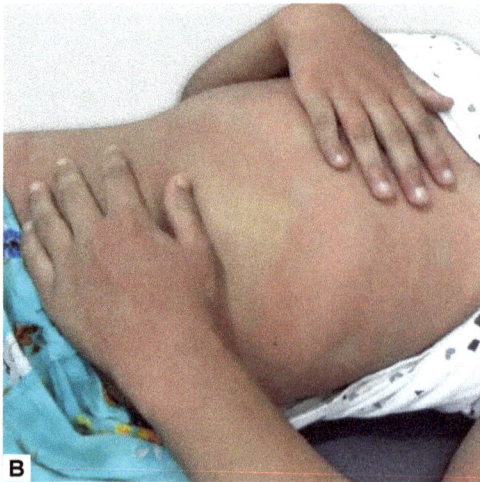

FIGS. 26A AND B: Urticaria.

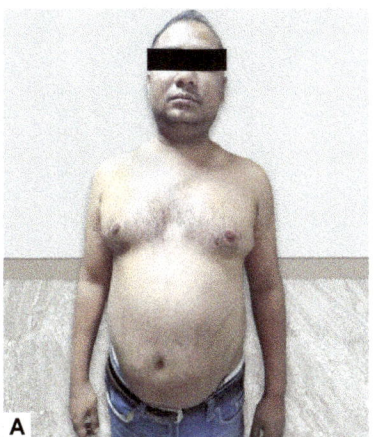 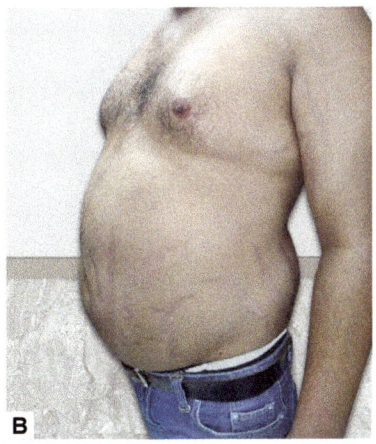

FIGS. 27A AND B: Cushingoid face.

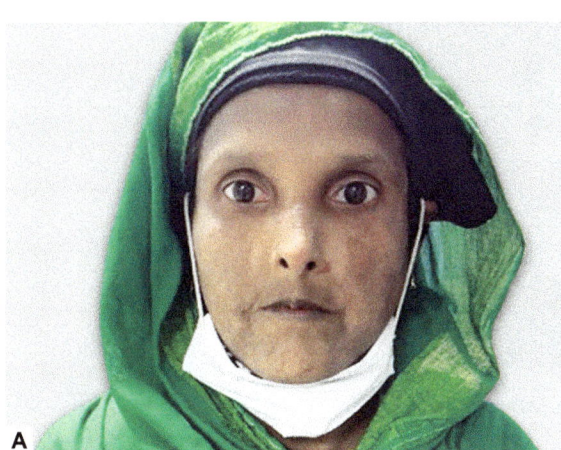 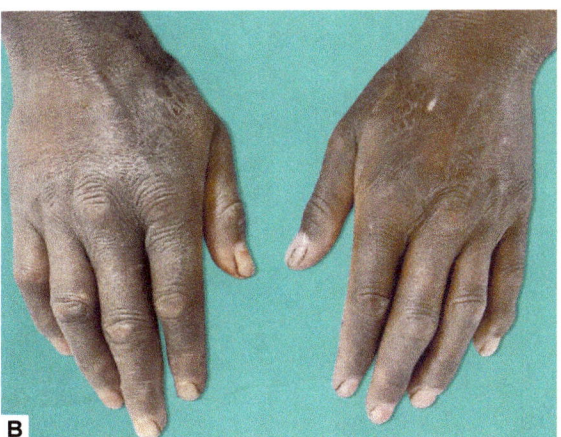

FIGS. 28A AND B: Systemic sclerosis.

Look for increased adipose tissue in the upper back and above the clavicle.

Lemon on stick appearance.

Now look for violaceous or purple striae in the abdomen, buttock, upper thigh, and upper arm.

Ask about steroid use (for bronchial asthma, rheumatoid arthritis, SLE), DM, hypertension, back pain (kyphosis with osteoporotic fracture).

Systemic Sclerosis (Figs. 28A and B)

- Smooth, shiny, and tight skin with hypo and hyperpigmented area in the skin.
- The nose is pinched up and tapered.
- Lips are thin, with perioral puckering of the skin.
- Microstomia.

Now look for—facial telangiectasia, indurated skin of the hands, sclerodactyly, Raynaud's phenomenon (± infarct or gangrene), dilated nail fold capillaries, and calcinosis cutis.

Look for distribution of skin involvement; limited cutaneous systemic sclerosis (LCSS), or diffuse cutaneous systemic sclerosis (DCSS).

Ask for dysphagia, chest pain, breathlessness, and cough.

Acromegaly (Figs. 29A to C)

Coarse facial feature with prominent supraorbital ridge, protruding lower jaw (prognathism) with malocclusion of the teeth when jaw clenched. Large lips, nose, and tongue.

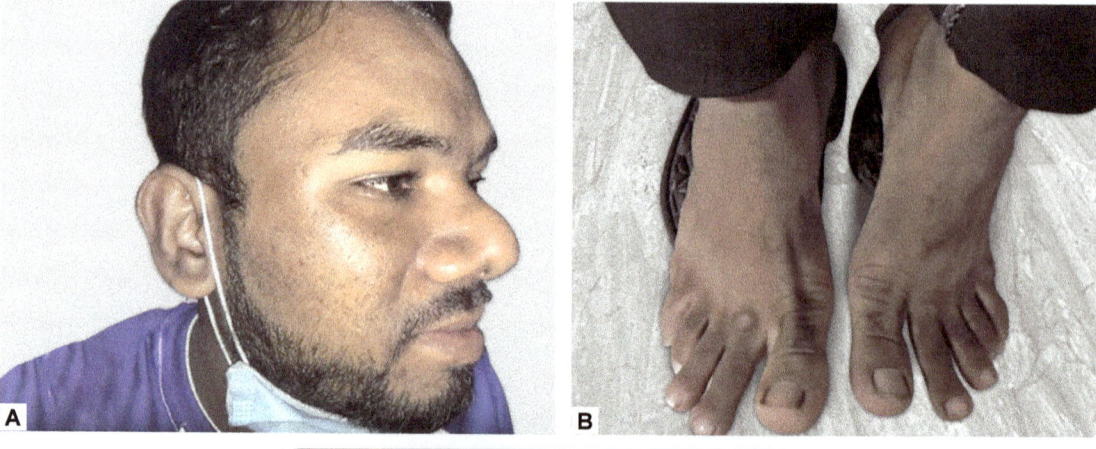

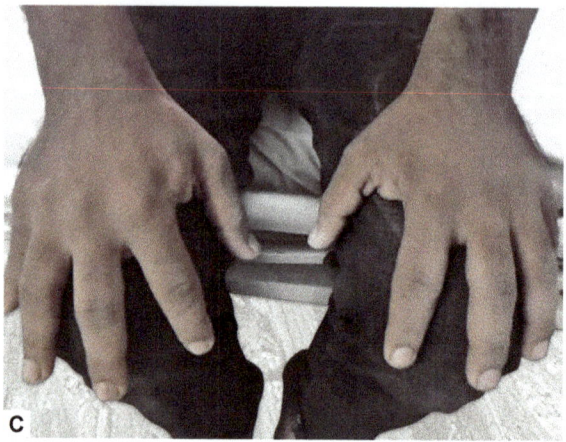

FIGS. 29A TO C: Acromegaly.

Ask about increasing size of fingers, shoes, hats; DM, hypertension, and visual impairment.

Look for disease activity—sweating, axillary skin tags, and glycosuria.

Look for evidence of pituitary tumor—bitemporal hemianopia with optic atrophy.

Facial Nerve Palsy (Figs. 30A and B)

- Inspect the patient's face at rest for asymmetry (forehead wrinkles, angle of the mouth, nasolabial folds).
- Ask the patient to perform the specific facial movement:
  - Raise your eyebrows as like you are surprised or can you do a wide smile for me?—note any asymmetry.
  - Close your eyes tightly and do not let me open them—note the power.
  - Blow out your cheeks and do not let me deflate them—note the power.
  - Can you try to whistle for me?
  - Close your lips tightly and do not let me open them—note the power.

Other things to check:
- Inspect external auditory meatus for herpes zoster rash (Ramsay Hunt syndrome)
- Have you noticed any change in hearing (hyperacusis)?
- Have you noticed any change in taste sensation to the front part (anterior two-thirds) of your tongue?

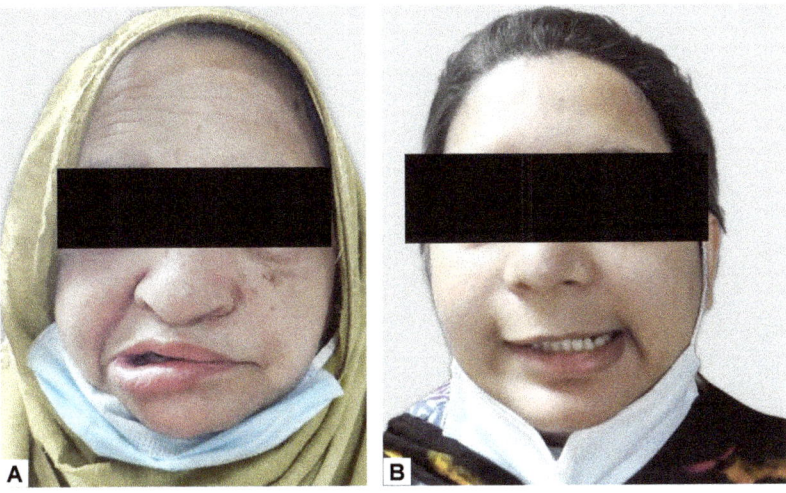

FIGS. 30A AND B: Facial nerve palsy.

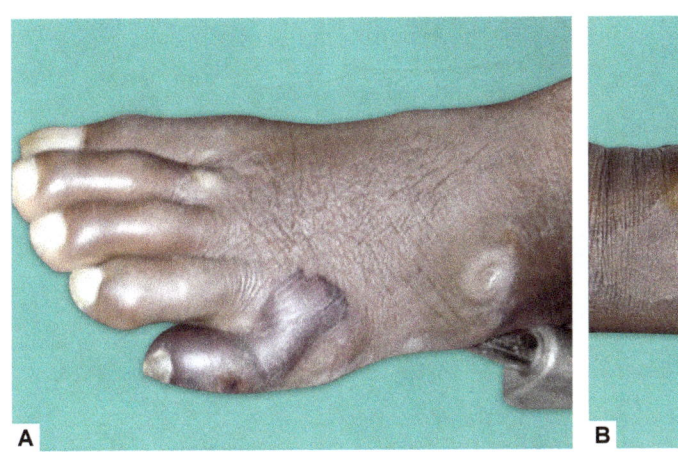
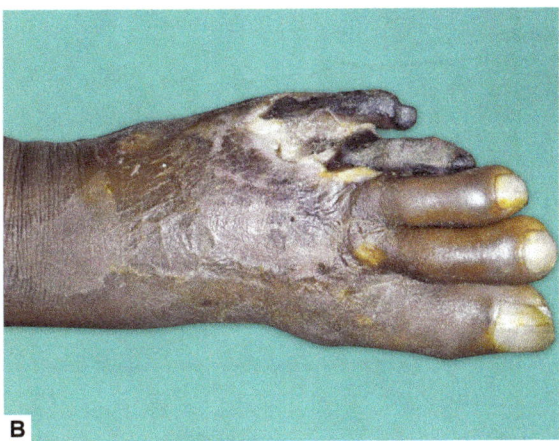

FIGS. 31A AND B: Diabetic foot.

- Have you noticed any weakness in your limbs (same side or opposite side of facial palsy)?

Diabetic Foot (Figs. 31A and B)

Picture illustrates dry gangrene (due to peripheral vascular disease) with evidence of cellulitis.

Look for evidence of neuropathic ulcer (weight bearing area), tinea pedis.

Examine the peripheral pulses and look for evidence of peripheral neuropathy.

Ask about fever, smoking history, hypertension, DM, dyslipidemia, and history of trauma.

Acute Hot Joint (Fig. 32)

- Septic arthritis
- Acute attack of gout

Other possibilities are:

- An acute attack of pseudogout
- Monoarticular presentation of oligo and polyarthritis (seronegative arthritis, RA)
- Trauma
- Hemarthrosis (coagulopathy—anticoagulant, hemophilia, leukemia)

Ask about speed of onset of the symptoms:

- *Within minutes*: Fracture or traumatic derangement of the joint.

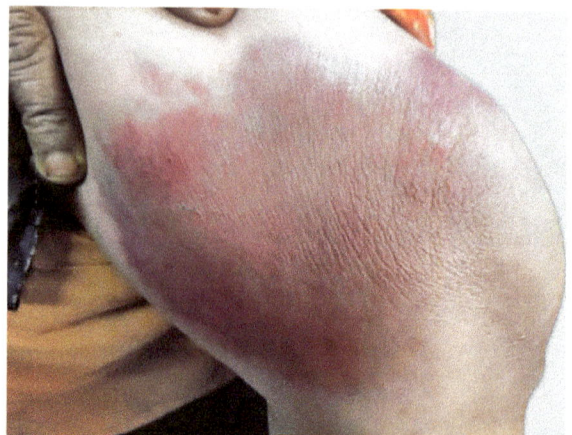

FIG. 32: Acute hot joint.

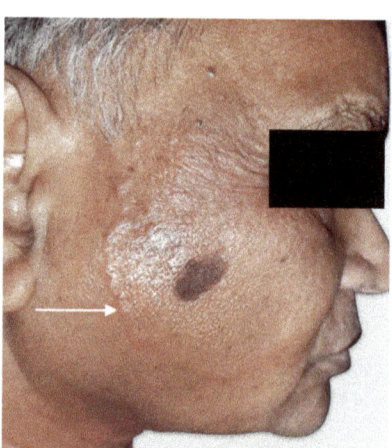

FIG. 33: Tinea corporis.

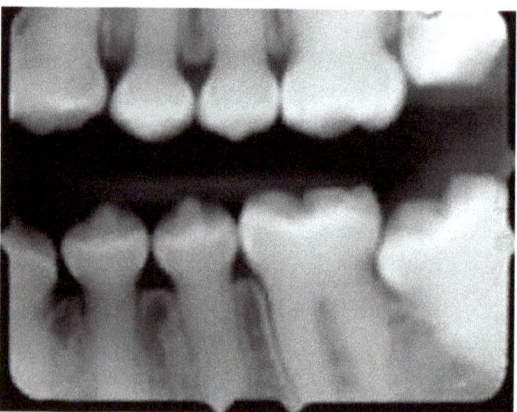

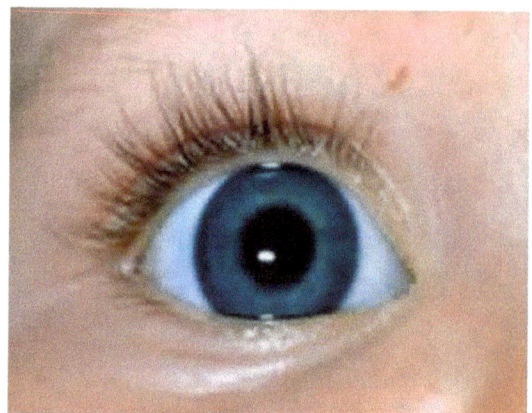

FIG. 34: Blue sclera and dentinogenesis imperfecta.

- *Several hours to 1–2 days*: Consider septic, crystal, or inflammatory arthritis.
- *Insidious onset over days to weeks*: Consider reactive arthritis, mycobacterial or fungal infection, osteoarthritis, tumor.

Any history of previous episode—gout/pseudogout, palindromic RA.

Any history of trauma or coagulopathy (? anticoagulant).

Any history of oral ulcer, colitis or psoriasis or FH of arthritis (seronegative).

Acute fever with chills and rigor or other systemic manifestations (septic).

Suggestive palindromic RA gout (drugs—aspirin, pyrazinamide, hydrochlorothiazide).

Tinea Corporis (Fig. 33)

Itchy, red, scaly, slightly raised ring (circular) shaped rash with central clearing in the face.

Look for other sites—buttock, trunk, arms, and legs.

- Athlete's foot (tinea pedis)
- Jock itch (tinea cruris)
- Scalp (tinea capitis)

Blue Sclera (Visible Choroidal Pigment) (Fig. 34)

Osteogenesis imperfecta (ask about the recurrent fracture, hearing aids, and look for dentinogenesis imperfecta)

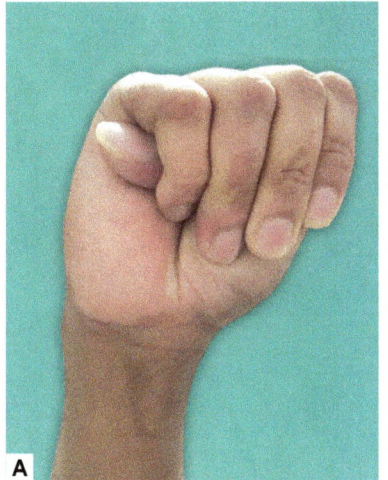 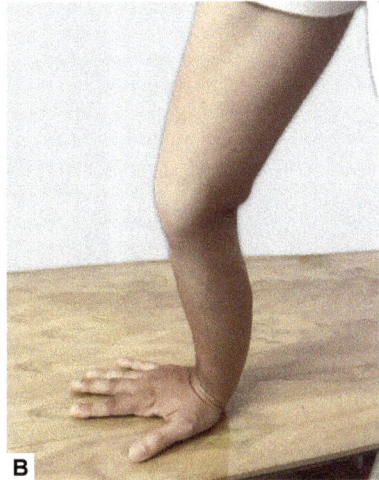 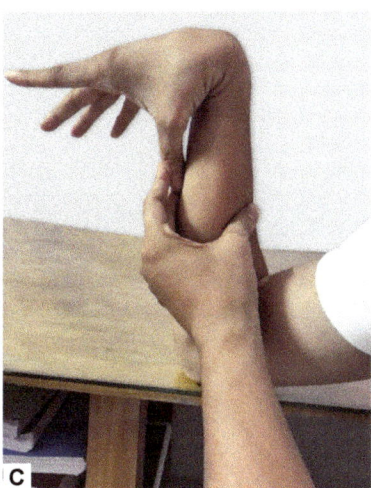

FIGS. 35A TO C: Ehlers–Danlos syndrome.

Differential diagnosis: Marfan syndrome, Ehlers–Danlos syndrome, pseudoxanthoma elasticum, and high myopia.

Ehlers–Danlos Syndrome (Joint Hypermobility) (Figs. 35A to C)

Differential diagnosis:
- Marfan syndrome (look for high arched palate with marfanoid habitus)
- Osteogenesis imperfecta (hearing aid, recurrent fracture)
- Down syndrome

Look for:
- Skin elasticity
- Fragility and texture change (thin and velvety skin) and signs of easy bruising
- Abnormal scar (atrophic scar that looks like cigarette paper)

Examine the cardiovascular (CVS) for the evidence of aortic regurgitation, mitral valve prolapse or mitral regurgitation (MR), and aortic root dilatation.

Ask for FH of similar illness. Ehlers–Danlos syndrome (EDS) is inherited in two ways:
1. Autosomal dominant inheritance (classical, hypermobile, and vascular EDS)
2. Autosomal recessive inheritance (kyphoscoliotic EDS)

Ask for joint pain and dislocation, suggestive history of aortic dissection, or osteoarthritis.

Turner Syndrome

Short and webbed neck, low hairline, and redundant skin fold on the back of the neck. Broad chest (shield chest) with a widely spaced nipple, small lower jaw (micrognathia), a small and fish-like mouth with the low set deformed ear.

Ask about menstrual history, DM, suggestive history of hypothyroidism, heart defect or vision, and hearing problem.

Now look for signs of congenital heart disease such as:
- Bicuspid aortic valve/aortic stenosis
- Coarctation of the aorta
- Partial anomalous venous drainage (PAVD)
- Hypertension or hypothyroidism

Diagnosis is confirmed by karyotype (45XO)

The further test includes ultrasonography (USG) of the kidney, ureter, and bladder (KUB) (for presence of horseshoe kidney), echocardiography, blood sugar, and thyroid function test (TFT).

Tuberous Sclerosis (Figs. 36A to C)

Multiple, small, reddish-brown, dome-shaped papules in the perinasal area, cheeks, and chin (adenoma sebaceum/angiofibroma).

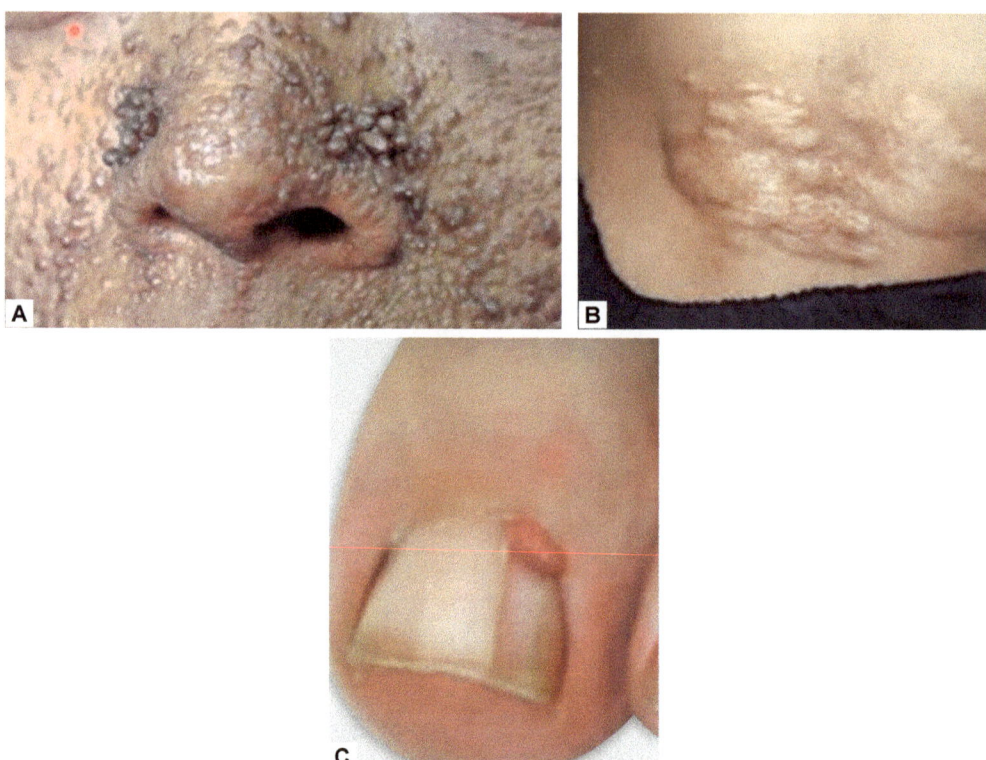

FIGS. 36A TO C: Tuberous sclerosis.

Now look for:
- Hypopigmented (off white), elliptical, or lance-shaped macules (ASH-Leaf macules) in the different sites of the body.
- Multiple firm yellowish-red or pink nodules are giving the texture of an orange peel (shagreen patches) on the buttock and back.
- Smooth, firm, flesh-colored (red) nodules that arise from the nail bed (periungual fibroma) in the toe and finger.

Now ask about:
- When it started (usually present since childhood)
- Family history (autosomal dominant—50% may have a positive FH)
- History of epilepsy or blackout (cardiac or neurological complications)
- Any learning difficulty?
- Any renal problem?

Now examine for mass in the abdomen (it usually associated with renal, hepatic, and gastrointestinal hamartomas).

Diagnosis is confirmed by a genetic test, and the further test would be CT or MRI of the brain for tuberous mass. Echocardiogram to exclude cardiac hamartoma. USG to identify renal tract cyst or hamartoma.

Clubbing (Figs. 37A and B)

Palpate the wrist for tenderness (hypertrophic pulmonary osteoarthopathy suggest bronchogenic carcinoma)

Look for cyanosis, cachexia, lymphadenopathy, nicotine stain, other symptoms of infective endocarditis or chronic liver disease (CLD).

Ask about FH (inherited) and suggestive history of respiratory, heart, and GIT disease.

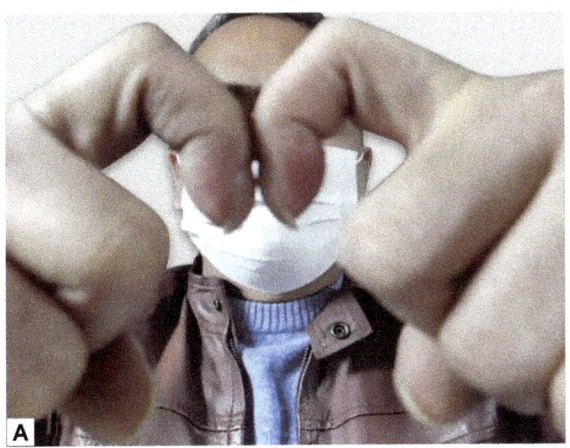 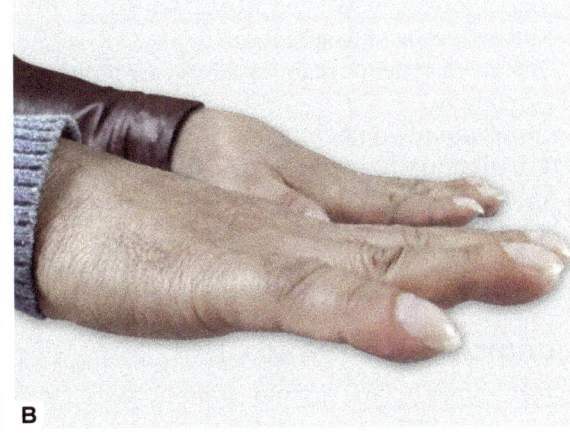

FIGS. 37A AND B: Clubbing.

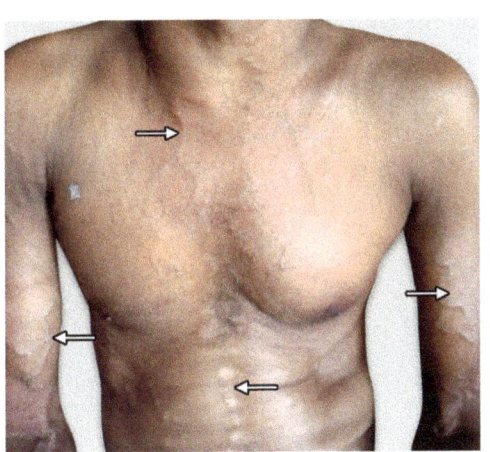

FIG. 38: Superior venacaval obstruction.

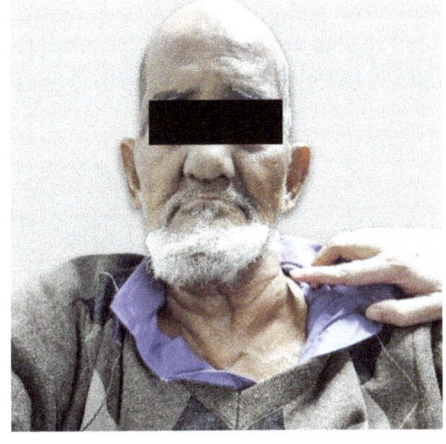

FIG. 39: Supraclavicular lymphadenopathy.

Examine the chest for evidence of bronchogenic carcinoma, DPLD, bronchiectasis, lung abscess, or empyema.

Examine the heart for congenital cyanotic heart disease or infective endocarditis.

Examine abdomen for evidence of IBD, CLD celiac disease.

Superior Venacaval Obstruction (Fig. 38)

Puffy, edematous, and plethoric face with congested conjunctival vessels and engorged nonpulsatile neck veins, dilated tortuous veins on head and chest.

Now look for suggestive findings of the underlying cause:
- Bronchogenic carcinoma (clubbing, lymph node, Horner syndrome, radiation tattoos, and chest sign)
- Lymphoma (generalized lymphadenopathy)

Supraclavicular Lymphadenopathy (Fig. 39)

Ask about generalized lymphadenopathy, hepatosplenomegaly (have you noticed any lumps or bumps in other parts like armpit, groin, or in your tummy?).

Ask about general symptoms—fever, night sweats, anorexia, or weight loss.

Ask about systemic manifestation—respiratory, GIT, or others.

Think about—Tuberculosis (TB), metastasis, lymphadenopathy, lymphoma, hematological malignancy [Chronic lymphocytic leukemia (CLL), acute lymphocytic leukemia (ALL)]

Ask and examine for evidence of pancytopenia (anemia, fever, or bleeding manifestation).

Jaundice (Figs. 40A to C)

Picture shows yellow discoloration of the sclera secondary to high serum bilirubin.

Look for clubbing, palmar erythema, anemia, Dupuytren's contracture, spider nevi, lymphadenopathy, gynecomastia, testicular atrophy, ascites, hepatosplenomegaly, and peripheral edema.

Ask about suggestive history of hematemesis and melena, hepatic encephalopathy, sore throat, rash (infectious mononucleosis), occupation (Weil's disease in sewage worker), intravenous (I/V) drug abuse, alcohol history, blood transfusion, previous surgery, abdominal pain, pale stool, and itching (obstructive jaundice) Dupuytren's contracture.

Bilateral Ptosis (Fig. 41)

Expressionless face with flat effect.

Differential diagnosis: Myasthenia gravis (MG), ocular myopathy, facioscapulohumeral myopathy, myotonic dystrophy, congenital or senile, very rarely—bilateral Horner's syndrome or 3rd nerve palsy.

Ask about diplopia: Onset, progression of the symptoms with diurnal variation with fatigability and examine for evidence of fatigability to establish your diagnosis of MG.

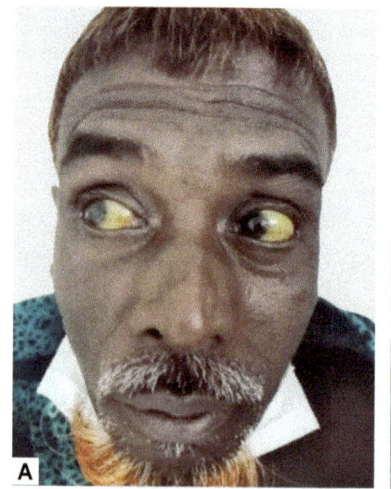
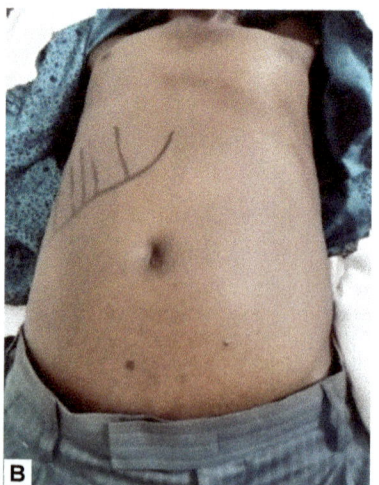
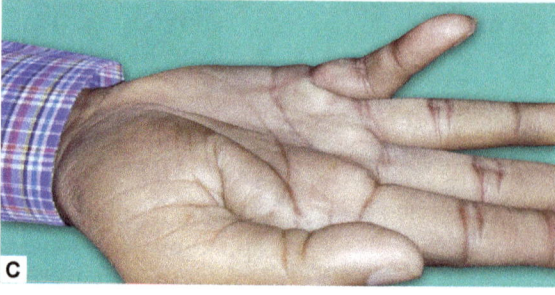

FIGS. 40A TO C: Jaundice, hepatomegaly, and Dupuytren's contracture.

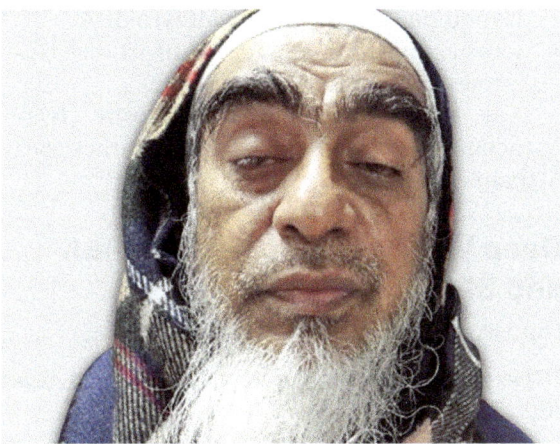

FIG. 41: Bilateral ptosis.

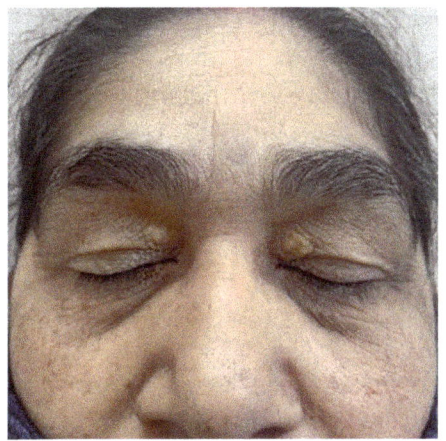

FIG. 43: Xanthelasma.

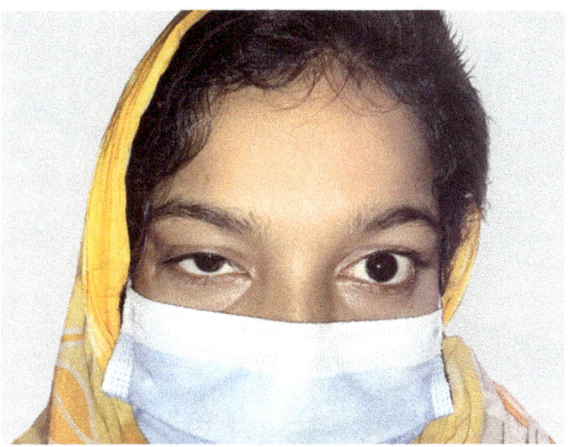

FIG. 42: Horner syndrome.

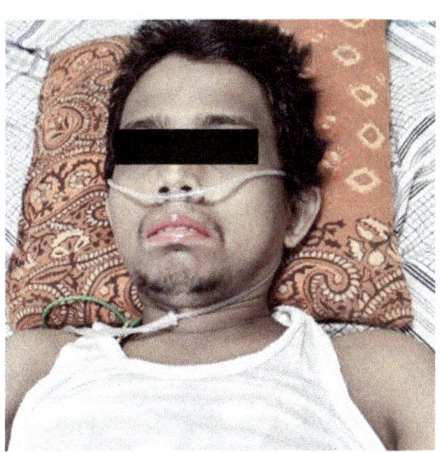

FIG. 44: Thalassemic face.

Horner Syndrome (Fig. 42)

Unilateral ptosis (partial), miosis, and enophthalmos.

Now look for—anhidrosis (lesion proximal to superior cervical ganglion).

Pancoast tumor (dullness in the apical lung zone, fullness in the supraclavicular area due to lymphadenopathy, tracheal deviation, clubbing), wasting and loss of sensation in hand with characteristic C8-T1 lesion in case Pancoast syndrome.

Ask about the history of a whiplash injury or neck pain (carotid dissection).

Xanthelasma (Fig. 43)

Sharply demarcated yellowish deposit of cholesterol underneath the skin.

Look for tendon xanthoma, eruptive xanthoma, and corneal arcus.

Ask about FH as suggestive history of liver disease [e.g., primary biliary cirrhosis (PBC)].

Ask about other cardiovascular risk factors or complications of hypertension, DM, myocardial infarction (MI), CVD.

Thalassemic Face (Fig. 44)

Large cheek bones, a depressed nasal breeze, protruding maxilla with a characteristic rodent or "squirrel-like" face.

Down Syndrome (Figs. 45A to C)

Flattened face, epicanthic fold (upsloping palpebral fissure), low set ears, collapsed nasal bridge, short neck, with excess skin at the back of the neck.

Look for:
- Wide, short hands, and short fingers
- A deep groove between the first and second toes
- A single, deep, crease across the palm of the hand
- Brushfield spots on the iris (yellow speckles)
- Short curved little finger
- Hypotonia and signs of hypothyroidism
- Cardiac murmur [congenital heart disease—atrial septal defect (ASD) or MR].

Ask about intelligence quotient (IQ)—Associated with acute leukemia, cataract, early Alzheimer disease.

Deep Vein Thrombosis (Figs. 46A and B)

Diffuse swelling in the left leg up to thigh.

Differential diagnosis: Cellulitis, trauma, and ruptured Baker's cyst.

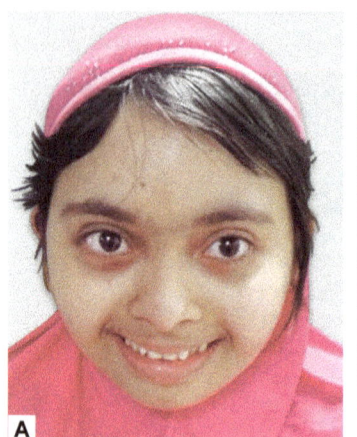 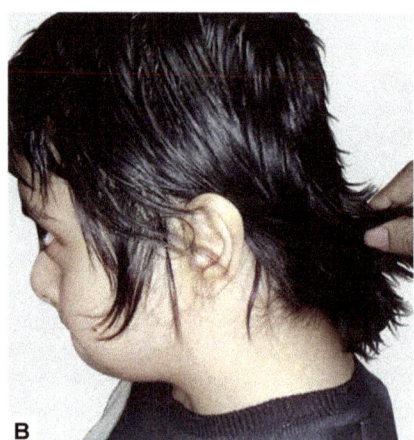 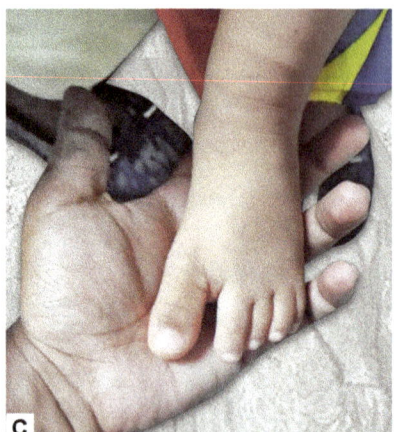

FIGS. 45A TO C: Down syndrome.

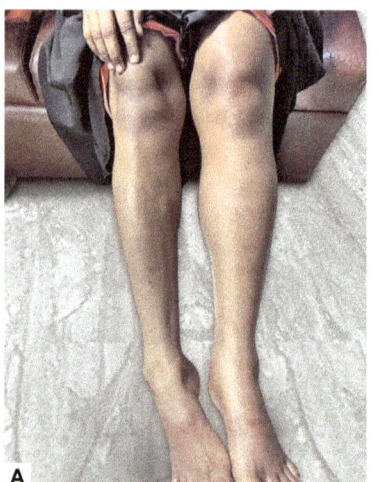 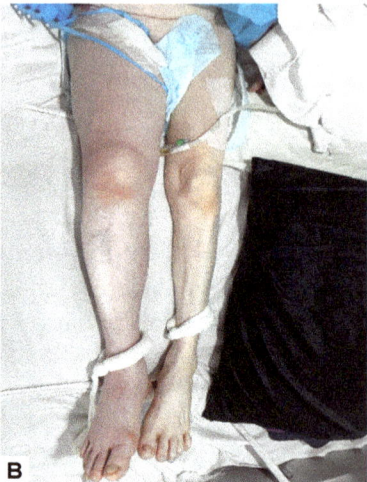

FIGS. 46A AND B: Deep vein thrombosis.

Ask about fever with chills, trauma, and diabetes (cellulitis).

Suggestive history of deep vein thrombosis (DVT)—recent surgery, FH of clot, long-haul flight, chest pain with breathlessness, hemoptysis (? pulmonary embolism).

Varicose Vein (Fig. 47)
Blue-purple colour, twisted, swollen and enlarged veins that usually occurs in the legs and feet.

Arsenicosis (Figs. 48A to C)
Diffuse hyperpigmented skin with rain-drop pigmentation.

Keratosis on the palm and sole with diffuse thickening.

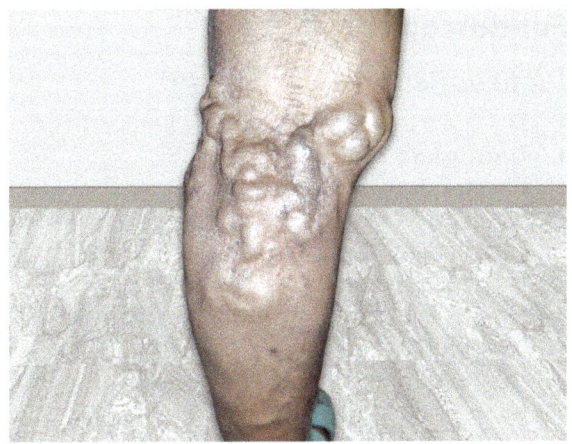

FIG. 47: Varicose vein.

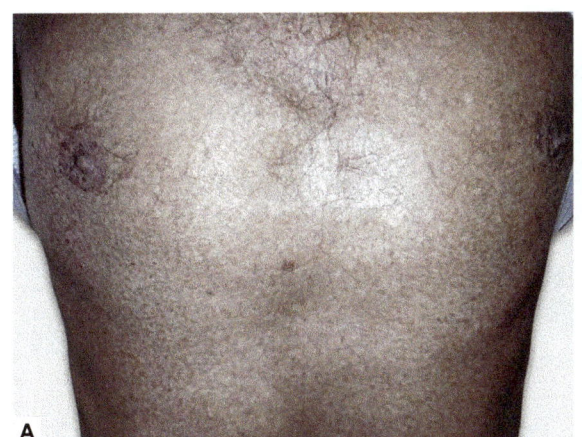
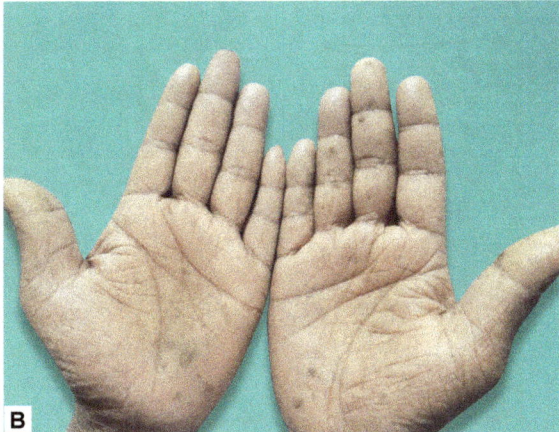
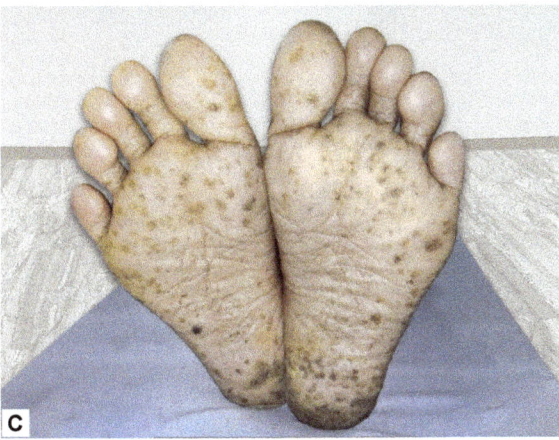

FIGS. 48A TO C: Arsenicosis.

Fundoscopy

Diabetic Retinopathy (Fig. 49)
- Dot (microaneurysm) and blot hemorrhage
- Hard exudate
- Flame-shaped hemorrhage and cotton wool spot (indicate retinal ischemia which stimulates new vessel formation)
- Neovascularization
- Hemorrhage and exudate at the maculae (maculopathy)
- Vitreous hemorrhage (large, dark floaters/red haze/no view to the retina at all)
- Photocoagulation scar

Hypertensive Retinopathy (Fig. 50)
Thin, irregular arterioles with an increased light reflex (copper or silver wiring).

Flame-shaped hemorrhage and cotton wool exudates (grade-3 hypertensive retinopathy).

Papilledema (grade-4 hypertensive retinopathy)—indicating cerebral edema, it may occur in malignant hypertension with or without flame-shaped hemorrhage and exudate.

Papilledema (Fig. 51)
The optic disc is swollen with blurred margin. Consider further examination for:
- Central scotoma

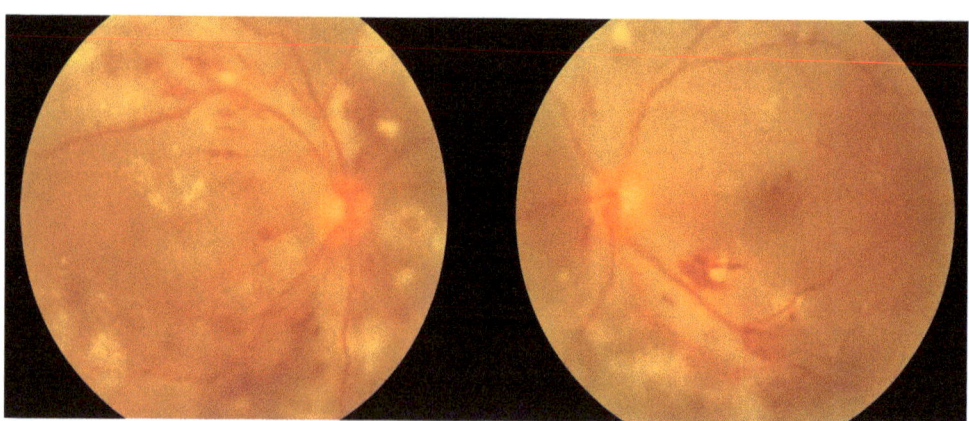

FIG. 49: Diabetic retinopathy.

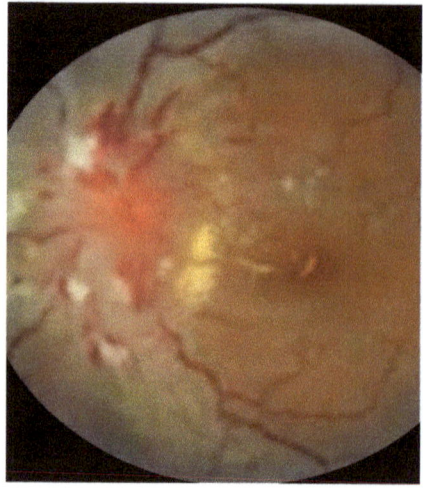

FIG. 50: Hypertensive retinopathy.

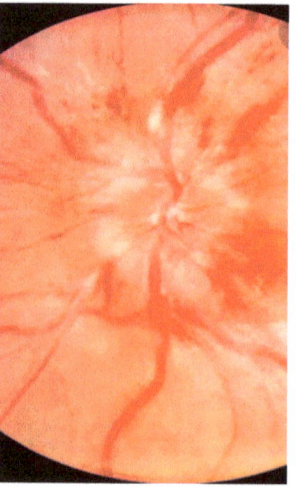

FIG. 51: Papilledema.

- Cranial nerve examination for false localizing signs
- Blood pressure
- Visual acuity and pupillary reactions are normal in papilledema (but in case of optic neuritis it will be affected)

Optic Atrophy (Fig. 52)

- The disc is pale and clearly delineated.
- In severe cases, the pupil reacts consensually to light but not directly.
- Field testing with the head of a hat pin reveals a central scotoma.

Foster Kennedy Syndrome (Fig. 53)

Evidence of optic atrophy possibly due to optic nerve compression due to frontal lobe tumor with contralateral papilledema due to raised intracranial pressure.

Retinal Vein Occlusion (Figs. 54A and B)

The veins are tortuous and enlarged, hemorrhage is scattered over the whole retina, irregular and superficial, like bundles of straw alongside the veins (central retinal vein occlusion) but if respecting horizontal raphe (confined to the sector) then suggest BRVO.

Underlying cause includes hypertension, DM, dyslipidaemia, hyperviscosity syndrome (e.g., Waldenström macroglobulinemia) or myeloma and CTD.

Glaucoma (Fig. 55)

Optic disc cupping but in case of advanced glaucoma large optic disc with sharply angulated vessels.

The visual field is grossly constricted, and the patient has an only central vision (tunnel vision—suggest advanced chronic glaucoma).

Retinitis Pigmentosa (Figs. 56A and B)

Pale optic disc attenuated retinal blood vessels and pigments spicules in the peripheries.

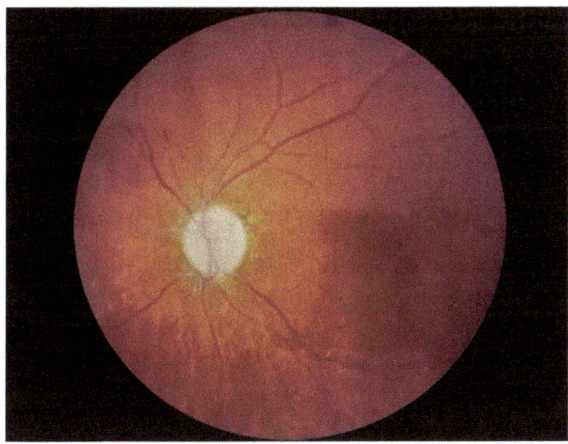

FIG. 52: Optic atrophy.

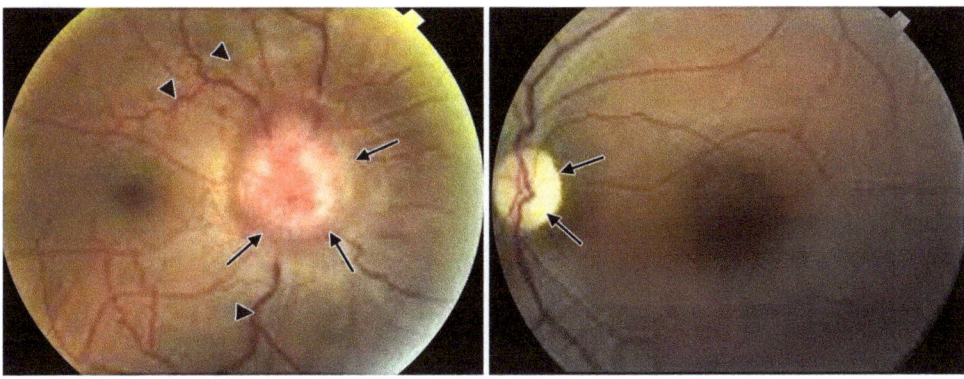

FIG. 53: Foster Kennedy syndrome.

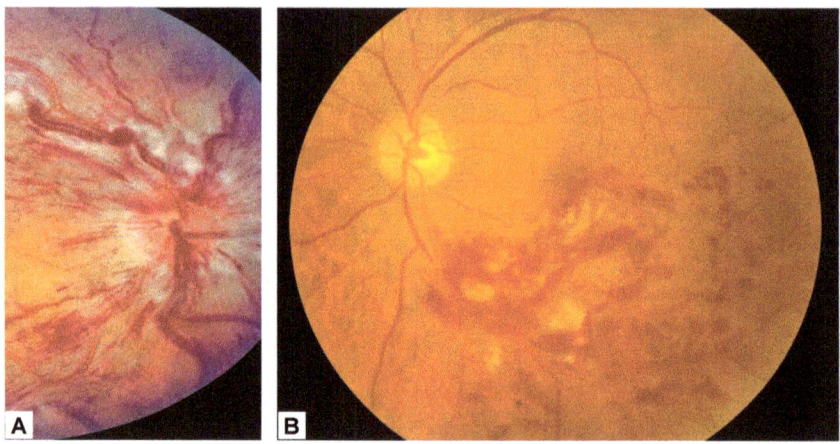

FIGS. 54A AND B: Retinal vein occlusion.

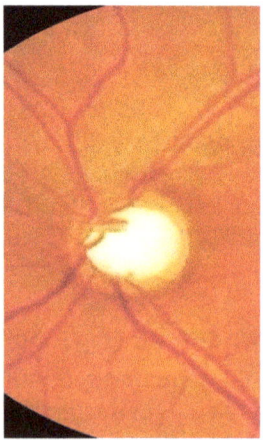

FIG. 55: Glaucoma.

The visual field is grossly constricted, and the patient has an only central vision (tunnel vision).

Look for underlying syndromes (e.g., truncal obesity, short stature, and polydactyly suggest—Laurence-Moon-Bardet-Biedl syndrome).

Cytomegalovirus Retinitis (Fig. 57)
Creamy retinal infiltrates with scattered retinal hemorrhage "scrambled egg and tomato ketchup."

Scars (Figs. 58 and 59)
Upper vertical midline incision that originates from the xiphoid process extend up to 1 cm above the umbilicus and then extends laterally to the right is called modified Makuuchi incision mainly used for hepatobiliary surgery and foregut procedure.

Kocher incision is right subcostal incision used to gain access for the gallbladder, the biliary tree (open cholecystectomy) but the extension of the incision to the other side of the abdomen called rooftop/chevron incision mainly used for upper GIT surgery (esophagectomy, bilateral adrenalectomy, hepatic resection, or liver transplant).
Modified Makuuchi Incision for liver lobectomy.

The rooftop incision with a vertical extension as breakthrough the xiphisternum is called Mercedes Benz incision classically seen in liver transplant.

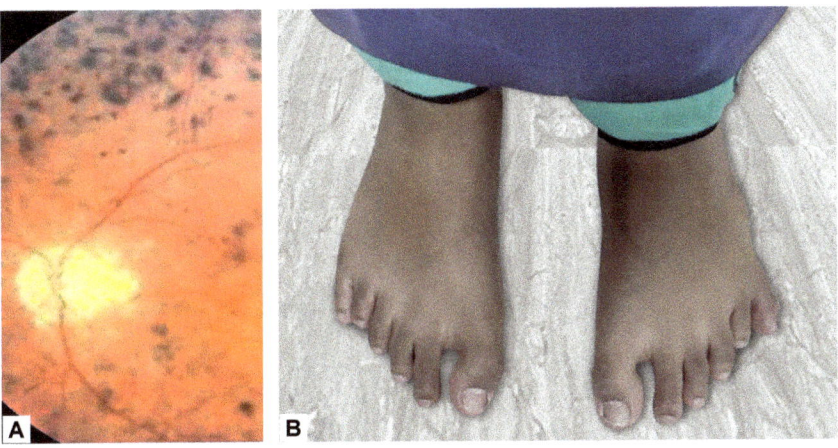

FIGS. 56A AND B: Retinitis pigmentosa and polydactyly.

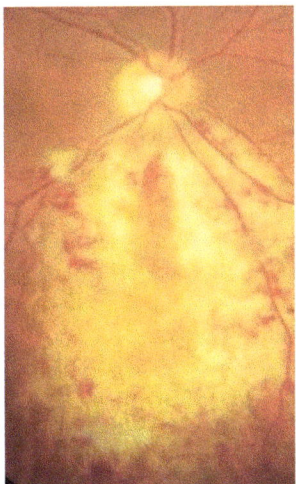

FIG. 57: Cytomegalovirus retinitis.

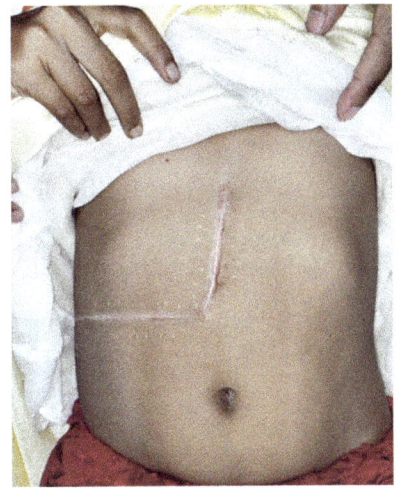

FIG. 58: Scars.

The Lanz incision is a transverse incision whilst the Gridiran incision is oblique incision are made at McBurney's point (two-thirds from the umbilicus to anterior superior iliac spine) mainly used for appendectomy.

Extension of Gridiran incision by division of the oblique fossa (Rutherford Morrison incision) mainly used for renal transplant but can be used for right or left-sided colonic resection, cecostomy, and sigmoid colostomy.

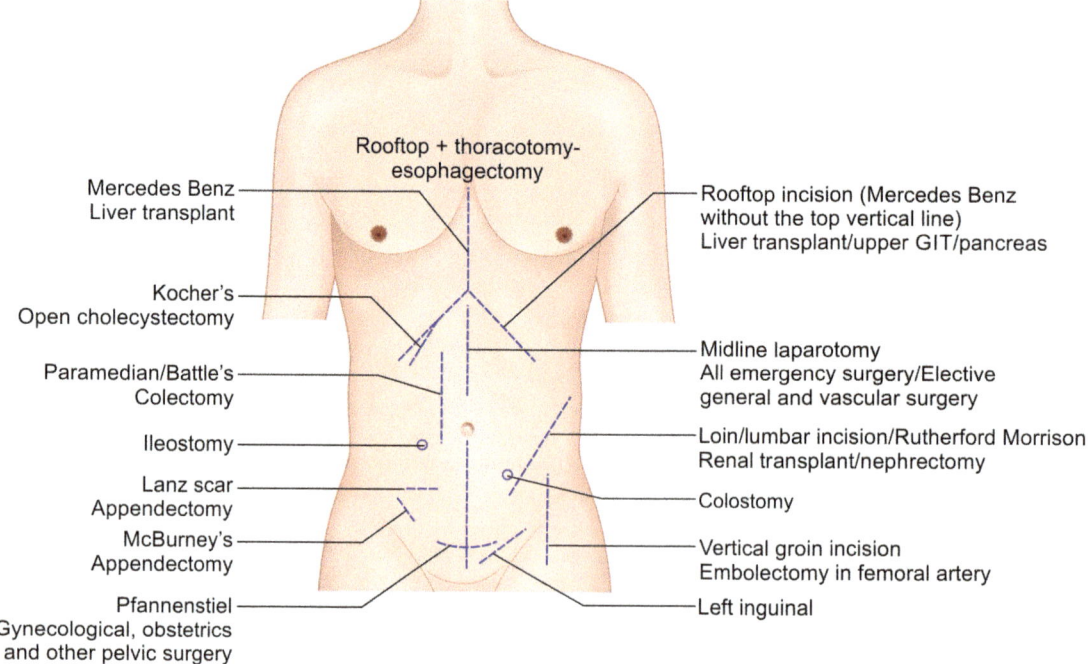

FIG. 59: Abdominal scar.

Chest Scars (Figs. 60A to C)

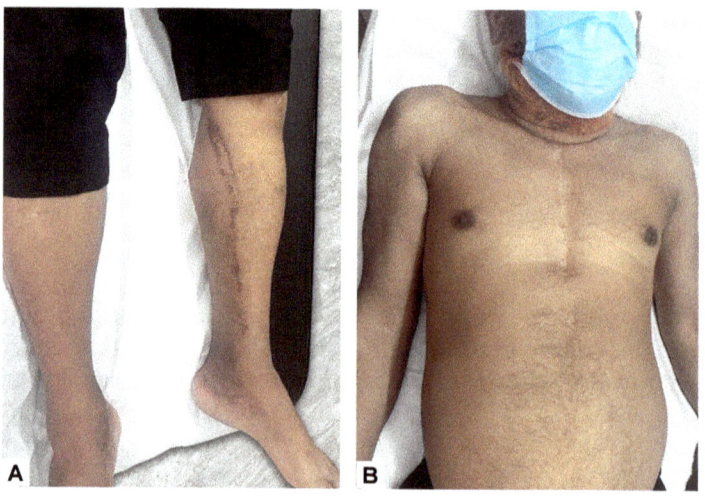

FIGS. 60A TO C: *Continued*

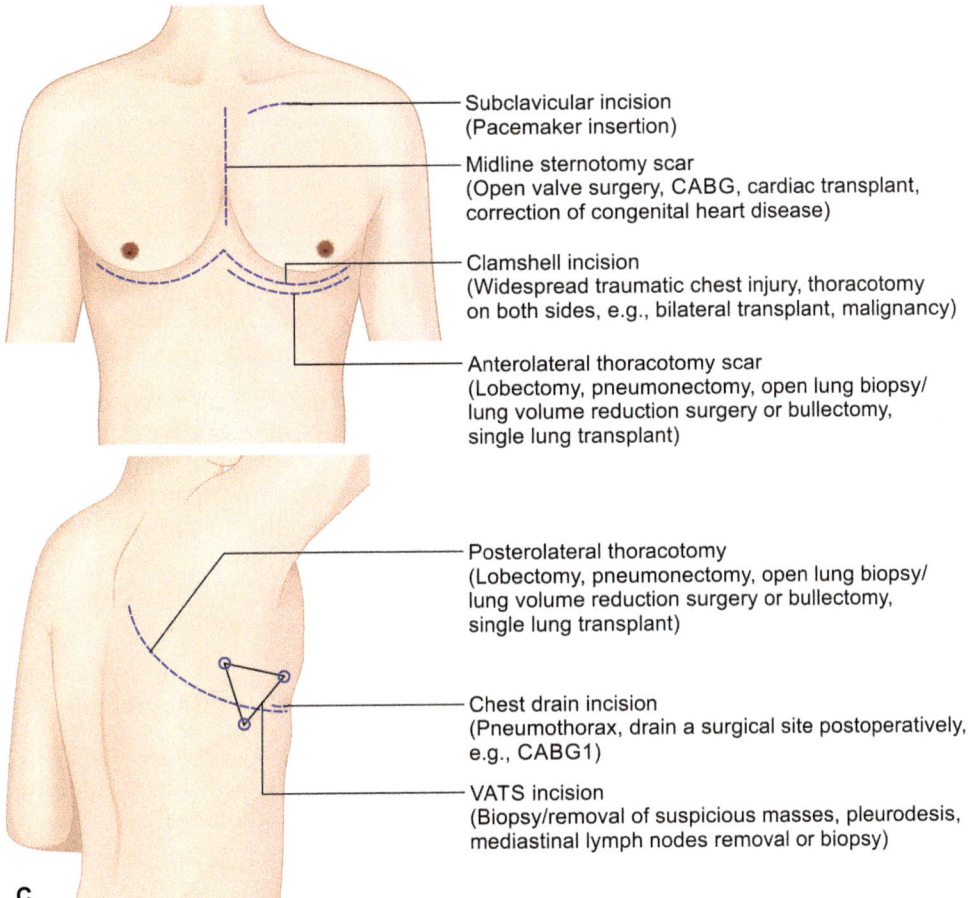

FIGS. 60A TO C: Chest scars.

Hypothyroidism

Your role: You are the Registrar in the Endocrinology Clinic.

Patient details: Mrs Elvia Gomez, a 45-year-old lady.

You have total 10 minutes with each patient. You will receive a warning after 6 minutes, and you will be stopped at 8 minutes. In the last 2 minutes, examiner will ask you to explain any abnormalities in the focused clinical history, abnormal clinical signs you may have elicited, and regarding your diagnosis or differential diagnoses including management plan (if this was not cleared from your consultation).

Referral

Clinical problem: Lethargy, weight gain with pain in both hands.

Baseline Observations

- *Pulse rate*: 58/minute
- *Blood pressure*: 125/80 mm Hg
- *Respiratory rate*: 18/minute
- *Oxygen saturation*: 99%
- *Temperature*: 37.2°C

Your task is to: Assess this problem by employing a brief focused clinical history and associated focused physical examination.

There is no need to finish the history prior to your physical examination.

Explain the patient of your possible diagnosis or differential diagnoses, including your investigation and management plan.

Address any concerns or specific questions which the patient may have.

At the end of the station, any notes you make must be handed to the examiners.

(*Once you get this clinical scenario, you will get 5 minutes to start this station for two scenarios. At that time, start to think about your diagnosis and differential diagnoses and plan for taking focused history as well as focused examination.*)

[*Differential diagnosis of weight gain*: Hypothyroidism, Cushing syndrome, insulinoma, polycystic ovary syndrome (PCOS), type-2 DM, hypothalamic insufficiency, fluid and salt retention due to chronic kidney disease (CKD), CLD, nephrotic syndrome, congestive cardiac failure (CCF), Drugs—antiepileptics, antipsychotics, or steroids.

Differential diagnosis of lethargy: Cushing syndrome, hypothyroidism, anemia

Differential diagnosis of hand pain: Rheumatoid arthritis, Carpal tunnel syndrome due to hypothyroidism, acromegaly.]

(*Once you enter the room search for a spot diagnosis; coarse hair; facial fullness; periorbital swelling; obesity; loss of outer one-third of eyebrow suggests hypothyroidism.*)

Introduction, Permission, and Identification

Candidate: Good morning, I am Mohammad Ali, one of the working doctors here today, I have been asked to examine you; is that okay with you?

Patient: Good morning, doctor …

Candidate: Thank you for coming, I would like to start by taking your full name, age, and where you have come from, please?

Patient: Yes, doctor………….. I am Mrs Elvia Gomez, 45-year-old, and from London.

Focus History

Candidate: Mrs Gomez, I understand you are having some problems; would you like to tell me more about this? Please tell me in your own words.

Patient: I have gained 12 kg in the last 6 months. I was 76 kg previously but now I am 88 kg. I am very conscious about my diet, and to be honest, my taste has not changed and maintained a healthy diet, but I am still gaining weight. I feel exhausted nowadays, particularly while carrying out household works such as washing, cleaning, and shopping. Recently, I have noticed that my face is swollen, and my skin is getting thicker. With all of these, I am anxious and depressed.

Analyze the Symptoms

Candidate: I am sorry to hear about your condition. I can see you are anxious, let me ask you some questions related to your symptoms for better understanding and see how we can help you.

Patient: Yes, sure ....

Candidate: Let us talk about weight gain:
- When the weight gain started exactly?
- Has it changed since started (is it increasing gradually or decreasing or the same)?
- How much weight have you put on?
- Did you put the weight all over the body, or specific areas like your trunk, back of the neck or legs?
- What about your diet and appetite?
- Do you take part in any physical activities? How many times in a day?
- Do you have a FH of obesity?

Patient: As I mentioned before, I have gained 12 kg, and I am taking a regular balanced meal with regular exercise as before, but I am gaining weight.

Candidate: Now tell me more about your tiredness...
- When did it start exactly? Is it increasing, decreasing day by day or the same?
- When you feel tired? Is there any particular time, such as in the evening or morning? Is it coming on and off or all the time with you?

Patient: I feel tired all the time especially with doing something.

Candidate: Mrs Gomez, you told me you have pain in both hands. Please tell me a little more about the pain like—where is the pain? Character? Grade? Relieving or aggravating factors?

Patient: Yes, doctor...... but, it is not just pain, there are some tingling and numbness in my both hands involving three and a half fingers, which increased at night and during physical activity (carpal tunnel syndrome).

Candidate: What about your menstruation? Is it regular or irregular? Amount of flow—increasing or decreasing? How many tampons do you change in a day? When was your last period day? What is the age of your last child?

Patient: In fact, I wanted to talk to you about this, Doctor. My menstruation is regular, but my menstrual flow has increased a lot in the last few months.

Other Important Targeted Histories
- Do you have any preference for hot or cold weather? Or do you feel the cold more when others are not?
- Any changes in your bowel habit? Are you constipated?
- Have you noticed any skin changes (dry) or hair loss?
- Have you noticed any snoring or early morning headache with daytime sleepiness [obstructive sleep apnea (OSA)]?
- Any chest pain, cough, breathing problem, or any racing in your heart?
- Any problem with memory and concentration? Sleeping more than usual? Hoarse voice?
- Loss of normal skin color (vitiligo)?
- Any shortness of breath, the difficulty in swallowing, change in voice (retrosternal extension)?
- Have you noticed any lump in your neck? Is it tender? Does it move upward during swallowing?
- Do you have any problems with your vision? Any eye pain, double vision, or diminished vision?

Patient: Yes, I feel cold when others are feeling hot, this happens even in summer when it is warm. My skin has become dry and thick. I have been noticing changes in voice for some time. And yes, I have constipation. However, doctor, I do not have any lump in my neck.

Quick Systemic Review, Past Medical History, Family History, Treatment, Social History According to Your Differentials

Quick Systemic Review

Candidate: Now I would like to ask some general questions that may or may not be related to your symptoms, just to know about your overall health (ask for those questions which were not asked yet).
- Do you have headache, nausea, vomiting, fever, any tummy pain, cough, or any other problems?
- What about your waterworks, amount, color, or frequency?

Patient: No. I do not have any of these...

Past Medical and Surgical History

Candidate: Mrs Gomez, now let us talk about your PMH....
- Do you have any similar condition in the past? Or any other illness, like any previous history of hormone disease such as thyroid, any high blood pressure, high blood sugar, any autoimmune diseases such as rheumatoid arthritis, keratoconjunctivitis sicca, or vitiligo?
- Do you have a history of previous surgery or radioiodine therapy for thyroid disease?

Patient: I had a history of thyroid disease 3 years back. At that time, I was sweating a lot, felt palpitation on my chest, and lost weight. The doctor first gave me some medicines, but there was no improvement, and later I was treated with radioiodine therapy.

Treatment History

Candidate:
- Are you on any regular medications [any particular drugs that are causing obesity such as steroids, tricyclic antidepressants (TCA), antipsychotic, anti-epileptics]?
- Do you take any over-the-counter medication or herbal remedies or any recreational drugs?
- Are you allergic to any medicine or anything else?

Patient: I am not taking any regular medications at this moment, and I do not have any known allergies.

Relevant Family History

Candidate: Is there anyone else in your family with this type of problem or any long-standing illness that runs in your families like thyroid disease, DM, hypertension, stroke, or any autoimmune disease or anything else?

Patient: Well... My mother has hypertension and taking medication for it.

Social History

Candidate:
- Do you smoke? If not—then ask, have you ever smoked? If yes—then how many years you were smoking? How many sticks per day?
- Do you drink alcohol? If yes—then how many drinks would you have in a week? (CAGE questionnaire if needed;
- Have you ever felt you needed to cut down on your drinking?
- Have people annoyed you by criticizing your drinking?
- Have you ever felt guilty about drinking?
- Have you ever felt you needed a drink first thing in the morning (eye-opener) to steady your nerves or to get rid of a hangover?)
- What are you doing for a living? How have these symptoms affected your job? (If not working—then ask....... are you finding it

difficult to cope with finance because you are missing work?)
- Are you married? Who is at home with you or who is supporting you now? Do you have any children?
- How are all of these symptoms affecting your life?

Patient: I am a housewife, and nowadays, I am having a hard time doing housework because of my physical weakness. I have two children; I am staying with my husband, and they are all healthy. I never smoke but drink 2/1 glass of wine on weekends with my friends.

Candidate: I can see this has affected your life. We are here to help you, before that is there anything I have missed or anything you want to tell me? Or, have I missed anything, or do you want to add anything more?

Patient: No….

Candidate: Would you mind if I go on to examine you?

Patient: It is all right.

Focused Examination

Here, focused examination would be as a whole general appearance including:

Face

- Obese or overweight, periorbital swelling with facial puffiness.
- Rough, dry skin, coarse facial feature with evidence of hair loss (brittle hair)

If evidence of Graves' ophthalmopathy (evidence of Grave's disease treatments—surgery or radio-iodine therapy).
- Then examine the eye properly for proptosis, chemosis, eye movement for diplopia or external ophthalmoplegia, and relative afferent pupillary defect (RAPD).

Hand

- Examine pulse for bradycardia
- Any nail changes (onycholysis, longitudinal ridging)
- Examination of median nerve including the presence of Tinel's (May I tap on your wrist? Do you feel any pain? or Phalen's signs) (Can you bend your wrist like this?)

Examination of the Neck for Thyroid Gland

- Any scars of previous surgeries
- If the thyroid gland is enlarged (goiter), then think about Hashimoto's thyroiditis/hypothyroid Graves' disease/drugs/transient hypothyroidism due to subacute thyroiditis (if it is tender)/postpartum thyroiditis (if there is a recent history of pregnancy).

Hypothyroidism can cause the proximal myopathy, peripheral neuropathy, cerebellar syndrome, or can be associated with other autoimmune diseases like pernicious anemia, vitiligo. So, examine for these, if possible.

It can also cause anasarca including ascites/effusion/pitting or nonpitting edema. So, examine for these if possible.

Finally, it can cause hyporeflexia with delayed relaxation.

Association for other autoimmune diseases—Vitiligo, addisonian features, alopecia areata/totalis.

So, ask the examiner that—I would like to complete my assessment by checking blood pressure, doing urine dipstick, examining CVS and neurological system, and delayed relaxation of the ankle jerk.

Feedback to the Patient and Respond to the Patient's Concern

Candidate: Thank you very much for letting me examine you. You said at the beginning that the main problems were tiredness, weight gain, cold intolerance, and pain in the hands. Is there anything else troubling you that we have missed or any questions to ask or any concerns?

Patient: I am really upset doctor, please tell me what is going on?

Candidate: Considering what you have told me and the signs I elicit on examination, I think you may have a condition known as hypothyroidism meaning that your thyroid gland is underactive and is not producing enough thyroxin hormone. The best way to treat your symptoms is by replacing the thyroxine that is not produced. Before starting treatment, we need to confirm the diagnosis by doing TFTs as well as other blood tests to exclude other possible causes of your symptoms. Is that okay? Is there anything, in particular, you are concerned about?

Patient: No.

Candidate: Okay, thank you for spending time with me.

Patient: Thank you.

Discussion with Examiner

Examiner: Please present your case.

Candidate:
This middle-aged lady presented with progressive unintentional weight gain with cold intolerance, lethargy, tingling and numbness in both hands.

On examination, the patient is overweight with myxedematous facies (thickened and coarse facial feature, periorbital puffiness with pallor).

The skin is dry, rough, cold, and there is generalized swelling of the feet which is nonpitting.

She has a hoarse and croaky voice.

There is thinning of the hair which is dry and brittle.

She has bradycardia; her pulse is 52 beats/minute and regular.

Phalen's test is positive bilaterally, and this would be in keeping with bilateral carpal tunnel syndrome.

So, in summary, my diagnosis would be Graves' disease with resultant hypothyroidism (as there is no scar in the neck—likely treated by radioiodine therapy previously) with bilateral carpal tunnel syndrome.

Examiner: How would you investigate this case?

Candidate: I would like first to do a set of the blood test most importantly, a thyroid function profile, including thyroid-stimulating hormone (TSH) level and T4 level. Other tests include CBC with ESR, urea and electrolyte (U&E), liver function tests (LFTs), lipid profile (since hypercholesterolemia can be a complication).

If I wanted a further investigation, I would like to check autoantibodies—anti-TSH receptor antibody, anti-thyroid peroxidase (TPO) antibody and antithyroglobulin antibody and potentially also a T3 level to get a further understanding of the thyroid function.

Note: If the thyroid gland is enlarged, I would also want to do an ultrasound scan of neck particularly looking at the thyroid gland to see if there is any evidence of malignancy within the thyroid gland or if there is any evidence of thyroid cysts or thyroglossal cysts. If thyroid ultrasound confirms the presence of goiter, then I would like to do a fine needle aspiration cytology (FNAC) test. Also, a chest X-ray to look for any retrosternal extension.

Examiner: How would you manage this case?

Candidate: The mainstay of management is thyroid hormone replacement with levothyroxine, typically 25–75 µg as a starting dose, titrated to response.

Following treatment initiation, TSH and T4 levels should be checked at 6–8 weeks with dose adjustments made accordingly.

Examiner: Please tell me some causes of hypothyroidism.

Candidate: Causes are:
- *Autoimmune cause*: Hashimoto's thyroiditis (most common, goiter present), primary atrophic hypothyroidism (no goiter).
- Following thyroid ablation by surgery or radioactive iodine therapy (in case of thyroid malignancy and thyrotoxic Graves' disease)
- Transient hypothyroidism due to postpartum or subacute thyroiditis
- *Drugs*: Antithyroid drugs, amiodarone, lithium, interferon therapy

Examiner: Tell me how would you initiate levothyroxine replacement therapy in an elderly patient with hypothyroidism or a patient with ischemic heart disease?

Candidate: As levothyroxine may precipitate angina or MI, it is, therefore, prudent to start with a low initial dose of levothyroxine, e.g., 12.5–25 μg/day and titrated up cautiously, by 25 μg every 2-4 weeks according to TSH level.

Examiner: Tell me about hypothyroidism in pregnancy.

Candidate: Hypothyroidism, particularly in the first trimester of pregnancy, has been shown to have harmful effects on fetal neurodevelopment. Thyroid hormone requirements usually increase substantially during pregnancy, with the range of dose increments being 25–50%. Women with pre-existing thyroid disease should have their TFT checked at least every trimester with a typical target range for TSH of 0.5–2.0 mU/L. After delivery, the patient can return to their prepregnancy dose, with immediate effect. Hypothyroidism in pregnancy increases the risk of anemia, toxemia of pregnancy, prematurity, low birth weight baby, stillbirth, and postpartum hemorrhage.

Graves' Disease

Your role: You are the Registrar in the Endocrinology clinic.

Patient profile: Mrs Lucy, a 35-year-old female.

Problem: Lump in the neck, weight loss, palpitation, and anxiety feelings.

(*Once you get this clinical scenario, you will get 5 minutes to start this station for two scenarios. At that time, start to think about your diagnosis and differential diagnoses and plan for taking focused history as well as focused examination.*)

Differential diagnosis:
- *For neck lump*: Thyroid swelling (Graves' disease, multinodular or solitary nodule, thyroid cancer); lymphadenopathy (lymphoma, sarcoidosis, and TB).
- *For weight loss*: Thyrotoxicosis; type-1 DM; chronic infection—TB; malignancy.
- *For palpitation*: Thyrotoxicosis, cardiac cause, or anemia.
- *For anxiety*: Thyrotoxicosis.

So, here most likely diagnosis would be thyrotoxicosis.

(*Once you enter the room search for a spot diagnosis; thin and appears fidgety with stare look; exophthalmos; enlarged thyroid gland suggests thyrotoxicosis.*)

Introduction, Permission, and Identification

Candidate: Good morning, I am Mohammad Ali, one of the working doctors here today, I have been asked to examine you; is that okay with you?

Patient: Good morning, doctor…

Candidate: Thank you for coming, I would like to start by taking your full name, age, and where you have come from, please?

Patient: I am Lucy, 35-year-old and from Liverpool.

Focused History

Candidate: Okay. Would you please tell me what brings you here today? Please tell me in your own words.

Patient: My main concern is the lump in my neck. I have lost weight, and also, I feel my heart beat quite faster than previous. I am getting irritable day by day, even my colleagues have commented that I am a little cranky at work, short-tempered and impatient.

Candidate: Let us talk about you lump..
- When did you first notice the lump?
- Has the lump changed in size over the time?
- How many lumps can you feel?
- Does the lump move when you swallow?
- Can you feel the lump beating (Pulsatile neck mass suggest carotid artery aneurysm)?
- Have you noticed similar lumps elsewhere—face, armpit, elbow, or groin (lymphadenopathy; lymphoma)?
- Do you have pain in the lump?
- Do you have any fever with night sweats or itching?

Patient: My husband first noticed the swelling of my neck 8 weeks ago. It is in the center of my neck, and not painful at all. I do not think it has grown in size, but I feel a little odd nowadays and wear scarves when going out. There is no lump in other parts of my body. No fever or night sweats.

Candidate: Now tell me more about your weight loss:
- How much weight have you lost? Over how long?
- Is the weight loss intentional or unintentional?
- Does it coincide with a change in diet, physical activity, or lifestyle?

- How is your appetite?
- Have you noticed any change in your bowels? Any diarrhea or constipation? How often do you open your bowels?

Patient: It is quite surprising that I have lost 5 kg weight in the last 4 months despite eating a little more than usual. And yes, my bowel frequency has increased more than usual but no loose stool.

Candidate: Okay........for palpitation:
- How long have you had the palpitation?
- Does palpitation occur gradually or suddenly?
- Do you feel racing or tapping heartbeat (suggest fast arrhythmia); missed or extra beat (ventricular ectopies)?
- Is there anything that triggers the palpitation or anything else that helps to stop the palpitation?

Patient: I feel that my heart is racing at work and even in bed at night. I do not know if something triggers it or not; I just feel it.

Candidate: Since, it suggests a case of Graves' disease, not lymphoma—by the patient's general look and history.

Other Important Targeted Histories

- Do you experience abnormal intolerance to hot weather more than usual, or are you sweating more than usual?
- Do you have shaking of the hands? Do you have these handshakes (tremor) at rest or with movement (usually all the time in thyrotoxicosis)?
- What about your menstrual history (last period, regularity, amount of blood—how many pads/day) ...are you planning for recent pregnancy? What is the age of your last child?
- Do you feel more anxious nowadays?
- Are you sleeping less? Nightmares?

Any symptoms related to Graves' ophthalmopathy:
- Do you have any pain or gritty sensation or watery eye? Any abnormality in your vision?

Any complications:
- Symptoms of goiter? Do you have any breathing difficulty (high cardiac output failure/part of AF/retrosternal extension)? Change in voice/hoarseness; difficulty in swallowing (retrosternal extension)?
- Do you have any long-standing disease like DM, hypertension, and cardiac problems?

Patient: Yes, Doctor, I cannot tolerate hot weather at all, my hands get sweaty all the time, and there is a tremor in my hands. My menstrual flow is decreased over the last couple of months. Besides, I feel agitated recently, and my sleep cycle is totally disrupted. I don't have pain in my eyes, but there are some abnormalities in my vision like sometimes I look double, also my eyes look bigger and prop out. But I do not have any other illness as you are talking about.

Quick Systemic Review, Past Medical History, Family History, Treatment, Social History According to Your Differentials

If it is not asked previously during initial history taking or incompletely asked then—take a full history of particular portion to make it complete.

Candidate: At this moment I would like to ask some general question which may or may not be related to your symptoms just to make sure everything is going okay with you.......
- Do you have joint pain, cough, breathlessness, chest pain, headache, vomiting, or any tummy pain?
- What about your waterworks?
- Do you have any similar condition or any other history of disease in your past?
- Have you attended any consultant or general physician or specialist for this problem? What was their impression? Did you receive any diagnosis? What treatment have you received? Did they work?
- Have you ever been admitted to the hospital in the past or any history of surgery?
- May I ask what medication you take? Do you take any over the counter medications or herbal medicine or any recreational drugs? Are you allergic to any medicine or anything else?
- Is there anyone else in your family with this type of problem or any long-standing illness that run in your families like DM, hypertension, stroke, thyroid, or other autoimmune disease or anything else?

- Do you smoke? Do you drink? What are you doing for a living? Are you married? Who is at home with you or who is supporting you now? Do you have children? Are you independent in activities of daily living?

Have I missed anything, or do you want to add anything more?

Okay, thank you. Would you mind if I go on to examine you now?

Focused Examination

Here focused examination would be:
- Examine for thyroid status
- Examination of the thyroid gland
- Evidence of Graves' disease (Graves' ophthalmopathy, pretibial myxedema)

Thyroid Status

- Ask the patient to hold the arms outstretched and assess for tremor—if no obvious tremor, then keep a paper on the hand and look for tremor.
- Examine the hand for clubbing with painful finger swelling due to periosteal reaction in limb bones (thyroid acropachy) and palmar erythema.
- Feel for warm and moist hand.
- Examine the pulse for tachycardia or atrial fibrillation (AF).
- Ask the patient to stand from sitting position with their arm crossed—for proximal myopathy.
- Lid lag or lid retraction (exposure of sclera above iris causing stare look).

Examine the Neck

Inspection: Carefully inspect the neck whilst the patient swallows a sip of water.

Any thyroidectomy scar—which typically forms a ring around the base of the neck.

Palpate from behind the patient's neck with slightly flexed position.... rest the fingers of both your hand over the gland and feel the lumps and isthmus if palpable, try to feel the lower border of the thyroid to see the retrosternal extension.
- Diffuse enlargement—Grave's disease
- Multiple nodule—Multinodular goiter
- *Single nodule*: adenoma, thyroid malignancy, lymphoma, and metastasis.

Assess for Lymphadenopathy

Percuss the chest (sternum) to assess for retrosternal goiter.

Auscultate the thyroid for a bruit (indicates hyperthyroidism most likely due to Graves' disease or malignancy).

Eye Examination

- Proptosis (an apparent lower rim of sclera; forward displacement) look from above and the side.
- Lid retraction.
- Soft tissue signs of active eye disease—red eye (scleral injection), chemosis (conjunctival swelling), periorbital edema.
- *Lid lag*: Ask the patient to follow your finger; eyelid lags behind the eyes descend as the patient watches your finger descend slowly.
- *Eye movement*: Ask the patient to report any double vision or complex ophthalmoplegia (especially on upward vertical gaze due to inferior rectus muscle involvement).
- *Visual acuity*: RAPD.
- *Fundoscopy*: Severe Graves' ophthalmopathy may result in optic nerve compression (papilledema) and optic atrophy (pale optic disc).

If possible—examine for proximal myopathy.

Jerks (brisk reflex), pretibial myxedema (edematous swelling above the lateral malleoli; the term myxedema is confusing here.)

Examine heart for evidence of heart failure.

Evidence of other autoimmune diseases (vitiligo, celiac disease, type 1 diabetes mellitus).

Feedback to the Patient and Respond to the Patient's Concern

Candidate: You said at the beginning that the main problems were neck swelling, palpitation, weight loss, and anxious feeling—is there anything else troubling you that we have missed or any questions or concerns?

Patient: I am really upset doctor; I want to know what exactly has happened to me, have you had any thoughts about what is going on?

Candidate: The lump you can feel in your neck is the thyroid gland and your signs and symptoms suggestive of it being overactive meaning that your gland is producing too much hormone. At this moment, we need to carry out some blood tests, particularly TFT, an ECG as well as USG of the neck and thyroid scan. These blood tests will confirm my suspicion. Then, we will refer you to a hormone specialist (endocrinology) clinic for further investigation and treatment.

Meanwhile, I will start a medication known as propranolol which will help with some of your symptoms such as tremor and palpitation. There are three main ways to treat an overactive thyroid—medications, surgery, and radiation. We will need to talk again once we have the test result to establish the most appropriate option for you.

Do you have any other concerns and questions? Thank you very much for spending time with me today.

Discussion with Examiner

Examiner: Would you please present your case?

Candidate:

This young lady presented with significant unintentional weight loss despite normal appetite, excessive sweating, palpitation, and thyroid swelling. The patient is thin and appears restless.

The hands are warm and moist with palmar erythema and fine tremor of an outstretched hand. The pulse is 108 beats/minute and regular. There are lid lag and lid retraction. There is also evidence of proximal myopathy.

She had bilateral exophthalmos and ophthalmoplegia with resultant diplopia, but there is no evidence of exposure keratitis, chemosis, or corneal ulceration.

The thyroid gland is diffusely enlarged, non-tender and no retrosternal extension.

There is evidence of pretibial myxedema and also evidence of digital clubbing consistent with thyroid acropathy.

So, in summary—my diagnosis is thyrotoxic Graves' disease.

Examiner: How will you investigate it?

Candidate: Initially, I would like to perform some blood tests, most importantly, TFT that includes free T3, free T4, TSH (raised T3, T4; and low TSH), as well as anti-TSH-receptor antibody (usually positive in Graves' disease >90% cases).

I would like to do an USG of the neck to identify any structural abnormality (such as goiter and nodule) and radioiodine uptake test with a thyroid scan to show the pattern of activity. (Homogenous increase uptake suggest a Graves' disease; focal area of activity is consistent with toxic nodule; absent or globally reduced uptake suggests thyroiditis).

Further test would be:
- FNAC, If nodule or suspected malignancy
- X-ray/CT scan of the chest to see the retrosternal extension

Examiner: How will you treat the case?

Candidate: If the final diagnosis is that of thyrotoxic Graves' disease; I would like to advice non-selective beta-blockers (propranolol) to control the symptoms of tremor and palpitation.

Then I would like to give the specific treatment of hyperthyroidism. Treatment options include:
- Medical therapy with antithyroid drugs such as carbimazole or propylthiouracil for 18-24 months, then withdraw (50% will relapse requiring radioiodine or surgery).
- Radioiodine therapy as an ablative therapy for thyrotoxicosis (most become hypothyroid post-treatment).
- The surgical option includes thyroidectomy.

Examiner: How would you manage a patient with Graves' ophthalmopathy?

Candidate: At first, I would like to stop smoking as soon as possible as it worse prognosis as well as want to involve eye specialists/ophthalmic surgeons urgently (if there is concern about optic nerve compression—reduced vision or papilledema).

Most have mild disease that can be treated symptomatically (artificial tear, sunglasses, avoid dust, elevate bed when sleeping to decrease periorbital edema).

- Diplopia may be managed with Fresnel prism stuck to one lens of a spectacle that aids easy changing as the exophthalmos change.
- In more severe disease may require high-dose steroids, surgical decompression, or orbital radiotherapy.

Examiner: What are the causes of hyperthyroidism?

Candidate:
- Graves' disease (most common)
- Toxic multinodular goiter or toxic adenoma

Other possibilities are:
- Thyroiditis (inflammation of the thyroid gland)
- Excessive intake of thyroid hormones
- Abnormal secretion of TSH
- Excessive iodine intake

Examiner: Do you know about the use of radioiodine?

Candidate: Recurrent hyperthyroidism patient may require definitive treatment with 131-iodine therapy. 131-iodine administered orally and then concentrated in the thyroid. It causes local tissue damage and a reduction in thyroid function over 6–8 weeks by releasing beta emission.

- Radioiodine therapy is contraindicated in pregnancy and breastfeeding.
- It can worsen the ophthalmopathy of Graves' disease (use steroid cover).
- Restrictions needed for a few weeks (roughly 3 weeks) after the dose is administered, including contact with the partner, household members, pregnant women, and children, depending on the dose administered.
- Pregnancy should be avoided for 6 months after the dose administered, to ensure that the radioactivity is fully cleared, hyperthyroidism is treated successfully, and any resultant hypothyroidism controlled.

Cushing Syndrome

Patient's details: Mrs Inshu Maria, a 45-year-old lady.

Clinical problem: Hypertension, weight gain, difficulty in climbing the stairs with extreme weakness. She has recently been diagnosed with diabetes.

(Once you get this clinical scenario, you will get 5 minutes to start this station for two scenarios. At that time, start to think about your diagnosis and differential diagnoses and plan for taking focused history as well as focused examination.)

[*Differential diagnosis of weight gain*:

Endocrine disease—Cushing, hypothyroidism, insulinoma, and PCOS.

Fluid retention—CCF, nephrotic syndrome, ascites due to liver cirrhosis [nonalcoholic steatohepatitis (NASH)]

Drugs—TCA, antiepileptics (Na-valproate, carbamazepine)

Others—Primary obesity, sedentary lifestyle.

As the patient is hypertensive and diabetic, presented with weight gain and proximal myopathy; here most important diagnosis would be Cushing syndrome, but CCF and cirrhosis due to NASH should be our strong differential diagnosis.]

(Once you enter the room search for a spot diagnosis; cushingoid appearance suggests Cushing syndrome.)

Introduction, Permission, and Identification

Candidate: Good morning, my name is Mohammad Ali. One of the working doctors here today. I have been asked to see you. Is that okay with you?

Patient: Good morning, doctor...

Candidate: Thank you for coming, I would like to start by taking your full name, age, and where you have come from, please?

Patient: Yes, doctor............. I am Inshu Maria, 45-year-old and from Dublin.

Focused History

Candidate: Ok, Mrs Maria. Would you please tell me what brings you here today? Please tell me your words.

Patient: I have gained weight rapidly, especially on my tummy and also on my face. I am feeling so weak and finding it difficult to climb the stairs at work. I am hypertensive for the last six months, and now I have diabetes also.

 (So here the main problem is weight gain with difficulty in performing a normal daily activity, hypertension and DM.)

Analyze the Symptoms

Candidate: I am sorry to hear about your condition, would you please tell me, a little bit more about your weight gain?

The important questions to be asked are:
- When this weight gain started exactly?
- Is it increasing or decreasing gradually?
- How much weight have you put on?
- Where have you put on the weight—abdomen? Trunk? Back of the neck or legs or ankle? Is the weight gain evenly distributed?
- What about your appetite or exercise?
- What about your diet? Please tell me what you would eat in a typical day—starting with breakfast? Enquire especially about the number of meals, frequency of snacks, types of food including fast food.
- How has this weight gain affected your daily activity of living or in your job or hobbies?

Patient: My key problem is weight gain of 8 kg from 72 to 80 kg over the last 8 months. Most of the weight has increased around my tummy and face. My diet and appetite have not changed, and I am very conscious of what I eat. I am feeling so tired during the daytime, especially when carrying out household work such as washing, shopping, and I struggle to climb the stairs at work.

Candidate: Now, please tell me more about hypertension? Are you taking any medication? Regularly or irregularly? Is it controlled or uncontrolled? What is your last BP record? Are you on regular follow up with your general physician? Do you have FH of hypertension?

Patient: As I told before, I am hypertensive for the last 6 months, and my current medication is ramipril 5 mg once daily, and it is well-controlled.

Candidate: Ok, would you please tell me more about your diabetes...
- For how long have you had diabetes? How was it detected first?
- How was it treated initially, and what is your current medication?
- Are you taking the medication regularly or irregularly? Is it controlled or uncontrolled?
- Have you ever monitored blood sugar? What is the usual range of blood sugar? What is your last blood sugar level and HbA1c?
- Are you on regular follow-up and where?
  (If the patient has a long history of DM, ask about the complications of DM; but in real life, 50% of first detected DM patient presents with at least one of the complications, so it is better to ask the following questions.)
- Do you have any history of hypoglycemic attacks like having palpitation, restlessness, excessive sweating, or dizziness with low blood sugar level which improved after taking a meal or sugar?
- Have you noticed pain in the calf during the walk and that relief with rest (intermittent claudication)?
- Have you had your eyes checked recently? What was his impression regarding your diabetic eye disease?
- Have you noticed tingling, numbness or burning sensation or loss of sensation in the feet?
- Have you noticed any change in your waterworks like amount, frequency, color, frothy urine, or any pain while passing urine (diabetic nephropathy)?
- Do you have chest pain or racing heartbeat, shortness of breath, or leg swelling?
- Have you ever been hospitalized for any complication and why?

Patient: My diabetes was detected incidentally 3 days back by general physician. He gave me the medicine metformin 500 mg twice daily, today I measured my blood sugar, and it is 12. My general physician informed me about the hypoglycemic attack, but I do not have any such attack till now. There is no one in my family with DM or hypertension.

Now ask to identify the cause of the weight gain, hypertension, and DM:

Candidate:
- Have you noticed any change in your appearance? Increased hair growth? Any change in menstruation? Any striae, acne, or hirsutism? Any change in the mood? Are you taking any (steroid) medication (? Cushing syndrome)?
- Have you noticed any intolerance to hot or cold weather, any menstrual change with the increased flow; dry, rough skin; constipation or change in voice (? hypothyroidism)?
- Have you noticed any chest pain, breathlessness, palpitation or cough (? cardio-respiratory cause of fluid retention)?
- Do you have any history of liver disease like jaundice, blood mixed vomiting, or black tarry loose stool (melena) or history of hepatitis-B virus (HBV) or hepatitis-C virus (HCV) infection in the past?

Patient: I have noticed a change in my appearance, especially with some acne on my face, excess hairy growth and also my face looking fuller. My period is more infrequent with scantier blood loss.

Quick Systemic Review, Past Medical History, Family History, Treatment, Social History According to Your Differentials

If it is not asked previously during initial history taking or incompletely asked then—take a full history of particular portion to make it complete.

Candidate: At this moment, I would like to ask some general questions just to make sure everything is going okay with you....
- Do you have headache, dizziness or loss of consciousness (LOC) or blurring of vision or weakness of limbs?
- Any nausea, vomiting, abdominal pain, or any changes in bowel habit?
- What about your waterworks? Any change in color, frequency, or any frothy urine, or any pain in passing urine or anything else?
- Do you have any similar condition or any other history of disease in your past?
- Have you attended any consultant or general physician or specialist for this problem? What was their impression? Did you receive any diagnosis? What treatment have you received? Did they work?
- Have you ever been admitted to the hospital in the past or any history of surgery?
- May I ask what medication you take? Do you take any over the counter medications or herbal medicine or any recreational drugs? Are you allergic to any medicine or anything else?
- Is there anyone else in your family with this type of problem or any long-standing illness that run in your families like DM, hypertension, stroke, thyroid or any autoimmune disease or anything else?
- Do you smoke? Do you drink? What are you doing for a living? Are you married? Who is at home with you or who is supporting you now? Do you have children? Are you independent in activities of daily living?

Have I missed anything, or do you want to add anything more?

Would you mind if in going on to examine you?

Focused Examination

From the history, we have got the impression of Cushing syndrome. Focused examination would be:
- The general appearance of Cushing
- Face
- Mouth
- Back
- Abdomen and chest
- Lower limb for proximal myopathy

Ask the examiner....I would like to complete my assessment by visual field examination (sometimes pituitary macroadenoma can cause bitemporal hemianopia), blood pressure measurement and urine dipstick for sugar.

General appearance:
- Increased adipose tissue in the face (moon face), upper back (at the base of the neck) and above the clavicle.
- Truncal/central obesity
- Steroid acne (papular or pustular lesion) over the face, chest, and back.
- Plethoric face, thin skin, and easy bruising.

Inspect the abdomen, buttocks, lower back, upper thigh, upper arm, and breast for violaceous striae.

Examine for proximal myopathy.

Sign related to an underling steroid responsive disease with SLE and rheumatoid arthritis.

Feedback to the Patient and Respond to the Patient's Concern

Candidate: You said at the beginning that the main problems were hypertension, DM, weight gain, acne with difficulty in climbing stairs. Is there anything else troubling you that we have missed or any questions to ask or any concerns?

Patient: Doctor, have you had any thoughts about what is going on?

Candidate: I think your symptoms may be because of an overproduction of steroid from the gland located above your kidneys. The condition is called Cushing syndrome. This is likely what has caused your weight gain, we are going to do some blood tests along with imaging of the brain and adrenal gland to confirm our diagnosis as well as want to exclude other conditions that may cause a similar problem.

If it is confirmed, then we will refer you to an endocrinologist (gland doctor) to give you the proper plan of management. Is that ok, Mrs Maria?

Do you have any concerns or worries? Thank you so much for spending time with me today.

Discussion with Examiner

Examiner: Would you please present your case?

Candidate:

This middle-aged lady presented with progressive unintentional weight gain, weakness, and difficulty in climbing stairs with DM and hypertension.

The patient has Cushingoid facies with centripetal obesity; interscapular and supraclavicular fat pads.

There is acne vulgaris on face and trunk. There are purpuric and petechial rashes with brushing on the skin. There are violaceous striae on the abdomen, and also there is evidence of proximal myopathy. There is no adrenalectomy scar.

So, in summary—these signs and symptoms consistent with Cushing syndrome.

Examiner: What are your differential diagnoses?

Candidate: Most important differential diagnosis includes adrenocorticotropic hormone (ACTH) secreting pituitary adenoma (Cushing disease); excess endogenous steroid from an adrenal gland (Cushing syndrome); exogenous steroid use (Iatrogenic Cushing); pseudo-Cushing syndrome such as alcoholism, obesity, and depression.

Examiner: How will you investigate this case?

Candidate: I would like to confirm my diagnosis by two steps approach; initially, I would like to confirm of hypercortisolism by doing:

- Overnight dexamethasone suppression test (1 mg dexamethasone at midnight and check, 9.00 am serum cortisol. This test is considered abnormal if the cortisol level is >50 nmol/L).
- 24-hour urine collection for free cortisol measurements.

Ideally, both tests should be done, and if negative, Cushing's is very unlikely; if positive, proceed to next step for identification of the cause of Cushing's syndrome by:

- Plasma ACTH level [ACTH levels should be undetectable in adrenal Cushing's but will be inappropriately normal or elevated in the pituitary (Cushing's disease) or ectopic Cushing's syndrome.]
- High dose dexamethasone suppression test (give 2 mg dexamethasone 6-hourly for 48 hours and measure baseline cortisol and at 48-hours.)

I would like to perform baseline investigation for complete management that includes CBC with ESR, fasting blood sugar (FBS), HbA1c, lipid profile, renal and liver function test.

Further tests would be imaging that includes MRI of the brain and CT scan of the adrenal gland to identify the cause as well.

Examiner: How would you treat this patient?

Candidate: The management of Cushing's syndrome depends on the underlying cause. If the cause is found to be exposure to an exogenous steroid, gradual withdrawal and stopping the steroid would be the appropriate treatment option.

If the final diagnosis is that of Cushing disease, options are including:

Treatment of pituitary Cushing's:
- Transsphenoidal resection
- Pituitary radiotherapy
- Bilateral adrenalectomy (rarely done)

Treatment of adrenal Cushing's is adrenalectomy.

Medical management includes:
- Ketoconazole
- Mitotane (if Cushing is caused by adrenal carcinoma)

Acromegaly

Your role: You are the medical doctor in the endocrine clinic.

Patient profile: Mr Mark, 45-year-old.

Problem: Headache, visual disturbance, and change in appearance.

(*Once you get this clinical scenario, you will get 5 minutes to start this station for two scenarios. At that time, start to think about your diagnosis and differential diagnoses and plan for taking focused history as well as focused examination.*)

[*Differential diagnosis*: In this case, as the patient has a history of headache with visual disturbance as well as a change in appearance (? acromegaly), So, here most likely diagnosis would be acromegaly due to growth hormone secreting pituitary macroadenoma with compressive symptoms.]

(Once you enter the room search for a spot diagnosis; prominent supraorbital ridge, coarse facies; prognathism; wrinkled forehead suggests acromegaly.)

Introduction, Permission, and Identification

Candidate: Good morning, I am Mohammad Ali, one of the working doctors here today, I have been asked to see you; is that okay with you?

Patient: Good morning, doctor...

Candidate: Thank you for coming, I would like to start by taking your full name, age, and where you have come from, please?

Patient: Yes, doctor............. I am Mark, 45-year-old, and from London.

Focused History

Candidate: Okay, Mr Mark, I understand you are troubled by some problems, would you like to tell me more about this?

Patient: I have had some problems with my vision for the last couple of months. I have headaches and recently noticed some changes in my appearance. Recently I felt so embarrassed when one of my friends commented that my appearance has changed a lot more than previous. I went to my general physician and he referred me to the hospital.

Analyze the Complaint

Candidate: I am sorry to hear about your sufferings......let me ask you some questions to find out what's been happening and to see how we can help you. Okay, Mr Mark?

Patient: Okay.

Candidate: At first, I would like to talk about visual disturbance.....
- When did you first notice the visual disturbance? Did it come on suddenly or gradually?
- Is it getting better, staying the same or getting worse overtimes?
- Is it affecting one eye or both? Which part of the vision is affected? All? Top half? Bottom half? Sides? Central? Is this same in both eyes? Do you see the wall of the room or the side of the road when looking straight forward?
- Do you have any pain in or around the eyes? Describe the type of pain you have?
- Do you have double vision?
- Have you noticed any graying of vision or loss of color vision?

- Have you noticed flashing lights? Zig-zag lines or any other pattern in your field of vision?

You also complained headache, now tell me:
- When the headache started exactly?
- Is it sudden or gradual in onset? Is it increasing or decreasing or the same when it first started?
- Where did the pain first start? Did the pain spread anywhere?
- Is it on one side or both side or central or frontal?
- What is the nature of the pain—is it throbbing? Tight? Shooting or stabbing?
- Is it coming on and off or all the time with you?
- Is the pain worse in the morning or at the end of the day?
- Does it worse by coughing, sneezing, and bending forward?
- Does light, noise, certain meals, and movement make the headache worse?
- What improves your headache like rest or any painkiller?

Patient: I have been noticing problems with my vision over the last 8 months, which I think causing a headache also. I usually wear glasses, and 6 months back, my eye doctor said that these were fine. Recently, I have had some problems with driving, particularly parking my car and being aware of what is around me exactly. I have found it is hard to change the lanes on the motorways. I also have a headache which gets worse when I am busy with my work.

Candidate: Please tell me—what do you mean by changing appearance?

Patient: My appearance has changed drastically—my hands have gotten bigger, so big that I had to change the size of my wedding ring twice. My feet have increased in size from 10 to 14, so I need to change the size of my shoes. My jaw is so big that it becomes difficult for me to eat and talk. I feel like I am growing out of my body size and becoming depressed at the same time. I remember a friend of mine who I met after a long time said, "You look so different."

Candidate: I am sorry to hear that—Do you have an old photo of you?

Patient: Not now, but it is true, my appearance has changed a lot.

Candidate: When the obvious appearance of acromegaly then targeted history to detect the complications and etiology of acromegaly.

Other Important Targeted Histories

- Have you noticed any tingling, numbness, or pain in the hands particularly three and a half fingers (Carpal tunnel syndrome—as a complication of acromegaly)?
- Do you have any problem in the private (intimate) relationship like decreased sexual desires or erectile dysfunction (associated hyperprolactinemia)?
- What about your shoe and ring size, do they fit (enlarge hand and feet)?
- Any difficulty in climbing stairs or getting up from the chair or standing from sitting position (proximal myopathy)?
- Any pain in your knee (osteoarthritis of the knee)?
- Have you noticed excessive sweating in your hands and feet?
- Have you noticed any snoring during sleep or daytime sleepiness and early morning headache (OSA)?
- Do you have any chest pain or racing heartbeats or breathlessness or leg swelling? (cardiomyopathy)
- Do you have HTN, DM (drinking more water than you used to, passing more urine than usual?)
- Constipation? Weight loss? bleeding with bowel motion? (Colon cancer).

Ask about Etiology

- Any headache, vomiting, blurring of vision [Usually, pituitary macroadenoma causing raised intracranial pressure (ICP)]? or,

- Are you passing more urine than usual? (hypercalcemia), watery diarrhea (pancreatic tumor)- MEN (multiple endocrine neoplasia)

Quick Systemic Review, Past Medical History, Family History, Treatment, Social History According to your Differentials

If it is not asked previously during initial history taking or incompletely asked then—take a full history of particular portion to make it complete.

Candidate: Now I would like to ask some general questions just to know about your overall health and your lifestyle, is that okay with you?
- Any history of LOC or dizziness?
- Do you have any altered speech?
- Do you have any history of shaking of the body with uncontrolled waterworks or bowel motion or tongue bite?
- Do you have any fever, weight loss, or loss of appetite?
- Do you have any similar condition or any other history of disease in your past?
- Have you attended any consultant or general physician or specialist for this problem? What was their impression? Did you receive any diagnosis? What treatment have you received? Did they work?
- Have you ever been admitted to the hospital in the past or any history of surgery?
- May I ask what medication you take? Do you take any over-the-counter medications or herbal medicine or any recreational drugs? Are you allergic to any medicine or anything else?
- Is there anyone else in your family with this type of problem or any long-standing illness that run in your families like DM, hypertension, stroke, thyroid, or any autoimmune disease or anything else?
- Do you smoke? Do you drink? What are you doing for a living? Are you married? Who is at home with you or who is supporting you now? Do you have children? Are you independent in activities of daily living?

Patient: My general physician diagnosed borderline DM 2 years ago, now I control it with diet only—at the last check it was 7.8. I am living with my wife.

Candidate: Have I missed anything, or do you want to add anything more?
Would you mind if I go on to examine you?

Focused Examination

Do a targeted examination according to the focused history and spot diagnosis that you noticed on the patient, mainly looking for confirming a diagnosis, rule out the differential diagnosis, looking for a complication, cause, and associated condition.

Here focused examination would be an examination of the eye and identification of features of acromegaly; if a suggestive history of carpal tunnel syndrome, then, examine the hand for median nerve palsy.

General appearance:
- Prominent supraorbital ridge, nose, and lips with coarse facial feature.
- Prognathism (pronounced jawline).
- Macroglossia (teeth impression in the tongue), with wide interdental space.
- Large spade-like fingers with thickened skin with sweaty hands.
- Husky voice, proximal myopathy, and acanthosis nigricans.

Examination of the eye:
- Visual acuity
- Visual field—Bitemporal hemianopia is an expected finding in acromegaly patient.
- Fundoscopy—for optic atrophy if the adenoma extends into the parasellar region.
- Eye movement and pupillary light reflex: III, IV, VI nerve palsies due to raised ICP.

I would like to complete my examination by measuring blood pressure, urine test for glycosuria as well as want to examine the CVS and GIT.

Feedback to the Patient and Respond to the Patient's Concern

Explain the condition briefly and sort out a plan for diagnosis, investigation, treatment, admission, advice, driving, prognosis if applicable.

Candidate: You said at the beginning that the main problems were headache, change in vision and appearance—Is there anything else troubling you that we have missed or any question to ask or any concern?

Patient: Doctor, what do you think what might be the cause of my problem? What happens to me?

Candidate: I think most probably you have a condition called acromegaly—a small area in your brain behind the nose, where the hormone-producing master gland is located called the pituitary gland. The gland is producing excess growth hormone which has caused your hands and bones grow.

The cause of this excess growth hormone production is a tumor in your master gland which is a noncancerous tumor that may compress your nerves for vision affecting your sight. At this time, we need to carry out some blood tests that include particularly growth hormone and blood sugar. We will also do an MRI scan of the brain to detect the tumor as early as possible. If it is confirmed, then it can be treated with mainly surgery or sometimes with medication or radiotherapy.

Do you have any other concerns?

Okay, thank you very much for spending time with me today.

Discussion with Examiner

Examiner: Would you please present your case?

Candidate:

This man presented with a history of headache, visual disturbance, and change in appearance.

The patient has large sweaty hands with broad palms and spatulate fingers. The skin over the dorsum of the hand is thickened. The patient has a prominent supraorbital ridge, enlarged nose, and lips with prognathism. There are wide-spaced teeth, and the tongue is enlarged.

He has a visual field defect—that is bitemporal hemianopia.

In summary—I think this gentleman has acromegaly in association with bitemporal hemianopia due to optic chiasma compression with underlying pituitary macroadenoma.

Examiner: How will you investigate it?

Candidate: At first, I would like to confirm our diagnosis by doing oral glucose tolerance test (OGTT) with measuring serial serum growth hormone (GH), insulin-like growth factor-1 (IGF-1) and blood sugar (normally GH secretion is inhibited by high glucose and hardly detectable. In the case of acromegaly, GH release fails to suppress. Here, samples for GH are collected at 0, 30, 60, 90, 120, and 150 minutes. The lowest GH value during OGTT >1 µg (>3 mIU/L) will confirm acromegaly.

Then, I would like to do other hormone tests to see the evidence of hypopituitarism, such as: fasting cortisol, ACTH, FT3, FT4, TSH, serum luteinizing hormone (LH), follicle-stimulating hormone (FSH), and testosterone. Also, I would like to see serum prolactin level (>30% patient with acromegaly may have hyperprolactinemia.)

My next step would be an MRI of the pituitary fossa to get the evidence of pituitary macroadenoma as well as serum calcium level to see the evidence of MEN1 as a cause of acromegaly.

Lastly, to see the complications of acromegaly, I would like to do some further tests such as:
- ECG and echocardiography to see the evidence of left ventricular hypertrophy (LVH), arrhythmia as well as cardiomyopathy.
- Nerve conduction study for Carpal tunnel syndrome (CTS).
- Colonoscopy to exclude colonic carcinoma
- Perimetry to see the visual defect.

Examiner: How will you treat the case?

Candidate: Here, the main aim to correct tumor compression by excising the lesion and to reduce IGF-1 and GH level to a safer range (<2 µg/L or 6 mIU/L).

Transsphenoidal hypophysectomy is considered as first-line therapy. If surgery fails to correct GH/IGF-1 hypersecretion, then we have to try somatostatin analogue (e.g., octreotide) and or radiotherapy.

The growth hormone antagonist pegvisomant is used in resistant or intolerant to a somatostatin analogue.

Examiner: Okay, now would you like to tell, what are the clinical signs of activity of acromegaly?

Candidate: Important clinical signs of activity of acromegaly include sweating, progressive enlargement of hands and feet, skin tags, worsening symptoms, DM, and hypertension.

Addison's Disease

Your role: You are the Registrar in the endocrine clinic.

Patient profile: Mrs Mathew, 38-year-old.

Problem: The patient has become increasingly tired and fatigued. Her husband has commented she becomes increasingly tanned.

(*Once you get this clinical scenario, you will get 5 minutes to start this station for two scenarios. At that time, start to think about your diagnosis, differential diagnoses, and plan for taking focused history as well as focused examination.*)

[*Differential diagnosis*:

For pigmentation:
- *Endocrine cause*: Addison's disease (autoimmune/TB), Nelson syndrome (scar of bilateral adrenalectomy ?), pituitary ACTH secreting tumor (Cushingoid appearance + HTN), ectopic ACTH (small cell carcinoma), and thyrotoxicosis.
- *Chronic disease*: CKD, CLD, haemochromatosis.
- *Chronic infection*: TB.
- *Others*: Racial/familiar, drugs (minocycline, phenothiazine, antimalarial, amiodarone)

For tiredness and fatigability: Anemia, DM, hypothyroidism/thyrotoxicosis, OSA, secondary/primary adrenal insufficiency, and depression.]

(Once you enter the room search for a spot diagnosis; generalized tanning, pigmentation of knuckles, palmar crease and buccal mucous and thin patient suggests Addison's disease.)

Greetings, Introduction, Permission, and Identification

Candidate: Good morning, I am Mohammad Ali. One of the working doctors here today. I have been asked to see you. Is that ok with you?

Patient: Okay....

Candidate: I will start by taking your full name; age, and where you have come from, please.

Patient: Mathew, I am 38 years old and from Dublin.

Focused History

Candidate: Ok, Mrs Mathew, would you please tell me what brings you here today. Please tell me in your own words.

Patient: Over the past few months, I have been feeling tired all the time, as well as feeling lightheaded on standing up or when I get out of bed in the morning. Recently my husband noticed I am getting tanned day-by-day.

Analyze the Symptoms

Candidate: Let us talk about your hyperpigmentation:
- When this tanned skin started exactly?
- Has it changed since it started? Is it gradually increasing or decreasing or the same?
- Where is it exactly? (Which parts are involved—is it only sun-exposed area or other parts of the body like private parts or within the mouth?)
- Is there any change in the pigment of any existing scars?

Patient: All over my body has been getting tanned (generalized pigmentation) for the last 6 months. It is here …… (skin creases, buccal mucosa, nipple, axilla, and all pressure points, involving both sun-exposed and nonexposed areas). I have also a scar on my hands which is getting darker day-by-day.

Candidate: Now please tell me a little bit more about your tiredness or fatigability? Like…
- When is it started exactly?
- Is it present all day or just toward the end of the day?

- Is it increasing day by day?
- How it affects your normal day to day activity?
- How is your sleep these days?
- How has been your mood recently? Can you score it on the scale of 1 to 10, 1 being the lowest mood and 10 being happiest?

Patient: It started 3 months back. My tiredness is all the time with me, and it is increasing. I feel exhausted particularly when carrying out household activities like shopping, washing, cooking, or cleaning, and also, I feel dizzy when standing from the sitting or the lying position. I am sleeping alright but still feeling tired. My mood is also fine.

Candidate: Now ask for other targeted histories, if our clinical diagnosis is obvious at this moment from the history and clinical appearance, then try to take targeted history to confirm our diagnosis, to exclude the differential diagnosis, and look for associated conditions.

Other Important Targeted Histories
- Any pain in your tummy? Vomiting? Diarrhea?
- Any lightheadedness or dizziness? Do you have any history of fainting attack or blackout whilst standing up from sitting position (orthostatic hypotension)?
- Any fever? Have you noticed weight loss? How much weight have you lost and over how long? What about your appetite?
- What about your menstruation? When is your last menstrual period? Is it regular or irregular? Amount of flow, is it increased or decreased?
- Do you have sweating, feeling cold, shaking, irritability, LOC (hypoglycemia)?
- Any neck swelling, do you tend to feel the hot or cold more than usual?
- Any changes in your bowel habit like constipation or diarrhea? Any excessive sweating or dryness of your skin, anxious, or irritable [thyroid disorder as a part of antiphospholipid syndrome (APS)]?
- Any part of your skin became lighter or lost color (vitiligo)?
- Any loss of hair (alopecia areata/totalis)?
- Shortness of breath (SOB), racing your heart, looking paler than usual (pernicious anemia)?
- Past history of human immunodeficiency virus (HIV), TB, meningitis?
- Drug history especially steroids, if the patient is on or used to take steroids, ask for the reason, dosage, duration, and gradual withdrawal (secondary hypoadrenalism but in that case, the patient will not have pigmentation).

Patient: I have a loss of appetite, and also, I am losing weight day by day, which is around 6 kg over the last 3 months. Also, I have not been menstruating for the last 3 months.

Quick Systemic Review, Past Medical History, Family History, Treatment, Social History According to Your Differentials

If it is not asked previously during initial history taking or incompletely asked then—take a full history of particular portion to make it complete.

Candidate: Now I would like to ask some general questions, just to make sure that everything is okay with you……
- Do you have a headache? Any cough? Do you have chest pain or shortness of breath?
- What about your waterworks, amount, color, or frequency?
- Do you have any similar condition or any other history of disease in your past?
- Have you attended any consultant or general physician or specialist for this problem? What was their impression? Did you receive any diagnosis? What treatment have you received? Did they work?
- Have you ever been admitted to the hospital in the past or any history of surgery?
- May I ask what medication you take? Do you take any over-the-counter medications or herbal medicines or any recreational drugs? Are you allergic to any medicine or anything else?
- Is there anyone else in your family with this type of problem or any long-standing illness that run in your families like DM, hypertension, stroke, thyroid or any autoimmune disease or anything else?

- Do you smoke? Do you drink? What are you doing for a living? Are you married? Who is at home with you or who is supporting you now? Do you have children? Are you independent in activities of daily living?

Have I missed anything, or do you want to add anything more?

Would you mind if I go on to examine you?

Focused Examination

Here focused examination would be:
- Distribution and nature of pigmentation.
- The abdomen for the scar of bilateral adrenalectomy.
- Vitiligo as well as check for any evidence of other autoimmune diseases, e.g., examine thyroid gland (Schmidt's syndrome—APS).
- Visual field defect.
- Request for assessment of BP lying and standing for postural hypotension.

Examine for hyperpigmentation particularly in:
- Palmar crease
- Lip and buccal mucosa
- Exposed and pressure areas such as feet and elbow; take off the patient's watch and also inspect around the belt and brasserie line. Non-sun exposed area such as nipple and axilla.

(Generalized pigmentation, bilateral adrenalectomy scar with evidence of bitemporal hemianopia suggest Nelson syndrome.)

Feedback to the Patient and Respond to the Patient's Concern

Candidate: You said at the beginning that the main problems were fatigue, tiredness, and generalized pigmentation. Is there anything else troubling you that we have not covered and any questions to ask or any concerns?

Patient: Doctor, what might be the cause of my problem? What happens to me?

Candidate: The symptoms you discussed and the signs I found on examination suggest you may have a condition called Addison's disease. Have you heard it before?

Patient: No.

Candidate: Well, let me explain it........it is a disease due to diminished secretion of a special protein in the body called steroid hormone secreted from glands located above your kidneys, mostly due to disturbance of your defensive system which supposed to attack the germs and bugs, in your condition, it unfortunately, attacks your own glands.

It is very important that we make a diagnosis so that we can start effective treatment, the mainstay of which is replacing those steroids. At this moment, we need to carry out some blood tests, especially hormone levels as well as other blood tests to confirm our diagnosis also to exclude other possibilities that may cause similar symptoms.

Do you have any concerns? Thank you for spending your time with me today.

Discussion between Examiner and Candidate

Examiner: Would you please present your case?

Candidate:

> *This middle-aged lady presented with generalized pigmentation, significant weight loss, tiredness, and postural dizziness.*
>
> *On examination, the patient has evidence of widespread pigmentation most marked in the buccal mucosa, skin creases, and pressure areas.*
>
> *There is no adrenalectomy scar.*
>
> *I would like to examine for postural hypotension and look for other autoimmune diseases (thyroid, vitiligo) and evidence of previous tuberculosis infection like apical lung sign. In summary—the diagnosis is Addison's disease.*

Examiner: How will you investigate the case?

Candidate: At first, I would like to do some basic blood tests that include CBC with ESR (eosinophilia), serum creatinine, serum electrolytes (hyponatremia with hyperkalemia), serum calcium (hypercalcemia), blood sugar (low or lower limit of the normal range) as well as liver function test.

Then I would like to check baseline cortisol level with ACTH level, here I would expect low cortisol with high ACTH in primary hypoadrenalism.

Finally, I would like to confirm my diagnosis by doing a short synacthen test (Blood cortisol levels are sampled before, and at 30 and 60 minutes after 250 μg of tetracosactide injection). To identify the etiology; I would like to do:
- Autoantibody (Anti-21-hydroxylase Ab)
- Chest X-ray (to exclude associated TB)
- CT scan of the chest and abdomen

Examiner: How will you treat the case?

Candidate: Here, glucocorticoid replacement is the mainstay of treatment. Hydrocortisone in divided dose classically 20 mg in the morning; 10 mg at evening.

Some patients may require fludrocortisone for postural hypotension. If the patient still not improving and having decreased libido, androgen replacement may help in that case.

I would like to offer a medic alert bracelet to the patient and want to explain the importance of close attention to steroid replacement and outline what to do when unwell (e.g., doubling hydrocortisone dose during an illness such as fever, injury, or stress. Give out syringes and in-date I/M hydrocortisone and educate how to inject 100 mg I/M if vomiting interferes with oral intake of steroids).

Examiner: Why does pigmentation occur in primary adrenal insufficiency?

Candidate: In case of primary adrenal insufficiency ACTH level will be high. Due to similarity in between ACTH and melanocyte-stimulating hormone (MSH), abnormally high concentrations of ACTH stimulate the melanocortin receptor, causing melanin deposition in skin by melanocytes.

Examiner: What are the differential diagnoses of buccal pigmentation?

Candidate:
- Addison's disease
- Leukoplakia (thickened white or grayish patches on the mucous membrane which is associated with increased risk of cancer)
- Peutz–Jegher's syndrome (autosomal dominant disorder; characterized by hyperpigmented macules on the lips and oral cavity with a benign hamartomatous polyp in the GIT)
- Melanoma
- Lichen planus

Examiner: What is the treatment of acute adrenal insufficiency?

Candidate: The management of acute hypoadrenalism involves rapid correction with steroid, glucose, I/V fluid replacement, and reversal of electrolyte abnormalities (mainly hyponatremia and hyperkalemia) as well as treatment of underlying cause such as infection or MI.

(If the diagnosis is not known but suspecting as a case of adrenal insufficiency, previously, dexamethasone is considered the preferred steroid since it is not measured in cortisol assay; therefore, it will not hamper subsequent diagnostic tests. However, hydrocortisone is the preferred steroid since it has both glucocorticoid and mineralocorticoid actions—subsequent diagnostic tests are not affected if done >12 hours after the last dose of hydrocortisone.)

Diabetic Foot

Your role: You are the Registrar in the endocrinology clinic.

Patient details: Mr John Alfrad, 50-year-old.

Clinical problem: This gentleman has cellulitis around a recent ulcer on the plantar surface of his right foot. He has had diabetes for the last 20 years and is on insulin. His last HbA1c was 10, 2 weeks back. He is also hypertensive for the last 5 years; taking amlodipine 5 mg OD and ramipril 5 mg OD.

[*Differential diagnosis*: As this middle-aged gentleman has long-standing, poorly controlled DM with hypertension and is now presented with cellulitis around a pre-existing ulcer; therefore, the most likely diagnosis is a diabetic foot that is usually associated with motor-sensory neuropathy, peripheral vascular disease as well as concomitant infections. So, during clinical consultation, we have to exclude these complications as well as other microvascular (retinopathy and nephropathy) and macrovascular (MI/CVD) complications.]

(*Once you enter the room search for a spot diagnosis; cellulitis with gangrene, charcot joint, peripheral edema suggest underlying nephropathy or CCF.*)

Introduction, Permission, and Identification

Candidate: Good morning, I am Mohammad Ali, one of the working doctors here today, I have been asked to see you; is that okay with you?

Patient: Good morning, doctor. Okay.

Candidate: Thank you for coming, I would like to start by taking your full name, age, and where you have come from, please?

Patient: Mr John Alfrad, I am 50-year-old and from Nottingham.

Focused History

Candidate: Okay, Mr Alfrad, would you please tell me what brings you here today. Please tell me in your own words.

Patient: I have had an ulcer under my big toe of the right foot for the last 6 months, recently, which is increasing in severity. I have had diabetes for the last 20 years and hypertension for the last 5 years.

Candidate: Please tell me a little bit more about your ulcer?
- When were you last well? How/when did you first notice the ulcer?
- Is it getting worse or getting improved or the same?
- Is there any pain in the ulcer? (Painless ulcer is usually neuropathic). Have you attended any consultant or general physician or specialist for this ulcer? What was their impression? Did you receive a diagnosis? What treatment have you received? Did they work? What investigations/scans were done?
- How it affected your daily activities or job?

Patient: I am facing difficulty with a painless ulcer under my right big toe for the past 6 months or so. I went to my general physician, and initially, he thought there was a narrowing of the arteries in my leg because of my smoking. After that, I had given an I/V course of Flucloxacillin, and the district's nurse came round several times per week to change the dressing. But recently, I noticed a strong smell coming from the ulcer, so I went back to the general physician who referred me to the hospital. These antibiotics caused little improvement.

Candidate: Okay, would you please tell me more about your diabetes?
- For how long have you had diabetes? How was it detected first?

- How it was treated initially, and what is your current medication?
- Are you taking the medication regularly or irregularly? Is it controlled or uncontrolled?
- Have you ever monitored blood sugar? What is the usual range of blood sugar? What is your last blood sugar level and HbA1c?
- Are you on regular follow-up and where?

(If the patient has a long history of DM, ask about the complications of DM.)

- Do you have any history of hypoglycemic attack that means palpitation, restlessness, excessive sweating, or dizziness with low blood sugar level which improved after taking meal or sugar?
- Have you noticed pain in the calf during a walk that relief with rest (intermittent claudication)?
- Have you had your eyes checked recently? What was his impression regarding your diabetic eye disease?
- Have you noticed tingling, numbness, or burning sensation or loss of sensation in the feet?
- Have you noticed any change in your waterworks like amount, frequency, color, frothy urine or any pain while passing urine? (Diabetic nephropathy)
- Do you have chest pain or racing heartbeat, shortness of breath, or leg swelling?
- Have you ever been hospitalized for any complication and why?

Patient: I have had DM for last the 20 years. Initially, it was treated by oral medications, but now I am on insulin for the last 2 years. My usual blood sugar levels are 11-14 mmol/L, and the last HbA1c was 10% 2 weeks ago. Since the last year, I have been feeling tingling, numbness and burning sensation in my feet more marked at night. I feel a little odd if my blood glucose is <6 as having a hypo, and I need to eat something. I have had MI in 2015 when I presented with central crushing chest pain and got streptokinase during the hospital stay. At that time, I made a good recovery, but I get occasional chest pain when walking up the stair.

Candidate: Now, please tell me about your hypertension:
- For how long you have hypertension?
- Are you taking medicine for it, and what is your current medication? It is controlled or uncontrolled? What is the usual recording of BP?
- Do you have a FH of hypertension or DM?
- What about your dietary habit and your exercise?
- *Do you smoke or drink alcohol?*

Patient: I am hypertensive for the last 5 years and on regular medication. It is usually well-controlled, and my last BP was 130/80 mm Hg. For hypertension, I am taking ramipril 5 mg and amlodipine 5 mg daily. I smoke 10 cigarettes per day for the last 20 years and drink occasionally.

Quick Systemic Review, Past Medical History, Family History, Treatment, Social History According to Your Differentials

If it is not asked previously during initial history taking or incompletely asked then—take a full history of particular portion to make it complete.

Candidate: Now I would like to ask some general question, is that okay with you?
- Do you have headache, dizziness, LOC, blurring of vision or shaking of the limbs?
- Do you have any fever, weight loss, or loss of appetite? Any cough? Any nausea, vomiting, or tummy pain? What about your bowel habit? Any constipation or diarrhea or the passing of blood in stool? Any joint pain or skin rash?
- Do you have any similar condition in your past?
- May I ask what medication you take? Do you take any over-the-counter medications or herbal medicine or any recreational drugs? Are you allergic to any medicine or anything else?
- Is there anyone else in your family with this type of problem or any longstanding illness that run in your families like DM, hypertension, stroke, thyroid or other autoimmune disease or anything else?

- What are you doing for a living? Are you married? Who is at home with you or who is supporting you now? Do you have children? Are you independent in activities of daily living?

Have I missed anything, or do you want to add anything more?

Would you mind if I go on to examine you?

Focused Examination

So, this patient presents with uncontrolled DM, diabetic foot with peripheral neuropathy and past history of MI, hypertension, and smoker.

So here focused examination would be.

Examination of Ulcer

- Neuropathic (weight-bearing areas as particularly metatarsal head area) versus arterial ulcer.
- The bone at the base of the ulcer suggests osteomyelitis.
- Look for evidence of infection/cellulitis/edema, erythema, and bad odors.
- Look for any evidence of tinea pedis in toe interspaces.

Vascular Examination of the Foot

Palpate the arterial dorsalis pedis and posterior tibial artery, if absent, check popliteal and femoral artery.

Evidence of Peripheral Neuropathy

Reduced muscle power and diminish reflex.

Assessment of Four Modalities of Sensation

- Pinprick
- Light touch
- Joint position
- Vibration sensation

I would like to complete my examination by doing CVS examination, urine dipstick for protein and sugar and fundoscopic examination for evidence of diabetic and hypertensive retinopathy, BP measurement.

Feedback to the Patient and Respond to the Patient's Concern

You said at the beginning that your main problems are a recurrent ulcer in the feet, hypertension and DM. Is there anything else that we have missed or any worries or concerns?

Patient: What might be the cause of my foot problem?

Candidate: I think your longstanding uncontrolled blood sugar has damaged your nerves that lead to ulcer in your feet. Now the ulcer is infected and takes an ugly look. At this moment, we would like to do some blood tests as well as duplex USG of the lower limb to exclude associated vascular insufficiency. It is vital to control your blood sugar as strictly as possible to reduce the risk of further damage to your body from diabetes. It is also important to take appropriate foot care to reduce the risk of complication or further damage. So, I will refer you to an MDT involving diabetic specialist and foot care specialist (podiatrist).

Patient: Will I need an amputation?

Candidate: I believe this is due to loss of sensation in the soles of the feet rather than vascular problems. At this point it is very important to control your blood sugar levels as strictly as possible as well as follow chiropody regularly and take care of your feet by wearing better shoes and socks. Therefore, we can avoid amputation.

Do you have any other concern?

Discussion between Examiner and Candidate

Examiner: Would you please present your case?

Candidate:

This middle-aged man presents with a recurrent ulcer, poorly controlled DM, hypertension, and a past history of MI. Examination of the lower limbs revealed evidence of diabetic peripheral sensory neuropathy.

There is impairment of sensation to light touch, pinprick, vibration, and joint position sense as stocking pattern. Peripheral pulses [anterior tibial artery (ADP) and posterior tibial artery (PTA)] are palpable.

There is an ulcer with associated cellulitis on the plantar surface of the right feet.

So, in summary, my diagnosis would be diabetic foot with associated peripheral neuropathy with Old MI with uncontrolled DM and hypertension.

Examiner: How will you investigate this patient?

Candidate: At first, I would like to do some basic blood tests that include FBC with ESR with CRP, urea and electrolytes, fasting lipids, blood sugar, HbA1c, and TFT.

Then most importantly, I would like to take a deep swab from the wound and sent for gram staining, culture, sensitivity, and fungal study. Other tests include:

- Duplex USG of the lower limbs to assess vascular supply.
- A plain X-ray of the foot to get the evidence of osteomyelitis. However, an MRI is often needed for the best assessment of osteomyelitis.

Finally, if the ongoing infection, then I would like to consider bone biopsy.

Examiner: How will you treat the case?

Candidate: At first, I would like to take some general measures that include most importantly optimal glycemic control, control of hypertension, and smoking cessation.

Then I would like to advise broad-spectrum antibiotics covering *Staphylococcus*, *Streptococcus*, and anaerobes. I would like to adjust antimicrobial therapy according to the blood and deep swab culture sensitivity. Antibiotic therapy should be continued for 3 months if bone visible or radiological evidence of osteomyelitis.

If there is evidence of deep tissue infection, a surgical review may require.

Ankylosing Spondylitis

Your role: You are a registrar in the rheumatology clinic.

Patient details: Mr Jimmy Brown, a 33-year-old man.

Clinical problem: Progressive severe back pain over the last 3 years following RTA, recently noticed painful red eye.

(*Once you get this clinical scenario, you will get 5 minutes to start this station for two scenarios. At that time, start to think about your diagnosis, differential diagnoses, and plan for taking focused history as well as focused examination.*)

[*Differential diagnosis of progressive back pain*: Ankylosing spondylitis, other seronegative arthritis, tumor or trauma of the spinal cord, a ruptured or herniated disc, and Pott's disease.

Differential diagnosis of a painful red eye: Uveitis, acute glaucoma, corneal ulcer, trauma, or infection.]

(*Once you enter the room, search for a spot diagnosis; question mark posture with restricted spinal movement, red eye suggests ankylosing spondylitis.*)

Greetings, Introduction, Permission, and Identification

Candidate: Good morning. I am Mohammad Ali, one of the working doctors here today. I have been asked to see you. Is that okay with you?

Patient: Good morning, doctor.....

Candidate: What is your name?

Patient: I am Jimmy Brown.

Candidate: Okay.... what may I call you?

Patient: You can call me Brown.

Focused History

Candidate: Nice to meet you Brown, thank you for taking this appointment. Would you please tell me what brings you here today? Please tell me in your own words.

Patient: I had a road traffic accident 3 years ago. I went to the accident and emergency (A&E) department and did an X-ray then, and fortunately, I did not have a fracture at that time. However, since then, I have been suffering from back pain which is increasing day-by-day. Most of the day, I take paracetamol and ibuprofen for my pain, but recently I have had red eye, which is painful, and I am having trouble looking at the light. So, my general physician sent me here for further assessment.

Analyze the Symptoms

Candidate: It is okay, would you please, tell me a little bit more about your back pain like:
The important questions to be asked:
- For how long you have had it? Is it constant or intermittent?
- Does it move anywhere else, like in your legs or anywhere?
- Is there any associated stiffness? Is it worse in the morning or evening?
- Is there anything that relieves your symptoms like rest, movement, or exercise or anything makes it worse?
- If I give you a pain scale of 0–10, where 0 is being no pain, and 10 is the highest pain, what is your score?
- Would you please tell me how this back pain has affected your daily life? What does it stop you from doing?
- Are there any other joints affected?
- Do you have any pain in the Achilles tendon or feet?

- Do you have any bowel problems like bloody diarrhea or any skin rash or nail changes like psoriasis?
- Do you have a similar type of back pain or psoriasis, or inflammatory bowel disease in your family?
- Do you smoke or drink alcohol? If yes, then for how long, what is the amount?

Patient: Over the last 5 months, I have noticed that my back pain is increasing in severity, and my pain score is around 8–9. It is mainly in the morning, and it is difficult to get out of bed nowadays. This improves considerably by the mid-morning after getting pain medication. So, I have now started taking painkillers regularly. However, recently I have had a similar type of pain in my both hips and right knee also. I do not have any diarrhea or skin problems, as you asked. My mother suffers from severe arthritis, diagnosed in her early 40, which I recall was presented initially in the same fashion. I do not smoke but drink alcohol occasionally.

Candidate: It is okay, so let us talk about your eye problem. You said at the beginning, you have pain and redness in your eyes but,
- Have you noticed any blurring of vision?
- Do you have a similar attack in the past?

Patient: Yes, Doctor, I have blurred vision, and it is hard for me to look at the light. I do not have any history of eye problems in the past.

Candidate: Since it suggests a case of ankylosing spondylitis—by the patient's general look and history)—then to check the extra-articular manifestations.

Other Important Targeted Histories

- Do you have any chest pain or racing heart [aortic regurgitation (AR)]?
- Do you have any shortness of breath (AR or lung fibrosis)?
- Do you have any pins and needle in your hands or pain in the hand joints or any frothy urine (amyloidosis)?

Quick Systemic Review, Past Medical History, Family History, Treatment, Social History According to Your Differentials

If it is not asked previously during initial history taking or incompletely asked—then take a full history of a particular part to make it complete.

Candidate: At this moment I would like to ask some general questions, is that okay with you?
- Do you have a headache, blurring of vision, any abnormal shakiness of the limb?
- Do you have any cough any fever? Any problem with your waterworks?
- Have you attended any consultant/general physician/specialist for these problems? Have you done any recent tests? Blood test and imaging? What was their impression? Did you receive any diagnosis? What treatment have you received? Did they work?
- Have you ever been admitted to the hospital in the past or any history of surgery?
- Are you taking any medication recently on a regular basis? Any over-the-counter medications/herbal medicine/any recreational drugs? Are you allergic to any medicine or anything else?
- Is there anyone else in your family with this type of problem or any long-standing illness that run in your families like DM, hypertension, stroke, thyroid, or any autoimmune disease or anything else?
- What are you doing for a living? Could you please tell me about your home condition? Who is at home with you, or who is supporting you now? Are you independent in activities of daily living?
- Are you sexually active? Tell me more about your partner.... Are you in a stable relationship (single/multiple)? Do you practice safe sex? If no, then ask... when was the last time you had unprotected sex? What is your sexual orientation? (gay/bisexual), what is your preferred route of sex (oral/vaginal/anal)?

Have I missed anything, or do you want to add anything more?

Okay, thank you. Would you mind if I go on to examine you now?

Focused Examination

(Targeted examination would be according to main complains and spot diagnosis.)

In this scenario, the most likely diagnosis is ankylosing spondylitis with uveitis as an extra-articular manifestation. So, the targeted examination would be evidence of ankylosing spondylitis and examination of eyes to see the evidence of uveitis as well.

If the patient complaining of breathlessness, then we have to examine the CVS to get evidence of AR (high volume collapsing pulse with early diastolic murmur) and mitral regurgitation (MR) [positive surgical margin (PSM) in apex] and bradycardia (? heart block).

Examination of the chest for evidence of apical lung fibrosis (shifting of the trachea to the same side with bronchial breath sounds).

Another important issue would be examined for evidence of psoriasis (skin rash or nail change).

- Eye examination
- *General inspection*: Circumlimbal injection (erythema around the limbus with dilated blood vessels).
- *Fundoscopy*: Cloudy fluid (flare) with white clumps of inflammatory cells and protein-rich fluid in the anterior chamber of the eye (hypopyon).
- Visual acuity may be reduced.
- *Pupil*: Often small, nonreacting, and irregular pupil.
- Evidence of ankylosing spondylitis (a most important part of examination)
- Ask the patient to get up from the chair and walk several meters, then turn and walk back; Observe for—absence for hyperextension of the cervical spine, kyphosis of the thoracic spine, and loss of normal lumbar lordosis (resulting in a protuberant abdomen; question mark posture).
- Note any stiffness and whether the patient turns with the torso and cervical spine fixed (ask the patient to look backward).

Active movement of the cervical spine in the six directions of movements—flexion, extension, lateral flexion (left and right), and lateral rotation (left and right).

Active low back movement (as for cervical spine):
- Forward flexion and extension
- Lateral flexion (right and left)
- Lateral rotation (left and right)

Palpate for tenderness over spine and sacroiliac joint (sacroiliitis); Achilles tendon and plantar fascia (plantar fasciitis, Achilles tendinitis).

The specific test for ankylosing spondylitis includes:
- Chest expansion at the 4th ICS (normal 2.5 cm)
- Finger to floor distance on forward bending (normal <10 cm)
- Occiput to wall distance (normal 0 cm)
- Perform Schober's test:
- Stand behind the patient and identify the dimples of venous with corresponding to the posterior superior iliac spine. Place a finger halfway between these points.
- Having asked the patient's permission, mark two lines, one 10 cm above and the other 5 cm below the point.
- Ask the patient to flex forward as far as possible and measure the increase in the distance between these two lines.
- A presence of <5 cm (e.g., <20 cm between the two marks) indicates a positive Schober's test result (50% increase would be expected in a normal healthy adult).

Feedback to the Patient and Respond to the Patient's Concern

Candidate: You said at the beginning that the main problem was increasing back pain, painful red eyes, blurred vision, and sensitivity to light. Is there anything else troubling you that we have not covered or any concerns?

Patient: I am really concerned with this recent progression in back pain and even more concerned with my recent eye problem too. I want to know what exactly happened to me. Have you had any thoughts about what is going on?

Candidate: The symptoms you discussed and the signs I have found on examination suggest you may have a condition known as ankylosing spondylitis. This condition is seen in young people and affects spine mobility as well as other joints. There is soreness in front of your eyes; it seems like a condition called acute anterior uveitis, and it may be associated with ankylosing spondylitis.

I will refer you immediately to an eye specialist for an urgent evaluation of your eyes (slit-lamp examination). It is important that you stay in the hospital for now to exclude other conditions that need urgent treatment, such as glaucoma and an ulcer of your cornea.

We will need to do some basic blood tests, X-ray spine, and MRI of the spine to establish our diagnosis of ankylosing spondylitis and exclude other causes that may cause similar symptoms. After that, you will be managed by an MDT involving a joint physician, eye physician, physiotherapist, and occupational therapist, to get the full care of management.

Do you have any concerns? Is there anything unclear you need me to clarify?

Patient: No.

Discussion with Examiner

Examiner: Would you please present your case?

Candidate:

This young man presented with increasing inflammatory back pain and right knee and hip joint pain for the last 3 years.

He also gave a history of painful red eyes and blurred vision with photophobia for the past 3 days.

The examination revealed a marked restriction in spinal movement almost in all directions, as well as increased wall occiput

distance and positive Schober's test. He has evidence of uveitis as well.

So, in summary, this is a case of ankylosing spondylitis with uveitis as an extra-articular manifestation.

Examiner: How will you investigate the case?

Candidate: Initially, I would want to perform some blood tests, and I would start by checking this patient's inflammatory markers (ESR and CRP), looking for evidence of disease activity in terms of the ankylosing spondylitis.

I would also want to check FBC and baseline urea, creatinine, electrolytes, and liver function tests, given this patient has been on nonsteroidal medication for some time and also thinking about future treatments.

After that, I would like to request an human leukocyte antigen (HLA) B27 (positive in 90–95% cases but only 5% patient HLA B27 positive have ankylosing spondylitis); besides, X-rays of his spine and sacroiliac joint looking for evidence of sacroiliitis (joint space narrowing or widening, erosions, sclerosis, and fusion), and fusion in the spine.

If these X-rays are normal, I may want to consider other imaging modalities such as an MRI scan of the spine (best test to detect early evidence of sacroiliitis when a plain X-ray is normal).

Examiner: How will you manage this case?

Candidate: As a part of general measures, it would be important for this patient to have a physiotherapist and occupational therapist review (exercise, not rest for backache, including intense exercise to maintain posture and mobility), and other treatments such as hydrotherapy have been proven to be effective in ankylosing spondylitis.

I would also want to ensure that any patient with ankylosing spondylitis who smokes receive appropriate smoking cessation counseling due to the close association with disease activity.

In terms of his medication, I want this patient to continue on his regular analgesia, and I may wish to escalate his regular ibuprofen to another nonsteroidal, such as naproxen [nonsteroidal anti-inflammatory drugs (NSAIDs) usually relieve symptoms within hours and may slow radiographic progression] as appropriate.

Following this, dependent on disease activity, I may wish to consider this patient for further immune-modulating therapy, such as sulfasalazine and methotrexate.

It may well be appropriate for patients with the refractory disease to consider further immune-modulating treatment in the form of anti-TNF agents or janus kinase (JAK) inhibitors such as tofacitinib or baricitinib.

Examiner: What advice should you give to a patient with ankylosing spondylitis who receives anti-TNF treatment (etanercept, adalimumab)?

Candidate: I would like to aware the patient of some matters, including:
- Always inform any doctor/dentist that they are on anti-TNF treatment.
- Stop the treatment if there is an intercurrent infection and seek urgent medical attention.
- Be up to date with vaccinations (Pneumovax, swine flu, influenza).
- Stop two treatment doses before any surgery.

Back Pain

Your role: You are a registrar in the General Medical Clinic.

Patient details: Mrs Jane, a 72-year-old lady.

Clinical problem: This elderly lady has been referred by her general physician with severe back pain. She lives alone and is struggling to cope at home. She has a history of osteoporosis, and her general physician is concerned that she may have had another vertebral fracture.

(Once you get this clinical scenario, you will get 5 minutes to start this station for two scenarios. At that time, start to think about your diagnosis, differential diagnoses, and plan for taking focused history as well as focused examination.)

[*Differential diagnosis of progressive back pain*: Collapsed vertebrae (osteoporotic, multiple myeloma, secondaries, trauma), ankylosing spondylitis, other seronegative arthritis, tumor or trauma of the spinal cord, a ruptured or herniated disc, and Pott's disease.]

(Once you enter the room, search for a spot diagnosis; kyphosis suggests collapsed vertebrae, question mark posture with restricted spinal movement, red eye suggests ankylosing spondylitis.)

Greetings, Introduction, Permission, and Identification

Candidate: Good morning. My name is Mohammad Ali, one of the working doctors here today. I have been asked to see you. Is that okay with you?

Patient: No problem.

Candidate: I will start by taking your full name, age, and where you have come from, please?

Patient: Mrs Jane, I am 72 and from London.

Focused History

Candidate: Okay, Mrs Jane, would you please tell me what brings you here today? Please tell me in your own words.

Patient: A week ago, I noticed back pain, and it is getting worse nowadays. I feel pain all the time, and all of the movement is now very painful. I have had a fracture in my back in the past and I am concerned that this may be related.

Analyze the Complaints

Candidate: It is okay, would you please, tell me a little bit more about your back pain.
The important questions to be asked are:
- For how long you have had it? Is it constant or intermittent?
- Does it move anywhere in your body, like your legs, tummy, or groin?
- Is it worse in the morning or evening? Any associated stiffness?
- Is there anything that increases or decreases your symptoms, like rest, movement, or exercise?
- If I give you a pain scale of 0–10, where 0 is being no pain, 5 is moderate, and 10 is the highest pain, what is your point?
- Are there any other joints affected?
- Would you please tell me how this back pain has affected your daily life or what does it stop you from doing?

Patient: I have back pain that started gradually around 1 week ago and is now present constantly. It wakes me up at night. It does not move anywhere and is not associated with morning stiffness. I just do not feel right in myself, and as I live alone, my daily activities such as washing, dressing, and cooking become increasingly difficult.

Other Important Targeted Histories

To detect the complications and etiology of back pain.

Candidate:
- Any history of trauma or fall?
- Do you have a fever or raised temperature, any changes in weight or appetite? Do you have any lumps and bumps in your body?
- What about your waterworks or bowel motion?
- Do you have any cough, chest pain, racing heartbeat, or breathing problem?
- Do you have a headache, blurring of vision, any abnormal shakiness of the limb, or anything else?

Patient: I do not have any history of falls recently. I have also been feeling feverish and sweaty and a bit shaky. I feel tired and exhausted. I have lost my appetite over the past week and lost a little weight over that period, but this is not significant weight loss.

Candidate: Do you have any other problems that we have missed?

Patient: No.

Quick Systemic Review, Treatment History, Past Medical History, Family History, Social History According to Your Differentials

Past Medical and Surgical History

Candidate: You mentioned a fracture in your past. Can you please tell me more about it?

Patient: I have osteoporosis and a broken bone in my back. About a month ago, I had a small cut on my toe, which caused pus to come out. My general physician gave me antibiotics, but I did not complete the course because they made me feel sick. Within a few days, my toes have improved and are now back to normal.

Candidate: Okay, Mrs Jane, thank you for sharing this with me. I need to ask you few more questions for a better understanding. Do you have any other medical illnesses like DM, hypertension or anything else other than osteoporosis? Have you ever been admitted to the hospital? Have you ever had any surgeries?

Patient: No.

Relevant Family History

Candidate: Is there anyone else in your family with this type of problem or any long-standing illness that runs in your family like DM, hypertension, stroke, thyroid, or any autoimmune disease or anything else?

Patient: Well... My mother broke her hip after a minor fall in her early seventies.

Candidate: I am sorry to hear about your mother.

Treatment History

Candidate: Tell me about your medication. Are you currently taking any medications? Do you take any over-the-counter medication or herbal remedies, or any recreational drugs? Are you allergic to any medicine or anything else?

Patient: I am taking alendronate 70 mg once weekly, calcium carbonate (Calcichew D3 Forte) two tablets daily.

Social History

Candidate: Mrs Jane, now tell me about your lifestyle,
- Do you smoke? If not—then ask, have you ever smoked? If yes—then how many years have you been smoking? How many sticks per day?
- Do you drink alcohol? If yes—then how many drinks would you have in a week? (CAGE questionnaire, if needed)
- You said you live alone. Do you have anybody else to support at your home?
- Do you work? How do you manage your finances?

Patient: I am a widower and a retired primary school teacher. I have never smoked but occasionally enjoy a glass of sherry. I am self-independent and live independently, but now I am facing difficulties in my daily activities such as washing and dressing due to this back pain.

Candidate: It is tough to manage everything by own when you are in pain, Mrs Jane, would you like me to arrange some social services for you?

Patient: Yes, please, doctor. I need some help.

Candidate: Sure. I will refer you to social services, which can help provide some carers who can come to your home and help you to manage your everyday life. I can also involve occupational therapists; they will assess your home condition and adjust according to your needs.

Have I missed anything, or do you want to add anything more?

Would you mind if I go on to examine you?

Focused Examination

In this scenario, the most likely diagnosis is infective discitis with features of sepsis. So, the targeted examination would be:
- Look at the observations to assess for septic shock (pulse—110, BP-90/70).
- Palpates spine looking for spinal tenderness.
- Conducts the focal neurological examination of lower limbs, assessing tone, power, and reflexes.
- Look for signs of endocarditis (skin lesions, murmur, etc.).

I would like to check sensation and perform a rectal exam to assess anal tone and perianal sensation.

Feedback to the Patient and Response to the Patient's Concern

Candidate: You said at the beginning that the main problems were increasing back pain, fever, and difficulty in doing daily activities. Is there anything else troubling you that we have not covered or any expectations or any concerns?

Patient: Why am I feeling so unwell?

Candidate: The most likely cause for back pain is an infection and the condition we can call infective discitis. This may be due to incomplete skin infection treatment, and now infection spread to your backbone through your blood, causing fever and back pain.

I would suggest getting admission so we can start your treatment with I/V antibiotics as early as possible, and also we will arrange some basic blood tests, X-ray spine and MRI of the spine to establish our diagnosis and exclude other causes that may cause similar symptoms. Is that okay with you?

Patient: Yes.

Candidate: After that, you will be managed by an MDT involving a bone doctor, specialist nurse, physiotherapist, occupational therapist, social workers to get the full care of management.

Do you have any other concerns? Is there anything unclear you need me to clarify?

Discussion with Examiner

Examiner: Would you please present your case?

Candidate:

This elderly lady presented with a short history of increasing back pain, pyrexia, hypotension, and a history of incompletely treated soft tissue infection.

She has spinal tenderness and establishes no signs of acute cord compression or other focal neurological signs.

So, I think this is a case of infective discitis presumed secondary to bacteremia following incompletely treated soft tissue infection.

Examiner: What would be your differential diagnosis?

Candidate: My differential diagnosis would be osteoporotic fracture with an alternative source of sepsis [e.g., urinary tract infection (UTI)]

Examiner: How will you investigate the case?

Candidate: I would want to do urgently an X-ray of the spine, MRI scan of the spine looking for evidence of discitis or cord compression.

After that, I would do some blood tests, including blood cultures, FBC, blood sugar, CRP, baseline urine, creatinine, and electrolytes.

Examiner: How will you manage this case?

Candidate: Immediate admission with close observation and assessing signs of sepsis syndrome and fluid balance.

I would like to start empirical antibiotics, e.g., I/V flucloxacillin, based on likely staphylococcal infection after sending a set of blood cultures.

Systemic Lupus Erythematosus

Your role: You are a Registrar in the Rheumatology Clinic.

Patient details: Mrs Samaira Khan, 29-year-old lady.

Clinical problem: Facial rash with right lower limb swelling.

(Once you get this clinical scenario, you will get 5 minutes to start this station for two scenarios. At that time, start to think about your diagnosis, differential diagnoses, and plan for taking focused history as well as focused examination.)

[*Differential diagnosis of facial rash*: SLE, dermatomyositis, MCTD, mitral stenosis, rosacea, sunburn, polymorphic light reaction, PKDL, herpes simplex/zoster, sarcoidosis, and tuberous sclerosis.

Differential diagnosis of unilateral lower limb swelling: DVT, cellulitis, trauma, ruptured baker's cyst, and bursitis]

(Once you enter the room, search for a spot diagnosis; here butterfly rash, discoid rash, hair loss, iatrogenic cushingoid appearance suggest SLE.)

Greetings, Introduction, Permission, and Identification

Candidate: Good morning; my name is Mohammad Ali, one of the working doctors here today. I have been asked to see you. Is that okay, Mrs Khan?

Patient: Okay.

Candidate: I will start by taking your full name, age, and where you have come from, please.

Patient: Mrs Samaira Khan, I am 29, and I am from Egypt.

Candidate: Would you mind if I take some notes?

Patient: Yes, sure.

Candidate: It would be confidential.

Patient: Thank you, Doctor.

Focused History

Candidate: Okay, Mrs Khan, what brings you here today? Please tell me in your own words.

Patient: Yes. I notice my right leg has been swollen since morning, and recently there is a rash on my face that I think may be due to sunburn.

Analyze the Symptom

Candidate: Would you please tell me more about your leg swelling?
Important questions to be asked are:
- When did you first notice swelling? Is it on one leg or both legs?
- Is it sudden or gradual onset? Is it increasing or decreasing?
- How extensive is the swelling? Is it below the knee or above the knee?
- Do you have any history of trauma?
- How it affects your activities of daily living?
- Do you have any fever or pain or numbness, or any changes in skin color?
- Do you have any history of recent surgery? Recent long-haul travel, pregnancy, any miscarriage or past history of a clot in your blood channel?
- Anyone in your family ever had a clot in the lungs or legs or does any clotting problem run in the families?
- Do you have any chest pain or breathlessness?

Patient: Since this morning, I have noticed pain in my right calf that is slowly increasing. I feel a little uncomfortable with my mobility and weight-bearing. There is no chest pain or shortness of breath, no history of recent long-distance travel or a history of clots previously, and no history of a clot in the family.

Candidate: Now, please tell me a little bit more about your facial rash?

Important questions to be asked are:
- When did you first notice this rash on your face?
- Are there any other areas affected (skin, scalp)?
- Is it sudden or gradual onset? Is it increasing or decreasing or static?
- Is it coming on and off or all the time with you?
- Is there anything that makes it worse (like sun exposure)?
- Is there anything that makes it better (like the use of sunblock)?
- Are there any associated pain or itching?
- Do you have any joint aches and pain? If so, which joints are affected? Is there any stiffness?
- Do you have any mouth ulcers? If so, is it painful or painless?
- Have you noticed any hair loss?

Patient: I have had this rash on my face for the last 1 year and have never noticed it. I like to go on vacation and enjoy sunbathing but have found that this rash gets worse when it comes in contact with the sun. It improves back from the holidays but has some degree of permanent scarring. Moreover, I get sunburn easily, and applying sunblock cream has helped. I do not have pain in any of the joints but have recently noticed mouth ulcers, especially on the roof of my mouth (hard palate), which is painful.

Candidate: Other targeted histories to confirm our diagnosis, rule out differential diagnosis such as MCTD, dermatomyositis, and look for the associated conditions such as Sjogren's syndrome or complications such as lupus nephritis.

Other Important Targeted Histories

- Have you noticed any changes in the color of your fingers on exposure to cold weather (Raynaud's phenomenon)?
- Have you noticed any dryness in your mouth or eyes or any gritty sensation in your eyes (Sjogren's syndrome)?
- Have you noticed any difficulty standing from a sitting position, climbing stairs, combing your hair due to weakness (dermatomyositis)?
- Have you noticed any difficulty swallowing or any skin change like being more tight, shiny, smooth than before (systemic sclerosis)?
- Have you noticed any change in your waterworks and blood, frothy urine, decreased amount, or burning sensation (lupus nephritis)?
- Do you have headaches, any dizzy spell/any blackout or the blurring of vision or shaky limbs and body (cerebral lupus)?
- Do you have any cough, breathing problem, chest pain, or palpitation (DPLD, pericarditis, pleuritis as extra-articular manifestations of SLE)?
- Are you on any medications recently (drug-induced lupus—diuretic, hydralazine, isoniazid, procainamide, anticonvulsants, etc.)?

Patient: No.

Quick Systemic Review, Past Medical History, Family History, Treatment, Social History According to Your Differentials

If it is not asked previously during initial history taking or incompletely asked then—take a full history of a particular portion to make it complete.

Candidate: Now I would like to ask some general questions just to make sure that everything is going okay with you....
- Do you have a fever, weight loss, or loss of appetite?
- Any nausea, vomiting, or tummy pain?
- Any abnormality in bowel motions? Any problem with waterworks?
- Do you have any similar condition or any other history of disease in your past?
- Have you attended any consultant or general physician or specialist for this problem? What was their impression? Did you receive any diagnosis? What treatment have you received? Did they work?
- Have you ever been admitted to the hospital in the past or any history of surgery?

- Do you take any over-the-counter medications or herbal medicine, or any recreational drugs? Are you allergic to any medicine or anything else?
- Is there anyone else in your family with this type of problem or any long-standing illness that run in your families like DM, hypertension, stroke, thyroid, or other autoimmune disease or anything else?
- Do you smoke? Do you drink? What are you doing for a living? Are you married? Who is at home with you, or who is supporting you now? Do you have children? Are you independent in activities of daily living?

Have I missed anything, or do you want to add anything more?

Would you mind if I go on to examine you?

Focused Examination

Here, history suggest, the most likely diagnosis is SLE or secondary APLA syndrome or MCTD presented with DVT, facial rash, and oral ulceration. So, here focused examination would be:
- Examination of the lower limb for DVT
- Examination of the facial rash and oral ulceration
- Examination of the other features for SLE or MCTD
- Other systemic examination such as CVS and respiratory system (if the patient has chest pain or breathlessness).

Examination of the Lower Limbs

- Establish asymmetrical leg swelling
- Assess the extent of leg swelling
- Pitting edema
- Establish no knee joint swelling
- Note any trophic changes (overlying erythema, blue or brown discoloration secondary to venous hypertension)
- Overlying temperature and calf tenderness
- If the patient has chest pain or breathlessness then examine the chest for:
  - Jugular venous pressure (JVP) and other signs of pulmonary hypertension (PHTN)
  - Any evidence of pulmonary embolus (consolidation, pleural rub)
  - Crackles (for pulmonary fibrosis)

Face/Head

- Photosensitive rash in the sun-exposed area (butterfly rash)
- Alopecia/scarring or discoid rash in the scalp
- Oral ulceration

Examination of the Skin and the Other Parts of the Body

- *Vasculitic lesion*: Mottled vasculitic rash on the palm frequently seen with active lupus
- Livedo reticularis [pink-blue mottling caused by capillary dilatation and stasis in skin venules sometimes are seen in APLA syndrome or polyarteritis nodosa (PAN), mainly in the legs]
- Discoid rash
- Tight shiny skin, particularly in the limbs when associated with scleroderma

Hand and Nail

- Raynaud's phenomenon, nail fold infarct, and palmar erythema
- Any evidence of rheumatoid arthritis, systemic sclerosis, or dermatomyositis (Gottron's papules)

Cardiac (if the Patient has Chest Pain and Breathlessness)

- Pericardial friction rub
- Cardiac murmur (Libman–Sacks endocarditis)
- Evidence of PHTN
- Crepitation for heart failure

Central Nervous System

If CNS manifestations present, then look for focal neurological deficit:
- Hemiparesis (due to stroke or as a complication of APLA)
- Paraparesis (transverse myelitis)
- Mononeuritis multiplex, or
- Evidence of peripheral neuropathy

I would like to complete my assessment by measuring blood pressure and urine dipstick for hematuria and proteinuria.

Feedback to the Patient and Respond to the Patient's Concern

Candidate: You said at the beginning that the main problems were rash on your face and right calf swelling. Is there anything else troubling you that we have missed or any concerns?

Patient: What actually happens to me, Doctor?

Candidate: The symptoms you discussed and the signs I found on examination suggest you may have a condition called systemic lupus erythematous with APLA syndrome. It is a disease due to disturbance in our defensive system, which supposed to attack bugs and germs. Sometimes, our defense system, instead of attacking germs and bugs, go crazy for an unknown reason, and it attacks our own tissues ....in your condition, it attacks your skin and blood vessels resulting formation of a clot in the blood channel of your lower leg as well as a facial rash.

At this time, we need to carry out some blood tests, urine tests, and USG of the lower limbs to establish our diagnosis and exclude other conditions that may give rise to similar problems.

The treatments may vary with time, depending on the severity of the disease or flare-up of symptoms and also which parts of your body are affected. Once we confirm the diagnosis, your treatment will start with medications such as steroids to reduce inflammation, hydroxychloroquine for your skin problem, and blood thinner medication for your clot in the leg.

It is important to protect your skin with clothing and sunscreen. Wear a hat to protect your face and wear a pair of ultraviolet (UV) protective sunglasses. Does it make sense for you, Mrs Khan?

Patient: Doctor, is it curable?

Candidate: Although, there is no cure for SLE, the condition can usually be controlled, and symptoms eased. Also, we will follow-up with you regularly by a specialist called a rheumatologist to see your recovery, disease activity, and prevent complications. Do you have any other concerns?

Patient: No.

Candidate: Okay, Mrs Khan, if you develop any sudden severe chest pain, breathlessness, limb weakness, slurred speech, or visual loss, then call 999 or come to us immediately (Safety-netting).

Thank you very much for spending time with me today.

Discussion with Examiner

Examiner: Would you please present your case?

Candidate:

This young lady presented with photo-sensitive rash, unilateral calf swelling as well as oral ulceration.

On examination, she has a sharply defined erythematous, confluent, a macular rash with scaling and follicular plugging (very close examination of the rash reveals that scale in many areas which appears as a dot) in the face affecting cheeks and nose; sparing the nasolabial fold (butterfly distribution).

There is swelling of the right leg up to the knee, which looks normal in appearance with an erythematous or cyanotic hue to the skin and mild tenderness to palpation in the calf. The affected calf feels indurated and is warmer than the other leg may suggest DVT.

She also has evidence of painless oral ulcers, particularly involving the hard palate.

So, in summary, my diagnosis would be SLE or secondary APLA syndrome.

Examiner: How will you investigate this case?

Candidate: These are largely determined by the pattern of disease. Initially, I would start by performing some blood tests to check inflammatory markers—ESR and CRP (ESR commonly elevated, CRP usually not elevated except during serositis or infection) looking for evidence of disease activity in terms of SLE.

I would also want to check FBC (it may show an array of hematological disorders including hemolytic anemia, thrombocytopenia, lymphopenia; thus, direct Coombs test and reticulocyte count is also helpful.).

Then I would like to do baseline blood urea, electrolyte, serum creatinine, LFTs, TFT, and urine examination (for proteinuria, hematuria, and red cell casts to see the evidence of renal involvement).

After that, I would like to request for autoantibody screen such as:

- Antinuclear antibodies (ANA) (positive in >95% cases, titer usually very high in SLE, i.e., >1:320)
- Anti-double stranded deoxyribonucleic acid (dsDNA) (usually positive, may rise during flares)
- Extractable nuclear antigens (ENA) (often positive, especially Ro, La, Sm, RNP)
- Complement (Low C4 and less commonly C3 associated with renal involvement, both may fall during active flares)
- Antiphospholipid antibodies (high titers associated with the secondary APS)
- Antihistone antibody (it is positive >95% cases of drug-induced SLE) as well as creatine kinase (CK)—if raised, suggests myositis.

I would like to perform other imaging modalities such as:

- *CXR*: Looking for evidence of fibrosis, effusions, cardiomegaly (can be a sign of pericardial effusion)
- *Echo*: Valvular incompetence or vegetations, pericardial effusion.
- Duplex USG of the lower limbs to get the evidence of DVT.
- Ventilation-perfusion (VQ) or computed tomography pulmonary angiography (CTPA) if concerns of pulmonary embolism (PE)

If we get evidence of renal involvement on routine blood and urine test, then I would consider renal biopsy, which may show glomerulonephritis with evidence of immune complex [immunoglobulin (Ig) and C3] deposition or microthrombotic disease.

I may well want to consider skin biopsy: It may show immune complex deposition (IgG/IgM and C3) at the dermal-epidermal junction.

Examiner: How would you treat a patient with SLE?

Candidate: The management of SLE is multidisciplinary. Management includes:

General measures
- Patient education
- Avoidance of precipitating drugs causing SLE
- Avoiding excessive sunlight, i.e., use of high factor sunblock, hats, and long sleeves to minimize the progression of the photosensitive rash.
- Physiotherapy and occupational therapy; useful to aid mobility and help to patient return to normal functional abilities.
- SLE itself is a strong risk factor for ischemic heart disease, so risk factors modifications for cardiovascular disease by controlling BP, dyslipidemia, smoking cessation etc., is crucial.

Pharmacological

Analgesics: NSAIDs (unless renal disease) have particular efficacy for tackling the pain and inflammation associated with arthritis and serositis but may worsen lupus nephritis.

Hydroxychloroquine (unless contraindicated; it reduces disease activity and improves survival) is particularly useful for treating skin disease and joint symptoms associated with lupus (A potential complication of using antimalarials is retinopathy; the patient should have a visual assessment, with a subsequent review at regular intervals).

Corticosteroids: These may be used topically (for skin disease), orally (to treat mild flare systemic disease, e.g., arthritis) or intravenously for severe flare (e.g., pulsed methylprednisolone for treatment of flares of lupus nephritis).

Immunosuppressants: Agents including cyclophosphamide, azathioprine, mycophenolate mofetil as steroid-sparing agent, and monoclonal antibody therapies (e.g., rituximab, belimumab) may all be used in severe systemic disease.

Aspirin and warfarin for APLA syndrome.

Other specific treatments will depend on the exact clinical features of the disease, e.g., renal replacement therapy or transplantation is indicated for patients with end-stage renal failure secondary to lupus nephritis.

Examiner: What investigations are helpful to determine if this patient's lupus is active?

Candidate: These are including:
- Urine cytology for red cell casts
- Urinalysis for blood and protein, urinary protein–creatinine ratio or ACR.
- U&E
- ESR, FBC to look for cytopenias
- Anti dsDNA antibodies
- Complement C3 and C4

Examiner: Tell me the causes of breathlessness in SLE and connective tissue disease (CTD).

Candidate: Causes are including:
- PE
- Pleural effusion, pericarditis
- Pneumonia (maybe opportunistic due to immunosuppression)
- Pulmonary fibrosis
- Reaction to biologics therapy (mimics ARDS)
- Acute MI
- Cardiomyopathy
- Renal failure causing pulmonary edema
- Neuromuscular-myositis causing ventilator muscle weakness or Guillain-Barre syndrome (very rare)

Examiner: Tell me the ACR criteria for SLE.

Candidate: ACR criteria include:
- Malar rash
- Discoid rash
- Photosensitive rash
- Oral ulcers
- Nonerosive arthritis in two or more joints
- Pleuritis or pericarditis
- Glomerulonephritis or proteinuria
- Seizures or psychosis
- Hemolytic anemia, leukopenia, lymphopenia, or thrombocytopenia
- Immunologic laboratory abnormalities, such as antibodies to dsDNA or the SM antigen or a false-positive serologic test for syphilis
- Positive ANA test that is not caused by a medication

Note: Four out of 11 criteria suggest SLE.

Systemic Sclerosis

Your role: You are a Registrar in the Rheumatology Clinic.

Patient profile: Mrs Jessica, a 48-year-old lady.

Problem: Painful cold hand with a chronic ulcer on her fingertips and difficulty swallowing over the past year.

(Once you get this clinical scenario, you will get 5 minutes to start this station for two scenarios. At that time, start to think about your diagnosis, differential diagnoses, and plan for taking focused history as well as focused examination.)

[This middle-aged lady having a history of Reynaud's phenomenon and dysphagia most likely diagnosis would be systemic sclerosis (SS), or it may be the part of MCTD such as SS with SLE or myositis overlapped. So here, focused history would be Raynaud's phenomenon, dysphagia and other symptoms and signs are related to underlying CTD.

Other causes of cold hand include peripheral arterial disease, hypothyroidism, Raynaud's disease (bilateral, age < 40, female sex, ergots, BB, OCP, chemotherapy)]

(Once you enter the room, search for a spot diagnosis; shiny tight skin, perioral puckering, sclerodactyly, calcinosis, Raynaud's phenomenon suggests systemic sclerosis.)

Introduction, Permission, and Identification

Candidate: Good morning; I am Mohammad Ali, one of the working doctors here today. I have been asked to see you. Is that okay with you?

Patient: Good morning, doctor...

Candidate: Thank you for coming; I would like to start by taking your full name, age and where you have come from, please?

Patient: Yes, doctor............. Mrs Jessica, I am 48-year-old and from London.

Focused History

Candidate: Okay, Mrs Jessica, what brings you here today? Please tell me in your own words.

Patient: I have had pain in my hands for the last 5–6 weeks, worsening day by day. Another major problem is that my fingers change their color in the cold.

Analyze the Symptoms

Candidate: Tell me more about your pain and color changes.....
- Since when you have these symptoms?
- Has it changed since it started, or is it increasing or decreasing?
- When does this happen, and what are the colors?
- Is there anything that makes it better? Does anything make it worse?
- Is the pain in your whole hand or just at your fingertips?
- Have you noticed involvement in the other part of the body, like the nose, ears?
- Is there any ulceration in your fingertips?

Patient: Over the past few years, my fingers have changed their color in the cold, first white, then blue, and finally red, which is sometimes very painful. The tips of my fingers were extremely painful, and an accidental cut 4 weeks back took almost 3 weeks to settle even with antibiotics. I have some ulcers on my fingertips nowadays, but I cannot find any cause for them.

Candidate: Do you have any other problems apart from this?

Patient: I have been having trouble swallowing particularly solid food for the last few months.

Candidate: Now tell me,
- When the difficulty of swallowing started exactly?
- Is it increasing, decreasing over time or the same?
- Is it more solid or liquid or both?
- Is it at starting of swallowing or after food pass to your food pipe (to differentiate between oropharyngeal and esophageal dysphagia) Is it worse at the end of the meal (? MG or the beginning [? Lambert–Eaton myasthenic syndrome (LEMS)]?
- Do you feel the food particles stuck to your food pipe? If yes, then, at which site?
- Any associated loss of weight? How much? For how long? What about your appetite?

Patient: It has been for the last couple of months, and I am scared as it is gradually worsening. Initially, it was for solid food, but now it is even on liquid food. My general physician referred me to my local hospital 6 months ago, and a camera test was done, which was entirely normal. Then another scan test (barium swallow X-ray) was also done, and the doctor told me that it was probably just the food pipe not pumping as well as it used to, and he put me on some antacid medicines. They helped to rid my swallowing problem a bit, but I still have to avoid a larger piece of meat or dry bread.

Candidate: Okay, let me ask you just a few more questions.......

Other Important Targeted Histories

- Do you have any skin changes like being more tight, shiny, smooth than before?
- Do you have joint pain or swelling?
- Do you have a skin rash? If so, does it worse on sun exposure?
- Are you losing hair? Do you have any mouth ulcer?
- Have you noticed dry mouth or dry eye (suggests associated Sjogren's syndrome)?
- Do you have diarrhea or weight loss?
- Do you have any breathlessness or cough (associated with lung fibrosis)?
- Have you noticed any chest pain or racing heartbeat, leg swelling, difficulty breathing with rest or exertion (suggest primary or secondary PHTN, myocardial fibrosis, and pericarditis)?
- Do you have difficulty rising from a chair or getting in and out of the car (proximal myopathy suggests associated myositis as a part of MCTD)?

Patient: Yes, recently, I have noticed some skin changes like tight shiny skin than before, particularly involving distal to the knee and elbow also in the face but not in the chest LCSS. I have had diarrhea and cramping tummy pain for the last few months, I was told this was irritable bowel syndrome (IBS). I am concerned about my weight loss; however, my appetite is pretty good, and I am trying to eat more than usual (It indicates bowel bacterial overgrowth and malabsorption secondary hypomotility of the bowel in systemic sclerosis patients).

Quick Systemic Review, Past Medical History, Family History, Treatment, Social History According to your Differentials

If it is not asked previously during initial history taking or incompletely asked then—take a full history of a particular portion to make it complete.

Candidate: Mrs Jessica, now let me ask you some specific questions so that I can get a clear picture of your overall health.

- Do you have headache, dizziness or LOC or blurring of vision or weakness of limbs?
- Any nausea, vomiting, abdominal pain, or any changes in bowel habit?
- What about your waterworks? Any change in color, frequency or any frothy urine, or any pain in passing urine or anything else?
- Do you have any similar condition or any other history of disease in your past? Have you ever admitted to the hospital?
- Have you attended any consultant or general physician or specialist for this problem? What was their impression? Did you receive any diagnosis? What treatment have you received? Did they work?

- Have you ever been admitted to the hospital in the past or any history of surgery?
- May I ask what medication you take? Do you take any over-the-counter medications or herbal medicine, or any recreational drugs? Are you allergic to any medicine or anything else?
- Is there anyone else in your family with this type of problem or any long-standing illness that run in your families like DM, hypertension, stroke, thyroid or any autoimmune disease or anything else?
- Do you smoke? Do you drink? What are you doing for a living? Are you married? Who is at home with you, or who is supporting you now? Do you have children? Are you independent in activities of daily living?

Have I missed anything, or do you want to add anything more?

Would you mind if I go on to examine you?

Focused Examination

As the clinical history suggestive of systemic sclerosis as well as she has a manifestation of GIT (diarrhea and dysphagia) condition. So, here focused examination would be an examination of the hands and face to detect SS's features and GIT. If the patient has respiratory symptoms or cardiovascular symptoms—then it should be examined as well.

Hand: Should be examined systemically as look, feel, move, functional status, an approach which was discussed in rheumatoid arthritis.

In the case of SS, we will get:
- Tight shiny skin (sclerodactyly) with flexion deformity and atrophy of the finger pulps.
- Dilated capillaries in nail fold, digital ulceration, or infarction/gangrenous fingertips.
- Firm, whitish dermal plaque, papules or nodules (calcinosis).

Face
- Tight skin around the lips (perioral puckering)
- Pinched or beaked nose
- Microstomia (reduced mouth opening; put three fingers in your mouth)
- Telangiectasia (widened vessels causes thread-like red line or pattern on the skin)
- Butterfly rash and an oral ulcer (associated SLE)
- Heliotrope rash (associated dermatomyositis)

Examination of the abdomen: It is appropriate in given symptoms, although the examination is often normal in systemic sclerosis.

I would like to complete my examination by measuring blood pressure (SS usually associated with malignant hypertension).

Respiratory system: For a sign of ILD (NSIP), the cardiovascular system for a sign of PHTN [due to development of interstitial lung disease (ILD) or primary pulmonary hypertension (PPH)] or heart failure as well as urine dipstick.

Feedback to the Patient and Respond to the Patient's Concern

Candidate: You said at the beginning that the main problem was a painful cold hand, dysphagia and diarrhea, is there anything else that we have missed or any concerns?

Patient: Have you had any thoughts about what is going on?

Candidate: The symptoms you described, together with changes in the color of the fingers, swallowing difficulty, tightening of the skin, point to a diagnosis called systemic sclerosis, a multisystem disease involving your food pipes causing dysmotility and difficulty of swallowing. It is causing narrowing of the small blood channels of your fingers, resulting in pain and color changes when exposed to cold weather. Sometimes, it affects the lung causing scarring and shortness of breath and maybe your kidney causing high BP, which can be remarkably high.

I would like to organize some tests to confirm our diagnosis and assess for any wider involvement of the organs I have just mentioned. The tests include a basic blood test, autoantibodies, CXR, and camera tests such as endoscopy and colonoscopy.

The management of the clinical condition would depend on the test results. Most importantly, general measures include avoiding cold exposure and wearing hand gloves that will help your hand symptoms. It is vital to stop smoking, as it will significantly help your symptoms. Additionally, I can prescribe some painkillers that can also help to reduce your pain. Do you have anything you would like to ask?

Patient: Is it curable, doctor?

Candidate: I am sorry to tell you that it is not curable, but it can be controlled. Treatment is directed mainly toward the symptoms control, such as for your diarrhea, we will give antibiotics. Disease progression is less responsive to immunosuppression than the other autoimmune arthritis or vasculitis.

Do you have any other concerns? Thank you so much for spending time with me.

Discussion with Examiner

Examiner: Would you please present your case?

Candidate:

This middle-aged lady has had a long history of Reynaud's phenomenon with dysphagia as well as diarrhea of prolonged duration.

On examination, the skin over the fingers and face is smooth, shiny, and tight.

There is sclerodactyly, and the nails are atrophic with evidence of Raynaud's phenomenon (the fingers are cold and cyanosed with atrophy of the finger pulps), there are telangiectases in the face and pigmentation. There are palpable nodules of calcinosis in some finger.

So, in summary, my diagnosis is systemic sclerosis.

Examiner: How will you investigate the case?

Candidate: I would like to do a basic blood test such as CBC, ESR, CRP, serum urea, serum creatinine, serum electrolytes, blood sugar, and urine routine examination.

Nail-fold capillaroscopy: To see the evidence of enlarged capillaries, microhemorrhage and dropout. Autoantibody screen such as ANA (90% case it will be positive), anticentromere antibody (80% patient with LCSS will be positive) and SCL-70 (40% patient with dc SSc will be positive).

As the patient has dysphagia, I would like to do a barium meal X-ray and upper GI endoscopy.

For the evaluation of diarrhea, I would like to do stool R/E and C/S, glucose breath test, and colonoscopy.

In case of respiratory involvement, I would like to do CXR, pulmonary function test, transfer factor, and HRCT of the chest.

In case of cardiac involvement—I would like to do ECG, color Doppler echocardiography, particularly for evidence of PHTN.

Examiner: How will you manage the patient?

Candidate: There is no proven effective treatment to prevent disease progression. The patient should be managed with an MDT approach involving a rheumatologist, physiotherapist, Occupational therapist as well as gastro, cardio, and respiratory physician.

For Raynaud's, we have to take some general measures such as wearing hand gloves (to keep the hand warm), smoking cessation, avoiding any precipitating drugs such as ergot derivatives or beta-blockers.

Pharmacological measure, including CCB, particularly nifedipine, is the drug of choice.
- For pulmonary hypertension (endothelin receptor antagonist; bosentan)
- Nebulized iloprost or infusion is helpful in the healing of a digital ulcer
- Methotrexate and mycophenolate mofetil (MMF) may be beneficial in treating skin thickening (disease progression is less responsive to immunosuppression than other autoimmune diseases such as vasculitis).
- For renal crisis (malignant hypertension), ACE inhibitors, or angiotensin receptor blockers (ARBs) are the drugs of choice.

Rheumatoid Arthritis

Your role: You are the medical doctor in the general medicine clinic.

Patient details: Mr John Thomas, a 58-year-old man.

Clinical problem: 3 years history of pain, swelling, and stiffness in his hands.

(Once you get this clinical scenario, you will get 5 minutes to start this station for two scenarios. At that time, start to think about your diagnosis, differential diagnoses, and plan for taking focused history as well as focused examination.)

[So, in this clinical scenario, the differential diagnosis would be:
- Rheumatoid arthritis
- Seronegative arthritis
- CTD such as SLE, MCTD (rheumatoid arthritis with SLE/systemic sclerosis/myositis)

So, history and examination should be made to establish my diagnosis, to exclude differential diagnoses, extra-articular manifestations of the disease, functional status of the patient, any physiotherapist, or occupational therapist input.]

(Once you enter the room, search for a spot diagnosis; rheumatoid hand, joint deformity, pyoderma gangrenosum suggest rheumatoid arthritis.)

Introduction, Permission, and Identification

Candidate: Hello, is it John Thomas?

Patient: Yes.

Candidate: Nice to meet you. I am Mohammad Ali, one of the doctors working here today. I have been asked to see you. May I confirm your date of birth, please?

Patient: Well, it is 15/02/1962.

Focused History

Candidate: Okay, that makes you 58-year-old. I understand the problem with your joints. Would you please tell me a little bit more about your problem?

Patient: Yeah, sure, doctor, I have had pain, stiffness, and swollen joints in both hands for the past 3 years. However, over the last 2 months, the pain and stiffness have been progressively worsening. Now, it is tough to do my usual activities.

Analyze the Symptom

Candidate: It is okay; I will do my best. Before that, let me ask you a few more questions to understand what has been happening with you and how can we help you. Is that okay with you?

Patient: Yes. Okay.

Candidate: Well, you have already told me that you are struggling with some daily activities, could you please tell me what sort of difficulties are you facing?

Patient: In terms of my hands, such as opening the jar, using cutlery or difficulty in cooking, dressing, writing, washing, and any kind of movement which required circular motion, I find it difficult to do so.

Candidate: I am sorry to hear that. Have you ever seen an occupational therapist and physiotherapist, and what were the recommendations, or any aids have you been instilled for it?

Patient: No.

Candidate: It is okay. I will refer you to an occupational therapist and physiotherapist, which will help you maintain your daily living activities.
   I understand the pain and stiffness in your joint has hurt you so much that you are struggling

to do your normal work. Would you please tell me when and how it progressed?

Patient: Basically, in the beginning, it was in my right-hand joints, then gradually it involved my left hand, and surprisingly it involved almost all joints in my body. So, I went to my general physician, and he referred me to a rheumatologist for his assessment.

Candidate: Some more questions about your symptoms, do these symptoms worsen at certain times of the day, such as at night or in the morning?

Patient: Yes, doctor, actually it is worse, particularly in the morning.

Candidate: Is there anything that relieves your pain or makes you feel better?

Patient: I think it improves with the usage of my hands.

Candidate: Okay, regarding your medication, are you currently taking any medication?

Patient: Initially, I took methotrexate, sulfasalazine, a steroid with some pain-relieving medications like indomethacin. However, due to some side effects of sulfasalazine, it was withdrawn; currently, I am taking methotrexate 20 milligram once weekly, folison 10 milligram once weekly, leflunomide and hydroxychloroquine 400 milligram daily.

Candidate: What type of side effects with sulfasalazine? And how it was managed?

Patient: I had some skin rash, tiredness, vertigo just after taking sulfasalazine; that is why it was stopped 2 years back.

Candidate: Have you ever received any injectable medicines like steroids or biologics?

Patient: A year ago, I was given steroid injections when I had a lot of pain in my joints.

Candidate: Okay, are you allergic to any medications or anything else other than this sulfasalazine?

Patient: Not so.

Candidate: Have you had any joint surgeries (laminectomy, arthrodesis, ulnar styloidectomy, CTS decompression or joint replacement)?

Patient: No.

Candidate: Well, Mr Thomas, let me ask you some specific questions just to assess your overall health. Okay?

To detect extra-articular manifestations or complications:
- Do you have any pins and needle sensation or burning sensation in the feet and hand (peripheral neuropathy or CTS)?
- Have you had any trouble with your eyes, particularly any sore or redness, dry eyes, or gritty sensation (episcleritis, scleritis, keratoconjunctival Sicca, scleromalacia, Sjogren's syndrome)?
- Do you have any cough, phlegm, breathlessness, or noisy chest (rheumatoid lung)?
- Do you have any chest pain, racing in your heart (palpitation) or dizzy spell (may represent a cardiovascular complication of rheumatoid disease)?
- Have you noticed any changes in your waterworks, amount, color, frequency or any frothy urine (glomerulonephritis or amyloid)?

Some questions to exclude differential diagnosis:
- Is there any oral ulcer, tummy pain, loose motion (enteropathic arthritis)?
- Any burning waterworks, eye pain, or redness (reactive arthritis)?
- Any skin rash (to exclude psoriasis/SLE/secondary vasculitis due to rheumatoid arthritis/primary vasculitis/dermatomyositis)?
- Have you noticed any color changes in your finger when it is exposed to cold weather (Raynaud's phenomenon as a manifestation of systemic sclerosis)?
- Any tight shiny skin or is there any difficulty in swallowing? (to exclude systemic sclerosis as a part of MCTD)?
- Do you have any difficulties in standing from a sitting position or any difficulties with combing hair (to exclude associated polymyositis as a part of MCTD)?

Candidate: It is okay, so let us talk about your lifestyle.......
- What are you doing for a living now?
- With whom you are living or who is supporting you at home?

- Do you smoke, or have you ever smoked?
- Do you drink alcohol?

Candidate: Regarding your personal and FH:
- Do you have any other medical problems or any long-standing diseases such as diabetes, hypertension, or any heart problems?
- Do you have any similar condition or long-standing disease in your family?

Patient: I live with my wife. I never smoke but occasionally drink alcohol. Nothing significant in my FH.

Focused Examination

Target
- Evidence of rheumatoid arthritis, particularly signs of active disease, functional status of the hand and the lower limb if possible.
- Evidence of extra-articular manifestations depending on suggestive history.

Would you mind if I examine your hand, please (we have to examine the hand—look, feel, move and functional status)?

Look
- Look for joint swelling, deformity, muscle wasting, scar, and rheumatoid nodule (symmetrical involvement in joint swelling and tenderness with sparing of the DIP joint suggests rheumatoid arthritis).
- Joint deformities are including (patient may not have any deformity due to surgical correction, so look for scars).
- Ulnar deviation of the metacarpophalangeal (MCP) joint
- Boutonniere or Swan neck deformity
- Z deformity of the thumb

Scars: The most common surgical scars are including:
- CTS compression scar
- Swanson's arthroplasty
- Wrist arthrodesis
- Ulnar styloidectomy
- Wrist synovectomy
- Tendon transfer (follow the line of a tendon)

Wasting may be due to disease (disuse atrophy) or polyneuropathy, or entrapment neuropathy:
- If there is wasting only in thenar eminence, then think for CTS -medial nerve palsy, then looks for other signs like characteristic sensory loss and power of the abductor pollicis brevis along with Phalen's and Tinel's signs (may I tap on your wrist, any pain?) for CTS.
- If generalized wasting except for thenar eminence, then think about ulnar nerve palsy and look for characteristic sensory loss and muscle Power.

Rheumatoid nodule (mainly found on extensor surface, especially over the elbows).

Feel
Feel the tenderness in all joints after taking permission (tenderness and swelling are key to determining whether inflammatory arthritis is active).

Movement (both active and passive movement):
- Ask the patient to make a fist and now open the hand and spread your fingers apart
- Prayer sign (to see the wrist dorsiflexion), and
- Reverse prayer sign (to see palmar flexion of the wrist)

Functional Status
Ask the patient: Are you able to undo a button in your shirt?

Other Systemic Examination (To see the Evidence of Extra-articular Manifestations)

Chest examination: (If the patient gives a suggestive history of chest disease)
- Stony dull on percussion or absent breath sound due to pleural effusion
- Fine late inspiratory crackles for DPLD
- Coarse crackles for bronchiectasis

Cardiac examination: If the patient gives a suggestive history of heart disease.
- Pericarditis can cause pericardial rub
- A murmur may be due to associated mitral regurgitation

- Crepitations in the lung bases may be due to heart failure

Skin: Pyoderma gangrenosum and vasculitic rash.

Eye: Red-eye suggests episcleritis or uveitis, scleritis, or scleromalacia perforans.

Abdomen:
- The patient may have anemia or
- Signs of infection due to neutropenia
- Splenomegaly may suggest Felty's syndrome.
 I would like to check BP and do a urine dipstick to get the evidence of glomerulonephritis.

Feedback to the Patient and Respond to the Patient's Concern

Candidate: You said at the beginning that the main problem was the increasingly severe pain, swelling, and stiffness in your hands. It sounds like this is affecting you considerably. Is there anything else that we have missed, like any questions, expectations or concerns?

Patient: Doctor……. I am struggling to perform my daily activities. So, I certainly want to reduce my pain and stiffness as much as possible to return to my normal activity.

Candidate: In fact, Mr Thomas, at this moment, you have presented with the flare of rheumatoid arthritis. Now I would like to do some blood tests and imaging to see the status of the flare of it and start steroid treatment (called prednisolone), which will help you a lot to reduce your pain and stiffness. Then I will arrange a consultation with one of my rheumatology colleagues to modify your present treatment regimen. We need to ask the occupational therapist in the rheumatology department to assess you and provide advice and equipment to improve your ability to carry out your activities of daily living at home. We will also ask the physiotherapist to see you, and he will give you some exercise techniques for maintaining a range of movement and muscle strength.

As a whole, we will refer you to an MDT involving a joint doctor, social worker, rheumatology clinic specialist nurse, physiotherapist, and occupational therapist to give you a proper plan of management and outpatient follow-up.

Patient: Are there any medicines like injections (biologics) that will cure my disease?

Candidate: Indeed, rheumatoid arthritis cannot be cured. A significant proportion of patients may attain remission using DMARDs such as methotrexate with or without biological agents like infliximab.
Do you have any other questions or concern?

Patient: No. Thank you.
Thank you for spending time with me today.

Discussion with Examiner

Examiner: Would you please present your case?

Candidate:

This middle-aged gentleman presented with inflammatory symmetrical polyarthritis involving both small and large joints of both upper and lower limbs with significant morning stiffness (>1 hour) for the last 3 years.

On examination, there is symmetrical deforming arthropathy of the small joints of the hands involving proximal interphalangeal (PIP) and MCP joints with sparing of the DIP joints. There is a spindling of the fingers due to soft tissue swelling at the PIP and MCP joints. There is palmar subluxation at the MCP joints and ulnar deviation of the finger. The deformities are including:

Swan neck deformity, Boutonniere's deformity and Z-deformity of the thumb. There are rheumatoid nodules present on the extensor surface of the forearm.

There are palmar erythema and generalized wasting of the small muscles of the hand. There are nail fold infarct and vasculitis skin lesions—however, no evidence of entrapment neuropathy.

The affected joints are warm, erythematous, and tender. The patient is unable to unbutton his clothes.

So my diagnosis is RA with evidence of active inflammation associated with deformity and secondary vasculitis.

Examiner: How will you investigate this patient?

Candidate: I would like to start the investigation by doing some basic blood tests such as:
- FBC with ESR with CRP; that may show normocytic normochromic anemia due to chronic disease with high ESR and CRP (due to active inflammation), low white blood cell (WBC) count may be due to associated Felty's syndrome or as a side effect of disease-modifying antirheumatic drugs (DMARDs) (due to bone marrow suppression).
- Blood U&Es, serum creatinine, and LFTs (for management of the patient or to see the side effects of the drugs and also before starting new treatment to see the contraindications).

I would like to do rheumatoid arthritis factor and anti-CCP antibody not only for diagnosis but, most importantly, to see the patient's prognosis.

X-ray of the hand to see the periarticular osteopenia, marginal erosion, joint space narrowing, and deformity.

If clinically suggest—then many investigations can be done to see the extra-articular complications such as ECG, CXR, echo, lung function tests, HRCT of the chest, nerve conduction study to see entrapment/peripheral neuropathy, power Doppler USG or MRI of the joints may be done to see active synovitis.

Examiner: How will you manage a patient with rheumatoid arthritis?

Candidate: This patient should be managed with the MDT approach involving a rheumatologist, rheumatologist specialist nurse, social worker, physiotherapist, and occupational therapist to modify the daily activity of living and mobility and dexterity aids.

During flare or early active disease, we can use steroids (prednisolone 30 mg daily for 6 weeks then gradual withdrawal over the 6 weeks) and NSAIDs to reduce pain and stiffness.

Early introduction of DMARDs is vital to get the maximum benefit of the patient to prevent deformity and extra-articular complications of rheumatoid arthritis.

The most common regimen would be:
- Methotrexate either alone or in combination with sulfasalazine or hydroxychloroquine.

If the patient is a case of refractory rheumatoid arthritis, then we can use biologics. Most importantly:
- TNF blockage:
  - Infliximab, adalimumab (anti TNF monoclonal antibody)
  - Etanercept (soluble TNF receptor antagonist)
- Newer biologics are:
  - Rituximab (anti-CD20 monoclonal antibody which depletes B cells)
  - Abatacept
  - Tocilizumab (anti-IL-6 receptor monoclonal antibody)
- JAK inhibitors (alternative to biologics):
  - Tofacitinib
  - Baricitinib

Examiner: Let us think, a patient of refractory rheumatoid arthritis [disease activity score (DAS 28) remains high (>5.1) despite triple therapy] is getting anti-TNF therapy for the last 2 months who presents to A&E with a minor infection such as cellulitis. How will you manage the case?

Candidate: The patient should be admitted immediately, and we have to stop the anti-TNF treatment; at the same time, we will give I/V antibiotics and seek specialist advice.

Examiner: How would you monitor a patient on DMARD therapy or anti-TNF?

Candidate: In fact, both DMARD and biologic therapies require regular specialist review.
- *Clinically*: Regular history and examination, looking for evidence of infection, especially TB or complications including pulmonary fibrosis (methotrexate, anti-TNF)
- Blood tests include FBC with ESR with CRP, U&E, LFTs (it should be done at regular

intervals, usually monthly for most DMARDs) for early detection of the drugs' adverse effects, especially cytopenia transaminitis.

Examiner: Tell me about the 2010 ACR/Eular classification criteria for rheumatoid arthritis.

Candidate: The ACR/EULAR classification system is a score-based algorithm for rheumatoid arthritis that includes the following four factors:
1. Joint Involvement
2. Serological tests
3. Acute-phase reactant
4. Duration of signs and symptoms reported by the patient

Here, 10 is the maximum number of points. A classification of definitive rheumatoid arthritis requires a score of 6/10 or more.

Joint involvement:
- 1 large joint (shoulders, elbows, hips, knees, ankles) = 0 points
- 2–10 large joints = 1 point
- 1–3 small joints (with/without the involvement of large joints), such as MCP, PIP, second to the fifth MTP, thumb interphalangeal (IP), and wrist joints = 2 points
- 4–10 small joints (with/without the involvement of large joints) = 3 points
- More than 10 joints (at least 1 small joint, plus any combination of large and additional small joints or joints such as the temporomandibular, acromioclavicular, or sternoclavicular) = 5 points

Serology test:
- Negative rheumatoid factor (RF) and negative anti-CCP ab = 0 points
- Low-positive RF or low-positive anti-CCP ab = 2 points
- High-positive RF or high-positive anti-CCP ab = 3 points

Acute-phase reactant:
- Normal CRP and normal ESR = 0 points
- Abnormal CRP or abnormal ESR = 1 point

Duration of signs or symptoms:
- Shorter than 6 weeks = 0 points
- 6 weeks or longer = 1 point

Examiner: What is the DAS 28 score? What is the significance of it?

Candidate: The DAS 28 measures the disease activity in rheumatoid arthritis. To calculate the DAS 28, we need to:
- Count the number of swollen joints (out of the 28)
- Count the number of tender joints (out of the 28)
- Measure the ESR or CRP
- Ask the patient to make a "global assessment of health" (indicated by marking a 10 cm line between very good and very bad).

To get the overall disease activity score, these results are then fed into a complex mathematical formula.
- A DAS 28 of >5.1 implies active disease,
- A DAS 28 of <3.2 implies low disease activity, and
- A DAS 28 of <2.6 implies remission.

If disease activity remains high (DAS 28 score >5.1) despite triple therapy in an adequate dose and duration, after that, it is usual to progress to biologic therapy.

Examiner: How do you distinguish active from inactive arthritis?

Candidate: It can be done by symptoms (increased pain, fatigue), swelling, joint tenderness, the warmth of joints and raised ESR. Sometimes, disease activity may be masked in a patient taking NSAIDs.

Examiner: List the possible causes of anemia in rheumatoid arthritis.

Candidate: Causes are:
- Anemia of chronic disease
- Iron deficiency (gastrointestinal blood loss due to NSAIDs or steroids)
- Felty's syndrome
- Bone marrow suppression (methotrexate or other DMARDs)
- Autoimmune hemolytic anemia
- Associated pernicious anemia
- Renal amyloid

Examiner: Could you please tell me some extra-articular manifestations of rheumatoid arthritis?

Candidate: Extra-articular manifestations are less commonly seen nowadays with the more

aggressive and early treatment of rheumatoid arthritis. However, it includes:
- *Cardiovascular*: Coronary artery disease, MI, and pericarditis.
- *Hematologic*: Anemia, thrombocytosis, Felty's syndrome, large granulocytic leukemia, and non-Hodgkin's lymphoma.
- *Pulmonary*: Pleural effusion, nodules, interstitial lung disease, and bronchiolitis obliterans.
- *Vascular*: Vasculitis and neuropathy.
- *Skin*: Rheumatoid nodules, vasculitic rash and pyoderma gangrenosum.
- *Eye*: Episcleritis, scleritis, and scleromalacia perforans.
- *Renal*: Amyloidosis.
- *Neurological*: Mononeuritis multiplex, peripheral neuropathy, compression neuropathy. Compression neuropathies include cervical myelopathy (atlantoaxial subluxation, signs include spastic paraparesis, hyperreflexia, upgoing plantar response with or without scar from previous surgery), ulnar neuropathy (elbow involvement), carpal tunnel syndrome (wrist involvement).

Gout

Your role: You are a Registrar in General Medical Clinic.

Patient details: Mr William, a 52-year-old man.

Clinical problem: Mr William, aged 52, has come to you with the complaint of pain in the big toe. He is hypertensive, diabetic, dyslipidemic and has a history of old MI 3 years back. His current medications are aspirin, atorvastatin, metformin, ramipril, and bendroflumethiazide.

(Once you get this clinical scenario, you will get 5 minutes to start this station for two scenarios. At that time, start to think about your diagnosis, differential diagnoses, and plan for taking focused history as well as focused examination.)

[*Differential diagnosis*: Crystal arthritis (gout/pseudogout), septic arthritis (gonococcal/nongonococcal), monoarticular presentation of polyarthritis (seronegative arthritis, rheumatoid arthritis), osteoarthritis, mycobacterial or fungal infection, Lyme disease, post-traumatic]

(*Once you enter the room, search for a spot diagnosis; here, any visible tophi in feet, hand or ear lobule suggest gout*)

Greetings, Introduction, Permission, and Identification

Candidate: Good morning. My name is Mohammad Ali, one of the working doctors here today. I have been asked to see you. Is that okay with you?

Patient: No problem.

Candidate: I will start by taking your full name, age, and where you have come from, please?

Patient: Mr William, I am 52.

Focused History

Candidate: Okay, Mr William, would you please tell me what brings you here today? Please tell me in your own words.

Patient: I was completely fine, but I have had severe pain in my big toe since last night. My pain was so severe that even I cannot touch my toe. After taking a painkiller, it has slightly reduced my pain, but I still have pain.

Analyze the Complaints

Candidate: Oh! I am so sorry to hear all; please tell me a little bit more about your pain so that I can be in a position to help you. Is that okay?
The important questions to be asked:
- You said you have this pain since last night; how did the pain start?
- Did it come suddenly or gradually?
- What were you doing when the pain started?
- Is the pain always there or comes and goes? Is it increasing, decreasing, or remain static?
- Can you describe the pain?
- Anything making it worse/better?
- Can you score the pain on a scale of 1–10?
- Does it affect both the feet?
- Do you have had any similar attacks in the past?
- Would you please tell me how this pain affected your daily life or what does it stop you from doing?

Patient: Yesterday, I was just watching TV and suddenly got this pain! The pain was so severe, and still, there is a lot of pain here. Last month, I had a similar type of pain in my right toe, but that was resolved after taking the painkiller. This time it is in my left toe with some swelling and redness.

Candidate: You said you took some medications; what did you take? How much did you take? Did they work?

Patient: I took ibuprofen 1 tablet at night and 1 in the morning but it did not help much.

Other Important Targeted Histories

To detect the complications and etiology of back pain.
- Any other symptoms like any redness or swelling? Any fever or raised temperature?
- Do you have pain in other joints like your knee, wrist, or shoulder?
- Do you have any skin rashes, nail changes, any oral ulcers, or an ulcer in your foot?
- Any history of trauma or have you ever injured your foot recently?
- Any pain or burning sensation while passing urine? Any bleeding or discharge from the end of your penis? Any redness, hotness, or swelling around your private part?
- Any diarrhea or altered bowel habit, tummy pain, nausea, or vomiting?
- Any cough, chest pain or breathing difficulty?
- Any headache, eye problem, tingling, or numbness in limbs or any weakness?
- Have you traveled anywhere recently?

Patient: No.

Quick Systemic Review, Past Medical History, Family History, Treatment, Social History According to Your Differentials

Candidate: Well, do you have any other medical conditions such as hypertension, DM, and any heart/liver/kidney disease?

Patient: Yes, 3 years ago, I had a heart attack. I have had hypertension and DM for the last 5 years. I am taking medications for it.

Candidate: May I know what symptoms did you have and how your heart attack had been managed at that time?

Patient: At that time, I had chest pain and breathing difficulty, mainly when I tried to do any physical activity. I was treated with angioplasty and a stent followed by some medications.

Candidate: Do you have any chest pain or breathing difficulties now?

Patient: No.

Candidate: It is all right, you said you have DM and hypertension, and you are taking medication for it. Have you checked your blood pressure and sugar level? Are these well controlled?

Patient: Yes, I checked it. My blood sugar level is well-controlled, but my BP has been slightly higher over the last few months, so my general physician added some more medication.

Candidate: Okay, please tell me what are the medications recently you are taking?

Patient: I am taking aspirin, atorvastatin, metformin, ramipril, and bendroflumethiazide. The last one added my general physician for my BP management.

Candidate: Okay, Mr William, I will measure your BP and further review your medications. Are you allergic to any medicine or anything else?

Patient: No.

Candidate: Tell me about your family members, is there anyone else in your family with this type of problem or any long-standing illness that run in your families like any arthritis, DM, hypertension, stroke, or anything else?

Patient: My mum has old-age arthritis.

Candidate: How is she now? How has it been managed?

Patient: She is taking medications for it.

Candidate: Let me ask you some questions about your lifestyle.......
- Do you smoke?
- Do you drink alcohol? What do you drink? How often and how much?
- Tell me about your diet? Does it include meat or dairy products? Do you do exercise?
- What do you do for a living? Is this pain affecting your work?

- Who is at home with you, or who is supporting you now?

Patient: I never smoke, but I drink three glasses of beer every evening. I love to eat meat and dairy products. I am an office worker, because of this pain, I had to take off day-to-day. I live with my wife and two children.

Candidate: Mr William, would you mind if I ask you some personal question? Are you sexually active? Are you in a stable relationship (single/multiple)? Do you practice safe sex?

Patient: Yes. I practice safe sex.

Thank you so much for answering my questions, is there anything that I have missed, or do you want to add anything more?

Would you mind if I go on to examine you?

Focused Examination

In this scenario, the most likely diagnosis is acute gout. So, the targeted examination would be:
- Examination of affected joint for any redness, hotness, tenderness, and movement restriction and any effusion in the joint.
- Examination of the hands and knees, and also offers to examine other joints.
- Checks ears for gout tophi.
- Check for observation charts, including pyrexia.
- If time favors, check for any evidence of heart failure by examining the heart and checking peripheral edema as well as any complications of diabetes (micro/macrovascular).

Feedback to the Patient and Respond to the Patient's Concerns

Candidate: You said at the beginning that the main problem was sudden severe pain, swelling, and redness in your great toe, is there anything else troubling you that we have not covered or any expectations or any concerns?

Patient: Why did it happen?

Candidate: From my assessment, you seem to have a condition called gout. It is a type of arthritis that causes sudden severe pain and commonly affects the big toe as you have. Other joints such as the knee, elbow, and wrists can also be affected. It can be caused by many factors; in your case, your BP medication, alcohol consumption, and diet can be the reason. First, we will do some blood tests and X-ray of your joint to find out the exact cause. Then, we will review your medications and make some necessary changes, if needed.

To prevent future attacks, lifestyle modification is the main part of treatment. I advise you to drink in moderation, and sometimes drinking alcohol other than beer also helps. I also advise you to maintain healthy body weight and avoid meat products and fatty foods in your diet.

At this moment, we would give you some painkillers to relieve your pain. Later on, according to your blood test result, we will give you some medication to prevent future attacks.

Do you have any other concerns?

Is there anything unclear you need me to clarify?

Discussion with Examiner

Examiner: Would you please present your case?

Candidate:

This middle-aged gentleman presented with a single, inflamed joint for the last 24 hours with a background history of a similar attack last month. He is diabetic, hypertensive, dyslipidemic, postpercutaneous transluminal coronary angioplasty (PTCA) status with old MI, obese, and heavy alcoholic.

On examination, the MCP joint of the great toe is erythematous, swollen, and tender.

There are no other joints affected and no signs of infection.

In summary, my diagnosis would be a recurrent attack of gout with hypertension, DM, post-PTCA status with old MI with obesity.

Examiner: How will you investigate the case?

Candidate: At first, I would do some blood tests, including uric acid, FBC, CRP, blood cultures, baseline urine, creatinine, and electrolytes.

I would also want to do an X-ray of the affected joint. If there is a significant amount of effusion, then joint aspiration would be my next investigation of choice to see the evidence of crystal under polarized light microscopy and exclude infection by leukocyte count, gram stain, and culture.

Examiner: How will you manage this case?

Candidate: As the patient already tried NSAIDs, I would choose colchicine as an alternative with some general advice, including rest and rehydration. Meanwhile, I would change bendroflumethiazide with a suitable one such as a calcium channel blocker—losartan.

The most important part of the management is lifestyle modification to prevent future attacks. Therefore, dietary modification, maintaining a healthy weight and drinking alcohol in moderation with avoidance of beer would be highly appreciated.

After checking uric acid level, I would commence him uric acid-lowering therapy with allopurinol or febuxostat.

Optic Atrophy

Your role: You are the Registrar in the General Medical Clinic.

Patient profile: Mr Simon Anderson, 45-year-old.

Present problem: Progressive reduction of color vision with visual disturbance.

(Once you get this clinical scenario, you will get 5 minutes to start this station for two scenarios. At that time, start to think about your diagnosis and differential diagnoses and plan for taking focused history as well as focused examination.)

Differential diagnosis: Optic atrophy (OA)/optic neuritis (ON) and retinitis pigmentosa (RP).

(Once you enter the room, search for a spot diagnosis for visual loss; the sign of DM suggest diabetic retinopathy; Cushing syndrome and acromegaly with bitemporal hemianopia with OA; Graves' ophthalmopathy; walking aid with OA suggest multiple sclerosis (MS); hearing aid with RP suggest Usher syndrome.)

Introduction, Permission, and Identification

Candidate: Good morning. I am Mohammad Ali, one of the working doctors here today. I have been asked to see you. Is that okay with you?

Patient: Good morning, Doctor…

Candidate: Thank you for coming. I would like to start by taking your full name, age, and where you have come from, please?

Patient: Yes, Doctor…………. Mr Simon Anderson, I am 45, and I am from London.

Focused History

Candidate: Okay, Mr Anderson. Would you please tell me what brings you here today? Please tell me in your own words.

Patient: I have been experiencing vision problems for the last few months, which is progressing now. While driving, I notice the most. I cannot differentiate the traffic light's colors while driving.

Analyze the Symptoms

Candidate: Would you please tell me a little bit more about your vision problem?
The important questions to ask are:
- Can you explain it to me? What do you mean by vision problem? Is it blurring of vision or loss of vision?
- When did you first notice visual disturbance?
- Is it affecting one eye or both eyes [unilateral OA may be ischemic, compressive or traumatic, glaucomatous, demyelinating; whilst bilateral involvement suggests demyelinating (MS), nutritional deficiency (B12 deficiency), toxic (tobacco, methanol, drugs like isoniazid, ethambutol, sulfasalazine, quinine, chloramphenicol), inflammatory sarcoidosis, Wegener's granulomatosis (WG) or infective (tuberculosis, syphilis, Lyme disease, measles, mumps, varicella)]?
- Is it getting worse, staying the same or getting better?
- Does it come on suddenly or gradually?
- Sudden loss suggests ischemic cause [giant cell arteritis (GCA)]
- Subacute loss suggests demyelinating (MS), Leber's hereditary optic atrophy
- Gradual loss suggests compressive lesion (pituitary tumor), toxic, and nutritional deficiency
- Very slowly progressive suggest inherited cause
- Do you have pain during eye movement (optic neuritis or glaucoma (angle-closure) or constant periocular pain indicate localized inflammatory process such as sarcoidosis or WG)?

- Which part of the vision is affected? Is it all or top half or bottom half or is it sides or central? Is this the same in both eyes?
- How it affects your day-to-day activity or job?
- Can you see the walls of the room or side of the road when looking straight forward (difficulty suggests peripheral vision is affected—bitemporal hemianopia/RP)?
- Can you read the newspaper (difficulty suggest central vision is affected likely to be OA or other cause like diabetic maculopathy, cataract, glaucoma, age-related macular degeneration, and cataract)?
- Have you noticed any change in color vision? Can you distinguish the traffic light's color during driving (it suggests optic neuritis/OA)?
- Do you have a similar problem in the family [suggest Autosomal dominant hereditary OA, Friedreich's ataxia, Leber's hereditary optic atrophy, diabetes insipidus, diabetes mellitus, optic atrophy, and deafness (DIDMOAD) syndrome, RP]?
- Have you noticed any change in night vision or any hearing loss (RP/any syndromic diagnosis of RP)?
- Do you have DM, glaucoma, any history of trauma, or infection in the eye?
- Do you have a headache or any history of LOC or shaking limbs or body (suggests SOL leading to compressive OA)?
- Do you have any unsteadiness in the gait (cerebellar or posterior column involvement) or hemiparesis or paraparesis (MS)?
- Does it hurt to brush your hair (scalp tenderness)? Do you get tired of chewing your food (jaw claudication) (temporal arteritis)?

Patient: I have had trouble seeing for the last 8/9 months. Recently I am facing difficulties when driving and stopping at the traffic lights. Remarkably the red light and also I find it difficult to choose my clothes or paint color. I went to an eye specialist but did not improve after getting treatment. I do not have double vision, headache, LOC, weakness, or any problem with my gait. I do not have a FH of similar illness or no past history of infection/trauma to my eyes or any other disease as well. But in the past, I had lung tuberculosis.

Candidate: When you had it? And how it was managed?

Patient: It was 1 year back, and I was treated with antituberculosis drugs (such as rifampicin, isoniazid, ethambutol, and pyrazinamide) for the first 2 months, then next 4 months I was treated by isoniazid and rifampicin and completed the full course of treatment.

Candidate: Okay, that is fine, you completed your course. Have you had any symptoms of tuberculosis like any cough, fever, weight loss, chest pain, or shortness of breath?

Patient: No.

Candidate: Has your eye problem started since your TB treatment? Have you noticed anything like this?

Patient: Yes, Doctor. I have noticed progressive changes in my vision since being on treatment.

Quick Systemic Review, Past Medical History, Family History, Treatment, Social History According to your Differentials

If it is not asked previously during initial history taking or incompletely asked, then take a full history of a particular portion to make it complete.

Candidate: At this moment, I would like to ask some general questions, is that okay with you?
- Do you have nausea, vomiting, tummy pain, limb swelling, and difficulty in the waterworks? What about your bowel habit, any constipation or diarrhea?
- Do you have any similar condition or any other history of disease in your past? Have you ever been admitted to the hospital or had any surgery?
- Have you attended any consultant or general physician or specialist for this problem? What was their impression? Did you receive any diagnosis? What treatment have you received? Did they work?
- May I ask what medication you take? Do you take any over-the-counter medications or

herbal medicine, or any recreational drugs? Are you allergic to any medicine or anything else?
- Any long-standing illness that runs in your family like DM, hypertension, stroke, thyroid, or other autoimmune disease or anything else?
- Do you drive? If yes, then ask, do you drive for a living? Do you smoke? Do you drink? What are you doing for a living? Are you married? Who is at home with you, or who is supporting you now? Do you have children? Are you independent in activities of daily living?

Patient: I am a banker, and I drive to my office. I never smoke or drink alcohol.

Candidate: Have I missed anything, or do you want to add anything more?
Would you mind if I go on to examine you?

Focused Examination

The patient has a history of subacute loss of vision as well as color vision. He had a past history of pulmonary tuberculosis (PTB) and got category-1 antituberculosis regimen. So, most likely diagnosis would be optic neuritis/optic atrophy due to drugs.

A most important part of examination would be examining the eye and examination of other cranial nerves as well as upper and lower limb neurological examination.

Examination of the Eye

Visual acuity: ON/OA frequently present with loss of central vision leading to reduce visual acuity.

Pupillary light response: Test for RAPD…in case of unilateral OA frequently produces RAPD, but it will be absent in the case of bilateral OA.

Fundoscopy: Optic disc change may be in OA
- Total pallor
- Temporal pallor (sometimes seen in demyelination, toxic, or nutritional deficiency)
- *Bow-tie pallor*: Compression of the optic chiasma
- *Cupping*: Glaucomatous OA

Further assessment if OA is detected, may involve:
- *Color vision*: may be reduced

Eye movement: Inflammatory and compressive lesion may also involve oculomotor nerves, particularly at the orbital apex (superior orbital fissure syndrome), so here external ophthalmoplegia, diplopia, or ptosis may be detected.
- Internuclear ophthalmoplegia or cerebellar nystagmus suggests MS.

Visual field detects: In OA, a central visual field defect will be present, but the pituitary tumor compressing optic chiasma may have prominent bitemporal hemianopia.

Presence of cerebellar sign: Hemiparesis or paraparesis may suggest MS as well.

Feedback to the Patient and Respond to the Patient's Concerns

Candidate: You said at the beginning that you had noticed progressive disturbance of vision and difficulties when driving and stopping at the traffic light. Is there anything else that we have missed or any concerns?

Patient: What is my problem, Doctor?

Candidate: I suspect you have optic atrophy due to degeneration of the nerve cable in the back of your eyes. It is possibly due to your previous tuberculosis or tuberculosis treatment. We need to carry out some investigations to find out the underlying cause for the changes to your vision, and this will include a blood test and a brain/orbital scan. Hence, I will refer you to an MDT involving a brain physician, eye physician, physiotherapist, and social worker to give you proper care and management plan.

Since you drive, you have to inform driver and vehicle licensing agency (DVLA) about your condition, and I will write in my notes that I have asked you to inform DVLA. This is because driving may carry the risk on your life and the others as well.

Candidate: Do you have any concerns?

Patient: Will it get better, Doctor?

Candidate: Difficult to say at this stage, whilst investigation is ongoing. However, let me assure you that we will give you full support in every step of your management.

Discussion with Examiner

Examiner: Would you please present your case?

Candidate:

This middle-aged gentleman presented with subacute loss of vision and color vision. Importantly, he had a past history of PTB and got category-1 antituberculosis regimen.

Examination of the eye revealed; The optic disc is pale and has a distinct margin on both sides of the eyes. No RAPD.

Visual field testing (using a red hat pin) reveals central scotoma on both sides. No sign of cerebellar dysfunction or INO

Other cranial nerves, upper limb, and lower limb examinations are entirely normal.

So, in summary, my diagnosis would be bilateral OA, most likely toxic origin (antituberculosis drug).

Examiner: How will you investigate this case?

Candidate: At first, I would like to do the basic blood tests such as FBC and ESR, glucose, vitamin B12 levels, ANA, antiphospholipid antibodies, and syphilis serology.
As the patient had progressive loss of vision, so, I would like to do neuroimaging that includes:
- Retinal photography and formal perimetry (e.g., Humphrey 30-2 or 60-2)
- *Electrophysiology*: Visual-evoked potentials
- MRI of the brain and orbits with contrast or CT scan of the orbits with contrast (if bony involvement suspected)

However, in case of sudden onset, I would like to do a cardiovascular assessment that includes ECG, echocardiography, carotid Doppler, and temporal artery biopsy, if required.

Examiner: How will you treat a case of optic atrophy?

Candidate: Management depends entirely on the etiology of optic neuropathy. In some cases, optic nerve damage may be partially reversible, e.g., visual recovery is often seen following the removal of a pituitary macroadenoma. However, after an ischemic optic neuropathy, visual recovery is usually minimal, and management centers on preventing further cardiovascular events.

Steroid treatment may be used in optic neuritis, where it accelerates visual recovery but does not affect the eventual visual outcome.

In case of arteritic anterior ischemic optic neuropathy, steroids are an essential treatment part to prevent further vascular occlusions.

In case of vitamin B12 deficiency, replacement is required.

Examiner: Tell some cause of optic atrophy?

Candidate: Here, the most common cause is MS. Other may include raised intracranial pressure (ICP) due to any cause, raised intraocular pressure (glaucoma), hereditary (such as Friedreich's ataxia, Leber's optic atrophy), vitamin B12 deficiency, and ischemic (GCA, WG, CSS).

[(If we get optic atrophy in one eye and papilloedema in another eye, then it is called Foster–Kennedy syndrome (optic nerve compression with raised ICP)]

Diplopia

Your role: You are the Registrar in the General Medical Clinic.

Patient profile: Mr Fred, 65-year-old.

Present problem: This gentleman is a known case of DM and hypertension presented with double vision and drooping of the eyelid for 10 days.

(Once you get this clinical scenario, you will get 5 minutes to start this station for two scenarios. At that time, start to think about your diagnosis and differential diagnoses and plan for taking focused history as well as focused examination.)

Differential diagnoses:
- 3rd nerve palsy with or without IV and VI nerve palsy due to:
- Mononeuritis multiplex (DM; hypertension; CTD—RA, SLE, Sjogren's syndrome; Vasculitis—WG, polyarteritis nodosa (PAN); rarely sarcoidosis)
- Multiple sclerosis (brainstem demyelination)
- Compressive lesion [posterior communication artery (PCA)/Internal carotid artery aneurysm, meningioma, parasellar tumor], brainstem malignancy
- *Brainstem infarction*: Weber, Benedikt syndrome
- Subacute or chronic meningitis; Malignant—lymphoma, carcinoma; Infection— tuberculosis, fungal
- Idiopathic
- Myasthenia gravis

(Once you enter the room, search for a spot diagnosis; ptosis with divergent squint suggests 3rd nerve palsy.)

Introduction, Permission, and Identification

Candidate: Good morning. My name is Mohammad Ali. One of the working doctors here today. I have been asked to see you. Is that okay?

Patient: Good morning, Doctor...

Candidate: Thank you for coming. I would like to start by taking your full name, age, and where you have come from, please?

Patient: Yes, doctor............. I am Fred, 45-year-old and from Bristol.

Focused History

Candidate: Okay, Mr Fred. Would you please tell me what brings you here today? Please tell me in your own words.

Patient: My left eyelid has drooped down, and I see double. Recently, my wife noticed my eye is pointing outward. I also have diabetes and hypertension.

Analyze the Symptoms

Candidate: Would you please tell me a little bit more about your double vision and drooping of the left eyelid?
Important questions to be asked are:
- When and how did you first notice the double vision?
- Did it come on suddenly or gradually [sudden (minutes)—vascular or trauma; rapid (days)—demyelinating; gradually (weeks)—compressive, myasthenia gravis (MG), SOL]
- Is it affecting one or both eyes?
- Do you have any pain in your eyes? Any blurred vision/loss of vision?
- Is it getting better or staying the same or getting worse over time?
- Is it coming on and off or all the time with you (diplopia and weakness of the other parts of the body worse toward the end of the day suggest MG)?
- Have you noticed any weakness or sensory disturbance (tingling and numbness) on the

right side of the body [crossed paralysis; sudden onset with this presentation suggests brainstem (midbrain) stroke; weber syndrome]?
- Have you noticed any unsteadiness in the gait (suggest cerebellar/posterior column involvement, maybe due to MS or if it is sudden onset with right-sided cerebellar involvement, then it is likely to be brainstem stroke—Benedikt's syndrome)?
- Do you have any fever, headache or any sensitivity to light or sound (suggest subacute meningitis, tuberculosis)?
- Do you have any fever, loss of weight, or appetite (suggest underlying malignancy)?
- Do you have joint pain and oral ulceration, skin rash, or any autoimmune disease (Mononeuritis multiplex/autoimmune disease induced transverse myelitis involving brainstem)?
- Please tell me how it affects your day-to-day activity?

Patient: When I woke up in the morning 10 days ago, I noticed my eyelid drooped off. It was slight at first, but it is getting worse. I see double, it is more when I look to the right side, particularly when looking with both eyes. I work in a multinational company, and I have to do lots of paperwork, because of this double vision I cannot work. I have taken sick leave for the last 7 days, now I am so scared that I will lose my job. I do not have any eye pain but have a headache.

Candidate: Mr Fred, I can see your worriedness. I will inform occupational health team, they will assess your workability and advise you regarding this. You said you have a headache, and please tell me more about it like:
- Since when you have had it? Was it sudden or gradual?
- Where exactly is the pain (unilateral/bilateral)? Is it continuous or comes and goes?
- What type of pain is it? How will you score it?
- Does the pain go anywhere? Is there anything that makes the pain better or worse?
- Does the pain increase on combing your hair and any jaw pain? Is there anything else with it like nausea, vomiting, or sensitivity to light?

Patient: I have a mild persistent headache on the left side of the head, which came on at the same time as the double vision. I do not have anything else with it.

Candidate: Okay, would you please tell me more about your diabetes?
- How long have you had diabetes? How was it detected first?
- How it was treated initially, and what is your current medication?
- Are you taking the medication regularly or irregularly? Is it controlled or uncontrolled?
- Have you ever monitored blood sugar? What is the usual range of blood sugar? What is your last blood sugar level and HbA1c?
- Are you on regular follow-up and where?
- Do you have any history of hypoglycemic attacks?
- Do you have any complications of DM like any heart, kidney, leg or eye problem?

Patient: I have had diabetes for the last 6 years; initially, it was controlled with diet only, then I started metformin for 4 years ago. My last HbA1c was 6.5.

Candidate: Now, please tell me about your hypertension?
- For how long you have hypertension?
- Are you taking medicine for it? What is your current medication for it?
- It is controlled or uncontrolled? What is the usual recording of BP?
- Do you have a FH of hypertension?
- What about your dietary habit and your exercise?

Patient: I have hypertension and taking amlodipine 5 mg daily, but sometimes it is not so well-controlled. My mother has hypertension taking medication for it.

Quick Systemic Review, Past Medical History, Family History, Treatment, Social History According to Your Differentials

If it is not asked previously during initial history taking or incompletely asked then—take a full history of a particular portion to make it complete.

Candidate: At this moment I would like to ask some general questions, is that okay with you?
- Do you have any nausea, vomiting, or tummy pain?
- Do you have any chest pain, breathlessness, palpitation or any cough?
- Any problem with your waterworks? What about your bowel habit? Do you have constipation? Do you have diarrhea, the passage of blood in stool?
- Do you have any similar condition or any other history of disease in your past? Have you ever been admitted to the hospital?
- Have you attended any consultant or general physician or specialist for this problem? What was their impression? Did you receive any diagnosis? What treatment have you received? Did they work?
- Have you ever been admitted to the hospital in the past or had any history of surgery?
- May I ask what medication you take? Do you take any over-the-counter medications or herbal medicine, or any recreational drugs? Are you allergic to any medicine or anything else?
- Is there anyone else in your family with this type of problem or any long-standing illness that run in your family like DM, hypertension, stroke, thyroid, or other autoimmune disease or anything else?
- Do you smoke? Do you drink?
- What are you doing for a living? Do you drive? If yes, then ask, do you drive for a living? Are you married? Who is at home with you, or who is supporting you now? Do you have children? Are you independent in activities of daily living?

Have I missed anything, or do you want to add anything more?

Would you mind if I go on to examine you?

Focused Examination

Here, the patient has a history of 3rd nerve palsy with significant vascular risk factors (DM, hypertension, smoking history). So, the examination should be done to identify whether it is complete (compressive/surgical) or partial (incomplete/medical) 3rd nerve palsy.

- Is there any association of II, IV, or other cranial nerve palsies?
- Is there any long tract sign (hemiparesis, hemianesthesia) or cerebellar involvement?]

Examination

Visual acuity: Typically normal but may be decreased due to macular damage (diabetic eye patient).

Pupil: Compressive lesions (PCA or internal carotid artery aneurysm, meningioma, parasellar tumor) affect both the superficial pupillary fiber and the deep motor fiber. So, here complete 3rd nerve palsy will occur whereas (microvascular disease) ischemic lesions (DM, hypertension, RA, SLE, or vasculitis) tend only to affect the motor nerves (the pupil will be unaffected).

If the ophthalmoplegia is predominant compared to the ptosis/pupil dilation, the cause is more likely to be vascular (ischemic). Conversely, if the ophthalmoplegia is minimal compared to the ptosis or pupil dilation, the cause is more likely to be extrinsic compression by an aneurysm, pituitary tumor or meningioma.

Movement

- In cranial nerve (CN) III palsy, the eyeball will deviate downward and laterally (divergent squint) and fail to elevate or move medially.
- In CN IV palsy, the affected eye will fail to adduct and look down (the eye will be intorted).
- In CN VI palsy, the affected eye will fail to adduct.

Use the cover test: Cover each eye in turn at the point of maximum diplopia; it will be the outer image that will disappear when the involved eye is covered.

Fundoscopy: Papilloedema suggest raised ICP due to SOL in the brain or optic neuritis or optic atrophy with evidence of diabetic and hypertensive retinopathy.

I would like to complete my examination doing cerebellar function tests, upper limb and lower limb examinations, other cranial nerves examinations, urine for glycosuria, proteinuria, and measuring blood pressure.

Feedback to the Patient and Respond to the Patient's Concern

Candidate: You said at the beginning that your main problem was double vision and drooping of the eyelid. Is there anything else that we have missed or any concerns?

Patient: What has happened to me, Doctor?

Candidate: I suspect the double vision and drooping of the eyelid may be caused by one of the nerves that control the muscles in the eye not working properly is called a 3rd nerve palsy. Most likely, it is due to the nerve damage from the toxic effect of diabetes, but stroke is a possibility. So, we need to exclude this (stroke) by doing further investigation, including blood tests and brain imaging, to help your diplopia, we can put a patch over your eyes/glasses temporarily, and you need to stop driving for the time being.

Hopefully, it will be better over the next few weeks; this might be a good time to help you to improve your blood sugar and blood pressure. I will refer you to see the diabetes team, who can give you more advice.

Patient: Doctor, will it affect my driving? I used to drive to my office.

Candidate: I am sorry to say, you cannot drive now. As you see double, it is dangerous to drive at this time. You have to inform DVLA about your condition, and I will write in my notes that I have asked you to inform DVLA.

Patient: But, Doctor, my workplace is far away. I have to drive. Otherwise, it will be difficult for me.

Candidate: I can understand your situation. In that case, you can explain your situation to your employer, and I hope they would arrange your transport.

Do you have any other concerns?
Thank you for spending time with me today.

Discussion with Examiner

Examiner: Would you please present your case?

Candidate:

This elderly man presented with acute onset of double vision and drooping of the left eyelid with a background history of uncontrolled DM and hypertension.

On examination of the eye revealed:
There is ptosis; lifting the eyelid reveals the left eye is deviated down and out (divergent squint); fails to elevate and move medially; there is angulated diplopia. Both pupils react usually.

So far, I examine, there is no evidence of long tract signs or cerebellar signs.

In summary, my diagnosis would be partial 3rd nerve palsy, possibly due to microvascular disease caused by DM and hypertension here.

Examiner: How do you investigate a case of diplopia?

Candidate: As the patient presented with incomplete 3rd nerve palsy with important cardiovascular risk factors suggest microvascular origin. However, at first, I would like to do baseline tests including:
- CBC with ESR with CRP
- Random blood sugar with HbA1c
- ECG, lipid profile, urine R/M/E, serum electrolytes, serum creatinine, TFTs and LFTs.

As the patient has a history of a headache, I would like to exclude posterior communicating artery aneurysm (although very unlikely here as these patients usually presented with complete 3rd nerve palsy) and stroke by doing magnetic resonance angiography (MRA) and MRI (brainstem stroke)/CT scan of the brain.

Examiner: How do you treat the case?

Candidate: Here, the most important steps of management would be optimizing cardiovascular risk factors by controlling blood sugar, blood pressure, as well as smoking cessation.

If there is radiological evidence of compressive or complex lesion (e.g., aneurysm, meningioma), then it may require urgent neurosurgical intervention.

Retinitis Pigmentosa

Your role: You are the SHO in General Medical Clinic.

Patient name: Mrs Anne Nelson, 35-year-old.

Patient problem: Progressive loss of vision.

(Once you get this clinical scenario, you will get 5 minutes to start this station for two scenarios. At that time, start to think about your diagnosis, differential diagnoses, and plan for taking focused history as well as focused examination.)

Differential diagnosis:
- Retinitis pigmentosa (painless slowly progressive peripheral vision loss, usually bilateral, night blindness, positive FH is the clue to diagnosis)
- Cataract
- Diabetic maculopathy
- Glaucoma (painless/painful)
- Age-related macular degeneration (2-5 is a progressive loss of vision that mainly affect the central vision) (difficulty in the reading newspaper)
- Optic atrophy (causes—compressive, toxic, nutritional; usually both central and peripheral loss of vision)]

[*Once you enter the room, search for a spot diagnosis for visual loss; the signs of DM suggest diabetic retinopathy; Cushing syndrome and acromegaly with bitemporal hemianopia with optic atrophy; Graves' ophthalmopathy; walking aid with optic atrophy suggest MS; hearing aid with RP suggest Usher syndrome*]

Introduction, Permission, and Identification

Candidate: Good morning. I am Mohammad Ali, one of the working doctors here today. I have been asked to see you. Is that okay with you?

Patient: Good morning, Doctor...

Candidate: Thank you for coming. I would like to start by taking your full name, age, and where you have come from, please?

Patient: Yes, Doctor............ Mrs Anne Nelson, I am 35, and from Liverpool.

Focused History

Candidate: Okay, Mrs Nelson, would you please tell me what brings you here today?

Patient: My vision has become progressively worse, particularly at night over the last few years.

Analyze the Symptom

Candidate: Would you please tell me a little bit more about your visual disturbance?
Important questions to be asked are:
- What do you mean by visual disturbance? Is it blurring of vision or loss of vision? If loss of vision, then ask, is it central/peripheral/upper or lower part?
- When did you first notice the loss of vision? Can you describe the onset of visual disturbance? Was it sudden or gradual onset?
- Is it increasing or decreasing day by day or the same?
- Does it affect one or both eyes?
- How it affects your normal day-to-day activity for a living?
- Do you see the walls of the room or side of the road when looking straight forward (difficulty suggest peripheral vision is affected by either retinitis pigmentosa or bitemporal hemianopia)?
- Can you read the newspaper (difficulty suggest central vision is affected)?
- Any change in night vision? Like....do you bump into things while walking outside at night/do you need to sleep with the lights on?
- Any change in color vision? Can you distinguish between the traffic light colors?

- Have you noticed double vision? Any flashes of light in your vision?
- Do you have a headache or any pain in the eye?
- Do you have diabetes?
- Any hearing difficulty (Usher, Refsum disease, Alport syndrome)?
- Has anyone in your family with a vision problem?
- Do you drive? If yes, then ask, do you drive for a living?

Patient: For the past 2 years, it has been challenging to see with both eyes, mainly when I go out for a walk in the evening and stay in a dimly lit room. I do not get to notice my surroundings very well and often bump into the furniture in the house. However, I have no headache, redness of the eye, double vision, pain, or sensitivity to light. No weakness or tingling sensation in the limbs or no hearing loss, no flashes of light in my vision, no difficulty in reading the newspaper. I am a driver; I broke the mirror of my truck in an accident last month; after that, I got scared and sought medical attention immediately. There is no one in my family with a visual problem.

(In history, the patient has progressive bilateral painless loss of vision, significantly affecting peripheral vision and night blindness. Here, most likely diagnosis would be retinitis pigmentosa. It may be primary or secondary to many syndromes. In that case, we should take history to exclude other syndromes associated with retinitis pigmentosa. Deafness is an important associated feature of Usher syndrome, Refsum's disease, Laurence-Moon-Bardet-Biedl syndrome. Therefore, it is essential to ask the patient about hearing loss.)

Other Important Targeted Histories

For Usher syndrome—ask the patient:
- Do you have any history of hearing loss (sensory-neural deafness) or any deafness in your family?

For Refsum's syndrome—ask the patient:
- Do you have any tingling or numbness in the limbs (peripheral neuropathy)?
- Do you have any skin change or rash (ichthyosis)?
- Do you have any unsteady gait (cerebellar ataxia)?
- Do you have any chest pain, palpitation, breathlessness, or limb swelling (cardiomyopathy)?

For Laurence-Moon-Bardet-Biedl syndrome—ask the patient:
- Do you have any finger deformity (polydactyly/syndactyly)?
- Do you have any change in waterworks, such as a change in color, amount, frequency or frothy urine (for DM and kidney problem)?

For Kearns-Sayre syndrome (mitochondrial disease):
- Do you have any awareness of your heartbeat or slow heartbeat (AV conduction block)?
- Have you noticed any unsteadiness in your gait (cerebellar ataxia)?
- Any double vision (ophthalmoplegia)?

For abetalipoproteinemia:
- Do you have any tummy pain or loose motion (steatorrhea)?
- Have you noticed any unsteadiness in your gait (cerebellar or sensory ataxia due to vitamin E deficiency)?

Quick Systemic Review, Past Medical History, Family History, Treatment, Social History According to Your Differentials

If it is not asked previously during initial history taking or incompletely asked then—take a full history of a particular portion to make it complete.

Candidate: At this moment, I would like to ask some general questions to know about your overall health. Is that okay with you?
- Do you have a fever, weight loss, loss of appetite? What about your waterworks/bowel habit?
- Do you have any history of other diseases in your past? Have you ever admitted to the hospital/any surgery?
- Have you attended any eye specialist for this problem? What was their impression? Did you receive any diagnosis? What treatment have you received? Did they work?

- Are you taking any medications currently on a regular basis? Any over-the-counter medications or herbal medicine, or any recreational drugs? Are you allergic to any medicine/anything else?
- Is there anyone else in your family with this type of problem or any long-standing illness that run in your families like DM, hypertension, stroke, thyroid, or other autoimmune disease or anything else?
- Do you smoke? Do you drink? What are you doing for a living? Are you married? Who is at home with you, or who is supporting you now? Do you have children?

Have I missed anything, or do you want to add anything more?

Would you mind if I go on to examine you?

Focused Examination

Here, the most important part of the examination would be eye examination, and for any syndromic diagnosis, examine the following:
- Ear examination for deafness (? Hearing aid)
- CVS for evidence of cardiomyopathy, bradycardia (AV block) or arrhythmia.
- CNS for peripheral neuropathy, cerebellar ataxia, and sensory ataxia.

For eye examination include:
- Visual acuity
- Eye movement—for diplopia
- Visual field
- Fundoscopy

Feedback to the Patient and Respond to the Patient's Concern

Candidate: You said at the beginning that your main problem was a progressive loss of vision. Is there anything else that we have missed, or do you want to add anything more? Do you have any concerns?

Patient: What has happened to me, Doctor?

Candidate: It is possible that you may have a condition called retinitis pigmentosa, meaning that there is an increased pigmentation in the back of your eyes, which is the sensor of the vision. These pigmentations obscure its ability to sense normally, which is an inherited condition.

Unfortunately, this is a progressive condition that leads to a gradual worsening of the vision, mainly in the periphery. There is no treatment at this moment, although some proposed treatments can delay it (vitamin A reduces progression). There is much research going on in this area, but nothing that likely to be helpful in the near future.

We will refer you to an MDT involving a brain physician, eye doctor, physiotherapist, and social worker (to give financial support) to give you the proper care and management plan.

As this is an inherited condition, I am going to refer you for genetic counseling. This will be particularly useful if you are thinking of having children.

Candidate: Do you have any other concerns or questions?

Patient: Can I still drive my truck?

Candidate: Unfortunately, your vision is below what is required from a legal point of view for both your car and heavy goods vehicle (HGV) licenses, and you should stop driving now as it is no longer safe to continue. You will need to inform the DVLA about this, then DVLA may want to arrange their own tests. Moreover, I am sorry to say; your insurance would not be valid if you had an accident.

Discussion with Examiner

Examiner: Would you please present your case?

Candidate:

This young lady presented with progressive reduced visual acuity, which was now 6/18 bilaterally. She also complained of trouble seeing at night and decreased peripheral vision, resulting in tunnel vision.

On fundoscopic examination, she had retinal pigmentation with a characteristic bone spicule pattern and evidence of waxy pallor over her optic disc.

So, in summary, my diagnosis would be retinitis pigmentosa, inherited rod dystrome which is likely to be primary rather than a secondary syndrome.

Examiner: How will you investigate it?

Candidate:
- Electroretinogram (most important test here)
- Optical coherence tomography (OCT)
- Electrooculogram
- Genetic test

Examiner: In this case, we do not have a FH, but it is an inherited condition. Can you tell me a little more about the modes of inheritance?

Candidate: There are several modes of inheritance. The condition can be autosomal dominant/autosomal recessive/X-linked recessive.

I am aware that there is also a risk of spontaneous mutation, which can occur in 30% of patients.

Examiner: How will you treat the patient if this lady is confirmed to have retinitis pigmentosa? How would she be managed?

Candidate: After confirmation through an ophthalmologic review, I would wish this patient to be referred to a geneticist for genetic counseling, and they may wish to perform genetic studies thereafter.

Unfortunately, there is no current treatment for retinitis pigmentosa (vitamin A reduces progression), and rest of the management is mainly supportive.

I would like to signpost this patient to appropriate charities and ensure that she received appropriate occupational therapy in the form of visual aids.

Vitreous Hemorrhage

Your role: You are the Registrar in the General Medical Clinic.

Patient profile: Mrs Lara House, 55-year-old.

Present problem: Sudden onset of visual disturbance with DM.

(*Once you get this clinical scenario, you will get 5 minutes to start this station for two scenarios. At that time, start to think about your diagnosis, differential diagnoses, and plan for taking focused history as well as focused examination.*)

Differential diagnosis:
Cause of sudden loss of vision:
- CVD (usually bilateral homonymous hemianopia)
- Amaurosis fugax/transient loss of vision (TIA)
- Vitreous hemorrhage (diabetic patient–unilateral, painless)
- Retinal artery occlusion (unilateral, painless)
- Pituitary apoplexy (bilateral loss of vision with shock)

Subacute/rapid onset but not sudden (usually over hour or days)
- Optic neuritis (painful)
- Retinal detachment (flushing of light and the appearance of floaters typically precede retinal detachment)
- Anterior uveitis (painful visual disturbance with the red eye with photophobia)
- Acute angle-closure glaucoma]

(*Once you enter the room, search for a spot diagnosis for visual loss; the sign of DM suggests diabetic retinopathy; Cushing syndrome and acromegaly with bitemporal hemianopia suggest optic atrophy; Graves' ophthalmopathy, walking aid with optic atrophy suggest MS; hearing aid with retinitis pigmentosa suggest Usher syndrome.*)

Introduction, Permission, and Identification

Candidate: Good morning. My name is Mohammad Ali. One of the working doctors here today. I have been asked to see you. Is that okay?

Patient: Good morning, doctor...

Candidate: Thank you for coming. I would like to start by taking your full name, age, and where you have come from, please?

Patient: Yes, doctor............. I am Lara House, 55-year-old and from Ireland.

Focused History

Candidate: Okay, Mrs House. Would you please tell me what brings you here today? Please tell me in your words.

Patient: I am diabetic for the last 12 years, and today morning when I woke up, I noticed almost no sight in my right eye. I got scared and came to the hospital.

Analyze the Symptoms

Candidate: I am sorry to hear about it. You look scary, but we are here to help you. Please tell me a little bit more about it.
Important questions to be asked are:
- What do you mean by no sight?
- When did you first notice it? Did it come on suddenly or gradually?
- Has it changed since it started? Is it affecting one or both eyes?
- Which part of the vision is affected? Is it all or top half or bottom half or sides or central? Is this the same in both eyes?
- Did the visual loss begin on the outside and extend to the center? Have you noticed any

flushing of light or floaters in the visual field (retinal detachment)?
- Do you have any pain in or around the eye or any headache or pain during combing hair and painful chewing (GCA)?
- Have you noticed any halo around the light (acute glaucoma and cataract)?
- Have you noticed any graying of the vision or loss of color vision, or can you distinguish the color of the traffic light?
- Have you noticed any double vision?
- Do you drive (a vital part of history in this case)? If yes, then ask, do you drive for a living?

Patient: I cannot see anything in my right eye since I woke up this morning. The last time when I get eyes checked for diabetes, the optician told me that I have diabetic changes in my eyes; so far, I have had no problem with my vision. I drive to my office, but I do not drive for a living.

Candidate: Please tell me a little bit more about your diabetes:
- For how long have you had diabetes? How was it detected first?
- How it was treated initially, and what is your current medication?
- Are you taking the medication regularly or irregularly? Is it controlled or uncontrolled?
- Have you ever monitored blood sugar? What is the usual range of blood sugar? What is your last blood sugar level and HbA1c?
- Are you on regular follow-up and where?
- Do you have any history of hypoglycemic attacks?
- Do you have any other complications of DM like any heart, kidney, or leg problem?

Candidate: I have had diabetes for the last 12 years. My last HbA1c was 10; initially, I was treated with tablets, but I have been using insulin for the last 5 years. I am very busy in my professional life; it is hard to maintain a diabetic lifestyle and control my blood sugar level under these circumstances. Hence, I have failed to attend two recent appointments at the eye clinic.

Quick Systemic Review, Past Medical History, Family History, Treatment, Social History According to Your Differentials

If it is not asked previously during initial history taking or incompletely asked then—take a full history of a particular portion to make it complete.

Candidate: At this moment I would like to ask some general questions, is that okay with you?
- Do you have headaches, dizziness or LOC or blurring of vision or weakness of limbs?
- Any chest pain, breathlessness, or cough? Any fever, any recent changes in weight or appetite?
- Any nausea, vomiting, abdominal pain, or any changes in bowel habits?
- What about your waterworks? Any change in color, frequency, or frothy urine or any pain in passing urine or anything else?
- Do you have any similar condition or any other history of disease in your past? Have you ever been admitted to the hospital?
- Have you attended any consultant or general physician or specialist for this problem? What was their impression? Did you receive any diagnosis? What treatment have you received? Did they work?
- May I ask what medication you take? Do you take any over-the-counter medications or herbal medicine, or any recreational drugs? Are you allergic to any medicine or anything else?
- Is there anyone in your family with this type of problem or any long-standing illness that runs in your family like DM, hypertension, stroke, thyroid, or other autoimmune diseases, or anything else?
- Do you smoke? Do you drink? What are you doing for a living? Are you married? Who is at home with you, or who is supporting you now? Do you have children? Are you independent in activities of daily living?

Have I missed anything, or do you want to add anything more?

Okay, thank you. Would you mind if I go on to examine you now?

Focused Examination

The patient has no evidence of long tract signs such as hemiparesis, hemianesthesia, or cerebellar symptoms; so, CVD is unlikely here. However, since the patient has a painless, unilateral, nontraumatic loss of vision on the background history of uncontrolled DM with diabetic eye disease, here, the most likely diagnosis would be—vitreous hemorrhage/retinal hemorrhage.

Other possibilities would be:
- Central retinal vein occlusion (CRVO)/branch retinal vein occlusion (BVRVO).
- Retinal arterial occlusion

The focused examination would be:
- Examination of the eye
- *Visual acuity*: Visual acuity should always be assessed separately for each eye.
- *Visual field*: If the history suggests peripheral visual field loss, then it should be determined in each eye by confrontation. Confrontation visual testing should be performed in each of four quadrants (upper and lower, nasal and temporal). The central visual field, including the size of the blind spot, should be tested vertically and horizontally.
- *Pupil reaction to light*: RAPD indicates either optic nerve disease (optic atrophy, neuritis) or widespread retinal damage. In vitreous hemorrhage—pupillary response to light will be normal.
- *Eye movement*
- *Fundoscopy*: If the red reflex is reduced or absent, it suggests vitreous hemorrhage (cataracts also diminish the red reflex in the affected eye but cause very gradual visual loss). If the hemorrhage is dense, it may completely hide the retina. If there is a fundal view, retinal neovascularization may be found. The opposite eye should be carefully examined for diabetic retinopathy.
(Optic disc cupping suggests glaucoma; Pale optic disc suggests optic atrophy; Blurred disc margin suggests optic neuritis or papilloedema.)
- Upper limb, lower limb, and other cranial nerves examinations to get the evidence of pure sensory or sensory-motor or autonomic neuropathy due to associated diabetic peripheral neuropathy or mononeuritis multiplex.
- Urine examination for proteinuria and glycosuria (diabetic nephropathy).

Feedback to the Patient and Respond to the Patient's Concerns

Candidate: You said at the beginning that the main problem was the sudden painless loss of vision with known diabetic eye disease. Is there anything else that we have missed, or do you want to add anything more?

Patient: I am terrified, doctor. Will I be permanently blind?

Candidate: During my examination, I found small bleeding inside the eye that prevents you from seeing through it. It is a complication of advanced diabetic eye disease. I would like to refer you urgently to an eye specialist who may recommend laser treatment to prevent further bleeding and permanent vision loss. Hopefully, it will clear over the next few weeks. However, it is very important to have good control of blood sugar, and hypertension, as well as smoking cessation, to prevent or reduce any further deterioration. We can take help from the diabetes team, they can give you more advice.

Since you drive, you have to inform DVLA about your condition, and I am going to write in my notes that I have asked you to inform DVLA. This is because driving may carry a risk to your life and the others as well.

Do you have any worries or concerns?

Discussion with Examiner

Examiner: Would you please present your case?

Candidate: This middle-aged lady presented with sudden painless vision loss of the right eye with a background history of poorly controlled blood-sugar with diabetic eye disease.

Examination of the right eye shows significantly reduced visual acuity with absent red reflex with evidence of vitreous hemorrhage (large dark floaters/red haze/no view to the retina at all) during the fundoscopic examination.

Examination of the left eye shows normal visual acuity, a normal field of vision, normal eye movement with no diplopia (asymptomatic). Fundoscopy showed evidence of diabetic proliferative retinopathy—dot hemorrhage (microaneurysm), blot hemorrhage, and hard exudates (yellowish, shiny, well-circumscribed small multiple fat depositions). There is also evidence of retinal ischemia—soft exudates (cotton wool spots—fluffy white, well or ill-defined, not shiny, large, few) with flame-shaped hemorrhage and neovascularization (new vessel formation) in mesh or trabeculae.

So, in summary, the cause of sudden loss of vision of this middle-aged diabetic patient would be vitreous hemorrhage.

Examiner: How will you investigate the case?

Candidate: In terms of basic tests, Initially, I would want to perform some blood tests and urine tests; I would start by checking this patient's random blood sugar and HbA1c level, FBC, inflammatory markers (ESR and CRP), baseline urea, creatinine, electrolytes, urine R/M/E, lipid profile, and LFTs.

Then I would like to do retinal photography as well as ocular B-scan ultrasonography.

Examiner: How will you treat the patient?

Candidate: Treatment depends on the severity of the retinopathy with or without significant maculopathy. Patients with background diabetic retinopathy can frequently be reviewed in the community by annual retinal photographic screening (diabetic retinopathy screening service).

If there are preproliferative diabetic retinopathy or maculopathy, onward referral to the ophthalmology clinic is required [routine referral to an ophthalmologist within 13 weeks) (smoking cessation, blood pressure maintenance 130/80 with angiotensin-converting enzyme inhibitors (ACEIs)/angiotensin II receptor blockers (ARBs) along with tight glycemic control are important steps of management.]

In diabetic maculopathy (macular edema, exudates, hemorrhage) needs an urgent referral to the ophthalmologist.

In case of proliferative retinopathy, urgent referral to the ophthalmologist within 2 weeks for panretinal laser photocoagulation (vitrectomy, intraocular steroid injection, sometimes helpful).

Pyoderma Gangrenosum

Your role: You are the Registrar in the General Medical Clinic.

Patient's details: Mrs Alina Jones, a 35-year-old lady.

Clinical problem: Painful foul-smelling non-healing ulcer in the right leg.

(Once you get this clinical scenario, you will get 5 minutes to start this station for two scenarios. At that time, start to think about your diagnosis and differential diagnoses and plan for taking focused history as well as focused examination.)

Causes of pyoderma gangrenosum:

In 50% cases, it is associated with systemic disease such as:
- Inflammatory bowel disease (IBD) [mostly ulcerative colitis (UC)].
- Rheumatological disease (rheumatoid arthritis, AS or seronegative arthritis)
- Hematological malignancy—myeloproliferative disorder [chronic myeloid leukemia (CML) or polycythemia rubra vera (PRV)], acute myeloid leukemia (AML), lymphoma, or IgA monoclonal gammopathy.
- Rare causes (SLE, liver disease—autoimmune/viral hepatitis, sarcoidosis, and thyroid disease)

(Once you enter the room, search for a spot diagnosis; rheumatoid hand, and characteristic appearance of the ulcer suggests the underlying cause of the ulcer.)

Greetings, Introduction, Permission, and Identification

Candidate: Good morning. I am Mohammad Ali. One of the working doctors here today. I have been asked to see you. Is that okay?

Patient: Okay.

Candidate: I will start by taking your full name, age, and where you have come from, please.

Patient: Mrs Alina Jones, I am 35-year-old and from London.

Focused History

Candidate: Okay, Mrs Jones. Would you please tell me what brings you here today? Please tell me in your own words.

Patient: I have developed an ulcer on my leg which is getting bigger. I also have joint pain.

Analyze the Symptoms

Candidate: Please tell me a little bit more about your ulcer?
The important questions to be asked are:
- When did you first notice the ulcer?
- Has it changed since it started? Is it getting better or getting worse day by day or the same?
- Have you had any history of trauma or surgery to the leg?
- Is there anything else that is worse or improve the ulcer?
- Do you have any fever or pain in the ulcer?

Patient: I noticed a lump on my lower leg eight weeks ago, which was painful. I went to the general physician, who gave me an antibiotic, but I cannot recall the name of the antibiotic. The lump did not get any better; instead, they have become enlarged, more painful and ulcerated. My general physician took a swab and asked the district nurse to do daily dressing for the ulcer. The ulcer was not improving, and I had another course of antibiotics last week. I have no pain in my leg when walking.

Candidate: Now tell me more about your joint pain (symmetrical/asymmetrical, upper limbs/lower

limbs/both, arthritis/arthralgia, inflammatory/mechanical, morning stiffness)?
- How it affects your day-to-day activity?
- Do you have an oral ulcer or photosensitive rash in other parts of the body?
- Do you have a FH of arthritis?
- Have you noticed any change in the color of the hand on exposure to the cold (Reynaud's)?
- Have you noticed any skin changes or difficulty in swallowing (scleroderma)?
- Do you have any difficulty in standing from a sitting position (proximal myopathy)?
- Have you noticed any dry eye or dry mouth or any difficulty in vision with red eye (uveitis)?

Patient: I have had joint pain and swelling in my hands and legs for the last 6 months. In the morning, I feel stiffness in my joints. It is hard nowadays to do my usual household tasks like I have problems with putting on clothes, gripping cutlery, taking baths, and climbing stairs due to joint pain.

Other Important Targeted Histories

- Have you noticed any change in bowel habits like on-off (relapse and remission) diarrhea, tummy pain, weight loss, or blood in stool (IBD)?
- Have you noticed any lump or bump in the armpit, neck, groin or tummy (lymphoma, organomegaly for myeloproliferative disease or goiter)?
- Do you have weight loss, tremors, excessive sweating, or shaking of the limbs (thyroid disease)?
- Do you have any history of yellowish skin or sclera, bloody vomitus, black tarry loose stool, or scratch mark (liver diseases)?

Quick Systemic Review, Past Medical History, Family History, Treatment, Social History According to Your Differentials

If it is not asked previously during initial history taking or incompletely asked then—take a full history of a particular portion to make it complete.

Candidate: Now I would like to ask some general questions, is that okay with you?
- Do you have a headache, LOC or dizziness? Do you have any chest pain, cough, shortness of breath, or limb swelling? Do you have any loss of appetite or vomiting or any change in waterworks?
- Do you have any similar condition or any other history of disease in your past? Have you ever been admitted to the hospital?
- Have you attended any consultant or general physician or specialist for this problem? What was their impression? Did you receive any diagnosis? What treatment have you received? Did they work?
- May I ask what medication you take? Do you take any over-the-counter medications or herbal medicine, or any recreational drugs? Are you allergic to any medicine or anything else?
- Is there anyone in your family with this type of problem or any long-standing illness that runs in your family like DM, hypertension, stroke, thyroid, or other autoimmune diseases, or anything else?
- Do you smoke? Do you drink? What are you doing for a living? Are you married? Who is at home with you, or who is supporting you now? Do you have children? Are you independent in activities of daily living?

Have I missed anything, or do you want to add anything more?

Thank you, would you mind if I go on to examine you.

Focused Examination

Here, the diagnosis is pyoderma gangrenosum, and the underlying cause is rheumatoid arthritis. So your focused examination would be examination of the ulcer and hand (for the evidence of rheumatoid hand).

Examination of the skin:

Location: Lower limb, trunk, and occasionally face.

Description: Classically, pyoderma gangrenosum start with a nodulopustular lesion that has been down to form a tender ulcer, maybe up to 10 cm in diameter. This large necrotic ulcer with a ragged violaceous border overhangs the ulcer bed together with areas containing erythematous plaques and pustules.

If the underlying cause of pyoderma gangrenosum is not obvious from history, then work for the underlying cause.
- IBD—clubbing, laparotomy scar, stroma site, and arthropathy.
- RA—arthropathy, rheumatoid nodule, episcleritis, and scleritis.
- *Myeloproliferative disorder*: Hepatosplenomegaly.
- Lymphoma—lymphadenopathy.
- PRA—splenomegaly, facial plethora, and dusky cyanosis.
- *Thyroid disease*: Assess for thyroid status (hypo/hyperthyroidism), goiter, thyroid eye disease, thyroid acropachy, and pretibial myxoedema.
- *Sarcoidosis*: Erythema nodosum, lupus pernio and DPLD.
- *Diabetes*: Fingertip-glucose testing skin pricks and fundoscopy for retinopathy.
- *Primary biliary cholangitis*: Scratch marks, xanthelasma, and sign of CLD.

Feedback to the Patient and Respond to the Patient's Concern

Candidate: You said at the beginning that the main problems were a painful ulcer on your leg and joint pain. Is there anything else that we have missed or any concerns?

Patient: What might be the cause of my leg ulcer? Have you had any thoughts about what is going on?

Candidate: I suspect the painful ulcer on your leg is a condition called pyoderma gangrenosum. However, the multiple joints pain and swelling may be caused by rheumatoid arthritis, which can be associated with this type of ulcer. The ulcer is likely to heal with treatment for your rheumatoid arthritis, but if not, we have other options to consider.

To confirm our diagnosis, we would like to do some blood tests as well as taking a swab from the ulcer and examine it in the lab to rule out infections. I will refer you to a skin specialist to see if a skin biopsy is necessary and a joint specialist to investigate your joint pain. Is that okay with you?

Do you have any other concerns?

Patient: Why is it not being cured with antibiotics?

Candidate: This ulcer is actually not due to any infections; instead, it is an inflammation of the skin, and that is why not responding to treatment with antibiotics. The inflammation in the skin will need to be settled down in order to heal the ulcer. We will ask the dermatology team to see you and plan further tests and treatment of the ulcer. Okay, thank you for spending time with me.

Discussion between Examiner and Candidate

Examiner: Would you please present your case?

Candidate:

This young lady presented with a non-healing ulcer in combination with a background of inflammatory polyarthritis involving both small and large joints with significant morning stiffness.

A large necrotic ulcer with a ragged, violaceous border overhangs the ulcer bed, together with areas containing erythematous plaques with pustules.

There is symmetrical deforming arthropathy of the small joints of the hand involving PIP and MCP joints with sparing of the DIP joints. There is also swan neck deformity and Z-deformity of thumb.

So, in summary, my diagnosis would be pyoderma gangrenosum due to underlying rheumatoid arthritis.

Examiner: How will you investigate the case?

Candidate: At first, I would like to do baseline blood tests that include CBC with ESR with CRP, urea and electrolytes, serum creatinine, TFTs, and LFTs.

Then I would like to take a skin swab to rule out infections; if needed, a skin biopsy can be performed to confirm the diagnosis (pyoderma gangrenosum is often a diagnosis of exclusion as laboratory and histopathological findings are variable and nonspecific).

To establish the underlying cause, I would like to do autoantibodies such as rheumatoid arthritis, anti-CCP antibody, ANA, ANCAs, and APA.

Gastrointestinal studies including stool for occult blood, colonoscopy, biopsy, and radiography.

Hematological studies, including protein electrophoresis, and bone marrow examination.

Examiner: How will you treat the case?

Candidate: Here, the main step of management is treating underlying disease (e.g., DMARDs for RA) and topical and systemic treatment for the ulcer. Topical therapy includes; potent steroid ointment and intralesional steroids.

I would also involve a tissue viability nurse for help with dressing and consideration of supplementary treatment such as potassium permanganate.

Very rarely, high dose systemic corticosteroids and infliximab may be required in refractory cases.

Psoriasis

Your role: You are the Registrar in the General Medical Clinic.

Patient's details: Mr William, a 35-year-old man.

Clinical problem: Increasingly difficult to perform his job as a painter and decorator.

(*Once you get this clinical scenario, you will get 5 minutes to start this station for two scenarios. At that time, start to think about your diagnosis and differential diagnoses and plan for taking focused history as well as focused examination.*)

[*Differential diagnosis*: Difficulty to perform his job may be due to joint pain (arthritis—rheumatoid arthritis, psoriatic arthropathy), trauma, weakness (mono or polyneuropathy, myopathy), Raynaud's syndrome (? systemic sclerosis)]

(*Once you enter the room, search for a spot diagnosis; psoriatic plaques, nail change, arthropathy suggests psoriasis.*)

Introduction, Permission, and Identification

Candidate: Good morning. My name is Mohammad Ali. One of the working doctors here today. I have been asked to see you. Is that okay?

Patient: Good morning, doctor.

Candidate: Thank you for coming, May I know your name, please?

Patient: I am William.

Candidate: And may I confirm your age, please?

Patient: I am 35-year-old.

Focused History

Candidate: Okay, Mr William. Would you please tell me what brings you here today?

Patient: I am finding it more difficult to perform my job as a painter and decorator for the last few months, and it is increasing day-by-day.

Candidate: I am sorry to hear about your difficulties. Let me ask you some questions first and see how we can help you. Would you please tell me why are you facing difficulties to perform your job? (Is it due to weakness or due to joint or muscle pain, stiffness, or anything else?)

Patient: I have pain and swelling in my hand joints.

Candidate: So, you have joint pain. Please tell me more about your joint pain.
- Is it only joint pain or swelling, or both? When did it start exactly? Which joints are affected (small/large/upper limb/lower limb/symmetrical/asymmetrical)?
- Is it more in the morning or at night? Is it increasing or decreasing or the same? Is there any morning stiffness, for how long?
- Does anything make it worse, like rest, movement, or activity?
- Does anything make it better like rest, movement, or any painkiller?
- Do you have back or neck pain (suggests ? seronegative arthritis)
- Do you have any skin rash—if present, then analyze the rash (onset, progression, site, worsening factor, improving factor, photo-sensitivity)
- Have you noticed any change in the nails?
- How is it affecting your job and activity of daily living or hobbies?

Patient: Actually, I have pain and swelling in my right thumb. At first, I noticed the problem with my ring finger on the right hand about 3 years ago when it became swollen; at that time, I could not bend or straighten my finger. It was settled down over a few months. 6 months ago, I again noticed that I had pain and swelling of the left thumb. I took some ibuprofen for that, and it was settled at that time. But now I think it has been causing problems with my work and I am worried that it may prevent me from working in the future. My thumbs feel really stiff in the morning and takes time (30 minutes) to get back to normal. I have scalp and elbow psoriasis—I use topical calcitriol and occasional steroid to control it.

Candidate: Since, it suggests a case of psoriatic arthropathy—by the patient's general look and history.

Other Important Targeted Histories
- Do you have a painful red eye with a blurring of vision (uveitis)?
- Do you have a history of psoriasis or a similar type of joint pain and swelling in your family?
- Do you have any pain in the feet or the Achilles tendon?
- Do you have any tummy pain, on and off diarrhea, or passing of blood mixed loose stool recently or in the past?
- Do you have pain during waterworks or any change in amount, color, frequency, or frothy urine recently or in the past?
- Are you losing hair? Do you suffer from a mouth ulcer (SLE)?
- Have you noticed dry mouth or dry eye (suggest associated Sjogren's syndrome)?
- Have you noticed a change in the color of your hand on exposure to the cold? If so, what are the colors? When does this happen? Have you noticed involvement in the other part of the body, like the nose, ears? Is there any ulceration (Raynaud's)?

Quick Systemic Review, Past Medical History, Family History, Treatment, Social History According to your Differentials

If it is not asked previously during initial history taking or incompletely asked then—take a full history of a particular portion to make it complete.

Candidate: Now I would like to ask some general questions, is that okay with you?
- Any history of LOC, dizziness, any altered speech, any history of shaking of the body with uncontrolled waterworks or bowel motion or tongue bite?
- Do you have any fever, weight loss, or loss of appetite?
- Do you have any similar condition or any other history of disease in your past?
- Have you attended any consultant or general physician or specialist for this problem? What was their impression? Did you receive any diagnosis? What treatment have you received? Did they work?
- Have you ever been admitted to the hospital in the past or have any history of surgery?
- May I ask what medication you take? Do you take any over-the-counter medications or herbal medicine, or any recreational drugs? Are you allergic to any medicine or anything else?
- Is there anyone else in your family with this type of problem or any long-standing illness that run in your family like DM, hypertension, stroke, thyroid problem, arthritis or anything else?
- Do you smoke? Do you drink? What are you doing for a living? Who is at home with you, or who is supporting you now?
- Are you sexually active? Do you have any stable partners? Do you practice safe sex by using condoms?

Patient: I never smoked but occasionally drink alcohol, which worsens my psoriasis, and now I have stopped drinking. I live with my wife and always practice safe sex.

Candidate: Have I missed anything, or do you want to add anything more?

Thank you for answering my questions. Would you mind if I go on to examine you now?

Focused Neurological Examination

In this scenario, the patient is a known case of psoriasis and has a history of joint pain and swelling. Here, the most likely diagnosis would be psoriatic arthropathy. So targeted examination would be:
- Skin examination for psoriasis
- Nail change
- Examination of the hand

Skin: Look for single or multiple scattered lesions. Well-demarcated, an erythematous raised plaque with a silvery scale, usually found on extensor surfaces symmetrically, scalp, umbilicus, groin, and natal cleft (examine these areas carefully).

Nail change:
- Pitting (psoriatic pits are large, deep, irregularly scattered within nail plate)
- Onycholysis (detachment of the nail from nail bed usually starting at the tip and/or sides)
- Subangular hyperkeratosis (thickening of the nail plate)

Examination of the hand:
- Look, feel, move, and the functional status of the patient.
- Look for a skin rash of psoriasis or any muscle wasting, joint deformity, scar, or rheumatoid nodule.
- Feel for joint tenderness and swelling as well as overlying warmness.

Movement:
- Prayer sign
- Reversed prayer sign, Buttoning or unbuttoning and fest compression (functional status).

Characteristic findings in the psoriatic arthropathy are:
- Asymmetrical oligoarthritis with DIP joint involvement with or without characteristic nail changes.
- Symmetrical polyarthritis (like rheumatoid arthritis, persistently seronegative) with or without characteristic nail changes.
- Arthritis mutilans, deforming and destructive arthritis leading to shortened fingers.
- Evidence of dactylitis with sausage digit.

If the history suggests inflammatory back pain, the spine should be examined as well.

If there is a suggestive history of uveitis or iritis, then examine the eye.

If the patient has a history of chest pain or breathlessness, then examine the cardio-respiratory system.

Feedback to the Patient and Respond to the Patient's Concerns

Candidate: You said at the beginning that you have scalp and elbow psoriasis. Now you find it difficult to perform your job as a painter and decorator due to hand joint pain and swelling. Is there anything else or any concerns?

Patient: Can you tell me, what is wrong with me?

Candidate: The pattern of joint disease in hands, nail changes, and plaques on your scalp and elbow suggest you have a condition called psoriatic arthropathy. We will need to carry out some investigations to confirm our diagnosis and exclude other possibilities. This will include some blood tests and X-rays. If confirmed, we will refer you to an MDT involving a joint doctor, skin doctor, physiotherapist, occupational therapist, and social worker to give you the proper management plan.

As long as you are concerned about your job, our occupational therapist can help you in this matter. They can guide you on how to perform your activities and find more options for you.

I am glad to know that you stopped drinking, and also, you do not smoke. Actually, both of the factors can trigger psoriasis.

Do you have any other concerns? Thanks.

Discussion with Examiner

Examiner: Would you please represent your case?

Candidate:

This middle-aged man presented with inflammatory arthritis involving the hand joints, and he has a history of psoriasis under treatment.

On examination—he has asymmetrical arthropathy involving mainly DIP joints. There is pitting of the fingernails and onycholysis. Some of the nail plates are thickened, and there is a thick scale (hyperkeratosis).

There are characteristic lesions of psoriasis at the elbow and scalp. The plaque is circular with well-demarcated edges, redness with a silvery scaly surface.

So, in summary, my diagnosis would be psoriatic arthropathy.

Examiner: How will you investigate?

Candidate: At first, I would like to do some basic blood tests such as:
- CBC, ESR, and CRP looking for anemia and raised inflammatory markers.
- Urine R/M/E, serum creatinine, serum electrolytes, and LFTs.

Then I would perform autoantibodies such as rheumatoid arthritis, anti-CCP antibody, ANA (usually seronegative).

Other tests include:
- X-ray of the hand joints (to look for erosive change with a pencil-in-cup deformity in severe cases).
- USG and isotope bone scan if the plain X-ray is inconclusive.

Examiner: How will you treat this case?

Candidate: I would like to treat the case under an MDT, and the mainstay of treatment is methotrexate, which is effective against both skin disease and arthritis. Hydroxychloroquine is best avoided as it can exacerbate skin psoriasis.
- NSAIDs for pain relief as well as an intra-articular steroid.
- Local cortisone injections are very effective for enthesitis.
- Steroids are used with caution as a significant flare of skin disease usually occurs on their withdrawal.
- If the patient's disease is severe enough, then anti-TNF blockers (infliximab) can be prescribed, which effectively control joint and skin involvement.

Examiner: What is the precipitating factor of psoriasis?

Candidate:
- Drugs (e.g., beta-blockers, chloroquine, hydroxychloroquine, lithium, terbinafine, interferon, NSAIDs, and steroids).
- Physical trauma (Koebner phenomenon)
- Infections (mainly beta-hemolytic *Streptococcus*; guttate psoriasis)
- Psychological stress
- Alcohol
- Tobacco
- Climate (psoriasis tends to flare in cold temperatures, although some facial psoriasis is worsened by exposure to sunlight).

Pleural Effusion

Your role: You are the Doctor in General Medicine Outpatient.

Patient details: Mr Anna Sami, 60-year-old man.

Clinical problem: Increasingly breathlessness with chest discomfort for 2 months.

(*Once you get this clinical scenario, you will get 5 minutes to start this station for two scenarios. At that time, start to think about your diagnosis and differential diagnoses and plan for taking focused history as well as focused examination.*)

[*Differential diagnosis*: Ischemic heart disease with heart failure, chronic obstructive pulmonary disease (COPD) with bronchogenic carcinoma with pleurisy (pleural effusion), and COPD with empyema (pyogenic or tubercular).]

(*Once you enter the room, search for a spot diagnosis; cachexia, clubbing, tar staining, inhaler, sputum pot, breathlessness suggest COPD complicated by bronchogenic carcinoma.*)

Introduction, Permission, and Identification

Candidate: Hello Mr Sami, good morning. I am Mohammad Ali. I am one of the working doctors here today. I have been asked to see you. At first, I would like to take a history, after that I will examine you as well. Is that okay?

Patient: Good morning, yes…

Candidate: Thank you for coming. Please tell me your full name.

Patient: I am Anna Sami

Candidate: And may I confirm your age, please?

Patient: I am 60-year-old.

Focused History

Candidate: Okay, Mr Sami, may I ask you what brings you here today? Please tell me in your own words.

Patient: Over the last 2 months, I have experienced increased shortness of breath and currently, climbing the stairs is getting harder with some chest discomfort. I am also worried because I have lost 3 kg weight over this period.

Analyze the Symptoms

Candidate: Okay, would you please tell me a little bit more about your breathlessness?

- What about the onset and progression, and do you use extra pillows during sleep (orthopnea)?
- Do you ever wake up at night with a feeling of breathlessness [paroxysmal nocturnal dyspnea (PND)]?
- Functional status of the patient, exercise tolerance.
- Any aggravating factors or relieving factors.
- Do you have a cough?
- Do you have any industrial or occupational exposure to asbestosis or coal recently or in the past?
- Do you smoke or drink alcohol? If smoke, then how much, for how long?

Patient: My symptoms started 2 months ago with mild shortness of breath. I used to feel short of breath when working in my garden or when I went for a walk in the evening. Over the past week, I have also felt shortness of breath at rest. I have to use extra pillows at bedtime now for my breathing difficulty. Also, I have had a dry cough for the last 3 months, which is worse in the morning. I am a lifelong smoker but worked in a shipyard for 12 years when I was young.

Candidate: What about your chest discomfort? Please tell me more about it (onset, site, progression, severity, any aggravating or relieving factor)?

Patient: I have had mild left-sided chest pain for the last 1 week, which aggravates during deep breathing.

Candidate: It is okay, you have already told me about weight loss, please tell me more about it. (How long? How much? Intentional or unintentional? Appetite? Exercise, diet, and other systemic manifestation, particularly GIT or thyroid?)

Patient: I have lost 3 kg weight over this period and also lost my appetite.

Candidate: Do you have any fever? Do you have palpitation? Any swelling of the limbs? Any lumps or bumps anywhere in your body?

Patient: No.

Quick Systemic Review, Past Medical History, Family History, Treatment, Social History According to Your Differentials

If it is not asked previously during initial history taking or incompletely asked, then take a full history of a particular portion to make it complete.

Candidate: Now I would like to ask some general questions, is that okay with you?
- Do you have any history of LOC or dizziness? Do you have any abnormal shaking of the body?
- Do you have any similar condition or any other history of disease in your past?
- Have you attended any consultant or general physician or specialist for this problem? What was their impression? Did you receive any diagnosis? What treatment have you received? Did they work?
- Have you ever been admitted to the hospital in the past or have any history of surgery?
- May I ask what medication you take? Do you take any over-the-counter medications or herbal medicines, or any recreational drugs? Are you allergic to any medicine or anything else?
- Is there anyone else in your family with this type of problem or any long-standing illness that run in your family like DM, hypertension, stroke, thyroid problem, or anything else?
- Do you work at the moment? Are you independent in activities of daily living? Who is at home with you, or who is supporting you now? Do you have children?

Have I missed anything, or do you want to add anything more?

Would you mind if I go on to examine you?

Focused Examination

Here the patient is a heavy smoker, and he has a history of increasing breathlessness with dry cough and significant weight loss but no fever. He has had a history of asbestos exposure in his young life, so that most likely diagnosis would be:
- Bronchogenic carcinoma with COPD or mesothelioma.
- Cardiovascular disease, though it is unlikely to have because the patient has no cardiovascular risk factors.

The focused examination would be respiratory system then, CVS as well.

The expected findings would be:
- For bronchogenic carcinoma:
  - Clubbing, cachexia, lymphadenopathy, and anemia.
  - As well as evidence of Pancoast syndrome such as Horner's syndrome with wasting of the small muscles of the hand with dermatomal sensory loss (C8, T1 lesion).

Respiratory system examination is vital here to see:
- Evidence of pleural effusion or collapse or consolidation for the mass lesion.
- Any evidence of cor-pulmonale (increased JVP, edema).
- Respiratory failure (cyanosis, flapping tremors).
- Pulmonary hypertension [palpable P2, left parasternal heave, tricuspid regurgitation (TR) murmur].

- Evidence of COPD (vesicular breath sounds with prolonged expiration with Rhonchi with or without crepitation and tar staining).

Cardiovascular

Evidence of AF, heart failure, raised JVP, edema, or murmur as well.

Feedback to the Patient and Respond to the Patient's Concerns

Candidate: You said at the beginning that the main problem was increasing breathlessness, chest discomfort, and weight loss. Is there anything else troubling you that we have missed or any expectations or any concerns?

Patient: Why am I having this shortness of breath, Doctor?

Candidate: I suspect the cause of your shortness of breath may be because of a condition called pleural effusion, which means a collection of the fluids around your right lung, and we need to find out what might be the cause of it. We are also concerned about your unintentional weight loss and your smoking history, as well as asbestos exposure in your young life. To help with your shortness of breath, we may need to drain this fluid of your lung to make you feel better as well as we would like to investigate the fluid to find out the underlying cause.

I would suggest getting admission to carry out some basic blood tests, chest X-ray, CT scan of your chest, and will arrange an urgent appointment with the lung physician.

In addition, I strongly advise you to stop smoking immediately, which may worsen your condition more.

Do you have any other concerns? Thank you for spending time with me today.

Discussion with Examiner

Examiner: Please present your case.

Candidate:
_____

Mr Sami is a lifelong smoker and worked in a shipyard for 12 years when he was young. He has had a history of increasing breathlessness with chest discomfort and significant weight loss for the last 2 months.

On examination, Mr Sami is a skinny gentleman; he is clubbed and has positive findings, including decreased chest expansion, stony dull percussion note from base to mid-zone, decreased air entry, and vocal resonance in the right side of the chest.

Though, he did not have a voice specific neurological complaint, Mr Sami has a marked intention tremor, impaired finger nose coordination, and dysdiadochokinesia. These are suggestive of cerebellar syndrome.

Given that, this gentleman has a right-sided pleural effusion with no other signs of fluid overload.

_____

With these clinical scenarios, I suspect he has a right-sided exudative pleural effusion secondary to:

- Malignancy possibility of mesothelioma due to potential asbestosis exposure or bronchogenic carcinoma due to potentially smoking history.
- Less likely possibilities would be a chronic infection like tuberculous pleural effusion or pulmonary infarction as well.
- The cerebellar disease is likely to be paraneoplastic as he is nonalcoholic.

Examiner: How will you investigate the case?

Candidate: At first, I would like to go for routine blood tests which include CBC with ESR with CRP, U&E, and LFTs.

Then I would go for a chest X-ray to confirm the diagnosis with doubt from the clinical examination.

Next, I go for ultrasonography; useful primarily as guidance for aspirating effusions may also help provide more information about pleural effusion; e.g., loculated or not, areas of pleural thickening.

The most important step would be—pleural fluid aspiration and analysis; this is the key diagnostic investigation, and it should be analyzed for:

Appearance:
- Turbid fluid with a foul smell is suggestive of empyema.
- Hemorrhagic effusion suggests malignancy, pulmonary infarction, rarely infection (particularly tuberculosis).
- Cloudy white or yellow fluid suggests chylothorax.

Biochemistry:
- Establish whether the effusion is an exudate or transudate. Here light's criteria can help to differentiate exudative from the transudative effusions (<25 g/L = transudative; >35 g/L = exudative; in case of 25–35 g/L and pleural fluid protein + serum protein ratio >0.5, then effusion is an exudative).
- Reduced pH (<7.2) is strongly suggestive of empyema and indicates intercostal drain insertion.
- Very low glucose concentrations (<2.2 mmol/L) are suggestive of severe infection/empyema, autoimmune rheumatic disease (rheumatoid arthritis, SLE) or esophageal rupture.
- Very elevated lactate dehydrogenase (LDH) concentrations are suggestive of severe infection/empyema, malignancy or autoimmune disease (rheumatoid arthritis, SLE).
- Raised adenosine deaminase (ADA) suggests tuberculosis.
- Raised pleural fluid amylase is a feature of pancreatitis, although it may also be found in bacterial pneumonia, carcinoma, and esophageal rupture.

Cytology:
- Predominantly, neutrophilia suggests bacterial infection, whereas lymphocytosis is found most often in malignancy, lymphoproliferative disease (lymphoma), tuberculosis and autoimmune disease. Cytology will be positive in 60% of malignant effusions.

Microbiology:
- Sputum, pleural fluid, and blood should be sent for microscopy, culture and sensitivity, acid-fast bacteria (AFB) staining and gene expert test to exclude underlying TB or pyogenic infections.

The investigation following respiratory review (MDT) including:
- Staging CT chest
- Plural biopsy
- Thoracoscopy or video-assisted thoracoscopic surgery
- Bronchoscopy, if there is a central-obstructive lesion and CT guided FNAC for a peripheral lesion to establish the histological diagnosis of lung carcinoma.

Examiner: How would you manage this case?

Candidate: The patient has likely inoperable lung carcinoma, and it should be discussed at an MDT meeting concentrating on relieving symptoms and discussion of the possible chemotherapy.

As long as the underlying lung cancer is diagnosed, the effusion can be drained.

Subsequent management would include:
- Insertion of a long-term catheter to drain further pleural effusions.
- The patient may have pleurodesis, and pleurodesis could be performed medically at the bedside or via thoracoscopy.

Chronic Obstructive Pulmonary Disease

Your role: You are the Doctor in the General Medical Clinic.

Patient details: Mr Donald Tiverton, a 55-year-old man.

Clinical problem: Increasingly breathlessness recently with weight loss.

(Once you get this clinical scenario, you will get 5 minutes to start this station for two scenarios. At that time, start to think about your diagnosis and differential diagnoses and plan for taking focused history as well as focused examination.)

(*Differential diagnosis*: COPD; COPD with bronchogenic carcinoma; tuberculosis with pleural effusion or pneumothorax; lymphoma with pleural effusion; heart failure; severe anemia with underlying malignancy.)

(*Once you enter the room, search for a spot diagnosis; tar staining, sputum pot, inhaler, clubbing, cachexia, breathlessness suggests COPD or COPD with bronchogenic carcinoma or infections.*)

Introduction, Permission, and Identification

Candidate: Good morning. My name is Mohammad Ali. One of the working doctors here today. I have been asked to see you. Is that okay with you?

Patient: Good morning, doctor...

Candidate: Thank you for coming. I would like to start by taking your full name, please...

Patient: I am Donald Tiverton.

Candidate: May I confirm your age, please?

Patient: I am 55-year-old.

Focused History

Candidate: Okay, Mr Tiverton, may I ask you what brings you here today? Please tell me in your own words.

Patient: I am feeling shortness of breath which is gradually worsening for the past 2 months. I have also lost some weight. Last night, I felt more breathless and got admitted to this hospital.

Analyze the Symptoms

Candidate: I am sorry to hear about your condition. Would you please tell me more about your breathlessness?

The most important questions to be asked:

- When did you first notice breathlessness? Were you completely all right before this period or, when did you last felt well?
- Did it come on suddenly or gradually? Is it increasing, decreasing gradually, or it is the same?
- Do you feel breathlessness at rest, or it is exertional, e.g., when do you feel breathless, like during running or fast walking or climbing upstairs or just walking around the house or even at rest?
- How does this breathlessness affect your daily life? How far could you walk before you had this breathlessness?
- Do you struggle for sleep due to breathlessness, and do you use extra pillows for sleeping?
- Are you on any inhalers? What is the color of your inhaler? Is it blue or brown or pink? Do you use a nebulizer for breathlessness?
- Is there any particular time in the day when your symptoms (cough and breathlessness) getting worse (diurnal variation)?
- Does anything in the particular trigger or aggravate the cough such as dust, pollen, fumes, or anything else?

- Do you have any industrial or occupational exposures to coal or asbestosis?
- Do you have any chest pain, palpitation, leg swelling, or any history of heart disease?
- Do you smoke? How many sticks in a day? How many years are you smoking?

Patient: I have been suffering from chronic chest problems for the past 10–15 years. Doctors told me the condition is smoker's lung, and I am taking inhalers for this. My breathing has gotten noticeably worse over the past 2 months. I had to stop working as a cleaner because of my breathing problem. I used to climb stairs and go shopping without any difficulties, but now I have to stop 2–3 times. I do smoke and taking 30–40 cigarettes per day for 35 years.

Candidate: Do you have any fever, cough, or any other problems with your breathlessness?

Patient: I have no fever, but I have a cough.

Candidate: Okay, you have a cough. Is it dry or productive? If it is productive, then ask about the amount of sputum–scanty or copious? What is the color of sputum? Is it whitish, yellowish, or greenish? Have you noticed any blood in phlegm?

Patient: I have had a cough for several years, producing brown mucus, but have not been coughing up blood. I have needed antibiotics frequently from general physician over the past 4 months while I cough up green sputum.

Candidate: Now, tell me a little bit more about your weight loss?
- How much weight have you lost? Over how long? How is your appetite?
- Is the weight loss voluntarily or involuntarily?
- Does it coincide with your change in diet or physical activity, or lifestyle?
- Have you noticed any bowel changes, any diarrhea or constipation, or any blood in stool?

Patient: I have lost my appetite. Even I have lost some weight, and it is around 6 kg in the last 4 months. The weight loss has been unintentional, and I have never been dieting. My bowels are regular, no bleeding, no tummy pain.

Quick Systemic Review, Past Medical History, Family History, Treatment, Social History According to Your Differentials

If it is not asked previously during initial history taking or incompletely asked, then take a full history of a particular portion to make it complete.

Candidate: At this moment I would like to ask some general questions, is that okay with you?
- Do you have headaches, dizziness or LOC, blurring of vision, any abnormal shakiness or weakness of limbs?
- Do you have any joint pain, skin rash, nausea, vomiting, or abdominal pain?
- What about your waterworks? Do you have any change in color, frequency, or frothy urine or any pain in passing urine or anything else?
- Do you have any similar condition or any other history of disease in your past?
- Have you attended any consultant or general physician or specialist for this problem? What was their impression? Did you receive any diagnosis? What treatment have you received? Did they work?
- May I ask what medication you take? Do you take any over-the-counter medications or herbal medicines, or any recreational drugs? Are you allergic to any medicine or anything else?
- Is there anyone in your family with this type of problem or any long-standing illness that runs in your family such as DM, hypertension, stroke, thyroid, or other autoimmune diseases, or anything else?
- Do you drink? What are you doing for a living? Are you married? Who is at home with you, or who is supporting you now? Do you have children?

Is there anything else that I have missed, or do you want to add anything more? Okay. Thank you, would you mind if I go on to examine you?

Focused Examination

From the history patient has COPD but complaining of weight loss with increasing breathlessness and requiring antibiotics several times. So, underlying malignancy, as well as a chronic infection like tuberculosis, should be excluded first.

Here, most important part of the examination would be the respiratory system with important peripheral signs such as:
- Anemia
- Lymphadenopathy, particularly cervical, supraclavicular, or axillary (malignancy, tuberculosis)
- Evidence of weight loss
- Most importantly clubbing
- Evidence of Pancoast syndrome that includes Horner's syndrome as well as wasting of the small muscles of the hand and sensory loss (C8, T1 lesion)

Then examine for respiratory system particularly for:
- Respiratory rate and evidence of respiratory failures such as flapping tremor and cyanosis.
- Evidence of PHTN including raised JVP and parasternal heave, loud P2, and TR murmur.
- Any evidence of collapse, or pleural effusion, or signs of consolidation.
- The most important auscultation finding would be a vesicular breath sound with prolonged expiration with Rhonchi with or without crepitation.

Examine for peripheral edema to see the evidence of cor pulmonale.

Other important systems would be CVS as a differential of breathlessness, urine for protein and sugar, pulse oximetry, and bedside ECG as well.

Feedback to the Patient to Respond to the Patient's Concern

Candidate: You said at the beginning that the main problem were increasing cough with shortness of breath and weight loss, is there anything else troubling you that we have missed or do you have any concerns?

Patient: Why do I get become breathless, doctor?

Candidate: Okay, you have had COPD for several years, but recently it becomes worse with increasing breathlessness and cough. You also have had a history of some weight loss. This needs to be investigated urgently. So, we will start with some blood tests, sputum samples to look for infection, and a chest X-ray. Then, we will refer you for more detailed scans (CT) of your chest and arrange an appointment to see a chest specialist who may arrange further investigations.

Patient: Have I got a cancer doctor?

Candidate: May I know why you are worried about cancer?

Patient: Doctor, my eldest brother has recently been diagnosed with bowel cancer. I am afraid I also get cancer!

Candidate: There are several different possible causes for becoming more breathless and also losing weight. These vary from less serious problems such as infections to more serious problems. I am sorry to say that; unfortunately, lung cancer may also present this way. So, we need to carry out these tests to find out what is causing your problems.

Meanwhile, it is very important for you to stop smoking immediately that worsens your condition more.

Patient: Is it worth stopping smoking now? Is not it just too late?

Candidate: Lung damage due to smoking is indeed irreversible. However, as it reduces the ongoing damage to your lungs, it is always good to stop smoking. We can help you to stop smoking by referring you to the smoking cessation clinic.

Do you have any other concerns? Thank you for spending time with me.

Discussion with Examiner

Examiner: Please present your case.

Candidate:

Mr Tiverton is a heavy smoker and known COPD patient, now presented with chronic cough, increasing breathlessness, and significant weight loss.

The positive clinical findings are:

He is breathless at rest (RR–20 breaths/min) and has evidence of an oxygen concentrator by the side of the bed.

There is pursed-lip breathing during prolonged expiration.

There is nicotine staining on the fingers.

The trachea is centrally placed with a reduced cricoid-notch distance and tracheal tug.

The patient uses accessory muscles of respiration, and there is indrawing of the lower intercostal muscles on inspiration.

The percussion note is hyperresonant throughout both lungs field; breath sounds are vesicular with prolonged expiration with added sound Rhonchi.

- No signs of PHTN like palpable P2 or right parasternal heave.
- No evidence of respiratory failures like flapping tremor or cyanosis.
- No evidence of cor pulmonale like raised JVP or peripheral edema.

In summary, the diagnosis is an acute exacerbation of COPD but most importantly, associated lower respiratory tract infection or tuberculosis or malignancy needs to be excluded.

Examiner: How will you investigate this case?

Candidate: At first, I would like to do routine blood tests, including FBC, ESR, CRP, U&E, TFT, and arterial blood gas analysis.

Other investigations include:
- Chest X-ray, most importantly
- ECG; P-pulmonale (right atrium hypertrophy) and signs of right ventricular hypertrophy
- Lung function test
- Sputum for microscopy, Gram staining, AFB staining and culture and sensitivity, and gene expert test for tuberculosis.
- CT chest (HRCT) with or without staging for cancer
- Echo if clinical suspicion of PHTN, CCF, or cor pulmonale.

Examiner: How will you manage this case?

Candidate: Treatment depends on the cause. Most importantly, I will treat any infections, if found and also rule out any underlying malignancy.

The next step would be—stop smoking and refer to smoking cessation services (a combination of counseling and medical therapy).

Pulmonary rehabilitation and supplements include oxygen or other nutritional requirements, would also be considered for this patient.

Next, I will arrange a respiratory referral for consideration of further investigation based on the result of the above tests, e.g., bronchoscopy to exclude obstructing lesions.

Pulmonary Embolism

Your role: You are the Registrar in the General Medical Clinic

Patient details: Mrs Polin, a 30-year-old lady.

Clinical problem: 4-days history of chest pain with breathlessness.

(*Once you get this clinical scenario, you will get 5 minutes to start this station for two scenarios. At that time, start to think about your diagnosis and differential diagnoses and plan for taking focused history as well as focused examination.*)

[*Differential diagnosis:* As the patient is young, here differential diagnosis would be pulmonary embolism, pneumonia, pneumothorax, cardiac causes (valvular, congenital, myocarditis, pericarditis, rarely ischemic) or functional.]

(*Once you enter the room, search for a spot diagnosis; butterfly rash, arthropathy with evidence of DVT suggests secondary APLA syndrome.*)

Introduction, Permission, and Identification

Candidate: Good morning. I am Mohammad Ali, one of the working doctors here today. I have been asked to see you; is that okay with you?

Patient: Good morning, doctor...

Candidate: Thank you for coming. I would like to start by taking your full name, please...

Patient: I am Polin.

Candidate: May I confirm your age, please?

Patient: I am 30-year-old.

Focused History

Candidate: Okay, Mrs Polin, would you please tell me what brings you here today? Please tell me in your own words.

Patient: I gave birth to a healthy baby boy 10 days ago. After coming home, I am feeling right-sided chest pain, and I notice the pain increased with coughing and breathing. I feel breathless while climbing stairs, walking a few steps, or doing household activities.

Analyze the Complaints

Candidate: So, you are complaining of chest pain. Could you please tell me a little bit more about your chest pain?
- When did the chest pain start? Did it come on suddenly or gradually?
- Where is the pain–is it in the center or side of the chest? Please localize it. Does it move anywhere like jaw, neck, arm, or back?
- What is the nature of your pain- is it dull, sharp or band like shooting pain around the chest or burning in nature?
- Is it constant or intermittent? If intermittent, then how frequently do you experience chest pain?
- Is there anything else that increases your chest pain like walking, exertion, taking deep breaths, movement, taking a meal or any posture?
- Do you feel pain at rest? Or anything else that decrease your chest pain like painkiller, antacid, or sublingual nitrate?

Patient: I have persistent chest pain that came on suddenly on the right side of the chest, but it does not move anywhere. It increases during coughing or deep breathing and is slightly relieved after taking paracetamol.

Candidate: Now, please tell me a little bit more about your breathlessness?
- When did you notice the breathlessness at first?
- Did it come on suddenly or gradually?

- Is it constant/on and off (intermittent)? If intermittent, then how frequently do you experience breathlessness?
- Is there anything else that worse your breathlessness?
- Is it exertional, or is it present at rest? Does lying down make it worse (orthopnea)?
- Is there anything else that relieves your breathlessness, like relief with rest or any medications like sublingual GTN or inhaler?

Patient: I have on and off breathlessness that increases on exertion like climbing upstairs and relieves with rest.

Candidate: When the history suggests pulmonary embolism, then targeted history to identify the risk factors of pulmonary embolism.

Other Important Targeted Histories

- Have you noticed any changes in bowel motion or your waterworks or any blood in passing urine or stool (underlying malignancy)?
- Do you have any joint pain, skin rash, mouth ulcer (underlying SLE or APLA syndrome)? Do you have any difficulty in standing from a sitting position? Have you noticed any change in the color of the hands in cold weather or cold exposure (other CTD for APLA syndrome)?
- Do you have any history of recent surgery or recent long-haul travel, any clot previously or any history of miscarriages previously?
- Do you have anyone in the family who ever had a clot in the legs or lungs, or does any clotting problem run in your family (protein C and S deficiency, Factor V Leiden)?
- What about your medication history? Are you taking any regular medicines, any over-the-counter or oral contraceptive pills (OCPs) or any recreational drugs? Are you allergic to any medications or anything else?
- Do you have any calf pain or swelling in the limbs (DVT)?

Patient: I was on a blood thinner (Enoxaparin) injection daily in the later stage of my pregnancy because of my previous three miscarriages. I was advised to continue it after giving birth, but I have not taken anything since I left the hospital. I think this might be for stopping the medicines. I do not have any history of a clot in my lung or no one in my family with clots. I have nothing else whatever you asked.

Candidate: I am sorry to hear about your previous miscarriages. Would you like to tell me in which period of your pregnancy you got miscarriages?

Patient: It was during my early pregnancy.

Quick Systemic Review, Past Medical History, Family History, Treatment, Social History According to Your Differentials

If it is not asked previously during initial history taking or incompletely asked, then take a full history of a particular portion to make it complete.

Candidate: Okay. Now I would like to ask some general questions, is that okay with you?
- Do you have any cough, phlegm, or bloody sputum? Do you have any fever, weight loss, or loss of appetite?
- Do you have any heart racing, irregular beat, or swelling of the limbs?
- Any weakness, dizzy spell, LOC, headache, visual disturbance, shaking of the body, or anything else?
- Do you have any similar condition or any other history of disease in your past?
- Have you attended any consultant or general physician or specialist for this problem? What was their impression? Did you receive any diagnosis? What treatment have you received? Did they work?
- Have you ever been admitted to the hospital in the past or have any history of surgery?
- Is there anyone else in your family with this type of problem or any long-standing illness that run in your family like DM, hypertension, stroke, thyroid or any autoimmune disease or anything else?
- Do you smoke? Do you drink? What are you doing for a living?
- Who is at home with you, or who is supporting you now? Do you have any other children? How are you coping with this, or how do you

take care of yourself and your baby with this problem? Do you need any help?

Have I missed anything, or do you want to add anything more?

Thank you, would you mind if I go on to examine you?

Focused Examination

The focused examination would be—respiratory system, CVS and most importantly, look for evidence of DVT.

Cardiovascular: Pulse, blood pressure, SaO_2, cyanosis, clubbing, JVP, any evidence of PHTN, or any evidence of heart failure (crepitation), heart murmur, or rub.

Respiratory system: Any evidence of pleural rub, effusion, or consolidation for pulmonary embolism or any other evidence of respiratory diseases causing chest pain and breathlessness.

Evidence of Deep Vein Thrombosis in the Lower Limb

Unilateral leg swelling should be compared with the other normal leg, and proximal extension into the thigh should be assessed. The calf in DVT feels bulky and indurated and moves "en masse", causing discomfort when move side-to-side. Any evidence of superficial vein or overlying skin changes such as erythema, warmth, or cyanotic hue.

No evidence of knee joint pain or swelling or tenderness.

Evidence of underlying cause of pulmonary embolism (oral ulceration, joint deformity, bilateral limb swelling for nephritic syndrome).

Feedback to the Patient and Respond to the Patient's Concerns

Candidate: You said at the beginning that the main problem was chest pain and breathlessness developed just after delivery of a child, and you have had a history of three miscarriages. Is there anything else troubling you that we have not covered or any expectations or any concerns?

Patient: What is my problem?

Candidate: I suspect the cause of your symptoms is due to a condition called pulmonary embolism means a clot in the blood channels of your lungs. The obstetrician gave you blood thinning injections daily during your pregnancy for something called APLA syndrome. The condition leads to recurrent miscarriages that you have had in the past and makes clots more likely. You said you stopped the injection that also put you at more risk to have a clot. I would suggest getting admission to give you the full doses of injections and carry out a scan to confirm the presence of a clot in the lung. Moreover, I would like to do some blood tests to establish APLA syndrome and exclude other possibilities causing this type of symptom as well. Is that okay?

Patient: Can I take the pill?

Candidate: Well, some pills like combined OCPs can increase the risk of clot formation. If you have a confirmed clot, your obstetrician will be able to advise you further about contraception, and it is possible to go onto the progesterone-only pill whilst breastfeeding, and it is better in terms of clot risk. Other alternative contraceptives are available, including coils, Copper-T, and injections.

Patient: How long do I need treatment if it is a clot?

Candidate: This will depend on whether you have any provocating factors for developing clots. We need more information about why you were on blood thinning injections as this will affect the length of time you need the blood thinner medication. You will need treatment for at least 6 months, but you may need longer-term anticoagulation, and we will ask the blood doctor to see you in the clinic to advice about this. They will be able to decide how long they think you will need the treatment.

Patient: Can I go home tonight?

Candidate: I would advise staying in and having the scans as an inpatient. We will get in touch with the obstetricians to see if you can be admitted to their ward and keep your baby with you.

Discussion with Examiner

Examiner: Could you please present your case?

Candidate:

The young lady presented with an acute history of pleuritic chest pain and breathlessness shortly after giving birth to a baby. This was on the background of three miscarriages before 12 weeks in the past. But no FH of DVT.

Examination revealed chest wall tenderness, but there were no signs of PHTN, pleural effusion, pleuritis, or any obvious signs of DVT.

Given this most likely diagnosis, I would like to rule out pulmonary embolism.

Examiner: What would be your differential diagnosis?

Candidate:
- The differentials I would like to consider would be infection; however, the history was not consistent with this, nor was the examination.
- I would also like to consider a pneumothorax; however, the physical examination did not give any evidence of it.
- Furthermore, I would like to consider pericarditis, although the history was not of positional chest pain, and the examination did not reveal anything that would make me consider pericarditis.
  Lastly, I would like to consider musculoskeletal chest pain, given the chest wall tenderness.

Examiner: How would you investigate this case?

Candidate: Stratification of the probability of pulmonary embolism based on history, examination, investigations, and two-level Wells score.
- Initially, I would start by doing simple blood tests—CBC and inflammatory markers to look for any sign of infection and anemia.
- I would like to do baseline U&E and LFTs as well as a clotting profile (prothrombin time (PT) with international normalized ratio (INR) and activated partial thromboplastin time (APTT)].

Most importantly,
- An ECG; the most common ECG findings are a normal ECG or sinus tachycardia. I would also look for signs of right heart strain, non-specific changes in T-wave and ST segments.
- The chest X-ray can be normal (want to look for small effusions, segmental, or subsegmental collapse).
- Arterial blood gas (ABG) may be normal; I would like to check the alveolar-arterial (A-a) gradient to indicate a ventilation perfusion (V/Q) mismatch.

Then, I would like to use the NICE recommend two-level Wells score to decide on the following management steps.

If pulmonary embolism is likely according to Wells score, NICE recommends:
- *Computed tomography pulmonary angiogram (CTPA)*: If CTPA contraindicated (allergy to contrast media, renal impairment, or those in whom the radiation risk would be too high), then the VQ scan indicated. If this test (CTPA or VQ) is negative and DVT is suspected, I will arrange a Doppler ultrasound of the legs to confirm/exclude DVT.

If a two-level Wells score is unlikely pulmonary embolism, NICE advises to:
- Check D-dimer; if raised, arrange CTPA. If normal, excludes pulmonary embolism, but the patient needs to be aware of the symptoms and signs of pulmonary embolism and when to return to the hospital (safety-netting).

NICE advice considering alternative diagnosis if:
- Patient with an unlikely two-level Wells score and either a negative D-dimer test or a positive D-dimer test and a negative CTPA.
- Patient with a likely two-level Wells score and both a negative CTPA and no suspected DVT.

D-dimer is, however, unlikely to be helpful in this patient as it is likely to be elevated with recent childbirth and as she has a high clinical probability of pulmonary embolism, I will arrange a CTPA (scores 4+, an alternative diagnosis is less likely than pulmonary embolism).

Note: If unstable (massive pulmonary embolism/shock), urgent CTPA but if too unstable for CTPA, then bedside echo to look at right heart (assess for right ventricular dysfunction/dilation) and consider thrombolytic therapy (if no contraindication).

Role of thrombophilia screen while unanticoagulated; lupus anticoagulant in the meantime.

Examiner: If we think of a different scenario in a patient presenting with a suspected pulmonary embolism who is unwell (hemodynamically unstable, hypoxia, tachypnea), how would you manage that?

Candidate: I would approach any patient who was unwell in an airway, breathing, circulation, disability and exposure (ABCDE) manner, I might wish to consider thrombolytic therapy if there is no contraindication.

Examiner: If there is a contraindication to thrombolysis in such a patient with a massive pulmonary embolism who is hemodynamically unstable, is there any other treatment you could consider?

Candidate: Then I would consider a surgical thrombectomy.

Atrial Fibrillation

Your role: You are the Registrar in the General Medical Clinic.

Patient details: Mr Brown, 48-year-old.

Clinical problem: Episodic palpitation and chest pain for 6 months.

(Once you get this clinical scenario, you will get 5 minutes to start this station for two scenarios. At that time, start to think about your diagnosis and differential diagnoses and plan for taking focused history as well as focused examination.)

[*Differential diagnoses of episodic palpitation*:
- *Paroxysmal AF*: Rheumatic heart disease, ischemic heart disease, thyrotoxicosis, hypertension, and idiopathic.
- Supraventricular tachycardia (SVT)/atrio-ventricular node re-entrant tachycardia (AVNRT).
- Ventricular or atrial ectopics]

(Once you enter the room, search for a spot diagnosis; exophthalmos, goiter, pretibial myxedema, thyroid acropachy suggests AF due to thyrotoxic Graves' disease.)

Introduction, Permission, and Identification

Candidate: Good morning. My name is Mohammad Ali. One of the working doctors here today. I have been asked to see you. Is that, ok?

Patient: Good morning, doctor. Ok.

Candidate: Thank you for coming. I would like to start by taking your full name, please...

Patient: I am Adam Brown.

Candidate: May I confirm your age, please?

Patient: I am 40-year-old.

Focused History

Candidate: Ok. Mr Brown, would you please tell me what brings you here today. Please tell me in your own word.

Patient: I am getting several episodes of racing heartbeat. I feel like my heart is pumping in a very weird way. My heartbeat does not feel regular when this happens. I also get chest pain and sometimes feel short of breath too.

Analyze the Symptoms

Candidate: Would you please tell me a little bit more about your racing heartbeat? [If the patient uses the word "palpitation", then ask how does palpitation feel like? Is it racing/tapping heart–for fast arrhythmia; missed/extra beat–ventricular ectopics; pounding in the neck/everything stopped for a moment–for bradycardia/atrio-ventricular (AV) dissociation].

Important questions to be asked are:
- When did you first notice it?
- Do you have it all the time or on and off? Or, how often do you experience palpitation?
- How do they start and stop? Is it sudden or gradual onset? How long does this episode last?
- Did you take your pulse at that time? If so, was it fast or slow? Was it regular or irregular?
- Is there anything that triggers the episode like stress, caffeine, or exertion?
- Is there anything that helps to stop the episode?
- Do you have chest pain or breathlessness, or leg swelling (associated symptoms)?
- Have you noticed any dizziness or LOC?

- Take history suggestive of thyrotoxicosis by asking–do you have weight loss? Do you have any preference for cold or hot weather or excessive sweating or diarrhea? Do you have tremors or shaking of limbs?
- Take history regarding vascular risk factors [hypertension, DM, dyslipidemia, smoking and past history of transient ischemic attack (TIA)-Do you have any history of sudden onset of weakness or loss of sensation, slurring of speech, or loss of vision in the past?]
- How are these symptoms affecting your daily life?
- Do you smoke or drink alcohol? If yes, then for how long and what is the amount?

Patient: I am usually well, but over the past few months, I have noticed episodes of fast racing of my heart lasting few seconds, particularly at night. These episodes have become a little more frequent over the past 6 months, and I thought this was due to stress. However, while walking this morning, I noticed a longer episode lasting an hour, and it felt different from usual. I felt my pulse and counted the rate of 120 beats/minute, and irregular too. Meanwhile, I have been hypertensive for the last 5 years and diabetic for 2 years; taking ramipril 5 mg daily and metformin 500 mg 12 hourly. I never smoke or drink alcohol.

Candidate: What about your chest pain [Follow site onset character radiation association time exacerbating/relieving factor and severity (SOCRATES)]?
- For how long? How did it start–suddenly or gradually?
- Where is the pain exactly in your chest?
- Is it getting better or worse?
- Could you describe the pain? Is it stabbing/heaviness/tearing/burning?
- Does it move anywhere else?
- Do you have it all the time or on and off?
- What makes it better? What makes it worse?
- How would it be on a scale from 0–10?

Patient: I have been suffering from chest pain with occasional shortness of breath for the last 6 months. Especially, when I do any work, walk or climb stairs, my chest pain worsens, and it gets better when I rest.

Quick Systemic Review, Past Medical History, Family History, Treatment, Social History According to Your Differentials

If it is not asked previously during initial history taking or incompletely asked then—take a full history of a particular portion to make it complete.

Candidate: At this moment I would like to ask some general questions, is that ok with you?
- Do you have a fever, weight loss, nausea, vomiting, or tummy pain? Do you have any joint pain or skin rash?
- Have you noticed any change in your bowel habit or waterworks?
- Do you have any similar condition or any other history of disease in your past?
- Have you attended any consultant or general physician or specialist for this problem? What was their impression? Did you receive any diagnosis? What treatment have you received? Did they work?
- Have you ever been admitted to the hospital in the past or have any history of surgery?
- May I ask what medication you take? Do you take any over-the-counter medications or herbal medicine, or any recreational drugs? Are you allergic to any medicine or anything else?
- Is there anyone in your family with this type of problem or any long-standing illness that runs in your family like DM, hypertension, stroke, thyroid or other autoimmune diseases, or anything else?
- What are you doing for a living? Are you married? Who is at home with you, or who is supporting you now? Do you have children? Are you independent in activities of daily living?

Have I missed anything, or do you want to tell me anything more? Ok, thank you. Would you mind if I go on to examine you now?

Focused Examination

From the history, the clinical diagnosis is paroxysmal AF with hypertension, DM, and stable angina. Here, the focused examination would be the CVS system. If there is any evidence of thyrotoxicosis (weight loss, tremor, diarrhea,

thyroid gland enlargement, or thyroid faces), then examine for thyroid status as well as thyroid gland and eye.
- *General appearance*: Features of thyrotoxic eye disease and shortness of breath.
- *Pulse*: Irregularly irregular pulse.
- *Face and neck*: Malar flush (mitral stenosis), carotid bruit, and goiter.
- *Precordium*: Feature of PHTN, valvular heart disease (murmur), heart failure (shifting of apex beat or crepitation or raised JVP or peripheral edema).
- *Neurological examination*: Focal neurological deficit for the previous stroke.

Feedback to the Patient and Respond to the Patient's Concerns

Candidate: You said at the beginning that the main problem was palpitation, chest pain, and breathlessness. Is there anything else that we have not covered or any concern?

Patient: Doctor, what is wrong with me? Can you tell me?

Candidate: I suspect the cause of your heart racing is due to an irregular heartbeat, called AF. As you have chest pain and shortness of breath on exertion, it suggests that there may have problems with the blood supply to the heart itself.

Initially, I would like to organize some investigations, starting with tracing of your heart (ECG), USG of the heart (echocardiography) and 24-hour measurement of your heart rhythm (Holter-monitoring), as well as some basic blood tests, TFT. We may also need to perform other tests to check the blood supply to the heart, such as coronary angiogram; it is a procedure to take images of the blood vessels that supply the heart with the help of a dye that we inject either through your wrist or groin. If the ECG confirms AF, we can start treatment right away.

Do you have any other concerns? Thank you very much for spending time with me today.

Discussion between Examiner and Candidate

Examiner: Would you please present your case?

Candidate:

This middle-aged gentleman is a known case of hypertension and diabetes (DM) presented with an episodic attack of palpitation, exertional chest pain, and breathlessness.

At this moment, the patient is in sinus rhythm; his pulse is 76 beats/minute, regular in rhythm with normal volume.

No evidence of valvular heart disease or heart failure or infective endocarditis, or PHTN as well.

No evidence of AF at this moment.

So, in summary, my diagnosis would be paroxysmal AF with underlining ischemic heart disease with hypertension and DM.

Examiner: How will you investigate the case?

Candidate: Initially, I would like to do some basic blood tests that include FBC with ESR, random blood sugar (RBS), HbA1c, lipid profile, U&E, TFT, magnesium (Mg), calcium, phosphate, Troponin I and coagulation profile (PT with INR).

Then I would like to do an ECG, chest X-ray, echocardiography to exclude structural heart diseases such as ischemia, mitral valve disease, and ASD.

Most importantly, I would like to do 24 hours Holter monitoring (24 hours tapes will often miss significant events as only pick-up events which happen in that 24 hours period; a 7-day event recorder is more helpful).

Finally, I would like to consider a cardiology referral for a coronary angiogram.

Examiner: How will you manage the case?

Candidate: At first, I would like to take some general measures, most importantly lifestyle modification, including reducing caffeine and alcohol, regular exercise, dietary modification and control of hypertension, DM, dyslipidemia as well.

Then I would like to consider rate control by using rate limiting drugs with beta-blockers, rate-limiting calcium channel blockers, with or without digoxin. (If the patient is hemodynamically unstable or having evidence of heart failure, then we have to consider rhythm control approach by chemical or electrical cardioversion; however, it is not applicable in this case as he has paroxysmal AF and is in sinus rhythm now).

Finally, to prevent future strokes, I would like to calculate the CHA_2DS_2-VASc scoring system and consider anticoagulant or antiplatelet according to the score.

Examiner: How do you decide who need anticoagulation for AF (CHA_2DS_2-VASc score)?

Candidate:

Systemic embolic risk	Score
Congestive cardiac failure/left ventricular dysfunction	1
Hypertension	1
Age >75	2
Diabetes	1
Stroke/transient ischemic attack/thromboembolism	2
Vascular disease (prior myocardial infarction, peripheral arterial disease (PAD), aortic plaque)	1
Age 65–74	1
Sex (female)	1

The maximum score is 9.

Recommendation: (According to ESC guideline)

Score 0 = Low stroke risk; no anticoagulation

Score 1 = Medium stroke risk (1.3%/year); patient preference (aspirin or anticoagulant)

Score 2 or more = High risk of stroke (>2.2%/year); oral anticoagulation.

CHAPTER 1 Clinical Consultation

Congestive Cardiac Failure

Your role: You are the Medical Doctor in the General Medical Clinic.

Patient details: Mr Thomas Paul, a 65-year-old man.

Clinical problem: A known case of heart failure, has noticed increasingly shortness of breath, swollen ankle, and difficulty in sleeping.

(Once you get this clinical scenario, you will get 5 minutes to start this station for two scenarios. At that time, start to think about your diagnosis and differential diagnoses and plan for taking focused history as well as focused examination.)

(*Once you enter the room, search for a spot diagnosis-raised JVP, peripheral edema, and breathlessness suggest congestive cardiac failure.*)

Introduction, Permission, and Identification

Candidate: Good morning. I am Mohammad Ali, one of the working doctors here today. I have been asked to see you; is that okay with you?

Patient: Good morning, doctor...

Candidate: Thank you for coming. I would like to start by taking your full name, please...

Patient: I am Thomas Paul.

Candidate: May I confirm your age, please?

Patient: I am 65-year-old.

Focused History

Candidate: Okay, Mr Paul, I understand you have some problem with your breathing, would you like to tell me more about this?

Patient: I feel short of breath most of the time, even at rest, and my shoes are no longer fit. I cannot sleep at night, and I feel tired throughout the day. I cannot do anything at all.

Analyze the Complaint

Candidate: I am sorry to hear that. Would you please tell me more about your breathlessness and how this problem has affected your life?

Patient: I have been feeling breathlessness on exertion for several months, gradually worsening day by day. Now I feel breathless while walking around my house. And also feel breathless when I lie down in bed at night, so I use three pillows to sleep. I cannot do anything else.

Candidate: I understand you are having a lot of trouble with breathing. Do you remember when you last felt well?

Patient: I was doing well until the last 6 months. Then I just started getting progressively weaker and breathless.

Candidate: Do you have any other problems like chest pain or racing heartbeat, cough, fever, or anything else?

Patient: Yes, I have chest pain similar to my previous angina.

Candidate: I am sorry to hear that. You said that similar to your previous angina, and what do you mean by that?

Patient: About 8 years back, I felt chest pain while I used to do any activity, and after taking a rest for a while, I felt better. But one day, suddenly, I developed severe pain, and I was rushed to the hospital immediately. Doctors told me I had a heart attack, and two stentings were done in my heart at that time. After that, I was completely fine and stopped attending the heart clinic for the last 2 years. But recently, the pain has come again, and I do not know why all this happens.

Candidate: Well, let me ask you a few more general questions to find out why this is happening.
- Is your appetite gone? Have you lost weight?
- Do you have any tummy pain? Have you been feeling sick, or have you vomited?
- Do you have any changes in your bowel habit or any difficulties in waterworks?
- Do you have any headache or any visual disturbance? Do you have any history of LOC/dizziness?

Patient: Last month, I suddenly fainted while walking in the park. After a while, I regained consciousness. I did not have to go to the hospital. Instead, my friends brought me home.

Candidate: Do you have any other medical conditions, Mr Paul?

Patient: I have diabetes and high blood pressure.

Candidate: When were you diagnosed with diabetes?

Patient: I have had diabetes for 7 years.

Candidate: Do you check your blood sugar regularly or take medicine for it? Have you been seen by a diabetic specialist?

Patient: No, my general physician takes care of it. I have taken metformin 500 mg twice daily recently.

Candidate: Can you tell me about your current blood sugar level and recent level of HbA1c?

Patient: It was 8.4 mmol/L after the meal, and the last HbA1c was 7, 3 months back.

Candidate: Do you have any complications of DM, like any problem with your eyes, kidneys, or legs?

Patient: No, doctor.

Candidate: How about your blood pressure? Is it well-controlled? Do you take medicines for it regularly? Moreover, what is your current medication for it?

Patient: I take ramipril 2.5 mg once daily at night and bisoprolol 2.5 mg daily in the morning, and furosemide 40 mg twice daily.

Candidate: Have you had your thyroid function checked ever?

Patient: I must have, but I am not sure.

Candidate: Okay, a few more questions. Have you had any other problems, such as asthma or high cholesterol?

Patient: I have high cholesterol, and I take atorvastatin 10 mg once daily.

Candidate: Have you ever been admitted to the hospital in the past or any surgery?

Patient: Yes, one time for my past heart attack 8 years back, but no surgery.

Candidate: Do you regularly go to an outpatient clinic?

Patient: No

Candidate: So, you are taking medications for your high blood pressure, diabetes, and high cholesterol. May I ask you, is there any other medications that you are taking? Any herbal remedies or any over-the-counter medications? Are you allergic to any medications or anything else?

Patient: I take aspirin and clopidogrel with other medications.

Quick Systemic Review, Past Medical History, Family History, Treatment, Social History According to Your Differentials

If it is not asked previously during initial history taking or incompletely asked then—take a full history of a particular portion to make it complete.

Candidate: Do you smoke? If no, then have you ever smoked? How about alcohol? How many drinks would you have in a week?

Patient: I would drink about four glasses of red wine.

Candidate: Are you working at the moment?

Patient: No

Candidate: Okay, are you finding it difficult to cope with finances because you are not working now?

Patient: No

Candidate: Are you married? Do you have any children? Who is supporting you now?

Patient: I got divorced 20 years back, and I have three children living with me.

Candidate: I see…are your parents alive? Are they well?

Patient: No, they are not alive.

Candidate: Is there any other medical illness in your family?

Patient: My sister has diabetes; she was diagnosed 4 years ago and takes a tablet for it.

Candidate: I will just quickly go over what you have told me to make sure I have it right. You have diabetes, hypertension, and high cholesterol and have had a history of heart attack with stenting in your heart. For the last 6 months, you have been experiencing increasing breathlessness and chest pain, and you also fainted last month.
 Have I missed anything, or do you want to add anything more?

Patient: No, I think you have covered it all.

Candidate: Okay, I think I have been asked all the questions that I need for now. Would you mind if I go on to examine you?

Patient: No problem, please go ahead.

Focused Examination

Here the most important part of examination would be cardiovascular system followed by respiratory system.

General appearance:
- Dyspnea at rest
- Cyanosis
- Hands:
  - Maybe peripherally cyanosed and cool with clubbing or splinter hemorrhage.
  - Pulse: Irregularly irregular pulse is associated with AF or slow rising pulse in aortic stenosis (AS) or pulsus alternans in severe cardiac failure.
- *Neck*: Raised JVP
- *Precordium and chest*:
  - *Apex beat*: Not displaced, heaving apex beat in aortic stenosis (AS) (unless long-standing severe disease with left ventricular dilation or associated aortic regurgitation) or post-MI heart failure.
  - *Thrill*: Systolic thrill in the aortic area.
  - *Murmur*: Ejection systolic murmur radiating to the carotid, best heard in the aortic area.
- Auscultate the lung for crackles.
- Examine for sacral and peripheral edema.
- *For DM*: Fundoscopy and peripheral neuropathy.
- Finally, ask for a blood pressure reading as well as urine for sugar and protein.

Feedback to the Patient and Respond to the Patient's Concerns

Candidate: You said initially that the main problem was shortness of breath and swollen ankle, is there anything else troubling you that we have not covered? Or any concern?

Patient: What happened to me, doctor? Why have I become so breathless nowadays?

Candidate: I suspect the cause of your shortness of breath and swollen ankles is a condition called congestive heart failure, where your heart muscle is not pumping as effectively as it should. Therefore, fluid collects on the lungs and periphery. We need to start treatment right now—we need to increase your water tablets (diuretics) as well as alter some of your other medicines (ACEI; beta-blocker) to help your heart work more effectively. I would like to do several investigations to assess the function of your heart [echocardiogram (ECG)] and blood tests [FBC, U&E, brain natriuretic peptide (BNP), etc.] to ensure that no other factors causing your symptoms; is that okay with you?
Do you have any other concerns?

Patient: No, thanks.
Thank you for spending time with me today.

Discussion with Examiner

Examiner: Would you please present your case?

Candidate:

This elderly gentleman presented with increasing shortness of breath associated with chest pain on exertion with a fainting attack for the last 6 months.

He has a significant cardiac history; he had an MI 8 years ago that was treated with primary percutaneous coronary intervention (PCI) and intervention of 2 stents. He has a history of non-insulin-dependent diabetes mellitus (NIDDM) (5 years), hypertension, and hypercholesterolemia. Unfortunately, he stopped attending cardiology outpatient clinics as he was asymptomatic.

On examination, Mr Paul was sitting comfortably at 45° and was in no distress. He had a slow rising, low volume pulse, regular at 64 beats/minute and non-displaced apex beat, which was heaving in nature.

On auscultation, the first heart sound was normal, but the second one was very soft.

A harsh ejection systolic murmur was heard in the aortic area radiating to the carotids and increased with expiration.

I would like to complete my examination by doing fundoscopy, blood pressure measurement, checking for other evidence of peripheral vascular disease and peripheral neuropathy and also urine for glycosuria and proteinuria as well.

In summary, my diagnosis would be post PTCA status with CCF, possibly due to severe AS and occlusion myocardial infarction (OMI) with strong cardiovascular risk factors including hypertension, DM, and hypercholesterolemia.

Examiner: How would you investigate this gentleman?

Candidate: At first, I would like to do some blood tests:
- FBC with ESR (for anemia), serum urea, serum electrolyte, serum creatinine, TFT (anemia, deranged electrolytes, and abnormal thyroid function may all exacerbate heart failure)
- BNP is a protein released from the ventricles in cardiac failure, it is a relatively non-specific but highly sensitive marker for the condition, helping to differentiate dyspnea secondary to cardiac failure from that attributable to other causes.

Next, most importantly, I would like to do:
- ECG–This may show evidence of the cause of cardiac failure (e.g., ischemic changes) or some of the sequelae (e.g., left ventricular hypertrophy, AF)
- Chest radiograph–Classic changes seen in heart failure include diversion of blood to the upper lobes of the lungs, perihilar edema, cardiomegaly, pleural effusions, and Karley B lines (representing interstitial edema).
- An echocardiogram is a key test for diagnosing heart failure, helping to define an etiology of heart failure (valvular disease) and the degree of impairment of ventricular function.
- Further, functional imaging may also be contributory, e.g., dopamine stress echocardiogram and cardiac MRI.

Examiner: How would you treat him?

Candidate: This patient should treat under an MDT approach, and important measures include:

General measures:
- No added salt diet and restricted fluid intake
- Adjust modifiable risk factors, i.e., Smoking, hypertension, diabetes
- Stop medications promoting fluid retention where possible (e.g., NSAIDs, steroids, calcium channel blockers, etc.)
- Weight reduction and rehabilitation/exercise programs
- Seasonal influenza immunization

Pharmacological treatments:
- *Diuretics*: Predominantly loop diuretics (e.g., furosemide) but also some role of thiazide diuretics (e.g., metolazone). They are of symptomatic but no prognostic benefit.
- ACE inhibitors/angiotensin receptor blockers have been known to cause ventricular remodeling with impaired function. However, these are of both symptomatic and prognostic benefit.
- *Beta-blockers*: Beta 1 adrenergic receptor-selective blockers have prognostic benefit in NYHA 2-4 cardiac failure. They may be contraindicated for several reasons (e.g., asthma or severe COPD).
- *Spironolactone*: This is of prognostic benefit in NIHA Class 3-4 cardiac failure. The side effects of hyperkalemia may limit its use.
- *Digoxin*: Useful if symptoms are still uncontrolled after the above therapy (even if in sinus rhythm) through its role as a mild positive inotrope, but of no prognostic benefit.
- *Hydralazine/long-acting nitrates*: Symptomatic and prognostic benefit in black people or people intolerant of ACE inhibitors.
- *Ivabradine*: A funny current antagonist with a growing role in cardiac failure management.

- *Intervention/surgical*:
  - Implantable cardioverter-defibrillator (ICD): Prognostic benefit for patients with NYHA 2-3 cardiac failure and left ventricular ejection fraction <35%.
  - Cardiac resynchronization therapy (CRT): A dual-chamber pacemaker with an additional left ventricular lead. It has a prognostic benefit for patients with NYHA 2-4 cardiac failure, left ventricular ejection fraction <35% and QRS interval >120 ms.
- *Surgical*:
  - Coronary artery bypass graft (CABG) or valvular surgery, if indicated. In severe cases, cardiac transplantation may be considered; technological improvements mean that cardiac devices (e.g., left ventricular assist devices) are increasingly used as an adjunct while patients wait for transplants to become available.

Examiner: Tell me some differential of breathlessness for this patient.

Candidate: Differentials include:
- Chronic obstructive pulmonary disease
- Chronic thromboembolic disease
- Pulmonary fibrosis

Lambert–Eaton Myasthenic Syndrome

Your role: You are the Doctor in the General Medical Clinic.

Patient details: Mrs Muna Mariya, a 53-year-old woman.

Clinical problem: Intermittent limb weakness.

(Once you get this clinical scenario, you will get 5 minutes to start this station for two scenarios. At that time, start to think about your diagnosis and differential diagnoses and plan for taking focused history as well as focused examination.)

(Differential diagnosis: Myasthenia gravis, LEMS, and myopathy.)

(Once you enter the room, search for a spot diagnosis; bilateral ptosis suggests myasthenia gravis.)

Introduction, Permission, and Identification

Candidate: Good morning. My name is Mohammad Ali. One of the working doctors here today. I have been asked to see you. Is that ok with you?

Patient: Ok.

Candidate: Thank you for coming. I would like to start by taking your full name, please…

Patient: I am Muna Mariya.

Candidate: May I confirm your age, please?

Patient: I am 53-year-old.

Focused History

Candidate: Ok, Mrs Mariya, would you please tell me what brings you here today?

Patient: For the past 6 months, I have been feeling weak in both legs.

Analyze the Symptoms

Candidate: Please, tell me more about your weakness….
- When did you notice weakness?
- Did it affect one or both sides?
- Where did you feel weakness exactly? Do you have any weakness in your hand or arm? Do you have any problem with your hand movement or fingers grip?
- Did it come on suddenly, or has it been developing over a period?
- Is it getting better or staying the same or getting worse over time?
- Is it coming on and off or all the time with you?
- Are these symptoms worse at the beginning/the end of the day, or whether they are worse after a sustained period of exercise?
- Any history of similar weakness in the past?
- How it affects your day-to-day activity for a living?

Patient: The weakness in my legs is not always with me. It is usually at its worst when I first get up in the morning and then seems to get better after walking for a while. However, if I undertake housework or walk to the nearby shops, the weakness quickly returns. I have found recently that I have difficulty getting up from a chair, mainly if I have been seated for several minutes. I also feel some weakness in my arms, but this does not really trouble me.

Candidate: Since, it suggests a case of LEMS or MG–by the patient's general look and history.

Other Important Targeted Histories

- Have you noticed any difficulty in swallowing, chewing, or have you ever experienced regurgitation of your food (nasal regurgitation)?

- Do you have any slurring of speech or voice changes?
- Do you have any breathing difficulty?
- Do you have any drooping of your eyelids or double vision?

Patient: I have also noticed that chewing has become difficult nowadays.

Candidate: Please tell me more about it……
- For how long do you have it? How does it affect your eating?
- Does it difficult to chew at the beginning of your meal or during the whole period?

Patient: It is difficult to chew at the beginning of my meal and then get better for a while. However, it returns after some time of my eating. My husband has noticed that my voice fades, and my speech also becomes slurred from time-to-time.

Candidate: Do you have any other problems? Do you want to add anything more?

Patient: I feel dizzy on standing and also have a stubborn cough…

Candidate: Please tell me more about your dizziness:
- What exactly do you mean by dizzy? For how long?
- Does it occur all the time or at any particular time?
- Do you have any history of LOC, fainting attack, shaky limbs, abnormal sensation, or weakness in your limbs?

Patient: I have noticed that I feel dizzy on standing from a sitting position and also feel some light-headedness.

Candidate: Ok. And about your cough:
- How long have you had this?
- Is it dry or productive? If it is productive, then ask about the amount of sputum-scanty or copious? What is the color of sputum? Is it whitish, yellowish, or greenish?
- Have you noticed any blood in phlegm?
- Is there any particular time in the day when your symptoms (cough and breathlessness) getting worse (diurnal variation)?
- Does anything in particular trigger the cough like dust, pollen, fumes, or anything else?
- Do you have any fever or any history of weight loss?
- Do you have any chest pain or breathlessness?

Patient: I have a dry cough, which has been troublesome for the past 3-4 months. I have lost some weight too.

Candidate: So tell me about your weight loss:
- How much weight have you lost? Over how long? How is your appetite?
- Does it coincide with your change in diet or physical activity or lifestyle?

Patient: I have lost about 4 kg and I have lost my appetite too.

Candidate: Well! Now let me ask some general questions:
- Do you have any dryness in your mouth? Do you have any dryness in your private part?
- Have you experienced excessive sweating or not sweating enough?
- Have you noticed any bowel changes, bloating, diarrhea, or constipation?
- Do you have any difficulties with waterworks?

Patient: Everything is normal, but my mouth is often dry, making eating more difficult.

Quick Systemic Review, Treatment History, Past Medical History, Family History, Social History According to Your Differentials

Past Medical and Surgical History

Candidate: Do you have any other medical illnesses like high blood pressure or high blood sugar?

Patient: I have had high blood pressure and have been on treatment for this for 4-5 years.

Relevant Family History

Candidate: Is there anyone else in your family with this type of problem or any long-standing illness that runs in your family like DM, hypertension, stroke, thyroid, or any autoimmune disease or anything else?

Patient: My father died at the age of 62 from motor neuron disease. My mother is 76 and has had two hip replacement operations and is a bit unsteady on her feet. She had an overactive thyroid gland which I remember was treated with radioactive iodine. She is now taking levothyroxine tablets. She is also on treatment for high blood pressure.

Treatment History

Candidate: I am sorry to hear about your loss. You have had hypertension for the last 4–5 years. Are you currently taking any medication for your hypertension?

Patient: I am taking a tablet ramipril 10 mg daily.

Candidate: Anything else other than ramipril? Any over-the-counter medications or herbal remedies, or any recreational drugs? Are you allergic to any medicine or anything else?

Patient: No

Social history:
- Do you smoke? For how long and how many sticks per day?
- Do you drink alcohol?
- What are you doing for a living? How have these symptoms affected your job?
- Are you married? Who is at home with you, or who is supporting you now?

Patient: I work in an office as a secretary. I am married with two grown-up children, and they both live away from home. My husband is an electrician and often works away from home. Since the age of 16 years, I have smoked 20 cigarettes per day but do not drink any alcohol.

Candidate: Have I missed anything, or do you want to add anything more?
Would you mind if I go on to examine you?

Focused Examination

Targeted examination would be according to main complaints and spot diagnosis.

In this scenario, the most likely diagnosis is LEMS. So, the targeted examination would be:
- *Neurological examination:*
  - *Ocular*:
    - Inspection for bilateral ptosis
    - Light reflex to rule out bilateral Horner's syndrome
    - The extraocular movement to see bilateral extraocular palsies
  - *Limbs*:
    - Muscle power, reflex, wasting, and fasciculations
  - *Fatigability test*:
    - Repeated blinking
    - Sustained upward gaze (unmasked asymmetric partial ptosis)
    - Counting test (ask the patient to count 1–50)
    - Repeated arm abduction
- Respiratory system examination for any evidence of bronchogenic carcinoma.
- Postural hypotension for autonomic features.

Feedback to the Patient and Respond to the Patient's Concerns

Candidate: You said at the beginning that the main problem was weakness in your limbs, dizziness on standing, dry mouth, slurred speech, and dry cough—Is there anything else troubling you that we have missed or any question to ask or any concern?

Patient: Do I have motor neuron disease?

Candidate: From the history and examination, there are no features of motor neuron disease. It is unlikely that you have motor neuron disease.
   I think most probably you have a condition called LEMS which affects the signals sent from the nerves to the muscles and the muscles are unable to tighten (contract) properly, resulting in muscle weakness and a range of other symptoms.
   I am afraid about half of LEMS cases occur in middle-aged or older people with lung cancer. So, we need to rule it out first by doing an urgent scan of your chest. Then, we will also go for some specific blood tests and nerve studies for LEMS to confirm our diagnosis.

Patient: Is it going to get worse?

Candidate: It is far too early at this stage to say anything like this. We need to evaluate you more by doing some investigations before saying what might or might not happen in the future.

Do you have any other concerns? Ok, thank you very much for spending time with me today.

Discussion with Examiner

Examiner: Please present your case.

Candidate:

> This middle-aged, heavily smoker, hypertensive lady is presented with a 6-month history of fatigable muscle weakness, slurred speech, autonomic dysfunction with dry mouth and postural dizziness. She also has a long history of dry cough and significant weight loss.
>
> On examination, she has proximal muscle wasting, weakness, and fatigability; muscle power is initially increased by brief exercise (reversed myasthenic effect), and the tendon reflexes are depressed but increased soon after activity.
>
> Although chest examination is completely normal, my diagnosis is LEMS with autonomic dysfunction as the paraneoplastic manifestations of small cell lung cancer.

Examiner: How will you investigate the case?

Candidate: I would do first some basic tests that include FBC, ESR, CRP, U&E, serum creatinine, LFTs, Urine R/M/E, TFTs, creatine phosphokinase (CPK), and CXR.

In terms of confirming the diagnosis, I would send antibodies for voltage-gated calcium channel (for LEMS) and acetylcholine receptor (for MG), and I would also arrange for neurophysiological testing, including EMG with repetitive stimulation test. I would expect to see an incremental effect on the action potentials in EMG in LEMS and decremental effects in MG.

Finally, I would like to do a chest CT scan for a detailed appearance of the lung to exclude underlying small cell carcinoma.

Examiner: If you have confirmed the diagnosis of LEMS, then how will you treat this patient?

Candidate: I would like to manage the patient with an MDT approach involving a neurologist, chest specialist, physiotherapist, specialist nurse, occupational therapist, and oncologist if the underlying cause is malignancy.

There is no cure for LEMS, so symptomatic treatment for neuromuscular weakness is the mainstay of treatment, including potassium channel blockers. It allows the electrical activity that passes through the neuromuscular junction for a longer period, increasing calcium influx into the nerve endings. Two potassium channel blockers are approved by USFDA that includes:
- Firdapse (3,4 diaminopyridine)
- Ruzurgi (amifampridine)

The role of cholinesterase inhibitor (pyridostigmine) has minimal effects in LEMS.

The next step of management would be immune modulation that includes:
- Prednisolone, steroid, intravenous immune globulin (IVIg), and plasma exchange.

Transient Ischemic Attack

Your role: You are a Registrar in Accident and Emergency.

Patient details: Mr Endy Jebs, 49-year-old.

Clinical problem: Referred by his general physician after having just had a short episode of visual loss.

(Once you get this clinical scenario, you will get 5 minutes to start this station for two scenarios. At that time, start to think about your diagnosis and differential diagnoses and plan for taking focused history as well as focused examination.)

[Here, the most likely diagnosis would be transient ischemic attack. Other differential diagnoses are:
- Temporal arteritis
- Central retinal vein occlusion (CRVO) or branch retinal vein occlusion (BRVO)
- Retinal or vitreous hemorrhage
- Diabetic maculopathy]

(*Once you enter the room, search for a spot diagnosis, particularly evidence of DM with complications, dyslipidemia, and other cardiovascular diseases.*)

Introduction, Permission, and Identification

Candidate: Good morning. I am Mohammad Ali, one of the working doctors here today. I have been asked to see you; is that okay with you?

Patient: Good morning, Doctor...

Candidate: Thank you for coming. May I know your name, please?

Patient: I am Endy Jebs.

Candidate: May I confirm your age, please?

Patient: I am 49-year-old.

Focused History

Candidate: Okay, Mr Jebs, I understand you have been referred by your general physician with some visual problems. Would you like to tell me what happened exactly?

Patient: This morning, I could not see anything with my right eye for a while. I went to my general physician immediately, and he referred me to you.

Analyze the Symptoms

Candidate: You did the right thing. So, you lost your vision for a while, can you tell me a little bit more about it?
- When did you notice the visual disturbance? What were you doing at that time? Was it sudden or gradual?
- Did it affect one or both eyes? Was it partial or complete?
- How long did it last? Do you get a complete recovery? Did it recur?
- Any history of similar illness before?

Patient: It all came on suddenly whilst I was walking to work. There was something like shutters coming down on my right eye. My vision went black for about 20 minutes. Then my vision gradually returned over about few minutes. It was the first time I had experienced this type of problem.

Candidate: When the history suggests TIA then targeted history to detect the complications and etiology of TIA.

Other Important Targeted Histories
- Have you noticed any weakness in the face or limbs?
- Have you noticed any numbness, loss of feeling, or pins and needle sensation/tingling sensation at that moment?

- Have you noticed any speech disturbance or any double vision?
- Have you noticed any shaking of the body and LOC at that time?
- Do you have any chest pain, palpitation, breathlessness, or leg swelling (cardiac thromboembolism)?
- Do you have a headache or painful chewing, or temporal pain during combing hair [suggestive of GCA/polymyalgia rheumatica (PMR)]?
- Do you have any history of illness like DM, hypertension, or any cardiac disease?

Patient: I have been diabetic for the last 3 years and hypertensive for the last 5 years. Recently, I went to a cardiologist who told me that I have AF and prescribed me some drugs. I am taking these drugs regularly except-warfarin.

Candidate: So, what are the drugs you are taking currently? Are you allergic to any medication or anything else?

Patient: Metformin 1 g/day, simvastatin 40 mg at night, and losartan potassium 50 mg at night.

Candidate: What about your diabetes?
- Is it controlled or not? For how long?
- Are you on regular follow-up? What was your last blood sugar or HbA1c?
- Do you have any history of hypoglycemia attacks?
- Do you have any diabetes complications such as foot problems or eyes problem? Has any ophthalmologist seen you recently or previously?

Patient: I have had diabetes for the last 3 years, and it is well-controlled with metformin. My general physician is taking care of it. My last HbA1c was 6.

Candidate: You told that–you have AF and your heart doctor told you to take warfarin for AF, but may I know, why are you not taking warfarin?

Patient: I reviewed some literature, and I found it increases bleeding risk—so I did not take it.

Candidate: I appreciate your concern. It is true that it increases the risk of bleeding in the brain, but if AF is not adequately treated, it increases the risk of stroke (ischemic) several times. However, if you take warfarin regularly and are closely monitored by a blood test, then the risk of hemorrhage will significantly reduce—I suggest you take warfarin regularly.

Quick Systemic Review, Past Medical History, Family History, Treatment, Social History According to Your Differentials

If it is not asked previously during initial history taking or incompletely asked then—take a full history of a particular portion to make it complete.

Candidate: At this moment—I would like to ask you some general questions:
- Do you have any fever, weight loss, or loss of appetite? Do you have any nausea, vomiting, tummy pain, or any changes in bowel habits?
- What about your waterworks? Do you have any change in color or pain in passing urine, frequency, or frothy urine, or anything else?

Patient: No

Candidate: Do you have any long-standing disease or stroke or similar illness in your family?

Patient: My mother has DM and hypertension, taking medication for it.

Candidate: Do you drive?

Patient: Yes, I drive to my office regularly.

Candidate: I am sorry to say—you have to inform DVLA about your condition to be assessed by their team before driving. Driving may be risky for yourself and the public because of the possibility of recurrence of vision loss during driving. Is it okay with you?

Patient: Okay

Candidate: What are you doing for a living? With whom you are living? Who is supporting you at home? Do you smoke? Do you drink alcohol?

Patient: I smoked 25 sticks per day for the last 20 years but have given up. I do not drink alcohol. I am an accountant and lives with my wife.

Okay, thank you, have I missed anything, or do you want to add anything?

Would you mind if I go on to examine you?

Focused Examination

Check for a pulse, BP, carotid bruit, CVS, as well as full neurological examination.
- Cranial nerve examination particularly: Visual acuity, visual field, pupil and fundoscopy
- Pulse: Irregularly irregular suggests AF
- BP: 30/80 mm Hg
- Carotid bruit
- CVS—signs of infective endocarditis, murmur or LVH or PHTN
- Palpate the temporal artery for tenderness: GCA

I would like to complete my examination by doing upper and lower limbs neurological examination, and dipstick urine test for sugar and protein.

Feedback to the Patient and Respond to the Patient's Concerns

Candidate: You said at the beginning, the main problem was a sudden loss of vision for a short period, and you are hypertensive, diabetic and have had AF. Is there anything else that we have missed or any expectation or any concern?

Patient: What would be the cause of loss of vision, Doctor?

Candidate: I suspect your visual disturbance has been caused by a condition known as a TIA or mini stroke. AF is associated with an increased risk of clot formation in the heart. Therefore, it is likely that a small clot has formed in the heart then entered the circulation to block a small artery in the eye.

As you have AF and had a TIA recently, we need to admit you to the hospital because your stroke risk is high. We will do some blood tests, ECG tracing, and brain scans at this moment. After that, you will be reviewed by a brain doctor for specialist assessment. After getting the CT scan report, we will start aspirin as early as possible if not contraindicated. Is that okay with you?

Do you have any other concerns? Thank you so much for spending time with me today.

Discussion with Examiner

Examiner: Would you please present your case?

Candidate:

This middle-aged gentleman presented with isolated transient loss of vision with multiple cardiovascular risk factors such as DM, hypertension, dyslipidemia with significant smoking history.

On examination, his pulse is 86 beats/minute, normal volume with an irregularly irregular rhythm.

There was no obvious cardiac murmur or carotid bruit.

So far, I examine, there was no clear evidence of neurological deficit.

In summary—I think this patient has TIA (amaurosis fugax) as a complication of AF.

Examiner: How will you investigate the case?

Candidate: I would like to start by initial blood tests with CBC, ESR, CRP, blood sugar, HbA1c, serum creatinine, serum electrolyte, lipid profile, and CXR.

My next step would be looking for evidence of cerebral infarct or cerebrovascular disease by CT scan or MRI of the brain.

As the patient has AF, I would do an ECG and color Doppler echocardiography to see the evidence of structural heart disease, thrombus, or vegetations as part of infective endocarditis.

Moreover, I would like to go for carotid Doppler.

Examiner: How will you manage the case?

Candidate: Although ABCD2 score is low (score <4), but with the presence of AF, the patient is encountered for a high-risk TIA. We need to admit the patient and need urgent evaluation by a neurologist.

Since the patient has AF, I would like to treat the patient with warfarin after 2 weeks, but initially, I would give antiplatelet therapy with aspirin 300 mg daily for 2 weeks.

The next important management step would be risk factors modifications, particularly control of DM, hypertension, dyslipidemia, and smoking cessation. So, I would like to involve an MDT involving a neurologist, diabetologist, cardiologist, and vascular surgeon as well to control other risk factors and carotid endarterectomy, if needed.

Transient Ischemic Attack in Young Female

Your role: You are the Registrar in the General Medical Clinic.

Patient profile: Mrs Sirin Ahmed, a 28-year-old lady.

Problem: Right-sided weakness of the body for 30 minutes while working at the office.

[Once you get this clinical scenario, you will get 5 minutes to start this station for two scenarios. At that time, start to think about your diagnosis and differential diagnoses and plan for taking focused history as well as focused examination.]

[Differential diagnosis: (as the patient is young)
- TIA due to:
  - Cardioembolic [valvular heart disease, infective endocarditis, and AF]
  - Vasculitis [SLE, antiphospholipid antibody syndrome (APLA), Sjögren syndrome]
- Hereditary thrombophilia (protein C, protein S, antithrombin-3 deficiency, Factor V Leiden)
- Familiar hyperlipidemia
- Paradoxical embolism due to perforated foramen ovale (PFO) or ASD, particularly those patients having proven thrombophilia.
- Cerebral autosomal dominant arteriopathy with subcortical infarcts and leukoencephalopathy (CADASIL)
- Sickle cell anemia
- Todd's paresis
- Hemiplegic migraine
- Carotid dissection if evidence of neck hyperextension injury or trauma
- Functional]

(Once you enter the room, search for a spot diagnosis; butterfly rash, unilateral limb swelling, skin rash, arthropathy suggest secondary APLA with TIA)

Introduction, Permission, and Identification

Candidate: Good morning. I am Mohammad Ali, one of the working doctors here today. I have been asked to see you; is that OK with you?

Patient: Good morning, doctor...

Candidate: Thank you for coming. May I know your name, please?

Patient: I am Sirin Ahmed.

Candidate: May I confirm your age, please?

Patient: I am 28 years old.

Focused History

Candidate: Ok, Mrs Ahmed. Would you please tell me what brings you here today? Please tell me in your own words.

Patient: This morning, when I was working in my office, I suddenly felt a pain on the right side of my head. I was feeling sick also. I thought it would be ok to drink tea, so I asked my staff to give me a cup of tea. However, I could not lift the cup of tea, and I noticed the weakness in my hand. I got scared and called the ambulance immediately and came to the hospital. Now I am feeling better, and the weakness of the hand is gone away.

Analyze the Symptoms

Candidate: If the history is not clear, then ask the following questions to clear it.
- When did you notice weakness?
- Did it come on suddenly, or has it been developing over a period of time? How long did it last? Do you still feel any weakness? Did it resolve completely?

- Where did you feel weakness exactly? Was it only in your hand? Any weakness in your face or legs? Did it affect one or both sides?
- Was there any problem with your speech?
- Any history of similar weakness in the past?

Candidate: Please tell me a little bit more about headaches.
- Where is the pain? Is the headache one-sided or both?
- How did it start? Suddenly or gradually? Is it worsening or static?
- What type of pain is it? Is it dull ache/compressing/sharp?
- Does the pain move or go anywhere?
- Is this the first time you have had this headache, or have you had it before? If yes, then is this the same headache as the previous one?
- Does anything make it worse, like looking to the light, coughing, or straining?
- Does your headache come with anything such as lack of sleep, OCP, starvation, caffeine, alcohol, cheese, and exercise?
- Does anything make you feel better, like taking rest or medication? Have you tried anything for your headache?
- Anything with the headache like blurring of vision, feeling sick, vomiting or sensitivity to light?

Patient: Over the last 4 years, I have been having an on and off headache, which lasts for about 3–4 hours and if I go to bed headache settles overnight but often lasts longer. During the headache, I feel nauseous. I have noticed that the headache is before my menstruation in most cases. Today, my headache was the same as my usual headache, but it was painful to look in bright lights. Now the headache has improved after taking paracetamol.

Other Important Targeted Histories

- Have you noticed any shaking of the body, any dizziness, LOC, tongue biting, uncontrolled water work? (Seizure/epilepsy; Todd's paresis)
- By any chance, are you pregnant? Any history of miscarriage before or any history of blood clots before? (APLA syndrome)
- Any history of joint pain and swelling, hair fall, and oral ulceration or frothy urine? (SLE)
- Any history of chest pain, palpitation, breathlessness, or leg swelling? (Cardiac emboli)
- Do you have any FH of blood disease or any history of a blood clot in the family? (Hereditary thrombophilia or sickle cell anemia)
- Do you have DM, HTN, dyslipidemia, a FH of stroke, heart disease? (a risk factor for atherosclerosis)

Patient: I have a history of two miscarriages.

Candidate: I am sorry to hear about it. May I ask in which period of your pregnancy you had these miscarriages?

Patient: It was before 12 weeks of my pregnancy.

Quick systemic review, PMH, FH, treatment, and social history according to your differentials: If it is not asked previously during initial history taking or incompletely asked, then take a full history of a particular portion to make it complete.

Candidate: Now I would like to ask some general questions, is that ok with you?
- Do you have a fever, weight loss, or loss of appetite?
- Any nausea, vomiting, abdominal pain, or any changes in bowel habits?
- What about your waterworks? Any change in color or pain in passing urine, frequency, or frothy urine, or anything else?
- Do you have any similar condition or any other history of disease in your past?
- Have you ever been admitted to the hospital in the past or have any history of surgery?
- Are you taking any medication recently? Any hormonal pills, over-the-counter medications, herbal medicine, or any recreational drugs? Are you allergic to any medicine or anything else?
- Is there anyone else in your family with this type of problem or any long-standing illness that run in your family such as DM, HTN, stroke, thyroid or any autoimmune disease, or anything else?
- Do you drive? Do you drive for a living?

- Do you smoke? Do you drink? What are you doing for a living? Are you married? Who is at home with you, or who is supporting you now?

Patient: I drive to my office but don't drive for a living. I never smoked but occasionally drink alcohol.

Have I missed anything, or do you want to add anything more?

Would you mind if I go on to examine you?

Focused Examination

Neurological examination—as a whole, to see any neurological deficit:
- Weakness
- Sensory loss
- Cerebellar sign
- Cranial nerve examination

Carotid bruit: For carotid artery stenosis.

Pulse: Irregularly irregular pulse suggests underlying AF causing TIA/Stroke.

BP: (For ABCD-2 assessment)

CVS: For murmur or evidence of HF or any sign of infective endocarditis.

Evidence of DVT (for hereditary thrombophilia or paradoxical emboli)

Examine for any evidence of underlying CTD or vasculitis, or RA? (arthropathy, rash, bedside proteinuria, and hematuria)

Feedback to the Patient with Responding to the Patient's Concern

Candidate: You said at the beginning, the main problem was a sudden onset of weakness in the right side of the body following an episode of right-sided headache. You had a history of two miscarriages. Is there anything else that we have missed? Is there anything, in particular, you are concerned about?

Patient: Have you had any thoughts about what is going on? Is it a stroke?

Candidate: Considering what you tell me and the signs I elicit on examination, I think the most likely diagnosis is hemiplegic migraine, a rare type of migraine. In addition to a severe headache, symptoms include weakness of one side of the body as you had. Therefore, it is sometimes confused with a stroke. However, I am very concerned about your history of previous miscarriages. Sometimes, it can be the part of a condition called APLA syndrome where your blood can become abnormally sticky and often responsible for stroke or a mini stroke (TIA). That's why I would like to do some blood tests and brain imaging to rule out such a serious condition.

If it is confirmed that you have APLA syndrome, we will refer you to an MDT involving a brain doctor, blood doctor, joint doctor, and a specialist nurse to decide for you the plan of care and management. OCP may trigger your migraine and APLA syndrome, so we are going to stop it and refer you to an obstetrician to give you another safe method such as a progesterone-only pill or copper IUD. Is that ok with you, Mrs Ahmed?

I am sorry to say—you have to inform DVLA about your condition to be assessed by their team before driving. Driving may be risky for yourself and the public because of the possibility of recurrence of weakness during driving.

Do you have any other concerns? Thank you for spending time with me today.

Discussion with Examiner

Examiner: Would you please present your case?

Candidate:

This young woman presented with an isolated transient episode of right-sided weakness following an episode of right-sided headache. She had a suggestive history of migraine-like headaches and a history of miscarriage two times during her early pregnancy.

However, there was no vascular risk factor (HTN, DM, Dyslipidemia, positive FH).

Examination revealed a normal pulse which was regular. There was no apparent cardiac murmur, and there were no carotid bruits. Thus, there was no clear evidence of focal neurological deficit at this moment.

In summary, I think this patient had a hemiplegic migraine. However, my strong differential diagnosis would be TIA due to APLA syndrome.

Examiner: How will you investigate this case?

Candidate: I would like to request an initial blood test including full blood count and inflammatory marker (ESR, CRP), looking for any evidence of anemia, thrombocytopenia with high ESR, and CRP.

I would like to do a complete metabolic panel, including urea, serum creatinine, serum electrolytes, LFTS, as well as doing baseline clotting screen (e.g., APTT).

Furthermore, I would like to do an autoantibody screen such as ANA, Ds DNA, ENA, complement level, antiphospholipid and anticardiolipin antibodies to exclude APLA syndrome.

I would like to request a baseline ECG and Holter monitoring—looking for paroxysmal AF.

A CT or MRI scan of the brain would be the most important investigation today.

Then, I may wish to perform color Doppler echocardiography, and a carotid Doppler. If there is any stenosis, I would want to proceed with a CT or MR angiogram of the neck and head to check for an aneurysm, clot, or stenosis because of plaque.

Examiner: If you confirmed APLA as a cause of TIA in this young lady, how would you treat her?

Candidate: I would want to aggressively anticoagulated this patient; current evidence favors warfarin over direct oral anticoagulant (DOAC).

Examiner: Do you know any other complications of APLA?

Candidate: Aside from TIA and stroke being from a complication of APLA, other more frequent complications are:
- DVT and PE
- Thrombocytopenia
- Livedo reticularis (netlike/reticulated red to bluish discoloration of the skin)
- Moreover, as seen in this case, recurrent fetal loss.

Examiner: How does carotid dissection present?

Candidate: Neck pain, headache, focal weakness, or amaurosis fugax, reduced sensation of taste, partial Horner's syndrome (ptosis and miosis), neck swelling, migraine-like symptoms, pulsatile tinnitus, or audible bruit reported. The first manifestation of this condition may be a stroke or TIA due to a carotid embolus breaking off from the clot forming at the site of the dissection.

Marfan Syndrome

Your role: You are the SHO in the General Medical Clinic.

Patient details: Mr Paul Nelson, a 45-year-old man.

Clinical problem: This tall man presented with progressive breathlessness.

[Once you get this clinical scenario, you will get 5 minutes to start this station for two scenarios. At that time, start to think about your diagnosis and differential diagnoses and plan for taking focused history as well as focused examination.]

Differential diagnoses of breathlessness in Marfan Syndrome:
- Aortic regurgitation or dissecting aortic aneurysm
- Mitral valve prolapse
- Pneumothorax or can be due to other cardio-respiratory causes.
- Anemia

[Once you enter the room, search for a spot diagnosis; marfanoid appearance suggests Marfan syndrome or homocystinemia]

Introduction, Permission, and Identification

Candidate: Good morning. My name is Mohammad Ali, one of the working doctors here today. I have been asked to see you. Is that okay with you?

Patient: Good morning, doctor...

Candidate: Thank you for coming; May I know your name, please?

Patient: I am Nelson.

Candidate: Well, you are 45 years old, right?

Patient: Yes, doctor.

Focused History

Candidate: Okay, Mr Nelson, would you please tell me what brings you here today?

Patient: I am fine at this moment, but when I walk, I feel breathless, and I have a fever also.

Analyze the Symptom

Candidate: Would you please tell me a little bit more about your breathlessness?
- When did you first notice breathlessness?
- Were you completely all right before this period? Or when were you last felt well?
- Did it come on suddenly or gradually?
- Is it getting worse or getting improved day by day or static?
- How far can you walk before your breathlessness stop you? Or how many flights of stairs can you manage without stopping?
- Do you struggle for sleep due to breathlessness?
- Does lying down make it worse (orthopnea)?
- Do you use extra pillows during sleep (orthopnea)?
- Do you ever wake up at night feeling breathlessness PND?
- Is there anything else that makes it worse/improve, like an inhaler or GTN spray?
- How it affects your activity of daily living or job?

Patient: Three months ago, I was able to walk about a mile, but now I have shortness of breath on exertion and even on walking about 200 yards. My breathlessness gets worse when lying flat in the bed, and now I sleep on three pillows. I never wake up at night with breathlessness and no cough.

Candidate: Now tell me about your fever.
- Duration; acute or chronic? Intermittent, regular/irregular?

- Have you measured the temperature? Highest recorded temperature?
- Any night sweats? Weight loss? Loss of appetite?

Patient: I have had a low-grade fever with night sweats for the last 4 weeks and have lost 2 kg weight over this period.

Candidate: Since it suggests a case of Marfan syndrome by the patient's general look and history, then other important targeted histories would be:
- Do you have any eye problems? Any surgery in the eye (cataract/lens distortion/retinal detachment)
- Do you have any history of severe chest pain with acute breathlessness followed by chest drain (pneumothorax)?
- Do you have any history of sudden severe chest pain, tearing in nature with radiation to the back in the past? (aortic dissection)
- Do you have fever, cough, racing heartbeat, or swelling of the limbs? (heart failure)
- Do you have any industrial or occupational exposure to asbestos or coal, recent or in the past?
- Did you have any recent dental work? Or do you take any recreational IV drugs?
- Do you have a similar illness in your family? (Marfan syndrome is AD, defect in fibrillin gene on chromosome 15)
- Do you have any other history of disease in your past? Have you ever been admitted to the hospital or have any history of surgery?
- Have you attended any consultant or GP or specialist for this problem? What was their impression? Did you receive any diagnosis? What treatment have you received? Did they work?
- Do you smoke? Do you drink? If so, then ask for the amount and duration.

Patient: Recently, I have noticed some ankle swelling which is progressively developed over the last 3 months. I was diagnosed with Marfan syndrome 8 years back, and I have a history of heart surgery [thoracoabdominal aortic aneurysm repair surgery with aortic valve replacement (AVR)] 5 years back. At the age of 8 years, I had a surgical lens removal to manage congenital myopia and an intraocular lens (IOL) implant. I am taking warfarin for my valve replacement. I am hypertensive and taking bisoprolol 5 mg once daily and losartan 50 mg once daily. My father is also a patient of a similar illness. I have no chest pain, palpitation, or cough currently. I am nondiabetic and nonsmoker but occasional alcoholic.

Quick systemic review, PMH, FH, treatment, and social history according to your differentials: (If it is not asked previously during initial history taking or incompletely asked, then take a full history of a particular portion to make it complete.)

Candidate: At this moment I would like to ask some general questions, is that okay with you?
- Do you have a headache, dizziness, any blackout, shaking limbs, loss/blurring of vision?
- Do you have nausea, vomiting, or tummy pain?
- What about your bowel habit? Do you have constipation, diarrhea or any blood in the back passage (hemorrhoids)?
- Have you noticed any change in waterworks such as amount, frequency, or pain while passing urine or frothiness in the urine?
- Are you allergic to any medicine or anything else?
- Any long-standing illness that runs in your family such as DM, HTN, stroke, thyroid, or other autoimmune disease or anything else?
- What are you doing for a living? Are you married? Who is at home with you, or who is supporting you now? Do you have children? Are you independent in activities of daily living?

Have I missed anything, or do you want to add anything more?

Would you mind if I go on to examine you?

Focused Examination

[So, this patient is a known case of Marfan syndrome, and he has a background history of AVR with repair surgery of thoracoabdominal aortic aneurysm and surgery for ectopia lentis, now complaining fever with progressive breathlessness. Here likely diagnosis would be infective endocarditis leading to the aortic regurgitation with heart failure. Hence focused examination would be cardiovascular system and identification of the features of Marfan syndrome.]

CVS

- Stigmata of infective endocarditis (splinter hemorrhage, clubbing, rash, Osler node, Jane way lesion).
- Evidence of pulmonary HTN and heart failure (both right and left).
- Evidence of aortic regurgitation (high volume collapsing pulse with wide pulse pressure and early diastolic murmur).

Evidence of Marfan Syndrome

- Tall stature with a long narrow face.
- Dolichostenomelia (disproportionately long arm—arm span >height)
- Arachnodactyly [wrist sign + thumb sign (can encircle the wrist with thumb and little finger)]
- Joint hyperextensibility (thumb able to touch ipsilateral wrist and adduct over the palm with its tip visible at the ulnar border)
- High arch palate
- Pectus carinatum or excavatum
- Kyphoscoliosis
- Flat feet

Eye Examination

- Tremor of the iris (iridodonesis) suggests upward lens dislocation.
- Retinal detachment; blue discoloration of the sclera, heterochromia iridis.

Chest

- A scar from previous surgery [repair of aortic aneurysm, AVR and chest drain (due to pneumothorax)
- Exclusion of the other causes of breathlessness (vesicular breath with prolonging expiration with wheeze due to COPD or bronchiectasis)
- Evidence of pneumothorax (absent breath sound with hyperresonant percussion note)

I would like to complete my examination by doing fundoscopy (to see Roth's spot) and urine dipstick test (for protein, RBC) and BP measurement.

Feedback to the Patient and Respond to the Patient's Concerns

Candidate: You said at the beginning, the main problem was progressive breathlessness and fever. Do you have any other problems that we have missed or any concerns?

Patient: What is the cause of my breathing problem? Why is this happening to me?

Candidate: As you have Marfan syndrome with a history of previous valve surgery, I suspect your breathlessness is due to heart failure as your valve is not working well. Since you have a fever, the condition may be due to an infection in your metallic valve, called infective endocarditis. To reach our diagnosis and rule out other causes, we will need to do some blood tests, USG of your heart (echocardiography), ECG, and chest X-ray.

In terms of your health condition, it's really important to admit you immediately and start the treatment with IV antibiotics as per protocol. Am I clear so far, Mr Nelson?

Do you have any other concerns or questions? Thank you for spending time with me.

Discussion with Examiner

Examiner: Would you please present your case?

Candidate:

This middle-aged gentleman presented with a subacute onset of breathlessness with evidence of infective endocarditis on a background of Marfan syndrome.

On cardiorespiratory examination, there is a major thoracoabdominal scar possibly due to repairing a thoracoabdominal aortic aneurysm with AVR.

There is a metallic click over the second heart sound, which may represent AVR, and there is also an early diastolic murmur associated with a mild collapsing pulse.

There is evidence of infective endocarditis, such as early clubbing with splinter hemorrhage. In addition, he has evidence of heart failure (raised JVP, basal crepitations, and edema).

The patient is tall with disproportionately long limbs compared to the trunk. His arm span is greater than the height. There is kyphoscoliosis of the spine and pectus excavatum of the chest wall.

The thumb and wrist signs are positive, confirming arachnodactyly. There is hypermobility of the joint, high arch palate, and flat feet. There are blue sclera and iridodonesis indicating lens dislocation.

In summary, my diagnosis would be heart failure due to aortic valve incompetence, possibly due to infective endocarditis.

Examiner: How would you investigate this gentleman?

Candidate: I would want to start with some baseline blood tests such as a full blood count looking for anemia as well as inflammatory markers (ESR, CRP) for any signs of infection.

I would want to check baseline urea, creatinine, and electrolytes, and LFTs and coagulation screen (PT with INR) to ensure that he is appropriately warfarinised.

I would like to do 2-3 sets of blood culture and echocardiography—to see the evidence of infective endocarditis; an ECG—to see the evidence of ischemia, and CXR—to exclude other differentials, particularly pneumothorax.

Other second-line investigations would be a CT scan of the chest and pulmonary function test.

Examiner: How will you treat the case?

Candidate: Here, the most important step of management would be general measures to improve symptoms and treatment of heart failure with diuretics (furosemide, spironolactone) and ACEI/ARBs.

As the patient has good clinical ground for diagnosing subacute bacterial endocarditis, I would like to start empiric treatment as soon as I have taken at least three sets of blood culture samples from different sites. Then, I would like to start benzylpenicillin (or vancomycin in a penicillin-allergic patient) plus low dose gentamicin.

Indeed, prosthetic valve endocarditis is very difficult to manage, and I would like to refer him to an MDT urgently involving a cardiologist and cardiothoracic surgeon. Many patients ultimately need surgical intervention (valve replacement).

Osteogenesis Imperfecta

Your role: You are the Registrar in the General Medical Clinic.

Patient details: Mr Leo, a 28-year-old man.

Clinical problem: Bluish discoloration of the eye.

[Once you get this clinical scenario, you will get 5 minutes to start this station for two scenarios. At that time, start to think about your diagnosis and differential diagnoses and plan for taking focused history as well as focused examination.]

[D/D of bluish discoloration of the eye:
- Osteogenesis imperfecta
- Marfan syndrome
- Ehlers–Danlos syndrome
- Pseudoxanthoma elasticum]

[Once you enter the room, search for a spot diagnosis; blue sclera, dentinogenesis imperfecta, hearing aid, scoliosis and evidence of recurrent fracture suggest osteogenesis imperfect.]

Introduction, Permission, and Identification

Candidate: Good morning. I am Mohammad Ali, one of the working doctors here today. I have been asked to talk with you and examine you. Is that ok with you?

Patient: Good morning, doctor…

Candidate: Thank you for coming. May I know your name, please?

Patient: I am Leo.

Candidate: Well, you are 28 years old, right?

Patient: Yes, doctor.

Focused History

Candidate: Ok, Mr Leo. Would you please tell me what brings you here today? Please tell me in your own words.

Patient: I went to an optician because of my eye color. Then she referred me to you because she thought it might be related to the fractures I have had since childhood.

Analyze the Complaint

Candidate: Would you please tell me a little bit more about eye color?
- When did you first notice it?
- Is it increasing or decreasing or the same?
- Do you have any visual problems or any pain in the eyes?

Patient: There has been a kind of bluish discoloration of my sclerae since childhood, but I have no pain in my eyes, and there is no problem with my vision.

Candidate: You mentioned fractures. Can you please tell me in detail about it? Like:
- How many fractures have you had?
- Which part is mainly involved?
- How the fracture occurred? (Is it low trauma fracture like just during playing and falling from a height or walking?)

Patient: I have recurrent fractures, and it's almost 20 times since childhood. I have had multiple fractures in my legs, arms, collar bone, and even a history of a hairline fracture in the spine. The fractures occurred due to simple trauma or while playing or falling, even while I walked.

Candidate: I am sorry to hear. It must be tough for you. Whom do you live with? How does it affect your day-to-day activity? How are you coping with your finances? Are you able to work?

Patient: I live with my family. They support me a lot, and I am managing everything with their help. I work in customer care service in an office, and I have to be very careful even while walking.

Candidate: That's nice to hear. You are working and managing your daily needs. However, at any point, if you need any help, we are always here to help you. Now tell me (when the obvious appearance of osteogenesis imperfecta then targeted history to detect the complications and other associated disorders):

- Do you have any other problems like hearing difficulty? (Hearing problem suggests middle ear bone involvement)
- Do you have any breathlessness, dizziness, palpitation, chest pain, or leg swelling? (May imply aortic incompetence)
- Do you have any other medical problems?
- Do you have any similar conditions in your family? (Mainly autosomal dominant but rarely it may be autosomal recessive.)

Patient: I have had hearing problems since childhood. I am recently using a hearing aid. My father had a similar illness, and he died in his early forties due to a heart problem.

Quick systemic review, PMH, FH, treatment, and social history according to your differentials: If it is not asked previously during initial history taking or incompletely asked, then take a full history of a particular portion to make it complete.

Candidate: I am sorry to hear about your loss. I would like to ask some general questions, is that ok with you?

- Any history of LOC, dizziness, or shaking of the body with uncontrolled waterworks or bowel motion or tongue bite?
- Do you have any altered speech?
- Do you have any fever, weight loss, or loss of appetite?
- Have you attended any consultant or GP or specialist for this problem? What was their impression? Did you receive any diagnosis? What treatment have you received? Did they work?
- Have you ever been admitted to the hospital in the past or have any history of surgery?
- May I ask what medication you take? Do you take any over-the-counter medications or herbal medicine, or any recreational drugs? Are you allergic to any medicine or anything else?
- Any long-standing illness that run in your families such as DM, HTN, stroke, thyroid or autoimmune disease, or anything else?
- Do you smoke? Do you drink?

Have I missed anything, or do you want to add anything more?

Would you mind if I go on to examine you?

Focused Examination

From the history (recurrent fracture, blue scleral, and hearing difficulty) likely diagnosis would be osteogenesis imperfecta. The focused examination would be:

Face
- Blue sclerae
- Dentinogenesis imperfecta (discoloration of translucent teeth)
- Hearing aids (due to involvement of the middle ear bones)

Locomotor
Evidence of multiple previous fractures (maybe patient in a wheelchair; have walking aids nearby or have the obvious scar)
- Bowing of the long bones
- Scoliosis
- Joint hyperextensibility (thumb able to touch ipsilateral wrist and adduct over the palm with its tip visible at the ulnar border)
- Pectus carinatum.

Skin
- Skin hyperlaxity

CVS: To see the evidence of aortic regurgitation (wide pulse pressure, high volume collapsing pulse, and early diastolic murmur).

Feedback to the Patient and Respond to the Patient's Concern

Candidate: You said at the beginning that your main problem was discoloration of the eyes with recurrent fractures in the past. What do you think? Why is this happening to you?

Patient: I also think all of this is related to my fractures, as my eye doctor said. I'm very fed up with the problem of my fracture. Can it be prevented in any way? Can you do something about it?

Candidate: I believe all of your symptoms and signs are due to a genetic condition called osteogenesis imperfecta. The blue discoloration of your eyes is a part of the condition, and there is no specific need to treat this. However, we can prevent further fractures with medications that increase your bone strength. We will need to plan some basic blood tests and X-rays of your bone to confirm the diagnosis.

As this is an inherited disorder, and there are implications for your (future) children that we need to discuss further if a diagnosis is confirmed. Therefore, I need to refer you to the genetic clinic. Is that ok, Mr Leo?

Meanwhile, to prevent your future fracture and improve your mobility, we will take an opinion from our occupational health team. They will assess you and make the necessary adjustments as you need.

Do you have any other concerns? Thank you for spending time with me today.

Discussion with Examiner

Examiner: Would you please present your case?

Candidate:

This man presented with bluish discoloration of the eyes and recurrent fractures, which have happened since childhood.

On examination, he was short stature with barrel shape chest, and he had an obvious deformity in both of his legs. In addition, he had multiple scars in different parts of his body indicated previous surgeries for his fractures.

He walked with an abnormal gait, and he also had joint hypermobility.

I believe all of these are in keeping with a diagnosis of osteogenesis imperfecta.

Examiner: How will you investigate?

Candidate: At first, I would like to start with some blood tests that include CBC with ESR, serum calcium, serum phosphate, serum alkaline phosphatase, vitamin D3 level, serum parathyroid hormone (PTH), as well as renal and liver function tests.

Then I would like to do X-rays of the involved bones and a DEXA bone density scan.

Finally, I would like to confirm the diagnosis by doing a genetic test (DNA blood test).

Examiner: How will you treat this case?

Candidate: There is no cure for osteogenesis imperfecta, but the main aim of the treatment is to correct and prevent fractures or deformities. Hence symptomatic improvement is the primary goal of currently available treatment options.

He should be managed under an MDT involving:
- Physiotherapy and rehabilitation with assistive devices such as wheelchair, braces, and other custom equipment.
- Orthopedic surgery to manage recurring fractures, bowing of the bone, scoliosis, and rodding is a minimally invasive procedure to insert a simple, telescopic metal rod (Fassier–Duval rod) in the length of a long bone to stabilize it and prevent deformity.

Medical therapy for pain and bone strength includes calcium, vitamin D, and bisphosphonate therapy.

Post-transplant Lymphoproliferative Disorder

Your role: You are the Registrar in the General Medical Clinic.

Patient details: Mr John, a 45-year-old male.

Clinical problem: Fever, weight loss, axillary lymphadenopathy, and swelling over the renal transplant.

[Once you get this clinical scenario, you will get 5 minutes to start this station for two scenarios. At that time, start to think about your diagnosis and differential diagnoses and plan for taking focused history as well as focused examination.]

Evaluation of post-transplant patients:
- Causes of renal transplant.
- *Functional status of the transplanted kidney*: Transplant dysfunction? (Acute/chronic rejection due to most commonly sub-therapeutic immunosuppression, secondary to infections or recurrence of the renal disease in the graft).
- Evidence of complication of immune suppression.
- *Infection*: Typical (lower respiratory tract infection, skin infection); atypical (CMV, pneumocystis jirovecii, EBV, BK virus, JC virus)
- *Malignancy*: Skin (SCC, BCC), lymphoproliferative (lymphoma, PTLD-post transplant lymphoproliferative disease)
- *Metabolic complication*: Post-transplant DM (steroid, tacrolimus)
- *Cardiovascular disease*: IHD, CVD, HTN
- *Drug-induced side-effect*:
  - Cyclosporin: Alopecia, tremor, gum hypertrophy, hirsutism
  - Tacrolimus: Nephrotoxicity, neurotoxicity (encephalopathy, tremor, seizure, blurring of vision), QT prolongation.
  - Azathioprine: Bone marrow suppression (anemia, neutropenia, thrombocytopenia), hepatitis/obstructive jaundice, pancreatitis, increase the risk of malignancy.
  - Steroid: Cushingoid appearance/Cushing syndrome, avascular necrosis of head of the femur, DM, proximal myopathy, osteoporosis]
- Evidence of renal replacement therapy (RRT) before the transplant.

[Once you enter the room, search for a spot diagnosis; Cushingoid appearance, hirsutism, transplant scar suggests post-transplant patient.]

Introduction, Permission, and Identification

Candidate: Good morning. My name is Mohammad Ali, one of the working doctors here today. I have been asked to see you. Is that okay with you?

Patient: Good morning, doctor...

Candidate: Thank you for coming. I would like to start by taking your name.

Patient: I am John.

Candidate: May I confirm your age?

Patient: I am 45 years old.

Focused History

Candidate: Okay, Mr John, would you please tell me what brings you here today? Please tell me in your own words.

Patient: I have had a fever for the last 2 weeks. I notice a swelling in my armpit. Recently I have noticed pain and swelling in my transplant kidney, and I have lost some weight.

Analyze the Symptoms

Candidate: Please tell me a little bit more about your fever?
- When did you first notice the fever? (duration)
- Is it coming on and off or all the time with you? (regular/irregular; intermittent/continuous)
- Have you measured the temperature? What was the highest recorded temperature?
- Any night sweats or focal symptoms such as cough, breathlessness, constipation, diarrhea, and difficulty passing urine?
- Have you travelled anywhere recently? Have you taken any antibiotics?

Patient: I have been suffering from fever, especially at night for the last 3 weeks. Last night it was 102°F. I took only paracetamol for my fever. I have a sore throat with this fever.

Candidate: What about your weight loss?
- How much weight have you lost? Over how long?
- Is the weight loss intentional or unintentional? How is your appetite?
- Have you noticed any bowel changes such as constipation/diarrhea or any blood in the stool?

Patient: I have lost 4 kg weight in the last 3 weeks, and also I have lost my appetite—no changes in bowel habit, no loose stool.

Candidate:
What about your armpit swelling?
- When did you first notice the swelling?
- Is it increasing or decreasing or the same in size?
- Does it painful? Is it fixed or mobile?
- Have you noticed any lumps or bumps in the other body parts such as in the neck, groin or tummy?

Patient: Since last week, I have noticed a swelling in my right axilla. There is no pain, but the swelling is movable.

Candidate:
You said at the beginning that you have swelling over the renal transplant.
- Is there any pain here? Is it warm or cold?
- Is it increasing in size or decreasing or the same?
- Is there any change in your waterworks such as amount/volume of urine, pain in passing urine, frothiness, or blood in the urine?

Patient: There is swelling over my transplant. It has been for the last few days. But I don't have any pain there. My waterworks go normal, and no other changes in the urine.

Candidate: Now tell me about your transplant (ask about his pre-transplant and post-transplant status).
- Do you know why a kidney transplant was done?
- How was it managed before the transplant? (hemodialysis or peritoneal dialysis)
- What about your transplant kidney? Is it a deceased or living donor transplant? Where and when it was performed?
- Do you have any history of post-transplant infection or rejection in transplant and how it was managed?
- What are the drugs you are taking currently? Do you have any side effects or complications of taking these drugs recently or in the past? *Like*:
    o Have you noticed any shaking limbs, confusion, dizziness, headache, or LOC?
    o Any difficulty in standing from a sitting position? Any changes in the skin? Any tremor? Any history of jaundice or bleeding?
    o Any history of fracture (avascular necrosis of the head of the femur)?
    o Do you have diabetes or HTN, or any illness?
    o Are you allergic to any medicine or anything else?

Patient: I had a cadaveric transplant 12 months ago for kidney failure. Before that, I was on dialysis via a fistula in my left hand. I had gout, and I took painkillers for a long time. Finally, doctors told me that it was the reason for my kidney failure. After 6-weeks of my transplant, I suffered an episode of rejection. Doctors did a snip test (biopsy) and treated me with IV steroids. I was last seen in the clinic 6 weeks ago and told that overall progress was satisfactory. My current medications include tacrolimus 1 mg 12 hourly, mycophenolate mofetil

500 mg 12 hourly, prednisolone 5 mg once daily, ganciclovir 1,000 mg 8 hourly, calcium carbonate 12 hourly, and ramipril 2.5 mg once daily.

Quick systemic review, PMH, FH, treatment, and social history according to your differentials: If it is not asked previously during initial history taking or incompletely asked, then take a full history of a particular portion to make it complete.

Candidate: At this moment I would like to ask some general questions, is that okay with you?
- Is there anyone in your family with this type of problem or any long-standing illness that runs in your family such as DM, HTN, stroke, thyroid or other autoimmune diseases, or anything else?
- Do you smoke? Do you drink?
- What are you doing for a living? Are you married? Who is at home with you, or who is supporting you now? Do you have children? Are you independent in activities of daily living?

Patient: I am a computer programmer, married with two healthy children, do not smoke but drink alcohol occasionally.

Candidate: Have I missed anything, or do you want to add anything more?
Would you mind if I go on to examine you?

Focused Examination

Here the patient with post-renal transplant status, now presented with fever and generalized lymphadenopathy. So focused examination would be:
- Any evidence of transplant failure such as a sign of fluid overload (raised JVP, sacral or peripheral edema, basal crepitation, HTN, and most importantly, history of urine output-oliguria, suggest renal failure) or any evidence of recent needling in the A-V fistula or tunneled line for hemodialysis.
- Sign of uremia (skin excoriation in response to pruritus, distal sensory-motor neuropathy)
- *Cushingoid feature*: (Evidence of recent high dose steroid therapy to manage a period of rejection)
- Tenderness over the graft suggests chronic graft rejection.

Past Evidence of Renal Replacement Therapy
- A-V fistula (wrist or cubital fossa)—the presence of thrill and bruit suggests functioning fistula.
- Recent puncture marks suggest recent hemodialysis
- Previous peritoneal dialysis scar marks in the abdomen (midline)

Evidence of Side Effects of the Drugs
- A tremor in outstretched hand (tacrolimus and cyclosporine)
- Gum hypertrophy (cyclosporine)
- Cushingoid facies, striae, thin skin with easy bruising or oropharyngeal candidiasis for oral steroid use.

Abdomen
- The scar for previous peritoneal dialysis or nephrectomy scar or transplant scar.
- Examine renal allograft (note any masses, tenderness, and bruit), hepatosplenomegaly.

Neck and Chest
- Para thyroidectomy scar.
- Hemodialysis catheter scar.
- *Lymphadenopathy*: Most important part of this patient's examination.

Cardiorespiratory: If there is evidence of infection due to chronic immune suppression from history.
Search for any evidence of skin malignancy as well.

Feedback to the Patient and Respond to the Patient's Concerns

Candidate: You said at the beginning that the main problems were fever, weight loss, and axillary lump with swelling over the renal transplant. Is there anything else that we have missed?

Patient: No. Can you please tell me why I have this problem? I am worried about whether my kidney fails again!

Candidate: As far you told, and I examined, it seems your transplant kidney is working well as you are passing normal urine, and there is no other evidence of transplant failure at this moment.

However, I am concerned about your fever, recent weight loss, and armpit swellings, which can be due to a complication of different drugs used to suppress your defense system that can be responsible for getting infections like TB, CMV, EMV, etc.

Although it is rare, but post-transplant lymphoproliferative disease (PTLD) is another possibility in a post-transplant patient with similar symptoms. PTLD is classified as lymphoma, a group of related cancers that affect your lymphatic system.

I would suggest getting admission so we can carry out further blood tests and imaging, taking a snip from your armpit swelling (lymph node biopsy) after getting your consent to know the nature of that growth. After getting the result, we will refer you to an MDT involving a renal transplant team, kidney doctor, blood doctor, specialist nurse, and a social worker and psychiatrist.

Do you have any other concerns, please? Thank you for spending time with me today.

Discussion with Examiner

Examiner: Would you please present your case?

Candidate: This middle-aged man presented with fever, weight loss, axillary lymphadenopathy, and swelling in the renal transplant.

Positive findings include:

A large "J" shaped scar with a palpable mass below it; a smooth, non-tender (3 × 4 cm) mass on the renal graft. There is lymphadenopathy involving the right axilla and both-sided submandibular regions. The lymph node is firm in consistency, discrete, nontender, and freely mobile.

He has a palpable AV fistula with a palpable thrill in the left arm and no evidence of recent needling here.

He also has two scars in his abdomen consistent with previous peritoneal dialysis.

No evidence of other access points for hemodialysis.

No evidence of volume overload (raised JVP, peripheral or sacral edema).

There is no evidence of the toxicity of immune suppression such as gum hypertrophy, tremor, skin malignancies, thinning of the skin, or other signs related to chronic steroid use.

So, in summary, the patient has a functioning renal transplant, and for his recent presentation, my differentials would be:
- Post-transplant lymphoproliferative disease
- Post-transplant infectious mononucleosis, CMV, and disseminated TB

Examiner: How will you investigate the case?

Candidate: I would like to start with basic blood tests include inflammatory markers and FBC, to look for evidence of sepsis (leukocytosis, raised CRP), serum urea, and creatinine, which will be elevated in the context of graft failure, serum electrolytes, blood sugar, lipid profile, LFT's, and very importantly immunosuppressive levels (cyclosporine or tacrolimus usually to rule out toxic or sub-therapeutic levels).

Then I would like to do a full septic screen including blood culture, urine R/M/E with cultures and stool cultures, and CXR, renal ultrasounds to look renal transplant mass, obstruction or perinephric collection; color flow Doppler of the renal transplant to look at vasculature and perfusion. I would also consider a CT scan of the abdomen.

Finally, I would like to do a lymph node biopsy; most importantly, PTLD lesion should be biopsied to established cell clonality, malignancy, and presence or absence of EBV virus.

Examiner: How will you treat the patient?

Candidate: The management will depend on the etiology of the presentation. I would like to involve an MDT, including the renal transplant team, nephrologist, and hematologist, for his proper management plan.

… CHAPTER 1 Clinical Consultation

Sexually Transmitted Infection

Your role: You are the Doctor in the General Medical Clinic.

Patient details: Mr Pitter Smith, a 25-year-old man.

Clinical problem: Dysuria

[Once you get this clinical scenario, you will get 5 minutes to start this station for two scenarios. At that time, start to think about your diagnosis and differential diagnoses and plan for taking focused history as well as focused examination.]

D/D of dysuria:
- UTI (upper or lower)
- STI (if dysuria is associated with urethral discharge)

[Once you enter the room, search for a spot diagnosis; petechial and lace-like rash in the trunk, limbs, palm, and sole with sparing the face, scalp, and neck suggests gonococcal urethritis.]

Introduction, Permission, and Identification

Candidate: Good morning. My name is Mohammad Ali, one of the working doctors here today. I have been asked to see you. Is that ok with you?

Patient: Good morning, Doctor…

Candidate: Thank you for coming. I would like to start by taking your name.

Patient: I am Pitter Smith.

Candidate: May I confirm your age?

Patient: I am 25 years old.

Focused History

Candidate: Ok, Mr Smith. Would you please tell me what brings you here today?

Patient: I have a burning sensation when passing urine. I have noticed a white discharge from the penis for the last 5 days.

Analyze the Symptoms

Candidate: Would you please tell me a little bit more about your waterworks?
- Since when you noticed pain while passing urine?
- Have you noticed any changes in color or amount or any frothiness in the urine?
- Have you noticed any blood during waterworks?
- Have you noticed any pain in the lower part of your tummy, flank, or loin?
- Do you have any fever with or without chills?
- Do you have any nausea, vomiting, or any other problems?

Patient: It has been for the last 5 days. I have to go to the loo more often these days, and I have to wake up during the night 2–3 times. I don't have any fever, chills, or tummy pain. But I am worried about the creamy white discharge from the penis.

Other Important Targeted Histories

Sexual History

Candidate: I can see your worriedness. Let me assess you first, and hopefully, we will be able to help you. Ok, Mr Smith?

Patient: Ok

Candidate: I am going to ask you some questions about your sexual health and sexual practice. I believe these questions are very personal, but they are very important for your overall health. Is that ok, Mr Smith? Just saying, I ask these questions to all my adult patients, regardless of age, gender, or marital status. These questions are important as the questions about other areas of your physical health, like the rest of our visits. This information will be kept strictly confidential. Is that ok with you, or do you have any questions before we get started? [The 5Ps of sexual history include partner, practice, protection from STD, past history of STD, and prevention of pregnancy.]

- **P**artner:
  - Are you presently sexually active (are you having sex)? If not, have you ever been sexually active?
  - In current months, how many sex partners have you had?
  - In the last 1 year, how many sex partners have you had?
  - Are your sex partner women, men, or both?
- **P**ractice: I will be more specific here about the kind of sex you have had over the last year to understand better if you are at risk for STD. Is that ok, Smith?
  - What kind of sexual contact have you had? Is it genital (insertion of penis in vagina), anal (insertion of penis in anus) or oral (insertion of penis in mouth)?
- **P**rotection:
  - Do you and your partner(s) take any protection against STD? If not, would you like me to tell the reason? If so, what type of protection do you use?
  - How often do you use this protection?
- **P**ast history of STD:
  - Have you ever been diagnosed with an STD? When and how were you treated?
  - Have you ever been tested for HIV or other STD? If yes, when were you tested? What was the diagnosis? How was it treated?
  - Has your current partner or any former partner ever been diagnosed or treated for an STD?
- **P**revention of pregnancy:
  - Are you currently trying to be the father of a child?
  - Are you concerned about getting your partner pregnant?
  - Are you using contraception?

Patient: I have had 14 sexual partners in total, all protected except for the recent two and Angela. Angela and I were in a long-term relationship, but we separated for 6 months. At that time, I had multiple partners. I was on a recent trip 1 month ago with friends, where I had unprotected sex with two partners, both were females. That was vaginal intercourse, no anal, no oral sex, no sex with men; I have no idea of their background sexual history. The penile discharge actually started 5 days ago after sex on holiday with one of my office colleagues. Last week, I noticed a faint red, lacy rash over my wrist, which has now gone away. Recently Angela and I have been together again, and I never use condoms with her. Angela is unaware of my urine problems and discharge.

Associated Arthritis

Candidate:
- Have you noticed gritty or painful red eye with or without blurring of vision? (conjunctivitis/uveitis for reactive arthritis)
- Do you have any joint pain or back pain (reactive arthritis)?

Patient: No

Quick systemic review, PMH, FH, treatment, and social history according to your differentials: If it is not asked previously during initial history taking or incompletely asked, then take a full history of a particular portion to make it complete.

Candidate: At this moment I would like to ask some general questions, is that ok with you?
- Do you have a headache, dizziness, or shaking limbs? Do you have chest pain, breathlessness, or swelling of limbs?
- Do you have any similar condition or any other history of disease in your past? Have you ever been admitted to the hospital?
- Have you attended any consultant or GP or specialist for this problem? What was their impression? Did you receive any diagnosis? What treatment have you received? Did they work?
- May I ask what medication you take? Do you take any over-the-counter medications or herbal medicine, or any recreational drugs?

Are you allergic to any medicine or anything else?
- Is there anyone in your family with this type of problem or any long-standing illness that runs in your family such as DM, HTN, stroke, thyroid, or other autoimmune diseases, or anything else?
- Do you smoke? Do you drink? What are you doing for a living?

Have I missed anything, or do you want to add anything more?

Would you mind if I go on to examine you?

Focused Examination

- *Overall inspection*: Look for rash (petechial, lacy rash of gonococcus, a maculopapular rash can be seen in HIV seroconversion).
- *Eye*: Evidence of uveitis/conjunctivitis.
- *Abdomen*: Look for supra-pubic tenderness or flank tenderness for cystitis or pyelonephritis.
- *Genitourinary*: Examine the testis, penis/external genitalia. Check for any evidence of discharge, balanitis/epididymitis.
- Any evidence of arthropathy (reactive arthritis)

Feedback to the Patient and Respond to the Patient's Concerns

Candidate: You said at the beginning, the main problem was dysuria and urethral discharge. Is there anything else that we have missed? Any concerns or expectations, or questions?

Patient: What's wrong with me, doctor?

Candidate: The combination of urethral discharge and burning while passing urine in a young man makes us concerned about sexually transmitted infection (STI), particularly given your recent unprotected sex with your casual partners. We will need to test the discharge for gonococcus and carry out a full check-up, including checking for other possible infections such as chlamydia and trichomonas. We will also recommend a blood test for HBV, HCV, HIV, and syphilis. Is that ok with you?

You should avoid any kind of sexual activity until your treatment finishes or completely cure the infection. As it is a sexually transmitted condition, Angela can get the infection from you. Therefore, it is very important to complete treatment by bringing your partner and treating her as well if she has got the infection.

Patient: How will I tell Angela?

Candidate: An honest approach is best. I suggest you explain to Angela that you had sexual partners while separated from her, and your doctors think you've caught an infection from that partner on holiday. I suggest you explain to her that the doctors have given you treatment and advice that she gets a full check-up. Please explain that it is important to get a check-up and receive any necessary treatment as there are potential risks to her future fertility if certain infections are left untreated.

Do you have any other concerns? Thank you for spending time with me today.

Discussion with Examiner

Examiner: Would you please present your case?

Candidate:

This young man presented with dysuria and urethral discharge on the background history of unprotected sex with a new partner.

He also has had a history of a faint red lacy rash over his wrist 7 days ago, which is now gone away.

In summary, my diagnosis would be gonococcal urethritis, but other causes of STI need to be excluded.

Examiner: How will you investigate this case?

Candidate: At first, I would like to do a urethral discharge swab for Gram staining and C/S looking for gram-negative gonococci and polymorphonuclear leukocytes (>25/HPF). If no gram-negative diplococci, a level of nonspecific urethritis is applied.

Then, I would like to take first void urine (FVU) samples for nucleic acid amplification test (NAAT) for gonorrhea, chlamydia, and trichomonas vaginalis.

As the patient has had multiple sexual partners, I would like to do a blood test for HBV, HCV, HIV, and syphilis (VDRL, TPHA).

Examiner: How will you treat this patient?

Candidate: The most important step of management would be to give antibiotics. The best regimen would be ceftriaxone 500 mg IM stat plus azithromycin 1 gm orally stat to treat concomitant other infections (50% of patients with gonorrhea may have a concomitant infection). In case of complicated disease, I would like to add doxycycline with or without metronidazole.

At the same time, I would like to advise the patient to avoid sexual contact until it is confirmed that any infection has resolved, and whenever possible, recent sexual contact should be treated.

CHAPTER 1 Clinical Consultation

Crohn's Disease

Your role: You are the Registrar in the General Medical Clinic.

Patient details: Mr Paul John, a 25-year-old man.

Clinical problem: This young man, referred by his GP, presented with recurrent abdominal pain and diarrhea for 2 months.

[Once you get this clinical scenario, you will get 5 minutes to start this station for two scenarios. At that time, start to think about your diagnosis and differential diagnoses and plan for taking focused history as well as focused examination.]

[Differential diagnoses: IBD (Crohn's disease), chronic pancreatitis, abdominal tuberculosis, giardiasis, GIT malignancy including lymphoma, malabsorption syndrome, e.g., Celiac disease.]

[Once you enter the room, search for a spot diagnosis; clubbing, pyoderma gangrenosum, and evidence of recurrent abdominal surgeries including stoma in situ suggest Crohn's disease]

Introduction, Permission, and Identification

Candidate: Good morning. My name is Mohammad Ali, one of the working doctors here today. I have been asked to see you. Is that ok?

Patient: Good morning, Doctor…

Candidate: Thank you for coming. I would like to start by taking your name.

Patient: I am Paul John.

Candidate: What would you like me to call you?

Patient: John.

Candidate: May I confirm your age?

Patient: I am 25 years old.

Focused History

Candidate: I gather from your GP's note that you haven't been so well over the past 2 months. Can you tell me what has been happening?

Patient: I have had recurrent pain in my tummy and diarrhea for the last 2 months. I have lost weight around 2 kg over the period.

Analyze the Symptom

Candidate: Ok, Mr John. Would you please tell me a little bit more about your tummy pain?
(The important questions to be asked.)
- When were you last well?
- When did you first notice the tummy pain? Did it come on gradually or suddenly?
- Where exactly does the pain come on? Can you show me?
- Is the pain constant, or does it come and go in waves?
- What sort of pain is it? Can you describe it? Is it sharp, dull, or cramping in nature?
- Does the pain move anywhere from your tummy? Does it go through to your back?
- How severe is the pain?
- Is there anything else that makes it better or worse while taking a meal, movement, or opening bowel?

Patient: I have had pain in the right lower area of my tummy for the last 3 months, which starts about 1 hour after eating. Along with this, I feel bloated and full. My partner told me that she could hear my bowel rumbling. I had severe pain last night, which came on about an hour after eating. It felt like a cramping and gripping pain in the right lower part of my tummy. I tried a hot water bottle and paracetamol to ease my pain, but it did not help. I vomited last night for the first time, and this did ease the tummy pain for a few hours.

Candidate: Ok, can you tell me more about your diarrhea?
- When did you first notice the diarrhea?
- Is it getting better or worse day-by-day or the same?
- How many times do you open your bowel a day?
- Amount or volume of the stool? Color and consistency of the stool?
- Is there any blood in the stool (dysentery, proctitis, and sigmoiditis)? Or any undigested food particles in the stool (malabsorption)?
- Is there any difficulty to flush away stool?
- Is there anything else that makes it worse or better such as diet, drugs, and foods? (Related to gluten-containing food such as wheat, barley, oats in Celiac disease/fatty food in case of chronic pancreatitis).
- Do you tend to feel hot more than usual? Any racing heartbeat, excessive sweating, irritability? (thyrotoxicosis)
- Do you wake up from sleep to open your bowel? (rule out IBS)
- Sexual history (HIV)
- Family history (IBD, Celiac)
- Any itchy rash, usually in the elbow and buttock (dermatitis herpetiformis) or any history of autoimmune disease (Celiac disease)?
- Do you smoke or drink alcohol? If yes, then for how long and what is the amount?

Patient: I have loose stool with custard consistency up to three times per day. I have not been opening my bowels at night. No blood in the stool or no rush to the toilet. Before this all started, I was opening my bowels once per day with formed motion. I am active, and I thought it might be due to stress initially, but now I think it might be related to the pain. My grandmother had bowel cancer at age 75 years and died shorter afterwards. I am a smoker; smoked 20 sticks per day for the last 6 years. I never drink alcohol.

Candidate: You said at the beginning that you have weight loss. Please tell me about your weight loss (intentional/unintentional, amount/duration, appetite, food habit, and exercise).

Patient: I have lost 2 kg over the last 2 months, despite a regular balanced meal. However, my appetite is good, and I am doing exercise regularly as before.

Candidate: (Since it suggests a case of Crohn's disease—by the patient's general look and history)—then to check the extra-articular manifestations,

Other Important Targeted Histories
- Please tell me how the symptoms affected your day-to-day activity or jobs?
- Do you have nausea, vomiting, difficulty in swallowing?
- Do you have a fever with night sweats?
- Do you have any recent foreign travel history?
- Have you noticed any mouth ulcers?
- Have you noticed any painful red-eye, blurred vision, or gritty sensation in the eye (uveitis)?
- Do you have joint pain or back pain (enteropathic arthritis)?
- Do you have any skin rash (erythema nodosum, pyoderma gangrenosum)?
- Have you noticed your eye white (sclerae) turned yellow with generalized itching (jaundice with PSC in UC)?
- Severe abdominal pain, systemic inflammatory response syndrome (SIRS) (e.g., fever), distended abdomen (rule out toxic megacolon)?

Patient: I have lower back pain.

Candidate: Since when have you had back pain? Any morning stiffness; or does the pain increase in the morning? Any other joints pain?

Patient: For the last 3 weeks. And yes, the pain increases in the morning. I don't have pain in other joints.

Quick systemic review, PMH, FH, treatment, and social history according to your differentials: If it is not asked previously during initial history taking or incompletely asked, then take a full history of a particular portion to make it complete.

Candidate: At this moment I would like to ask some general questions, is that ok with you?

- Do you have a headache, dizziness, LOC, or shaking limbs?
- Any chest pain, cough, breathlessness, or limb swelling?
- What about your waterworks? Have you noticed any change in waterworks?
- Do you have any similar condition or any other history of disease in your past? Have you ever been admitted to the hospital?
- Have you attended any consultant or specialist for this problem? What was their impression? Did you receive any diagnosis? What treatment have you received? Did they work?
- May I ask what medication you take? Do you take any over-the-counter medications or herbal medicines, or any recreational drugs? Are you allergic to any medicine or anything else?
- Is there anyone in your family with this type of problem or any long-standing illness that runs in your family such as DM, HTN, stroke, thyroid or other autoimmune diseases, or anything else?
- What are you doing for a living? Are you married? Who is at home with you, or who is supporting you now? Do you have children? Are you independent in activities of daily living?

Have I missed anything, or do you want to add anything more?

Ok, thank you. Would you mind if I go on to examine you now?

Focused Examination

From history, the most likely diagnosis is Crohn's disease with seronegative arthritis. So focused examination would be.

Peripheral Signs

Anemia, clubbing, erythema nodosum, pyoderma gangrenosum, mouth ulcer, angular stomatitis, and glossitis.

Abdomen

- Visible peristalsis (obstruction), any scar from previous surgery (due to obstruction, perforation, stricture, and fistula) or any stoma.
- Tenderness in the right iliac fossa with or without palpable mass, high pitched bowel sound (obstruction).

Examination in the spine: Just like ankylosing spondylitis (spinal movement) + evidence of sacroiliitis

I would like to complete my assessment by doing per rectal digital examination, urine dipstick for sugar and protein, BP measurement, as well as eye examination (for uveitis).

Feedback to the Patient and Respond to the Patient's Concerns

Candidate: You said at the beginning, the main problem was recurrent abdominal pain, back pain, diarrhea, and weight loss. Is there anything else that we have missed or any worries or concerns?

Patient: What's wrong with me, doctor? Do I have cancer like my grandmother?

Candidate: Your symptoms and signs raise the possibility that there is inflammation of the bowel lining called inflammatory bowel disease. It is less likely to get cancer at your age. However, we will do further tests to rule out cancer.

I would suggest getting admission so we can carry out some blood tests, stool tests, and camera tests (endoscopy/colonoscopy) to confirm our diagnosis as well as to exclude other possibilities that may cause similar symptoms. IBD is usually readily managed with medication. Occasionally, surgery may need to remove the affected bowel; once we exclude infectious cause, we can start treatment immediately.

Patient: Will I still be able to go to the University exam coming up in a couple of months?

Candidate: We will need to carry out the investigations and refer you to the tummy doctor. Then they will start treatment once a diagnosis has been made. The treatment will aim to get you well so that you can attend university and sit your exam as planned.

Do you have any other concerns or questions? Ok, thank you for spending time with me today.

Discussion with Examiner

Examiner: Would you please present your case?

Candidate:

This young man has been suffering with a subacute history of abdominal symptoms spanning for over the last 2 months with abdominal cramping, chronic diarrhea, and significant weight loss. This is on the background of extraintestinal symptoms of inflammatory back pain.

On examination—he is mildly anemic and has oral ulceration with evidence of uveitis. The abdomen is mildly tender in the right iliac fossa.

I feel the underlying diagnosis here is one of the IBDs, and because of these extra gastrointestinal symptoms, I suspect the diagnosis may be Crohn's disease with spondylitis.

Examiner: What is your differential diagnosis?

Candidate: Ileocecal TB, giardiasis, chronic pancreatitis. Because of his young age, malignancy is unlikely here.

Examiner: How will you investigate the case?

Candidate: I would like to start with basic blood tests that include CBC, ESR, CRP, U/E, serum creatinine, iron profile, B12, folate, LFT's including INR, and TFT's.

Then, I would like to do stool microscopy and culture with sensitivity as well as *Clostridium difficile* toxin assay to rule out infective gastroenteritis. Finally, to check for GI inflammation, fecal calprotectin (a simple, non-invasive test for GI inflammation with high sensitivity) may be helpful.

Moreover, I would like to do an additional X-ray to look for evidence of mucosal edema, bowel dilatation (in toxic dilatation; colon >5 cm dilates) or perforation.

Finally, I would like to refer the patient for endoscopies, particularly colonoscopy, to perform biopsies of the large bowel to determine whether this is Crohn's or ulcerative colitis. Other tests include:
- Capsule endoscopy to detect isolated proximal disease.
- MRI scans are increasingly used to assess pelvic disease, fistula, small bowel disease activity, and strictures.

Examiner: Now tell me, how will you treat a case of Crohn's disease?

Candidate: During an acute attack, to induce remission, we have to use steroids. In case of mild-to-moderate Crohn's disease (symptomatic but systemically well), prednisolone 40 mg/day for 1 week, then tapered by 5 mg every week for the next 7 weeks. Azathioprine (2–2.5 mg/kg/day orally) is used if refractory to steroids, relapsing on steroid taper, or requiring >2 steroids courses per year.

However, in case of severe disease, the patient requires IV hydration or electrolytes replacement; thromboprophylaxis; IV steroids, e.g., hydrocortisone 100 mg 6 hourly after excluding concomitant infections. If improving, switches to oral prednisolone (40 mg/day); if not, biologics (anti-TNF alpha-infliximab) have a role in combating such situation.

About 50–80% of cases need one or more surgical interventions in their lifetime. The indication includes:
- Most commonly, drug failure.
- GIT obstruction from stricture, perforation, fistulae, and abscess.

Other measures include enteral nutrition (polymorphic diet is preferred) if needed and smoking cessation.

CHAPTER 2

History Taking

- ❏ Hemoptysis
- ❏ Headache
- ❏ Joint Pain
- ❏ Abdominal Bloating
- ❏ Night Sweats

Hemoptysis

Your role: You are the doctor in the respiratory clinic.

Patient profile: Mr Alex Blacksmith, 65-year-old.

Problem: Chronic cough and hemoptysis.

Please read the referral letter printed here. You have 14 minutes to take a history from the patient. You will have 1 minute to collect your thoughts. In the last 5 minutes, examiner will ask you to explain any abnormalities in the detailed clinical history and regarding your diagnosis or differential diagnoses including management plan (if this was not cleared from your consultation).

Referral

"Dear Doctor,

Thank you for seeing Mr Alex Blacksmith who has had chronic cough and hemoptysis for the past few weeks. He has been treated for chest infections six times in the last 2 years but has no other lung problems. A chest X-ray has been done which shows changes consistent with bronchiectasis.

Please see the patient and advise on further investigation and management.

Yours Sincerely,
General Practitioner"

Your task is to: Take a detailed history, construct a diagnosis, differential diagnosis, and plan for further investigation and management. Explain your possible diagnosis or differential diagnoses, including your investigation and management plan to the patient. Address any concerns or specific questions that the patient may have.

Do not examine the patient.

At the end of the station, any notes you make must be handed to the examiners.

[Once you enter the room search for a spot diagnosis; dyspnea, using the accessory muscle of respiration, raised jugular venous pressure (JVP), cachexia, sputum pot, inhalers, nebulizer, and oxygen mask suggest respiratory illnesses]

Introduction, Permission, and Identification

Candidate: Good morning, I am Dr Ali, one of the working doctors here today, I have been asked to talk to you; is that okay with you?

Patient: Good morning. Yes, doctor ...

Candidate: Thank you for coming, I would like to start by taking your full name, age, and where you have come from, please?

Patient: Yes, doctor ... I am Alex Blacksmith, I am 65 and from London.

Candidate: What would you like me to call you?

Patient: Alex is fine.

Detailed History

Candidate: Okay, Alex, I understand you have been referred by your general practitioner (GP) and a chest X-ray has been done for you. Would you please tell me more about what exactly has happened to you?

Patient: I have had a cough for a long time, but recently I have been coughing up blood. First, I noticed blood 3 weeks ago that was a very little amount, but now it is occurring several times a day for the last 2 weeks. I got scared and went to my GP, and then GP did an X-ray and send me here.

Analyze the Complaint

Candidate: Alex, I can see you are worried, let me ask you some questions to find out what has been happening and to see how we can help you. Is that, ok?

Patient: Okay.

Candidate: At first, tell me more about your cough.
- Since when did you have a cough? Is it increasing, decreasing gradually, or is it the same?
- Is it on and off or all over the day? Or any particular time in the day like in the morning?
- Does anything in the particular trigger or aggravate the cough like dust, pollen, fumes, or anything else?
- Anything makes it better like taking inhalers? Or have you tried anything for it?
- Does it contain any phlegm? If yes—how much? Cupful/spoonful? What is the color of your phlegm—white, green, or brown?
- You told me that you have been coughing up blood, is this the first time you noticed blood?

Patient: For the last 2 years, I have had this cough, which usually contains white phlegm, I have this cough all day, but it increases in the morning. I feel that I have to clear my chest every morning, and can cough up a cupful of sputum. This is the first time I have noticed blood on phlegm, but I have had greenish phlegm on several occasions over the last 2 years. And this time happen the worst thing; I have been noticing the blood. I do not know what has been happening, now I am tired of this cough, Doctor!

Candidate: I can see you are suffering for a long time and it is quite reasonable to become exhausted. We are here to help you, hopefully, we can find a proper solution for you. Along with this cough do you have any other symptoms such as:
- Breathlessness? Wheeze? Chest pain? Heart racing? Any swelling in your limbs?
- Any fever? Night sweats? Weight loss? Changes in your appetite?
- Have you noticed any lumps or bumps anywhere in your body?

Patient: Oh yes, Doctor. I have breathing problems, particularly while I climb stairs and walk faster. Otherwise, nothing else actually.

Candidate: Please tell me more about your breathing problem.
- When did you first notice it? Was it come on suddenly or gradually? Is it increasing, decreasing gradually, or is it the same?
- Is there any particular time in the day when your breathlessness gets worse? (Diurnal variation)
- You told me that you feel breathless while climbing stairs and fast walking. How about while just walking around the house or at rest?
- How does this breathlessness affect your daily life? How far could you walk before you had this breathlessness?
- Do you struggle to sleep due to breathlessness, and do you use extra pillows for sleeping?
- Does anything in the particular trigger or aggravate it? Does anything make it better like taking rest, inhaler, or nebulizer?

Patient: I have had this breathing problem for the last 6 months. I feel that this is getting worse nowadays, but I am ok with my daily activities. I am ok when I walk slowly and just take some rest while fast walking it resolves.

Candidate: Well, you told me that you have had greenish phlegm on several occasions, can you tell me more about what happened and how it was managed?

Patient: Yes, in the last 2 years I have had six episodes of chest infection, I have got greenish phlegm along with this cough and every time I needed a course of antibiotics.

Candidate: Any other symptoms apart from this cough and breathlessness?

Patient: No.

Quick Systemic Review, Past Medical History, Family History, Treatment, and Social History According to Your Differentials

Quick Systemic Review

Candidate: Now I would like to ask some general questions that may or may not be related to your

symptoms, just to know about your overall health (ask for those questions which were not asked yet).
- Any history of loss of consciousness or dizziness? Any abnormal shaking of the body?
- Do you have any headache, nausea, vomiting, or any tummy pain?
- Any alteration in your bowel habit? Any diarrhea or constipation?
- What about your waterworks, amount, color, or frequency?

Patient: No. I do not have any of these...

Past Medical and Surgical History

Candidate: Alex, now let us talk about your past medical history....
- Do you have had any similar conditions in the past? Or any other illness? Like any high blood pressure or high blood sugar, lung condition, heart disease, or anything you want to mention?
- Have you ever been admitted to the hospital in the past or have any history of surgery?

Patient: No. I had only chest infections multiple times nothing else.

Treatment History

Candidate:
- Are you on any regular medications? Do you take any over-the-counter medication or herbal remedies or recreational drugs?
- Are you allergic to any medicine or anything else?

Patient: I am not taking any regular medications at this moment, and I do not have any known allergies.

Relevant Family History

Candidate: Is there anyone else in your family with similar symptoms? Or, is there any long-standing illness that runs in your family like asthma, diabetes mellitus (DM), hypertension (HTN), stroke, or any autoimmune disease or anything else?

Patient: No.

Social History
- Do you smoke? If not—then ask, have you ever smoked? If yes—then how many years have you been smoking? How many sticks per day?
- Do you drink alcohol? If yes—then how many drinks would you have in a week? (CAGE questionnaire if needed—discussed in clinical consultation)
- What are you doing for a living?
- Do you have any industrial or occupational exposures to coal or asbestosis?
- How have these symptoms affected your job? (If not working—then ask....... are you finding it difficult to cope with finance because you are missing work?)
- Are you married? Who is at home with you or who is supporting you now? Do you have any children?

Patient: I am a retired school teacher. I smoke a lot, 20 sticks a day for the last 15 years. I do not drink alcohol. I live with my wife and I have two children.

Travel History

Candidate: Have you recently traveled anywhere?

Patient: No.

Make Summary

Candidate: Thank you very much for giving me all the information. Just a quick recap of everything you have told me so far—you have had a chronic productive cough for the last 2 years and for the last 3 weeks you have been coughing up blood on several occasions. Over that period, you have had recurrent chest infections which were treated with antibiotics. You do not have any other medical conditions and you are not taking any medications currently. Have I missed anything or do you want to add anything more?

Patient: No....

Candidate: So, Alex, what do you think might be going on? Are you particularly concerned about anything?

Patient: Doctor, I do not know what is going on, but I am really concerned about lung cancer.

Candidate: Is there any particular reason you are concerned about cancer?

Patient: One of my friends was recently diagnosed with cancer and he smokes a lot. I am afraid as I also smoke a lot.

Candidate: I am sorry to hear about your friend, how he is doing now?

Patient: He is receiving chemotherapy now, not so well actually.

Feedback to the Patient and Respond to the Patient's Concern

Candidate: Hmm...I can understand why you are worried. From whatever you have told me about your symptoms and also your chest X-ray finding which shows some changes, I am suspecting you have most likely a condition called bronchiectasis or chronic obstructive pulmonary disease. Unfortunately, cancer could be another possibility. Therefore, we need to do some further tests to find out the exact cause and exclude anything serious like cancer. Do you know what is bronchiectasis?

Patient: What is it?

Candidate: In our lungs, airways are a bit like a tree, the tree trunk is the biggest bit, and it gradually splits off into tiny branching airways known as bronchi. Bronchiectasis is a condition where the airways of the lungs become abnormally widened, leading to a build-up of excess phlegm or sputum that can make the lungs more vulnerable to infection. Is that clear so far, Alex?

Patient: Yes.

Candidate: Would that be okay to have a little chat about what we are going to do for you now?

Patient: Yes, please.

Candidate: First of all, I will examine you and then we will arrange further investigations including routine blood tests, liver function tests, kidney function tests, urine tests, and a special scan called a high-resolution computed tomography (HRCT) scan of the chest, your lung function test called spirometry and bronchoscopy.

After confirming bronchiectasis, you will be offered chest physiotherapy and mucolytics, to help you clear mucus or phlegm out of your lungs. Bronchodilators help improve airflow within your lungs. Also, sometimes you might need antibiotics to treat any lung infections that develop.

In rare cases, surgery may consider for bronchiectasis where other treatments have not been effective, the damage to your bronchi is confined only to a small area, and you are in good overall health. Does it make sense for you?

Patient: Yes.

Candidate: Alex, you told me you smoke a lot and you know that smoking can cause cancer. Not only cancer even smoking can cause other lung diseases like bronchiectasis by damaging airways. It is highly advisable to stop smoking immediately. Have you ever tried to quit smoking?

Patient: No.

Candidate: Do you think you can do it on your own? We do have lots of available services to help you quit smoking if you need help. We can refer you smoking cessation clinic where you will meet peoples who have successfully stopped smoking. Shall I arrange a referral for you?

Patient: I think it will be helpful.

Candidate: Well, I will arrange a referral for you and I will also give you the NHS Smokefree helpline number where you can seek help if you find it difficult to cope with quitting. Do you have any other concerns?

Patient: No.

Candidate: Now I am going to discuss your condition with my seniors and arrange further investigations of whatever I have discussed, would that be okay with you?

Patient: Yes.

Candidate: In addition to that, I will give you some written information where you can read more about bronchiectasis. I will give you my contact details as well to contact me if you have any worries or queries...

Thank you so much for spending time with me.

Patient: Thank you.

Discussion with Examiner

Examiner: Would you please present your case?

Candidate:

Mr Alex, a 65-year-old gentleman heavily smoker, a retired school teacher has presented with chronic productive cough for the last 2 years and progressive exertional breathlessness for the last 6 months.

He had recurrent hemoptysis for the last 6 weeks. He had a history of recurrent chest infections and a history of taking antibiotics for six episodes over that period.

On the basis of this clinical scenario with the X-ray evidence, my strong provisional diagnosis would be bronchiectasis. However, my strong differential diagnosis that should be excluded would be bronchogenic carcinoma and chronic obstructive pulmonary disease (COPD).

Examiner: How will you investigate it?

Candidate: Before doing the investigation, I would like to examine my patient first. Then I would like to start my investigation by doing complete blood count (CBC), erythrocyte sedimentation rate (ESR), C-reactive protein (CRP), sputum for Gram staining, culture and smear (C/S), acid-fast bacilli (AFB) study, gene expert test as well as malignant cell. Here, the most important test for detailed assessment of the chest would be the HRCT chest. Depending on the HRCT chest report further tests would be bronchoscopy and bronchoscopy-directed biopsy and bronchoalveolar lavage (BAL) for infections screen and malignant cell or computed tomography (CT) guided fine needle aspiration cytology (FNAC), if required.

Other tests include spirometry, arterial blood gas (ABG), random blood sugar (RBS), liver function test, renal function test, electrocardiogram (ECG), Echo, and thyroid function test for full assessment and management. However, to identify the underlying cause of bronchiectasis other tests include:
- Immunoglobulin level (look for any evidence of immunodeficiency)
- Human immunodeficiency virus (HIV) serology
- Aspergillus serology for allergic broncho-pulmonary aspergillosis (ABPA)
- Autoimmune screen for connective tissue disease
- Sweat test and *CFTR* gene for cystic fibrosis
- Nasal biopsy (if suspected mucociliary dyskinesia—refer to a specialist)

Examiner: Let us think this is a case of idiopathic bronchiectasis, how will you manage the case?

Candidate: Management of idiopathic bronchiectasis would be guided by an multidisciplinary team (MDT). This would include:
- *Respiratory physician*: To treat any possible infections or complications by using appropriate antibiotics (according to bacterial sensitivity) and other drugs therapy (such as bronchodilators, inhaled corticosteroids, nebulized hypertonic saline-mucolytics, antifungals), vaccination (commonly influenza and pneumococcal).
- Smoking cessation and nutritional supplementation and long-term oxygen therapy (LTOT), if required.
- Chest physiotherapy for postural chest drainage and devices such as a flutter may aid sputum expectoration and mucus drainage.
- Chest surgeons should also be involved for any surgical resection (in case of localized bronchiectasis, which is poorly controlled with medical therapy), bronchial artery embolization for massive hemoptysis and lung transplantation in advanced bilateral disease.
- Specialist nurse and also with an occupational therapist.

Headache

Your role: You are the doctor in the Acute Medical Unit.

Patient profile: Mrs Elena Walker, 32-year-old.

Problem: Headache.

Referral

"Dear Doctor,

Thank you for seeing Mrs Elena Walker who has presented with a headache for the last 2 weeks. She has a previous history of migraine headaches. The headache this time is much worse and long-lasting than her typical headache.

She is clearly distressed by these headaches. Please see the patient and advise on further investigation and management.

Yours Sincerely,
General Practitioner"

Your task is to: Take a detailed history, construct a diagnosis, differential diagnosis, and plan for further investigation and management. Explain your possible diagnosis or differential diagnoses, including your investigation and management plan to the patient. Address any concerns or specific questions that the patient may have.

Do not examine the patient.

At the end of the station, any notes you make must be handed to the examiners.

Introduction, Permission, and Identification

Candidate: Good morning, I am Dr Ali, one of the working doctors here today, I have been asked to talk to you; is that okay with you?

Patient: Good morning. Yes, doctor…

Candidate: Thank you for coming, can I confirm your name and age, please?

Patient: Yes, doctor………… I am Elena Walker, I am 32.

Candidate: What would you like me to call you?

Patient: Elena is fine.

Detailed History

Candidate: Okay, Elena, I understand you have been referred by your GP. Would you please tell me more about what exactly has happened to you?

Patient: I have been suffering from headaches for the last 2 weeks. It started while warming up for my aerobics class 2 weeks back, but now every day after wakening up from bed I get this headache and heaviness in my head. It is so distressing, I feel nauseous and I am noticing some problems with my vision.

Analyze the Complaint

Candidate: I am sorry to hear about that. You are looking uncomfortable and distressed, are you comfortable talking now?

Patient: Yes, Doctor.

Candidate: Would that be okay with you if I ask some questions about your symptoms for a better understanding?

Patient: Okay.

Candidate: Tell me more about your headache.
- How was it started? Suddenly or gradually? Is it constant or on and off?
- Is it getting worse or remaining the same? Does it happen before?
- Where exactly is the pain? What type of pain is it—dull, throbbing, or stabbing?

- How severe they are on a scale of 0 to 10? Does the pain move anywhere else?
- Does anything trigger the headache? Anything makes it worse or better?
- How frequent are they? How long do they last in each episode?
- What do you do during a headache? Have you tried anything for it?
- Is this the worst headache in your life?

Patient: The pain is all over my head but more in the back of the head. It started suddenly and is getting worse day by day. As I said it is worse in the morning but remains all day. It is a dull pain and would be 5 out of 10 on severity scale. Nothing makes it worse, nothing makes it better. I have had a migraine headache for the last 5 years but this time the pain is worse. I went to my GP, and he referred me to the hospital.

Candidate: So, you have a migraine headache,
- How frequently do you get an attack of your migraine? How long does it persist each time?
- Do you get an aura like abnormal sensation or perception before attacks, any visual disturbance, or any numbness or weakness in limbs?
- How are you in between your attacks? How is it managed?
- Is this the same headache you get each time in your migraine attack?

Patient: I have had episodes of migraine very occasionally. I feel nauseous, vomited 1 or 2 times, and have light sensitivity while my attacks. Each time it persists for a few hours or a day only, but this time the pain is for the last couple of days. My headache usually goes away after taking ibuprofen and paracetamol but this time nothing is helping my headache.

Candidate: You told me about a visual problem, please tell me more about it, what do you mean by the visual problem?

Patient: For the last 1 week, I am noticing that I have lost vision in both eyes and everything on the right side of my sight is blurry.

Candidate: I see…

- Has it persisted? Has it happened before? Can you read a book or a newspaper?
- Have you noticed any double vision? Any changes in pupil size?
- Any pain, redness, watery eye, or discharge?
- Has this headache and vision problem affected your life anyway?

Patient: I had trouble finding the correct keys on my computer keyboard. There is no double vision, no redness, discharge, or pain. In the beginning, I was managing my job somehow, but now it is tough, I have taken off days for the last 3 days.

Candidate: I understand having a headache all time and vision problems can make anyone feeble and it is really tough to maintain daily life. Hope we can help you and things will get better.
- What do you do for a living? How is your working environment?
- Are you on under any stress? How is your mood recently?
- Whom do you live with? Is everything okay at home?

Patient: I am an accountant. It is stressful but manageable. My mood is fine. I live with my husband and my child. Everything is fine at home. My husband is also concerned about my headache and told me to visit my GP.

Candidate: Good to hear that your husband is supportive. Do you have any other symptoms?

Patient: No.

Quick Systemic Review, Past Medical History, Family History, Treatment, and Social History According to Your Differentials

Quick Systemic Review

Candidate: Elena, just a few more questions about your overall health.
- Do you have any weakness, numbness, or loss of sensation in your limbs or face? Any history of loss of consciousness? Abnormal shakiness of the body?

- Any dizziness or lightheadedness? Any problem with your balance or gait? Any tingling or buzzing in the ear? Any hearing loss?
- Any fever or flu-like symptoms? Any neck stiffness? Sensitivity to light? Any skin rashes?
- Any tenderness in your temple, and jaw pain?
- Do you feel tired or lethargic nowadays? Any joint pain or back pain?
- Any changes in your weight recently? How is your appetite? Have you noticed any lumps or bumps anywhere in your body?
- Any breathlessness? Cough? Wheeze? Chest pain? Heart racing? Any swelling in your limbs?
- Do you have any nausea, vomiting, or tummy pain? Have you noticed any change in your bowel habit or any diarrhea/constipation? Any problem with your waterworks?
- Are you menstruating regularly? When was your last menstrual period?

Patient: No.

Past Medical and Surgical History

Candidate: Elena, apart from this migraine headache, do you have any other medical conditions like any high blood pressure or high blood sugar, lung condition, heart disease, or any history of stroke? Have you ever been admitted to the hospital in the past or have any history of surgery?

Patient: No.

Treatment History

Candidate: Are you on any regular medication? Are you allergic to any medicine or anything else?

Patient: No.

Candidate: I am sorry to ask, by any chance are you taking any recreational drugs?

Patient: No.

Relevant Family History

Candidate: Is there anyone else in your family with similar symptoms? Or is there any long-standing illness that runs in your family like asthma, DM, HTN, stroke, or any autoimmune disease or anything else?

Patient: No.

Social History

- Do you smoke? If not—then ask, have you ever smoked? If yes—then how many years have you been smoking? How many sticks per day?
- Do you drink alcohol? If yes—then how many drinks would you have in a week? (CAGE questionnaire if needed—discussed in clinical consultation)
- Do you drive? Do you drive for your living?

Patient: I do not smoke. I do not drink alcohol. I drive to my office.

Travel History

Candidate: Have you recently traveled anywhere particularly to the tropics or to Africa, South America, or Asia?

Patient: No.

Make Summary

Candidate: Thank you very much for giving me all the information. Just a quick recap of everything you have told me so far—you have had progressive and continuous headaches for the last 2 weeks, which is worse in the morning. You have a history of migraine headaches, but this time's headache is completely different from your usual migraine headache. Along with this headache, you have nausea and visual problem. This has a significant impact on your job life and you have taken sick leave because of your symptoms. You do not have any other symptoms, and this is the first time you have had this long-lasting headache. You do not smoke and drink alcohol. You were generally fit and well, and do not have any other medical conditions. Have I missed anything, or do you want to add anything more?

Patient: No....

Candidate: So, Elena, what do you think might be going on? Are you particularly concerned about anything?

Patient: Doctor, I do not know what is going on, I am concerned about whether this is something more serious than my migraine attack.

Feedback to the Patient and Respond to the Patient's Concern

Candidate: Hmm... I understand why you are worried, anyone in your position would feel the same. But you are in the right place, and we will do our level best to help you. Well, actually from whatever you have told me there are multiple possibilities that can cause this type of headache. It could be an unusual attack on your migraine headache. However, I am concerned about your symptoms as your headaches are persisting and progressing and also you have lost your vision. We need to rule out anything serious like brain tumors or brain hemorrhages. For this, we need to run some investigations including some baseline blood tests, liver, and kidney function tests, urine tests, ECG, chest X-ray and most importantly brain imaging which is a CT scan and magnetic resonance imaging (MRI) of the brain. Would that be okay with you?

Patient: Yes.

Candidate: Well, in the meantime you will be reviewed by a brain specialist and treatment will depend on your investigation reports and the neurologist's opinion. Am I clear so far? Do you have any other concerns?

Patient: Will my vision be back, Doctor?

Candidate: Elena, I can sense what you are going through, unfortunately, I am not in a position to say anything about your vision right now, we need further evaluation and after that, I can tell you about the outcome of your condition. Do you have any other concerns?

One more thing I would like to discuss with you, as you have a vision problem, I would advise you to stop driving till we confirm your diagnosis and your vision comes back fully. Does it make sense, Elena?

Patient: Yes, ok.

Candidate: Do you have anyone with you who can take you home?

Patient: I will call my husband to come and drive me home.

Candidate: That is great. I will give you some written information where you can read more about headaches and vision problems.

Thank you so much for spending time with me.

Patient: Thank you.

Discussion with Examiner

Examiner: Would you please present your case?

Candidate:

Mrs Elena Walker, a 32-year-old lady presented with sudden onset of headache for the last 2 weeks. Her headache is persistent and gradually progressive in severity and is worse in the morning associated with nausea and vomiting. She also has had a history of right-sided vision problems in both eyes, but she does not give any history of right-sided weakness or paresthesia or any systemic symptoms like fever, weight loss, loss of consciousness, or convulsion. She had a past medical history of classical migraine for the last 5 years. However, for the recent onset of headaches with different character and severity, my most likely diagnosis would be posterior cerebral artery stroke (likely hemorrhagic). And my strong differential diagnosis would be space occupying lesions (SOL) in the occipital lobe.

Examiner: Okay, you mentioned that she has a visual field defect. Could you please tell me how the name of the visual field defect helped you to localize the lesion?

Candidate: I would like to examine the patient neurologically both upper and lower limbs and cranial nerves. If the patient has evidence of right-sided hemianopia with no evidence of macular sparing (complete visual field defect) suggests middle cerebral artery stroke. However, in this case, I would expect left hemisphere signs like right-sided sensory changes with or without evidence of motor signs (increased tone, reflex, weakness).

Examiner: Okay, your patient comes to your clinic in the outpatient with a chronic scenario, how would you proceed with your investigations?

Candidate: Here, the most important diagnostic test would be an MRI of the brain. If it suggests ischemic stroke, I will do carotid Doppler to see the evidence of carotid artery stenosis. Echocardiogram to look for evidence of cardiac thrombus, prolonged ECG monitoring to look for arrhythmias, specifically paroxysmal atrial fibrillation.

Examiner: Okay, let us move on and think if this lady comes into accident and emergency (A&E) with these presentations, how would you proceed for investigation?

Candidate: I would arrange an urgent CT scan of the brain, if it showed no evidence of hemorrhage, I would consider thrombolysis therapy.

Joint Pain

Your role: You are the doctor in Acute Medical Unit.

Patient profile: Mr James, 30-year-old.

Problem: Joint pain.

Referral

"Dear Doctor,

Thank you for seeing Mr James, who is a 30-year-old gentleman currently studying for a Postgraduate Certificate in Education (PGCE) in physical education. Over the past 10 days, he has had worsening back pain and knee pain. He has also experienced generalized body ache and for the last 3 days, has had red and gritty sore eyes.

About 6 weeks ago, he was admitted to the hospital with suspected appendicitis after 2 days of worsening pain in the right lower abdomen. The pain was severe initially but gradually resolved. It was associated with diarrhea but no blood for 3 days which settled on the antibiotics he was given in the hospital.

Please see the patient and advise on further investigation and management.

Yours Sincerely,
General Practitioner"

Your task is to: Take a detailed history, construct a diagnosis, differential diagnosis, and plan for further investigation and management. Explain your possible diagnosis or differential diagnoses, including your investigation and management plan to the patient. Address any concerns or specific questions that the patient may have.

Do not examine the patient.

At the end of the station, any notes you make must be handed to the examiners.

Introduction, Permission, and Identification

Candidate: Good morning, I am Dr Ali, one of the working doctors here today, I have been asked to talk to you; is that okay with you?

Patient: Good morning. Yes, doctor...

Candidate: Thank you for coming, I would like to start by taking your full name and age, please?

Patient: Yes, doctor............. I am James, 30-year-old.

Detailed History

Candidate: Okay, James, I understand you have been referred by your GP. Would you please tell me more about what exactly has happened to you?

Patient: I have back pain for 10 days. Also, I have pain all over my body. My eyes are red, watery, and sore.

Analyze the Complaint

Candidate: You have back pain and also some problem with your eyes, would that be okay with you if I ask some questions about your symptoms for a better understanding?

Patient: Okay.

Candidate: At first, tell me more about your back pain.
- For how long you have had it? Has this happened before?
- How was it started? Is it constant or intermittent?
- Does it move anywhere in your body, like your legs, tummy, or groin?
- Is it worse in the morning or evening? Any associated stiffness?

- Is there anything that increases or decreases your symptoms, like rest, movement, or exercise?
- If I give you a pain scale of 0 to 10, where 0 is being no pain, 5 is moderate, and 10 is the highest pain, what is your point?
- Are there any other joints affected? Do you have any pain in the Achilles tendon or feet?
- Would you please tell me how this back pain affected your daily life or what it stops you from doing?

Patient: For the last 10 days I have had this back pain, it started gradually and is now present constantly. It does not move anywhere but in the morning, I feel stiffness which improves after a while with some gentle movements. This is the first time I have had this type of back pain and I have also knee pain. I am managing my daily life with some restrictions.

Candidate: Can you tell me more about your knee pain?

Patient: I have left knee joint pain and swelling for the last few days. The pain and swelling are increasing day by day. This is also the first time it has happened to me.

Candidate: By any chance have you had any recent trauma? Any other joints involved? Is there any redness or hotness around the knee? Have you tried anything for it? Anything makes it worse or better?

Patient: No, only this left knee is painful and swollen. I tried paracetamol but did not help. There is redness around the joint.

Candidate: You mentioned eye problems, since when did you have these red eyes? You told me about watering and gritty sensation, is any pain in your eyes? Any changes in vision? Has it happened before?

Patient: I have pain in my eyes and it is hard for me to look at the light. I do not have any history of eye problems in the past. I have some blurring of vision also.

Quick Systemic Review, Past Medical History, Family History, Treatment, and Social History According to Your Differentials

Quick Systemic Review

Candidate: I see… just a few more questions about your overall health.
- Do you have any fever or flu symptoms?
- Do you have any pins and needles in your hands? Or pain in the hand joints? Any problem with urination like any urgency, increase frequency, pain while urination or any frothy urine? Do you have any bowel problems like bloody diarrhea?
- Any skin rash or nail changes like psoriasis?
- Do you feel tired or lethargic nowadays?
- Any changes in your weight recently? How is your appetite?
- Have you noticed any lumps or bumps anywhere in your body?
- Any breathlessness? Cough? Wheeze? Chest pain? Heart racing? Any swelling in your limbs?
- Do you have any nausea, vomiting, or tummy pain?
- Any headache? Dizziness, lightheadedness? Any history of loss of consciousness or dizziness? Abnormal shakiness of the body?

Patient: I have no fever or flu symptoms, but I have psoriasis. I do not have any diarrhea right now, but I was admitted to the hospital last time for tummy pain and diarrhea. I have had some burning pain while urination and also urinary urgency for the last few days, this is the first time I have had these urinary problems.

Candidate: Since when did you have psoriasis? How is it managed? Is it well-controlled?

Patient: For the last 5 years and it is well-controlled with creams that my skin specialist prescribed.

Candidate: Ok. James, you had diarrhea and you were admitted to the hospital, right? When was that? How were you managed at that time? Has it happened before?

Patient: Well, I had tummy pain and diarrhea for 3 days 6 weeks back and I got admitted to the hospital. Doctors first thought I had appendicitis but later on, I improved with antibiotic treatment.

Candidate: Do you have any other symptoms?

Patient: No.

Candidate: How have all of these symptoms affected your life? How are you coping with these?

Patient: It is tough, doctor, I can manage. I am just concerned about what is happening with me!

Past Medical and Surgical History

Candidate: James, apart from psoriasis, do you have any other medical conditions like any high blood pressure or high blood sugar, lung condition, heart disease, arthritis, or anything you want to mention? Have you ever been admitted to the hospital in the past or have any history of surgery?

Patient: No.

Treatment History

Candidate: Can you tell me which cream you are using for your psoriasis? Are you on any other regular medications? Are you allergic to any medicine or anything else?

Patient: I do not know the name of my creams. No other medications.

Candidate: I am sorry to ask, by any chance are you taking any recreational drugs?

Patient: No.

Relevant Family History

Candidate: Is there anyone else in your family with similar symptoms? Or is there any long-standing illness that runs in your family like arthritis, psoriasis, DM, HTN, stroke, or any autoimmune disease or anything else?

Patient: No.

Sexual History

Candidate: James, I need to ask you some personal questions about your sexual health, may I ask?
- Are you sexually active? Do you practice safe sex?
- Do you have any stable partners?
- How many partners do you have in the last 6 months?
- By any chance do you have any discharge from your penis or any rash or ulcer around your private part?

Patient: No. I have a wife and no other partners. I practice safe sex.

Social History

- Do you smoke? If not—then ask, have you ever smoked? If yes—then how many years have you been smoking? How many sticks per day?
- Do you drink alcohol? If yes—then how many drinks would you have in a week? (CAGE questionnaire if needed—discussed in clinical consultation)
- What are you doing for a living? How have these symptoms affected your job? (If not working—then ask....... are you finding it difficult to cope with finance because you are missing work?)
- Are you married? Who is at home with you or who is supporting you now? Do you have any children?

Patient: I am a school teacher. I do not smoke. I do not drink alcohol. I live with my wife.

Travel History

Candidate: Have you recently traveled anywhere?

Patient: No.

Make Summary

Candidate: Thank you very much for giving me all the information. Just a quick recap of everything you have told me so far—you have had back pain which is more in the morning and knee joint pain, redness and swelling for the last 10 days. You have eye pain and blurred vision, and also some urinary problems such as urgency and burning pain. You had a recent history of hospital admission for diarrhea which was treated with antibiotics. You have psoriasis well-controlled with topical creams. You practice safe sex and have no history of recent travel. You live with your wife, do not smoke and do not drink alcohol. Have I missed anything, or do you want to add anything more?

Patient: No....

Candidate: So, James, what do you think might be going on? Are you particularly concerned about anything?

Patient: Doctor, I do not know what is going on.

Feedback to the Patient and Respond to the Patient's Concern

Candidate: From whatever you have told me about your symptoms, there are multiple possibilities right now in my mind that could be the cause. It could be joint infections that we called septic arthritis, could be related to your psoriasis and also could be another disease called reactive arthritis which is commonly precipitated by diarrheal illness. To make a confirmed diagnosis, we need to do some investigations including your full blood count, infection markers, blood culture, your liver function tests, kidney function test, urine test, and also X-rays of your back and knee joints. Importantly, we may need to do a small procedure called joint fluid aspiration to take some fluid from your knee and test for any infections. Would that be okay with you?

Patient: Yes.

Candidate: Do you have any concerns till now?

Patient: How can you treat me?

Candidate: Well, that is a valid concern, depending on your diagnosis we will treat you. If we find any infection, then we will give you intravenous (IV) antibiotics for a long time and if it comes as arthritis-like psoriatic or reactive arthritis then we will treat you under a rheumatology joint Specialist with some medication called disease-modifying antirheumatic drugs (DMARDs). Do you have any other concerns?

Patient: No.

Candidate: Now I am going to arrange further investigations of whatever I have discussed, would that be okay with you? In addition to that, I will give you some written information where you can read more about arthritis.

Thank you very much for spending time with me.

Patient: Thank you.

Discussion with Examiner

Examiner: What are your differential diagnoses in this case?

Candidate:

In this case, he reported having generalized body ache and inflammatory back and knee joint pain. He also reported some urinary symptoms like dysuria and urinary urgency as well as painful red eye suggestive of uveitis.

In the context of a recent diarrheal illness, I believe this could be in keeping with reactive arthritis.

However, other differentials to consider would be:

He has an acutely inflamed left knee that could be a septic arthritis

In the context of the known psoriatic disease, this could be the first presentation of psoriatic arthritis.

He has had a history of an acute diarrheal illness with abdominal pain 6 weeks ago. So, there is a possibility of enteropathic arthritis, however, it was very short-lived.

Examiner: So, you have mentioned several differential diagnoses, which one of those mentioned would be the most important to exclude?

Candidate: I believe the priority is here to exclude septic arthritis.

Examiner: How will you manage this patient?

Candidate: At first, I would like to examine the joint and back for evidence of inflammations and sacroiliitis and examine for evidence of uveitis, plantar fasciitis, and Achilles tendinitis.

I would also want to have full sets of observations to make sure he is not febrile.

Then I would like to do some simple blood tests first including CBC with inflammatory markers such as ESR and CRP, renal function tests, and liver function tests.

If I am still concerned about it being septic arthritis, I would want to give some IV antibiotics.

I would also want to involve the orthopedic team to get a prompt review from them as to whether it needed an urgent washout or diagnostic aspiration for joint fluid assay.

However, the principal management of reactive arthritis is supportive. I would like to give simple analgesia and nonsteroidal anti-inflammatory drugs (NSAIDs) with some gastro-protection including proton pump inhibitors (PPIs). But if symptoms continue or deteriorate and I felt that rheumatology input would be valuable, given that in some rare cases there can be a role of immunosuppressive therapy that would be the best to lead by them.

Examiner: You asked about Mr James, sexual history, why was this relevant?

Candidate: Regarding reactive arthritis, the most common precipitant in the western world is a chlamydial infection which is commonly sexually transmitted.

However, the most common cause worldwide is diarrheal diseases such as *Shigella* and *Salmonella*. So, it would be interesting to know if a stool culture has been done at the time of the presentation.

CHAPTER 2 History Taking

Abdominal Bloating

Your role: You are the doctor in Medical Unit.

Patient profile: Mrs Enola Homes, 32-year-old.

Problem: Abdominal bloating.

Referral

"Dear Doctor,

Thank you for seeing Mrs Enola Homes who has presented with abdominal bloating for the last 8 weeks. She has had a history of altered bowel habits for the last 6 weeks.

Routine investigations were done, and microcytic anemia was the only finding. Please see the patient and advise on further investigation and management.

Yours Sincerely,
General Practitioner"

Your task is to: Take a detailed history, construct a diagnosis, differential diagnosis, and plan for further investigation and management. Explain your possible diagnosis or differential diagnoses, including your investigation and management plan to the patient. Address any concerns or specific questions that the patient may have.

Do not examine the patient.

At the end of the station, any notes you make must be handed to the examiners.

Introduction, Permission, and Identification

Candidate: Good morning, I am Dr Ali, one of the working doctors here today, I have been asked to talk to you; is that okay with you?

Patient: Good morning. Yes, doctor...

Candidate: Thank you for coming, can I confirm your name and age, please?

Patient: Yes, doctor............ I am Enola Homes, I am 32.

Candidate: What would you like me to call you?

Patient: Enola is fine.

Detailed History

Candidate: Okay, Enola, I understand you have been referred by your GP. Would you please tell me more about what exactly has happened to you?

Patient: I have had some tummy discomfort, bloating, feeling nauseous for the last 2 months, and diarrhea for the last 6 weeks. Then I went to my GP and did some tests, but GP said everything is normal except anemia. I am feeling tired and lethargic nowadays.

Analyze the Complaint

Candidate: I am sorry to hear about this. Would that be okay with you if I ask some questions about your symptoms for a better understanding?

Patient: Okay.

Candidate: Tell me more about your diarrhea and tummy discomfort.
- How was it started? Suddenly or gradually?
- Is it getting better or worse day by day or the same?
- How many times do you open your bowel a day?
- Do you wake up from sleep to open your bowel?
- Amount or volume of the stool? Color and consistency of the stool?
- Is there any blood or mucus in the stool (dysentery, proctitis, sigmoiditis)? Or any undigested food particles in the stool (malabsorption)?
- Is there any difficulty to flash away stool?

- Is there anything else that makes it worse or better like diet, drugs, or foods? (Related to gluten-containing food like wheat, barley, and oats in celiac disease/fatty food in case of chronic pancreatitis).
- How was your bowel habit before that?
- Do you have any tummy pain? Have you ever vomited?

Patient: I have loose mucoid stool 5/6 times a day, and never noticed any blood. It is getting worse for the last 2 months. I have not noticed anything that triggers or worse my diarrhea. This is the first time I have had this long-term diarrhea. I have bloating particularly 1 hour after taking a meal. I feel nauseous but never vomited.

Candidate: You told me about tiredness and lethargy—since when have you been feeling tired and lethargic?

Patient: For the last 2 months, I feel tired, always I lie down on my bed, and I do not have any energy to do my daily work. I have a 2-year-old child but it is difficult for me to take care of my baby.

Candidate: I can understand you are unable to do your daily activities. I am sorry to hear about that. Hopefully, we can help you to feel better. Just a few more questions about your general health.

Quick Systemic Review, Past Medical History, Family History, Treatment, and Social History According to Your Differentials

Quick Systemic Review
- Do you tend to feel hot more than usual? Any racing heartbeat, excessive sweating, irritability? (thyrotoxicosis)
- Any itchy rash, usually in the elbow and buttock (dermatitis herpetiformis) or any history of autoimmune disease (celiac disease)? Any mouth ulcers?
- Any dizziness or lightheadedness? Any problem with your balance or gait? Any tingling or numbness or weakness in your limbs? Any problem with your vision?
- Any fever or flu-like symptoms? Any changes in your weight recently? How is your appetite? Have you noticed any lumps or bumps anywhere in your body?
- Any breathlessness? Cough? Wheeze? Chest pain? Any swelling in your limbs? Any joint pain?
- Any problem with your waterworks?
- Are you menstruating regularly? When was your last menstrual period?
- How is your mood recently? Are you under any stress right now? How is everything going in your life?

Patient: I have lost 5 kg in the last 6 months. I had flu symptoms 6 weeks back, but they resolved after a few days, no antibiotics were needed.

Candidate: Regarding your weight loss, is it intentional? How is your appetite?

Patient: My appetite is normal. I eat as normal as before, but I have lost weight.

Past Medical and Surgical History

Candidate: Enola, do you have any other medical conditions like any high blood pressure or high blood sugar, lung condition, heart disease, or any history of stroke? Have you ever been admitted to the hospital in the past or have any history of surgery?

Patient: No.

Treatment History

Candidate: Are you on any regular medication? Are you allergic to any medicine or anything else?

Patient: No.

Candidate: I am sorry to ask, by any chance are you taking any recreational drugs?

Patient: No.

Relevant Family History

Candidate: Is there anyone else in your family with similar symptoms? Or is there any long-standing illness that runs in your family like DM,

HTN, stroke, bowel problem, any autoimmune disease or anything else?

Patient: My mother has bowel cancer I am really concerned about bowel cancer.

Candidate: I am sorry to hear about your mother. Your concern is reasonable. How is she doing now?

Patient: She is fine.

Sexual History

Candidate: Enola, I need to ask you some personal questions about your sexual health, may I ask?
- Are you sexually active? Do you practice safe sex?
- Do you have any stable partners?
- How many partners do you have in the last 6 months?
- By any chance do you have any discharge from your vagina? or any rash or ulcer around your private part?

Patient: Only my husband no other partners. I practice safe sex.

Social History

- Do you smoke? If not—then ask, have you ever smoked? If yes—then how many years have you been smoking? How many sticks per day?
- Do you drink alcohol? If yes—then how many drinks would you have in a week? (CAGE questionnaire if needed—discussed in clinical consultation)
- What do you do for a living? Who is at home? Is everything okay at home?

Patient: I do not smoke. I do not drink alcohol. I live with my husband and son. Everything is fine.

Travel History

Candidate: Have you recently traveled anywhere?

Patient: No.

Make Summary

Candidate: Thank you very much for giving me all the information. Just a quick recap of everything you have told me so far—you have had loose stool containing mucus but no blood for the last 6 weeks. You also have had bloating and nausea for the last 2 months. You have lost 5 kg weight over the last few days which is unintentional, and your appetite is normal. You feel tired and lethargic all the time and have difficulty coping with daily household tasks. Your mother has bowel cancer, and you do not have any other past medical history. Have I missed anything, or do you want to add anything more?

Patient: No....

Candidate: So, Enola, do you have any idea what might be going on?

Patient: Doctor, I do not know what is going on, I am concerned about whether this is something more serious like my mother!

Feedback to the Patient and Respond to the Patient's Concern

Candidate: Hmm... I understand why you are worried, anyone in your position would feel the same. But you are in the right place and we will do our level best to help you. Well, actually from whatever you have told me there are multiple possibilities that can cause these types of symptoms. It could be due to infections such as tuberculosis (TB) and giardiasis. It could be due to conditions like celiac disease or inflammatory bowel disease but as you are concerned and your mother has bowel cancer, we should exclude bowel cancer as well. So, we need to do some further tests including checking your vitamin level, iron levels, your liver and kidney function tests, autoantibodies and also a camera test called endoscopy and biopsy. Would that be okay with you?

Patient: Yes.

Candidate: That is great. I will give you some written information where you can read more about your symptoms.

Thank you so much for spending time with me.

Patient: Thank you.

Discussion with Examiner

Examiner: Would you please present your case?

Candidate:

> My patient Mrs Enola Homes, a 32-year-old young lady presented with chronic diarrhea containing mucus but no blood with significant unintentional weight loss for the last 6 weeks. She also gave a suggestive history of anemia, abdominal bloating, and nausea. However, she does not give any history of fever, loss of appetite, abdominal pain or any lump in the abdomen or neck or risky sexual behavior.
>
> From this clinical scenario, my strong differential diagnosis would be malabsorption syndrome (like celiac disease) and thyrotoxicosis. My other important differentials that need to exclude here are—any chronic infections like intestinal TB, giardiasis, or inflammatory conditions such as Crohn's disease and bowel cancer.
>
> However, to reach my diagnosis I would like to do a thorough clinical examination and relevant investigations.

Night Sweats

Your role: You are the medical doctor in Acute Medical Unit.

Patient profile: Mr Steven Jones, 62-year-old.

Problem: Fever and night sweats.

Referral

"Dear Doctor,

Thank you for seeing Mr Steven Jones who has a 6-week history of fever and night sweats. 5 months back he had a transurethral resection of the prostate (TURP). He has been treated with two courses of antibiotics for suspected urinary infection. He has a history of aortic valve disease and valve replacement was done 10 years back.

Please see the patient and advise on further investigation and management.

Yours Sincerely,
General Practitioner"

Your task is to: Take a detailed history, construct a diagnosis, differential diagnosis, and plan for further investigation and management. Explain your possible diagnosis or differential diagnoses, including your investigation and management plan to the patient. Address any concerns or specific questions that the patient may have.

Do not examine the patient.

At the end of the station, any notes you make must be handed to the examiners.

Introduction, Permission, and Identification

Candidate: Good morning, I am Dr Ali, one of the working doctors here today, I have been asked to talk to you; is that okay with you?

Patient: Good morning. Yes, doctor…

Candidate: Thank you for coming, I would like to start by taking your full name, age, and where you have come from, please?

Patient: Yes, doctor…………. I am Steven Jones, I am 62 and from London.

Candidate: What would you like me to call you?

Patient: Jones is fine.

Detailed History

Candidate: Okay, Jones, I understand you have been referred by your GP. Would you please tell me more about what exactly has happened to you?

Patient: I have been feeling unwell for the last 6 weeks. I have a fever and drenching night sweats and have been to my GP twice. I had prostate surgery and my GP told me that I had a urinary infection. I have taken two courses of antibiotics, but still, I am having this excessive sweating every night.

Analyze the Complaint

Candidate: So, you have been feeling unwell for the last 6 weeks. Jones, would that be okay with you if I ask some questions about your symptoms for a better understanding?

Patient: Okay.

Candidate: At first, tell me more about your fever and night sweats.
- Have you measured your temperature? If so, how high does it go?
- Is it constant or on and off?
- Does the fever ever disappear? How often does it peak?
- Tell me about night sweats, do you need to change your clothes at night?
- Does it happen before?

Patient: It is a low-grade fever, I have not measured the temperature but particularly it comes in the evening. I need to change my clothes at night because of excessive sweating. This is the first time I am feeling so unwell with these night sweats.

Candidate: I am sorry to hear about this. Hopefully, we can find a proper solution for you. You told me you had prostate surgery 5 months back, can you tell me more? Do you have any problem with your urination like:
- Do you need to go to the loo more often than usual?
- Any changes in your urine color? Any cloudy or frothy urine?
- Any pain while urination? Any urgency? Any problem with holding your urine?

Patient: Doctor, I had to go to the loo more often before my surgery but now it is fine. Although, I have been noticing for the last few days my urine becomes dark.

Candidate: You also told me you have taken two courses of antibiotics, which antibiotics have you been prescribed? Did you complete the courses? Any improvement after that?

Patient: I do not know the name of these antibiotics. The last course of antibiotics has made me feel slightly better, but not completely, still I have night sweats and fever.

Quick Systemic Review, Past Medical History, Family History, Treatment, and Social History According to Your Differentials

Quick Systemic Review

Candidate: I see… just a few more questions about your overall health.
- Do you feel tired or lethargic nowadays?
- Any changes in your weight recently? How is your appetite?
- Have you noticed any lumps or bumps anywhere in your body?
- Any breathlessness? Cough? Wheeze? Chest pain? Heart racing? Any swelling in your limbs?
- Any headache? Dizziness, lightheadedness? Any history of loss of consciousness or dizziness? Abnormal shakiness of the body?
- Do you have any nausea, vomiting, or tummy pain? Any joint pain or skin rash?
- Have you noticed any change in your bowel habit or any diarrhea/constipation?

Patient: I feel generally fatigued. Nowadays, I feel short of breath while exertion. My appetite has been reduced and I have lost about 6 kg in weight over the last 6 weeks. Nothing else.

Candidate: Since when have you been feeling fatigued? Is it getting worse? Is it all over the day or at a particular time a day? Has it happened before?

Patient: For the same duration, Doctor. I feel tired and lethargic all the time and it is getting worse.

Candidate: Do you have any other symptoms?

Patient: No.

Candidate: How have all of these symptoms affected your life? How are you coping with these?

Patient: It is tough, doctor, I cannot go anywhere now because of this tiredness, I was supposed to visit my grandson last week, but I did not go. I cannot sleep at night. I stay in the bed all day, feeling so tired and lethargic.

Candidate: I can sense things are really tough for you, coping with multiple symptoms are quite difficult. We will try our best to help you, Jones.

Past Medical and Surgical History

Candidate: Jones, apart from your prostate problem, do you have any other medical conditions like any high blood pressure or high blood sugar, lung condition, heart disease, or anything you want to mention? Have you ever been admitted to the hospital in the past or have any history of surgery?

Patient: I had valve replacement surgery 10 years back because one of my heart valves was narrowed. I have high blood pressure, but it is well-controlled with medication.

Candidate: How you were diagnosed with a valve problem? Do you know which valve was that? Is it a mechanical valve replacement or bioprosthesis? How have you been since then? Do you have any symptoms now?

Patient: I had syncope and breathlessness at that time and my heart doctor told me my aortic valve was become narrowed. Then I had valve replacement with a mechanical valve. Now I am ok, no problem at all. I am taking warfarin for my valve replacement since then.

Candidate: Well, you are taking warfarin, do you follow-up with your heart specialist regularly? When was your last blood clotting test? Is it well-controlled? Have you recently gone through any dental procedures or any other procedures? During your prostate operation had you received proper prophylaxis?

Patient: I get followed up annually. My blood clotting tests have been well-controlled and it was tested 2 months back. I am not sure if they gave me antibiotics at that time or not, but apart from my prostate surgery, there is no other surgery.

Treatment History

Candidate: Which medication are you taking for your high blood pressure?

Patient: Amlodipine.

Candidate: Apart from warfarin, are you on any other regular medications? Are you allergic to any medicine or anything else?

Patient: No.

Candidate: I am sorry to ask, by any chance are you taking any recreational drugs?

Patient: No.

Relevant Family History

Candidate: Is there anyone else in your family with similar symptoms? Or is there any long-standing illness that runs in your family like asthma, DM, HTN, stroke, or any autoimmune disease or anything else?

Patient: No.

Social History

- Do you smoke? If not—then ask, have you ever smoked? If yes—then how many years have you been smoking? How many sticks per day?
- Do you drink alcohol? If yes—then how many drinks would you have in a week? (CAGE questionnaire if needed—discussed in clinical consultation)
- What are you doing for a living? How have these symptoms affected your job? (If not working—then ask……. are you finding it difficult to cope with finance because you are missing work?)
- Are you married? Who is at home with you or who is supporting you now? Do you have any children?

Patient: I am a retired school teacher. I do not smoke. I do not drink alcohol. I live with my wife.

Travel History

Candidate: Have you recently traveled anywhere particularly to the tropics or to Africa, South America, or Asia.

Patient: No.

Make Summary

Candidate: Thank you very much for giving me all the information. Just a quick recap of everything you have told me so far—you have had fever and night sweats for the last 6 weeks, despite taking two courses of antibiotics because your GP thought it is a urinary tract infection. You feel generally fatigued and short of breath while exertion. Your appetite has been reduced and lost about 6 kg weight over the last 6 weeks. You had prostate surgery 6 months back, but you do not have any urinary problems except the darker color of urine. You have had an aortic valve replacement 10 years back and you are taking warfarin for this. You get followed up annually. Your HTN is well-controlled with amlodipine, you do not smoke and drink alcohol. Have I missed anything, or do you want to add anything more?

Patient: No....

Candidate: So, Jones, what do you think might be going on? Are you particularly concerned about anything?

Patient: Doctor, I do not know what is going on, why I am not getting better despite two courses of antibiotic treatment?

Feedback to the Patient and Respond to the Patient's Concern

Candidate: Hmm.... I understand all of these symptoms have really affected your life. Anyone in your position would be worried and would feel the same. Well, actually, from whatever you have told me about your symptoms, there are multiple possibilities right now in my mind that could be the cause. All of your symptoms are suggestive of a condition called infective endocarditis. However, this can be due to lymphoproliferative disease, infection like TB or other deep-seated infections. Have you ever heard about infective endocarditis?

Patient: No. What is it?

Candidate: Infective endocarditis is a serious infection of the inner lining of the heart chambers. The infection usually involves heart valves and particularly if you have a valve replacement. Unfortunately, it is a serious and life-threatening infection.

Patient: Doctor, what will happen now? You said life-threatening!

Candidate: I understand you are scared by my words, unfortunately, it is a potentially fatal condition and needs urgent treatment. Therefore, we need to admit you to the hospital and run further investigations to confirm the diagnosis and exclude other possible causes. Would that be ok with you?

Patient: Ok.

Candidate: That is fine, I will arrange admission for you. Before that, are you taking any antibiotics right now?

Patient: No, I finished my course 1 week back.

Candidate: Well, after admission, we will take three sets of blood cultures, and also some other tests including routine blood tests, liver function tests, kidney function tests, urine tests, chest X-ray, and ECG. You will be reviewed by a heart specialist to check your valve status and an echocardiogram will also be done.

After confirming infective endocarditis, we will give you antibiotics according to the local antibiotic guideline. As you have valve replacement you will be given IV antibiotics for at least 6 weeks. Sometimes, if the infection is severe then we might require valvular replacement. Does it make sense for you?

Patient: Yes.

Candidate: Do you have any other concerns?

Patient: No.

Candidate: Now I am going to discuss your condition with my seniors and arrange admission and further investigations of whatever I have discussed, would that be okay with you?

Patient: Yes.

Candidate: In addition to that, I will give you some written information where you can read more about infective endocarditis.

Thank you so much for spending time with me.

Patient: Thank you.

Discussion with Examiner

Examiner: Would you please present your case?

Candidate:

Mr Jones, a 62-year-old gentleman hypertensive, presented with low-grade intermittent fever with evening rise and night sweats.

For the last 6 weeks, he has had a history of exertional fatigability, anorexia, and significant weight loss of 6 kg over the period. He has had a past medical history of mechanical aortic valve replacement for which he is on warfarin therapy with regular follow-up. He also had a history of TURP surgery 6 months back for benign enlargement of prostate (BEP).

Based on the clinical scenario, the most likely diagnosis is subacute infective endocarditis. However, my strong differential diagnoses would be chronic infections such as TB and other deep-seated infections or lymphoproliferative disease (lymphoma).

Examiner: How will you investigate this patient?

Candidate: At first, I would like to examine the patient to get some clues to establish my diagnosis as well as exclude other differentials.

Then I would like to start my investigation by doing baseline blood tests including CBC, ESR, CRP, renal function tests, liver function tests, chest X-ray, ECG, and ultrasonography (USG) of the whole abdomen.

Here, the most important test would be three sets of blood cultures to identify the infection and guide antibiotic therapy which includes/ including an echocardiography 2D, M mode, and color Doppler to see the evidence of infective endocarditis (e.g., vegetation, abscess, new valvular regurgitation).

Examiner: Let us think the patient has infective endocarditis, how will you manage this patient?

Candidate: As the case fatality of infective endocarditis with prosthetic valve is very high, I would like to manage the patient with a multidisciplinary team (MDT) approach involving cardiologists, surgeons, and microbiologists to increase the chance of a successful outcome. After sending blood culture samples, I will start antibiotics urgently (blind treatment) with IV benzylpenicillin and gentamicin for 6 weeks. The antibiotic regime may need to be modified after getting the C/S result.

Some of the patients may require cardiac surgery if:
- Heart failure due to valve damage.
- Failure of antibiotic therapy.
- Abscess or large vegetation of the left-sided valves with evidence or high risk of systemic emboli.

CHAPTER 3

Clinical Examination: Cardiovascular System

- ❑ Cardiovascular System Examination
- ❑ Aortic Stenosis
- ❑ Aortic Regurgitation
- ❑ Mixed Aortic Valve Disease
- ❑ Mitral Stenosis
- ❑ Mitral Regurgitation
- ❑ Mitral Valve Prolapse
- ❑ Mixed Mitral Valve Disease
- ❑ Pulmonary Stenosis
- ❑ Prosthetic Aortic Valve
- ❑ Prosthetic Mitral Valve
- ❑ Atrial Septal Defect
- ❑ Ventricular Septal Defect
- ❑ Patent Ductus Arteriosus
- ❑ Intracardiac Device

Cardiovascular System Examination

1. Meticulously, read the clinical scenario; this shall help you predict what you are going to find and do only what you have been asked.
2. Carefully greet the examiners in a nice, decent, and balanced manner—this will definitely carry a positive impact on them.
3. Sanitize your hands with antiseptic liquid (antiseptic liquid is provided to you in the station).
4. Greet the patient, introduce yourself, confirm your patient identity, and take permission.
   (Hello, Mr X .... Good morning, I am Mohammad Ali....One of the working doctors here, today....I have been asked to examine you....Is that okay with you?).
5. Explain to the patient in easy yet precise terms about your procedure—this shall help to get required cooperation from the patient (I would like to examine your hands, face, neck, chest, and legs if that are okay with you?).
6. Ask about the pain and discomfort and reassure the patient (Do you have any pain or discomfort?......... I would be gentle during the examination, please let me know if you feel any pain or discomfort).
7. Adequately positioned (position the patient 45° in bed).
8. Sufficiently expose the patient appropriate to the examination (Please maintain dignity.... Expose the patient from head to the mid-abdomen).
   [Explain every subsequent step before doing it so that the patient will be more cooperative and this will help you score better in skill-7 (maintaining patient's welfare)]
9. A general survey of the patient from the end of the bed (see the patient as a whole, do not rush to examination, look for bedside clues and other clues in the patient).

Bedside Clues:
- Listen metallic click (Metallic valve replacement).
- Treatment adjunct: O_2 therapy (oxygen tank?); Any medication—GTN spray; Mobility aid.
- Check the patient: Comfortable/uncomfortable at test, does he breathing at a good rate?
- Any syndromic appearance: Marfan syndrome [?Aortic regurgitation (AR)]; Down syndrome (?VSD); Noonan syndrome (?PS); Turner syndrome [Coarctation of the aorta, AR, aortic stenosis (AS)].
- Head, neck, and face: Xanthelasma; Malar flush (rosy flushed checks and dilated capillaries—?MS); Vigorous neck pulsation (?AR); Cyanosis.
- Inspect chest (ask the patient for better exposure—"please keep your hand to waist")
  - Mid sternotomy scar: Valve replacement [mitral valve replacement (MVR), aortic valve replacement (AVR)] or repair; coronary artery bypass graft (CABG—usually associated with Saphenous vein graft harvest scar); Cardiac transplant.
  - Lateral thoracotomy scar:
    a. Cardiac cause: Mitral valvulotomy, coarctation repair, patent ductus arteriousus (PDA) ligation, Blalock-Thomas-Taussig shunt
    b. Respiratory cause: Lobectomy, pneumonectomy, lung transplant, bullectomy, previous thoracoplasty for TB
  - Signs of previous chest drain scar
  - Left subclavian scar [pacemaker/implantable cardioverter defibrillator (ICD)]

- Precordial bulge (suggest long-standing heart disease; e.g., congenital heart disease)
- Visible pulsation
  o Inspect leg:
    - Vein harvesting scars (?CABG); Pedal edema; Differential cyanosis and clubbing (PDA with reversed shunt); Diabetic change (necrobiosis lipoidica, diabetic dermopathy)
  o Inspect abdomen:
    - Distension (?ascites and hepato-megaly) suggests—?CCF (heart failure)
10. *Hands (Ask the patient to hand out with palm facing downwards)*:
    o Splinter hemorrhage (reddish/brown streaks on the nail bed; subacute bacterial endocarditis).
    o Clubbing (ask the patient to place the nails of his index finger back to back)—loss of the angle between nail fold and nail bed: Bacterial endocarditis; Cyanotic congenital heart disease; Eisenmenger syndrome.
      - Long fingers: Check for Marfan syndrome: AR or MVP
      - Press on the nail and observe for Quincke's sign (?AR)
      (Ask the patient to hand out with palms facing upwards)
      - Color (Dusky bluish discoloration; Cyanosis suggests hypoxia)
      - Temperature: Cool periphery may suggest poor cardiac output/hypovolemia
      - Osler's node (tender red nodules on finger pulps/thenar eminence)—infective endocarditis.
      - Janeway lesion (nontender maculopapular or nodular erythematous lesion on the palm and sole suggests bacterial endocarditis).
      - Tar staining
      - Xanthomata (raised yellow lesions often noted on the tendon of the wrist suggest hyperlipidemia).
      - Ecchymosis (?Warfarin treatment for AF or valve replacement)

11. *Examine the pulse*:
    o Radial pulse:
      - Asses for rate and rhythm—regular rhythms; irregularly irregular rhythm: AF; regularly irregular rhythm: Ventricular bigeminy or trigeminy.
      - Radio-radial delay (palpate both radial pulse simultaneously) suggests subclavian artery stenosis (e.g., compression by cervical rib) or aortic dissection.
      - Radiofemoral delay (usually not done but ask the examiner to see) suggests coarctation of the aorta.
      - Collapsing pulse (first confirm the patient has no pain in the shoulder—palpate the radial pulse with your hand wrapped around the wrist—and then elevate the arm above the head briskly whilst maintaining the position of your hand, feel for a tapping impulse as blood empties from the arm very quickly in diastole, resulting in a palpable sensation). It can occur in the normal physiological state (e.g., fever/pregnancy) or a cardiac problem (e.g., AR/PDA) or high output state (e.g., anemia/AV fistula/thyrotoxicosis).
      Examine the brachial and carotid pulse to assess volume and character.
    o Volume (low, average, large):
      - Low volume in stenotic lesion
      - Large volume in VSD and AR
    o Character:
      - Collapsing: AR, PDA
      - Pulsus bisferiens: Double aortic valve disease (AR with AS)
      - Slow-rising pulse: AS
12. *Ask him to look up and examine eyes*: Xanthelasma, corneal arcus, pallor.
13. Ask him to open his mouth and examine the mouth for the high arched palate (?Marfan) or cyanosis.
14. *Inspect the neck for vigorous pulsation*: AR (Corrigan sign).
15. Ask him to turn his head and examine JVP for elevation (distinct from the carotid artery by double impulse, cannot be palpated,

accentuated by performing hepatojugular reflux):
- Ask the patient to turn his head away from you.
- Observe the neck for the JVP (located in line between two heads of the sternocleidomastoid).
- Measure the JVP—number of centimeters from the sternal angle to the upper border of pulsation. Normally <5 cm, if it is raised, then it may indicate—fluid overload, right ventricular failure/pulmonary hypertension (PHTN), and tricuspid regurgitation.
- If prominent waves, then feel the opposite carotid pulse. If it is systolic, then it is the prominent "v-wave"—TR; if it is diastolic, then it is "a-wave"—PHTN, pulmonary stenosis (PS), right ventricular hypertrophy (RVH).
- If the patient is in AF and finds a prominent wave, then it suggests v-wave; as a-wave is absent in AF.
- Look for hepatojugular reflux—first, ensure the patient has no pain in the abdomen, apply pressure to the liver and observe the JVP for a rise.

16. *Close inspection of the chest*:
    - Scar:
      - Left lateral thoracotomy scar/submammary scar—minimal invasive valve surgery such as mitral valvuloplasty.
      - Mid sternotomy scar
      - Infraclavicular scar (both sides)—pacemaker
      - Left mid-axillary line: Subcutaneous implantable cardioverter defibrillator
    - Chest wall deformities (pectus excavatum, pectus carinatum)
    - Visible pulsation—forceful apex beat may be visible in HTN, LVH.
17. Palpate the apex for site, character (heaving—AS and HTN causing LVH; tapping—MS; thrusting—MR, AR) and thrills (diastolic—MS; systolic—MR).
18. Palpate left parasternal edge for thrill and heave (RVH due to PHTN or PS).
19. Palpate pulmonary area for palpable S2 (PHTN) and thrill (systolic—PS, diastolic—PR).
20. Palpate aortic area together with the neck for thrills (systolic—AS, diastolic—AR)
21. *Auscultate the four valves areas*:
    - Palpate the carotid pulse to determine the first heart sound.
    - Auscultate "upwards" through the valve area using the diaphragm of the stethoscope.

    Heart sound:
    - S1: Loud—MS, Muffled—MR, Variable intensity—AF, Clicky sound—MVR
    - S2: Accentuated—PHTN and systemic HTN; Muffled—AR and AS; Wide fixed splitting S2 in ASD; Clicky sound in valvular replacement (usually aortic).

    Murmur:
    - Low pitched localized mid-diastolic murmur with opening snap: MS.
    - Soft blowing pansystolic murmur in the apex that radiates to the axilla: MR.
    - Harsh ejection systolic murmur that radiates to neck: AS
    - Pan systolic murmur best heard in the left lower parasternal area suggests TR or VSD.
    - Ejection systolic murmur best heard in the pulmonary area suggests PS.

    - If you get a murmur (systolic) in the apex, then look for radiation to the axilla and in the aortic area, then look for radiation to the neck (by holding the breath in expiration).
    - During the procedure, ask the patient to take a deep breath in-breath out then hold ....., left-sided murmur increases its intensity with breath-hold in expiration. On the other hand, the right-sided murmur increases its intensity during breath-hold in inspiration.
    - Now...repeat auscultation across the four-valve area with the bell of the stethoscope...
    - Roll the patient on to his left side and listen over the mitral area with the bell during breath-hold in expiration (for mitral stenosis).

- Sit the patient forwards and auscultate over the left parasternal area (4th ICS) with breath-hold expiration (for AR).
22. Auscultate, the lung base for crackles, may suggest pulmonary edema secondary to left ventricular failure (consider chronic lung disease if the patient has no sign of fluid overload—pulmonary fibrosis or bronchiectasis).
23. *Check for sacral edema*: Ask if he has any pain in the back.
24. *Examine the legs for*:
    - Pitting edema at malleoli, then shins
    - Saphenous vein graft harvest scar
    - Ecchymosis (?anticoagulation)
25. *Formulate your comment and diagnosis*:
    - Diagnosis (MR, MS, AR, AS)
    - Complications (heart failure, PHTN, infective endocarditis, atrial fibrillation)
    - Causes (congenital, rheumatic fever, infective endocarditis, infarction)
26. Say thanks to the patient at the end of the examination and cover him up before turning around to the examiner.
27. Wash hands.
28. To complete the examination, offer the examiner to look at the patient's observation chart, measure blood pressure, doing a bedside urine dipstick, and bedside ECG.

Cardiology Case Presentation

[If you are confident of the diagnosis, it is far more impressive to state the diagnosis and justify it by presenting the important relevant positive and negative findings, otherwise presenting the case in a systemic manner mentioning the important positive and negative findings. Try to give a possible cause of the condition, e.g., AR most likely secondary to infective endocarditis. It is better to comment on the severity, any complications of the disease (e.g., heart failure) or of the treatment (e.g., purpura, ecchymosis secondary to warfarin use)]

I would like to complete my examination by measuring blood pressure, doing urine dipstick, looking at the patient's observation chart.

I believe this gentleman has.... (diagnosis).... (complication).... (cause).

This gentleman is lying comfortably in bed with an average built ... His pulse is...... Positive findings of the examination .....

He has (No) sign of infection endocarditis

(No) sign of PHTN

(No) sign of heart failure.

Aortic Stenosis

Mr Peterson, a 71-year-old man, complained of worsening shortness of breath on exertion. Examine the cardiovascular system.

(After finishing cardiovascular system examination within 6 minutes of time)

Candidate: I would like to complete my examination by looking at the full sets of clinical observations chart, measuring blood pressure, doing urine dipsticks, and checking for the radiofemoral delay.

Examiner: Would you like to present your case, please?

Candidate:

This patient is an elderly gentleman with signs of severe AS likely secondary to a degenerative disease given his age.

The physical signs are:

Pulse is 78 beats/min, regular, low volume, and slow-rising character.

The blood pressure is 110/90 with narrow pulse pressure.

Apex beat is normal in position with heaving in character.

A systolic thrill is palpable in the aortic area.

On auscultation:

A harsh ejection systolic murmur is heard throughout the pericardium but most prominent in the 2nd intercostal space, which is also louder on expiration and radiates to the carotids.

First heart sound is normal, but 2nd heart sound quiet.

No evidence of PHTN (loud P2 or parasternal heave).

He has no evidence of infective endocarditis such as pyrexia, clubbing, splinter's hemorrhage, Osler node, Janeway lesion.

No evidence of heart failure (crepitations, raised JVP or peripheral edema).

Several signs suggest this patient's AS could be severe:
- Soft second heart sound
- The long duration (not loud) of the murmur
- Heaving apex beat
- Low volume slow-rising pulse
- And narrow pulse pressure.

Examiner: Okay, now tell me, why is this not PS?

Candidate: In the case of PS, the site of the murmur would be different. I would expect to hear PS loudest over the pulmonary area. Moreover, I would expect there to be a right ventricular heave.

I might expect it in a different demographic analysis of the patient, such as a younger patient with PS.

Examiner: What would be the differential diagnosis of an ejection systolic murmur?

Candidate: My differential diagnoses would include:
- Aortic stenosis
- Aortic sclerosis (Here, murmur will be localized to the aortic area with no radiation. Pulse volume, character, and pulse pressure will be normal).
- Hypertrophic obstructive cardiomyopathy (jerky pulse with normal 2nd heart sound with no radiation to the neck).
- Supravalvular AS (no ejection click, normal 2nd heart sound).

Examiner: If you perform an ECG and an echocardiogram, and the ECG shows left ventricular hypertrophy, but the echo shows that he has severe AS with a valve area of 0.9 cm² and good LV function, how would you manage this patient?

Candidate: The echocardiogram has confirmed this patient has severe AS and we know already that he is symptomatic with exertional breathlessness. I would like to take the history of other symptoms such as chest pain, syncope, or any other symptoms of heart failure. Any symptoms (chest pain, breathlessness, and syncope) in the context of severe AS would prompt referral to the surgeons for consideration of valve replacement.

Examiner: Okay, let us think your patient is asymptomatic but has echocardiographic evidence of severe AS. When will you consider him for surgery?

Candidate: Asymptomatic patient with AS requires surgery where the MPG is 40 mm Hg or more and any of the following:
- Systolic dysfunction (LVEF <45%)
- Abnormal response to exercise (BP fall)
- VT
- LVH >15 mm
- Valve area <0.6 cm²

Examiner: Now, tell me about the medical management of AS. What drug options are you familiar with?

Candidate: The main would be beta-blockers.
- To slow the heart rate and hence increase ejection time.
- It can be used in symptomatic patients who are waiting for surgery or those unfit for surgery.
- It can also reduce cardiac workload by reducing the rate of rising of systolic pressure and thus effective valve gradient.

Some medications are very important to avoid in AS:
- Vasodilators (which can increase the gradient across the valve) may include ACE inhibitors, ARBs, CCB, nitrates, sildenafil.

Examiner: Well, you know about the medical management, now tell me in case of symptomatic severe AS, what surgical options are you aware of?

Candidate: Mechanical AVR would be more durable and will last longer; however, it does require lifelong anticoagulation.

A tissue AVR does not require life-long anticoagulation but is not as durable.

A transcatheter aortic valve intervention (TAVI) would be appropriate for those patients who are not fit for surgical intervention.

Examiner: Tell me the standard criteria for echocardiographic grading of the severity of AS.

Candidate: In case of mild AS: Valve area is >1.5–2 cm² and mean valve gradient is <20 mm Hg.

In case of moderate AS: Valve area is 1–1.5 cm² and mean valve gradient is 20–40 mm Hg.

In case of severe AS: Valve area is <1 cm² and mean valve gradient is >40 mm Hg.

Examiner: Would you like to tell me about the prognosis in AS by different types of presenting complaints?

Candidate: Patients of AS usually remain asymptomatic in the mild to moderate stages of severity. Later, they may develop angina, breathlessness, or syncope, indicating a worsening prognosis.
- The worst prognostic symptom of AS is breathlessness due to heart failure. Median survival time is only for 2 years here.
- In case of syncope, it is 3 years.
- Moreover, a patient with chest pain has 5 years median survival time.

Aortic Regurgitation

Mr Emrey, a 72-year-old man, complained of exertional breathlessness. Examine the cardiovascular system.

(After finishing cardiovascular system examination within 6 minutes of time)

Candidate: I would like to complete my examination by measuring blood pressure, checking for the radiofemoral delay, doing urine dipstick, and looking at the patient's observations chart.

Examiner: Would you like to present your case, please?

Candidate:

I believe this gentleman has AR.

The physical signs are:

Pulse is 76 beats/min, regular, and large volume with a collapsing character (water hammer pulse).

The blood pressure is 160/60 with wide pulse pressure.

Visible carotid pulsation is seen on the neck (Corrigan's sign)

Apex beat is displaced with thrusting in character.

On auscultation:

First and 2nd heart sounds are normal.

There is an early diastolic murmur at the lower left sternal edge loudest with the patient sitting forward in breath-hold expiration.

No evidence of PHTN (loud P2 or parasternal heave).

No stigmata of infective endocarditis such as pyrexia, clubbing, splinter's hemorrhage, Osler node, Janeway lesion.

No evidence of heart failure (crepitations, raised JVP or peripheral edema).

Several signs suggest this patient's AR could be severe:
- Clinically dilated heart (shifted apex beat)
- High volume collapsing pulse with very wide pulse pressure (notably low diastolic blood pressure)
- Shorter murmur
- Another criterion of severe AR is signs of left-sided heart failure, which is absent here.

Examiner: How will you manage this case?

Candidate: At first, I would like to take a full history from this patient, such as associated chest pain, breathlessness, palpitation, and other features of heart failure.

Then I would also like to do a further test of blood—CBC, CRP, U&E's, serum creatinine.

If there is any evidence of infective endocarditis, I would do three sets of blood cultures, an ECG, and chest X-ray.

Most importantly, I would request transthoracic echocardiography to confirm the diagnosis and grade it. Here I would look for LVEDD (left ventricular end diastolic diameter), LVESD (left ventricular end systolic diameter) EF, the width of AR jet, RF (regurgitant fraction).

As the patient is already symptomatic and has had features of severe AR, the patient should be planned for valve replacement. This can be surgical valve replacement, or if there are serious comorbidities and not fit for surgery, then we can plan for TAVI.

Examiner: Could you please tell me indications of surgery in an asymptomatic severe AR patient?

Candidate: If AR is severe, even in the absence of symptoms, the following features would indicate valve replacement.
- *LV dilatation*:
  - LVEDD >70 mm corrected for BSA (>35 mm/m^2)
  - LVESD > 50 mm corrected for BSA (>25 mm/m^2)
- EF <50%
- RF >50%—best assessed by cardiac MRI.

Examiner: Tell me some causes of AR?

Candidate: The causes of AR should be considered depending on the pattern of onset as being acute or chronic. In case of chronic AR, causes are:
- Bicuspid aortic valve
- Hypertension
- CRHD (chronic rheumatic heart disease; usually associated with mitral valve disease)
- Aortitis (syphilis, Takayasu's arteritis, ankylosing spondylitis)
- RA
- SLE
- CTD (Marfan syndrome, pseudoxanthoma elasticum, Ehlers-Danlos syndrome, osteogenesis imperfecta)
- Polycystic kidney disease
- VSD with prolapse of the right coronary cusp.

In case of acute AR—the most common cause is infective endocarditis.

Other causes include—aortic dissection or rupture sinus of Valsalva or prosthetic valve failure.

Examiner: What do you think? What is the cause of AR of this gentleman?

Candidate: So far, I examined this patient, I did not find ARP (Argyll Robertson pupil) for syphilitic arteritis.

No obvious signs of Marfan syndrome such as high-arched palate or arm span > height.

No evidence of arthropathy for RA, ankylosing spondylitis or SLE.

No evidence of connective tissue disease (CTD) such as:
- Blue sclerae, hearing aids, or evidence of recurrent fracture for osteogenesis imperfecta.
- Plucked chicken skin appearance, loose skin over the neck and axillae for pseudoxanthoma elasticum.
- Blue sclera, hyperextensible skin and joints, purpura and evidence of poor skin healing for Ehlers-Danlos syndrome.

No evidence of associated mitral valve disease that is an expected finding in rheumatic heart disease (CRHD).

Moreover, there are no obvious stigmata of infective endocarditis.

So, I believe this patient has a bicuspid aortic valve.

Mixed Aortic Valve Disease

Mr Robert, a 58-year-old man, complained of breathlessness. Examine the cardiovascular system.

(After finishing cardiovascular system examination within 6 minutes of time)

Candidate: I would like to complete my examination by measuring blood pressure, doing a urine dipstick, looking at the observations chart, and checking for the radiofemoral delay.

Examiner: Would you like to present your case, please?

Candidate:

I believe this gentleman has mixed aortic valve disease.

Positive findings are:

Pulse is 76 beats/min, regular, and slow rising.

Apex beat is displaced 1 cm to the left in the midclavicular line, which is forceful and heaving in character (pressure overload).

There is a systolic thrill palpable at the apex, aortic area, and also at the carotid.

On auscultation:

There is a harsh ejection systolic murmur in the aortic area, which radiates into the neck.

There is also an early diastolic murmur in the lower left sternal edge best heard in sitting forward with breath-hold expiration.

The aortic component of 2nd heart sound is soft.

No evidence of PHTN (loud and palpable P2 or parasternal heave).

No stigmata of infective endocarditis (pyrexia, clubbing, splinter hemorrhage, Osler node, Janeway lesion).

No evidence of heart failure (crepitations, raised JVP, or peripheral edema).

I would like to take a full history to establish his symptomatic status, and my investigations of choice would be an echocardiogram to confirm the diagnosis, quantify the severity.

Examiner: How would you classify the predominant lesion in this case?

Candidate: I believe AS would be the predominant lesion in this case.

Not just because of the character of the murmur heard with the radiation to the neck on the auscultation, but also for the:
- Slow-rising pulse rather than collapsing pulse.
- There is a systolic thrill, and the second heart sound is soft.
- Apex beat is heaving in nature.

I would like to record the BP. Here I expect systolic blood pressure will be low with narrow pulse pressure.

Examiner: Please tell me how will you manage this case?

Candidate: At first, I would like to take a full history from the patient, such as chest pain, breathlessness, palpitation, or any other symptoms suggestive of heart failure.

Then I would like to do a full set of blood tests that include CBC, CRP, U&E's, serum creatinine and three sets of blood cultures (if there was any evidence of infective endocarditis).

I would do next:
- An ECG—here, I expect left ventricular hypertrophy or LBBB.

- A chest X-ray for cardiomegaly or evidence of pulmonary congestion.
- Moreover, most importantly, echocardiography to confirm the diagnosis and grade it. Here I would look for pressure gradient, valve area, LVEDV, LVESV, EF, and the width of the AR jet.

As this patient is already symptomatic and has features of mixed aortic valve disease, the patient should be planned for surgical valve replacement or TAVI.

Examiner: Well said. Now, as a part of the preoperative assessment for surgery, what other important tests would you usually like to do?

Candidate: Most importantly, I would like to do a coronary angiogram. If there is significant coronary artery disease, CABG should be carried out at the same time as valve replacement.

Examiner: Tell me, what do you know about infective endocarditis prophylaxis?

Candidate: According to the National Institute for Health and Care Excellence (NICE) guideline, the following cardiac conditions are at increased risk of developing infective endocarditis:
- Acquired valvular heart diseases with stenosis or regurgitation
- Hypertrophic obstructive cardiomyopathy
- Past history of infective endocarditis
- Structural congenital heart disease includes surgically corrected or palliative surgery, but excluding isolated ASD, fully repaired VSD or fully repaired PDA, and closure devices that are judged to be endothelialized.
- Valve replacement.

Prophylactic antibiotic against infective endocarditis is not routinely recommended for people undergoing dental procedures and for people undergoing nondental procedures in the following areas:
- Upper and lower GIT procedures
- Genitourinary tract, which includes urological, gynecological, obstetric procedures, and childbirth
- Upper and lower respiratory tract that includes ear, nose, throat procedures, and bronchoscopy.

Any episodes of infection in a person at risk of infective endocarditis should be investigated and appropriately treated to lower the risk of developing infective endocarditis.

If a person at risk of endocarditis is undergoing genitourinary or gastrointestinal procedures at any site where there is a suspected infection, he/she should receive an appropriate antibiotic that covers organisms that cause infective endocarditis.

Examiner: Tell me which antibiotics are used on the high-risk dental procedure?

Candidate: Amoxicillin 3 g or clindamycin 600 mg orally 1 hour before is recommended for the high-risk dental procedure.

Mitral Stenosis

Mrs Polen, a 35-year-old lady, complained of breathlessness. Examine the cardiovascular system.

(After finishing cardiovascular system examination within 6 minutes of time)

Candidate: I would like to complete my examination by looking at the full sets of clinical observations chart, measuring blood pressure, doing urine dipsticks, and checking for the radiofemoral delay.

Examiner: Would you like to present your case, please?

Candidate:

I believe this middle-aged lady has mitral stenosis with signs of PHTN and atrial fibrillation.

The physical signs are:

Pulse is 84 beats/min, irregularly irregular rhythm.

JVP is not raised.

Apex is not displaced and in the 5th intercostal space, which is tapping in nature.

Left parasternal heave is also present here.

On auscultation:

First heart sound is loud and variable. There is a loud pulmonary component of 2nd heart sound, and an opening snap followed by a mid-diastolic rumbling murmur localized to the apex and heard most loudly in the left lateral position with breath-hold expiration with the bell of the stethoscope.

No evidence of pulmonary congestion (bibasal crepitations), right-sided heart failure or no stigmata of infective endocarditis.

Examiner: You mentioned this is a case of mitral stenosis. Can you please tell me what the severity of MS of this patient is?

Candidate: I think this patient has severe MS, which is suggested by:
- Presence of AF
- Signs of PHTN
- A long length of murmur
- And early opening snap (a short gap between S2 and opening snap)

Other features of severe MS, such as signs of pulmonary congestion and right heart failure, are absent here.

Examiner: Please tell me, how will you investigate this case?

Candidate: At first, I would like to take a full history from this patient, particularly focusing on the symptoms consistent with heart failure, such as fatigue, exertional dyspnea, orthopnea, fluid retention; or symptoms consistent with AF—palpitation, poor exercise tolerance, a history of stroke; or any history of fever due to infective endocarditis.

Then I would like to start with baseline blood tests, including:
- CBC and ESR, CRP, U&E/s, serum creatinine, and three sets of blood cultures (for infective endocarditis)

Then I would like to do:
- An ECG—here I would expect AF or if in sinus rhythm P-mitrale and RBBB with RVH.
- A chest X-ray—to identify pulmonary congestion, prominent pulmonary artery (PHTN) with evidence of LA enlargement (double right heart border with splaying of the carina).

The most important test would be transthoracic echocardiography:
- To assess the severity by looking mitral valve area (MVA) and mean pressure gradient.

- To assess the suitability for percutaneous balloon mitral valvoplasty (PBMV)
- To check pulmonary pressure and RV function.

A further test would be a transesophageal echocardiography:
- For a detailed assessment of valvular and supravalvular anatomy.
- Moreover, to assess LA appendage for thrombosis before PBMV.

Finally, right and left heart catheterization can be done, particularly important for patients >40 years:
- To assess coronary anatomy
- MVA (mitral valve area)
- PASP (pulmonary artery systolic pressure)
- PAWP (pulmonary artery wedge pressure)

Examiner: What are the causes of mitral stenosis?

Candidate: Most common cause of mitral stenosis is chronic rheumatic heart disease. Other causes are very rare, such as:
- *Congenital*: Isolated, cor triatriatum (a division of one atrium into two by a membrane), Fabry's disease, mucopolysaccharidoses
- *Degenerative*: Severe mitral annulus calcification
- *Nonvalvular causes*: LA myxoma, large vegetation in infective endocarditis, or LA thrombus.

Examiner: How will you treat this case?

Candidate: As this patient is already symptomatic and complaining of breathlessness, I want to assess her by the New York Heart Association (NYHA) dyspnea scale.

Symptomatic patients with NYHA II dyspnea and moderate (MVA: 1.0–1.5 cm^2, MPG 5–10 mm of Hg) or severe MS (MVA ≤1 cm^2, MPG >10 mm of Hg) should be offered for PBMV if the valve is amenable. If unsuitable, and presence of severe PHTN (PAP >60 mm of Hg) then surgical repair or valve replacement should be considered; otherwise, the patient should be subjected to a 6 monthly follow-up.

Symptomatic patient with NYHA III/IV dyspnea and moderate or severe MS is associated with poor prognosis without intervention.

- PBMV should be offered if the valve is amenable; otherwise, surgical repair or replacement should be undertaken.
- PBMV should be considered in any patient who is not fit for open-heart surgery.

Examiner: Now tell me which patient should be offered PBMV or surgery in an asymptomatic MS patient?

Candidate: Patients who are asymptomatic but have moderate or severe MS should assess for suitability for PBMV.

If suitable, the patient should be assessed for PASP and PAWP.

If, however, the PSAP >50 mm Hg, which rises to >60 mm Hg with exercise, and/or the PAWP on right heart catheterization is >25, or there is a new onset of AF, then PBMV should be offered. Moreover, if unsuitable for PBMV, then plan for valve surgery.

However, if PASP is <50 mm Hg and does not rise to >60 mm Hg or PAWP on right heart catheterization is <25 mm Hg, then the patient should follow up annually.

Examiner: What determines the suitability of a valve for PBMV?

Candidate: Patient should be assessed with Wilkins score, which includes:
- Leaflet mobility
- Thickening
- Subvalvular thickening and calcification are each separately assessed on a scale of 1–4. If the score is <8: the valve is likely to be amenable.

PBMV increases the severity of MR usually by one grade and, therefore, cannot be carried out if moderate or more severe MR is present.

PBMV cannot be undertaken in the presence of LA thrombus due to the risk of embolization. If this persists despite anticoagulation, PBMV is absolutely contraindicated.

Examiner: Tell me, what do you know about the medical management of MS?

Candidate: Medically, we can provide the patient:
- Rheumatic fever prophylaxis, e.g., penicillin (I/M or oral)

- Treatment of AF (warfarin, digoxin, and beta-blockers)
- Treatment of heart failure (diuretics including furosemide and spironolactone).

Examiner: How do you manage MS presenting in pregnancy?

Candidate: Symptomatic patients with severe MS should be advised against pregnancy without treatment.

Asymptomatic patients often present in the mid-trimester with symptoms as a result of the increased heart rate and intravascular volume associated with pregnancy.

Patients with severe MS and NYHA III or IV symptoms that develop during pregnancy should be treated with PBMV with TOE guidance to minimize radiation exposure.

Mitral Regurgitation

Mr John, a 40-year-old man, complained of breathlessness. Examine the cardiovascular system.

(After finishing cardiovascular system examination within 6 minutes of time)

Candidate: I would like to complete my examination by measuring blood pressure, checking for the radiofemoral delay, doing urine dipstick, and looking at the patient's observations chart.

Examiner: Would you like to present your case, please?

Candidate:

I believe this gentleman probably has had mitral valvotomy and now has severe mitral regurgitation with AF with signs of PHTN and pulmonary congestion.

On general examination: The patient is dyspneic at rest, the pulse is 84 beats/min with an irregularly irregular rhythm, JVP is elevated with a systolic V wave.

On examination of the precordium:

There is a lateral thoracotomy scar that suggests he has had previous mitral valvotomy. Apex is displaced and thrusting in nature. He has systolic thrill at the apex with left parasternal heave.

On auscultation:

First heart sound is soft, but the pulmonary component of 2nd heart sound is loud. There is a pansystolic murmur at the apex loudest in expiration, which radiates to axilla. Also, there is a pansystolic murmur at the lower left sternal edge, louder in inspiration (TR murmur for PHTN).

On auscultation of the lung field, there is bilateral basal crepitation, and peripheral edema is noted on his legs. There are no stigmata of infective endocarditis.

Examiner: How will you investigate this case?

Candidate: At first, I would like to take a full history from the patient, particularly focusing on if he has had any childhood infections such as rheumatic fever, which would lead me to the etiology of the condition.

I would also like to find out if he has had any recent procedures or has been having any pyrexia or feeling unwell recently to rule out an infective cause for the condition.

Then I would like to start with the baseline blood tests such as CBC and ESR, CRP, U&E'S, serum creatinine, and three sets of blood cultures. I would do next:
- An ECG—here, I expect any evidence of AF, or in case of sinus rhythm P-mitrale (broad bifid P-wave).
- A chest X-ray—to identify pulmonary congestion and assess cardiac size.

Most importantly, I would like to do an echocardiogram.
- To assess the site and size of the regurgitant jet and dimensions on the left atrium.
- It can help to distinguish the cause of MR (functional/structural).
- The severity of the MR is graded by measuring the LV ejection fraction and end-systolic dimension.

Finally, I would like to do right and left heart catheterization, including coronary angiography to assess pulmonary pressure and coronary anatomy.

All patients having valve surgery should have coronary angiography to exclude significant coronary artery disease that would require bypass grafting (CABG) at the same time as valve replacement.

Examiner: You have mentioned that this patient has severe mitral regurgitation. Please tell me what the features are indicating this is a case of severe MR?

Candidate: He had almost all the features of severe MR. Such as:
- He had atrial fibrillation, which had developed due to LA enlargement.
- He had features of PHTN such as loud and palpable P2, left parasternal heave, TR murmur.
- The apex beat was displaced grossly, and the presence of systolic thrill at the apex.
- Features of CCF include crepitations on both lung bases, raised JVP with systolic V wave, and peripheral edema.

Examiner: Tell me some other features that may indicate mild or moderate severity MR.

Candidate: Mild chronic MR is suggested by the presence of sinus rhythm, absence of LV dilatation, and absence of signs of CCF unless this is the etiology of the MR (functional). Moderate MR is characterized clinically by the absence of features of either mild or severe.

Examiner: Would you like me to tell some causes of MR?

Candidate: This should be considered depending on the pattern of onset as being acute or chronic. In case of chronic MR, causes include:
- *MV prolapse (affected 1-2.5% of the population)*: Marfan syndrome or other CTD (Ehlers–Danlos syndrome, Pseudoxanthoma elasticum, osteogenesis imperfecta), ADPKD, hereditary, or idiopathic.
- Chronic rheumatic heart disease
- *Papillary muscle dysfunction*: Ischemic, functional, degenerative or due to disease of chordae tendineae
- Degenerative mitral valve disease

- *Functional*: Secondary to LV dilatation due to any cause (e.g., ischemic cardiomyopathy or dilated cardiomyopathy) resulting in lateral displacement of the papillary muscles and dilatation of mitral annulus that is interfering with coaptation of the valve leaflets to produce MR.
- Previous valvoplasty for MS (left thoracotomy scar may present here)

In case of acute MR which is usually a medical emergency leading to a sudden onset of severe dyspnea and pulmonary edema. It is commonly caused by chordal rupture from ischemia or posterior papillary muscle dysfunction due to MI or more rarely, due to infective endocarditis.

Examiner: Well said. Now tell me, what actually is the cause of mitral regurgitation here?

Candidate: Here, this patient has had a lateral thoracotomy scar which indicates a previous mitral valvotomy scar. This patient possibly has a history of severe MS due to CRHD (as this is the leading cause of severe MS), which was treated by mitral valvotomy. Patients with previous valvotomy for MS may either develop restenosis or MR or a combination of both.

MR is a common complication of mitral valvotomy, so I believe this patient's MR is due to previous mitral valvotomy.

Examiner: So, you diagnosed this as a case of MR due to previous mitral valvotomy. How will you treat this gentleman?

Candidate: The patient is symptomatic (complaining of breathlessness) and clinically has had evidence of severe MR.

Indeed, no medical treatment ultimately has been shown to alter the prognosis of severe MR. The patient definitely requires valve surgery that can be valve repair or, more commonly, requires MVR. Before that, optimal medical management should be implemented that include:

Management of AF:
- Rate control by digoxin and or beta-blocker
- Anticoagulant therapy (warfarin if not contraindicated)

Management of heart failure:
- Diuretics for congestive symptoms
- ACEI or ARB
- Spironolactone
- Beta-blocker, according to heart failure guideline therapy.

Examiner: That's great! Finally, tell me the indication of surgery in an asymptomatic severe MR patient.

Candidate: Indications are:
- Asymptomatic patient with severe MR with EF 30–60% and LVESD >40 mm.
- Patients with chronic severe MR and new-onset AF or PASP >50 mm Hg at rest with preserved LV function (>60%).

Surgical options are:
- Mitral valve repair or MVR with chordal preservation.

For those patients who are not fit for conservative surgery and those with central MR due to mitral valve prolapse, percutaneous transthoracic mitral valve clip repair can be done.

Mitral Valve Prolapse

Mrs Pam, 34-year-old lady, is an asymptomatic case. Examine the cardiovascular system.

(After finishing cardiovascular system examination within 6 minutes of time)

Candidate: I would like to complete my examination by measuring blood pressure, checking the radiofemoral delay, doing urine dipstick, and looking at the patient's observation chart.

Examiner: Would you like to present your case, please?

Candidate:

I believe this patient has a mitral valve prolapse with a secondary connective tissue disorder, which is most likely to be Ehlers–Danlos syndrome.

The findings that I have elicited from this examination are:

A mid-systolic click is followed by a late systolic murmur loudest at the apex, which radiates to the axilla.

Apex beat is not displaced with normal in character.

Pulse is 76 beats/min, regular and normal in character.

No evidence of PHTN (palpable and loud P2, left parasternal heave)

No evidence of heart failure (raised JVP, peripheral edema, bilateral basal crepitations).

No stigmata of infective endocarditis.

Ehlers–Danlos syndrome was suggested by the classical phenotypic features of:
- Joint hypermobility
- Skin hyperelasticity and
- Blue sclerae

I would like to take a full history to establish her symptomatic status, and my investigation of choice would be an echocardiogram to confirm the diagnosis, quantify the severity.

Examiner: Would you like to tell me the severity of the murmur of MVP of this young lady?

Candidate: The patient is asymptomatic and healthy-looking. She has no features of severe MR, such as:
- Displaced apex beat with thrusting nature and thrill
- Features of PHTN
- Features of right and left-sided heart failure.

So, clinically this is a case of mild or mild to moderate severity MR.

Examiner: Okay, please tell me some causes of hypermobility.

Candidate: Most commonly, hypermobile joints are appeared without any underlying health condition and are termed benign hypermobility syndrome. Other causes include:
- Marfan syndrome
- Ehlers–Danlos syndrome
- Osteogenesis imperfecta
- Down syndrome
- Morquio syndrome

Examiner: You diagnosed this case as a mitral valve prolapse due to Ehlers–Danlos syndrome. Now tell me some other causes of the prolapsed mitral valve.

Candidate: The most common cause is:
- Sporadic myxomatous degeneration (primary)

Or, secondary to other CTDs such as:
- Marfan syndrome (high arched palate, arachnodactyly, arm span > height, hypermobility)
- Pseudoxanthoma elasticum (plucked chicken skin appearance, loose skin over the neck and axilla)
- Osteogenesis imperfecta (blue sclerae, hearing aids, recurrent fracture)

It may be associated with ADPKD—here, I expect HTN with bilateral palpable kidneys.

Or, SLE—where a butterfly rash, oral ulceration, hair loss, and arthropathy may be expected.

Examiner: Which mitral valve leaflet (anterior or posterior) is involved in this patient's case?

Candidate: As this patient has a mid-systolic click followed by late systolic crescendo-decrescendo murmur loudest at the apex with radiation to the axilla; it indicates floppy anterior mitral valve leaflet.

On the other hand, if there is a mid-systolic click (which is usually but not always) followed by a late systolic crescendo-decrescendo murmur loudest at the left sternal edge; then it indicates floppy posterior mitral valve leaflet.

Examiner: Tell me some complications of mitral valve prolapse?

Candidate: Complications include:
- Progression to severe MR where we will get pansystolic murmur.
- Infective endocarditis
- Stroke (embolic phenomenon)
- Arrhythmias (prolonged QTc interval)
- Sudden death.

Examiner: What are the differential diagnoses of MVP murmur, and how would you differentiate them?

Candidate: My differentials would be:
- AS—here I would expect ejection systolic murmur, usually louder in the aortic area with radiation to the neck.
- PS—ejection systolic murmur, louder in inspiration in the pulmonary area.
- Trivial mitral regurgitation—a short murmur that may not be pansystolic and no click.
- Hypertrophic obstructive cardiomyopathy—more marked in the aortic area and left parasternal area that diminished with squatting, intensifies with standing and Valsalva maneuver, and no radiation to the carotid.

Examiner: How would you manage this lady's long term follow-up?

Candidate: I would like this lady to follow up regularly in the cardiology clinic with regular Echocardiography to ensure that she does not have any signs of decompensation from her mitral valve prolapse.

Given her potential Ehlers–Danlos syndrome diagnosis, I would also follow up regularly with the ophthalmologists, as she is at risk of lens dislocation.

Mixed Mitral Valve Disease

Mr Mehta, a 45-year-old man, is complaining of breathlessness. Examine the cardiovascular system.

(After finishing full cardiovascular system examination within 6 minutes of time)

Candidate: I would like to complete my examination by measuring blood pressure, doing urine dipstick, looking at the observation sheet.

Examiner: Would you like to present your case, please?

Candidate:

I believe this middle-aged gentleman most likely has mixed mitral valve disease with signs of PHTN with atrial fibrillation. Here clinical signs favor mitral stenosis as being the predominant valvular lesion.

The physical signs are:

His pulse is 88 beats/min, irregularly irregular rhythm. JVP is not raised. Apex is not displaced and tapping in nature. Left parasternal heave and palpable P2 are also present here.

On auscultation:

There is a loud 1st heart sound, and the pulmonary component of the second heart sound (P2) is also loud. There is an opening snap followed by a mid-diastolic murmur localized to the apex. There is another pansystolic murmur that radiates to axillae.

No evidence of left or right-sided heart failure.

No signs of infective endocarditis such as splinter hemorrhage or clubbing.

No signs of warfarin therapy.

Because of his breathlessness, I would like to investigate him with:
- Complete blood count, ESR, and CRP, as well as three sets of blood cultures to exclude associated infective endocarditis.
- Chest X-ray, ECG, and most importantly, color Doppler echocardiography to assess the valve disease accurately.

Examiner: Why MS is a predominant lesion here, not mitral regurgitation?

Candidate: Because he has an undisplaced apex beat, which is tapping in character. His 1st heart sound is loud with the opening snap. So, I believe he has a predominant mitral stenosis lesion.

In case of predominant mitral regurgitation, I expect displaced and thrusting apex beat with soft 1st heart sound.

Examiner: Okay, now, think this patient has loud 1st heart sound but enlarged left ventricle with other features suggestive of mixed mitral valve disease. Then what is your opinion in that case?

Candidate: In fact, it is very difficult to say clinically, as the loud 1st heart sound would suggest predominant mitral stenosis; on the other hand, the enlarged left ventricle suggests mitral incompetence as the more important lesion.

In case of severe MR without MS, a mid-diastolic flow murmur may be heard without opening snap.

The presence of a 3rd heart sound (due to rapid ventricular filling in severe MR) is incompatible with a significant degree of MS.

I think color Doppler echocardiography would be required to resolve the issue.

Examiner: Could you talk to me a little bit about the treatment options for this patient?

Candidate: The treatment options can be split into medical and surgical.

From a medical point of view:
- If there was evidence of fluid overload, we have to use diuretics for offloading the patient.
- We need to control the heart rate with beta-blockers or other rate-limiting drugs.
- Moreover, ensuring optimal blood pressure control often with ACE-inhibitors or ARB's as well as warfarin for AF if not contraindicated.

We would also like to do serial color Doppler echocardiography to assess the progression of the lesion.

From a surgical point of view:
- Intervention would depend on how symptomatic a patient was and the findings on color Doppler echocardiography.

The surgical options would either be through valve replacement or valve repair.

Examiner: Tell me the indications of MVR for mitral stenosis.

Candidate: In case of severe mitral stenosis with associated PHTN (PASP >60 mm Hg) where valvotomy is contraindicated due to abnormal valve morphology or associated LA thrombus or associated with moderate-to-severe MR.

Pulmonary Stenosis

This 35-year-old man had an incidental finding detected on an insurance medical checkup, please examine his CVS.

(After finishing cardiovascular system examination within 6 minutes of time)

Candidate: I would like to complete my examination by looking at the full sets of clinical observations chart, measuring blood pressure, doing urine dipsticks, and checking for the radiofemoral delay.

Examiner: Would you like to present your case, please?

Candidate:

> I believe this gentleman had PS, and the most likely unifying diagnosis, which would explain the phenotypic features and PS in this instance, is Noonan's syndrome.
>
> The findings that I had elicited from the examination were:
>
> He had a loud ejection systolic murmur heard best in the pulmonary area, radiating to the left shoulder. The murmur was accentuated by inspiration.
>
> I believe that this was nonsevere PS because of the absence of a number of clinical findings—he did not have raised JVP with prominent A-wave or left parasternal heave, or pansystolic murmur of functional tricuspid regurgitation at the lower left sternal edge from right heart dilation. I could not see any evidence of right heart failure.
>
> Moreover, he had no evidence of infective endocarditis as well.

Noonan's syndrome was suggested by the classical phenotypic features of:
- Short stature
- Typical facies (webbed neck, ptosis, flat nasal breeze)
- Widely spaced nipple
- Cubitus valgus

Patients with Noonan syndrome may have mild intellectual disabilities and motor development delay; however, I did not assess for these.

I would like to take a full history to establish his symptomatic status, and my investigations of choice would be an echocardiogram to confirm the diagnosis, quantify the severity and its precise etiology (valvular, subvalvular or supravalvular) and whether there are any concomitant cardiac lesions of Noonan's syndrome such as a septal defect or hypertrophic cardiomyopathy.

Examiner: Would you like to tell me the differential diagnoses of this type of murmur?

Candidate: In terms of differential diagnoses of this type of ejection systolic murmur—the most important D/D would be AS or LV outflow tract obstruction. However, the murmur of AS would be ejection systolic character, which is loudest in expiration in the aortic area, radiates to the carotids with narrow pulse pressure and slow rising pulse.

Other differentials would include VSD and ASD; however, the location and character of the murmur may be different.

Examiner: Can you tell me the clinical symptoms of someone who may have severe PS?

Candidate: The symptoms would include:
- Effort intolerance
- Chest pain or breathlessness on exertion

- Presyncope and syncope as well as signs and symptoms of right-sided heart failure, including peripheral edema, and ascites.

Examiner: So, you said at the beginning you would like to do echocardiography but now tell me what other investigations would you like to perform?

Candidate: Other investigations include:
- 12-lead ECG—whilst an ECG may be normal in nonsevere PS; however, it may show RVH with or without strain and right atrial enlargement in severe PS.
- CXR—to look for dilated pulmonary arteries and reduce lung markings.
- Cardiac MRI for accurate quantification of pulmonary flow, RV size and function assessment, cardiac morphology, and associated lesions.

Examiner: How will you manage the case?

Candidate: If history and investigations suggest severe PS (if peak gradient >70 mm of Hg or evidence of right ventricular failure), then we have to consider pulmonary balloon valvoplasty or valve replacement (either surgical or percutaneous).

Medical management includes diuretics for symptomatic relief.

Prosthetic Aortic Valve

Mr Morison, a 61-year-old man, complained of breathlessness. Examine the cardiovascular system.

(After finishing full cardiovascular system examination within 6 minutes of time)

Candidate: To complete my examination, I would like to perform full sets of clinical observations, including blood pressure measurement and urine dipstick and check for the radiofemoral delay.

Examiner: Would you like to present your case, please?

Candidate:

I believe this gentleman has had an AVR, which appears to be functioning well... (suspect valve failure if decreased prosthetic clicks with a regurgitant murmur, evidence of heart failure with the peripheral signs of AR).

A prosthetic click was audible with the unaided ear.

There are two midline sternotomy scars.

Pulse is 64 beats/min; rhythm is regular with normal in volume and character.

On auscultation:

First hear sound is normal; however, there is an ejection systolic murmur (best heard in the tricuspid area) and a prosthetic click at the 2nd heart sound.

No evidence of oral anticoagulation (e.g., purpura or bruising of the skin).

No evidence of PHTN (e.g., palpable and loud P2 or left parasternal heave).

No stigmata of infective endocarditis such as pyrexia, clubbing, splinter hemorrhage, Osler node, or Janeway lesion.

No evidence of heart failure (bi-basal crepitations, raised JVP or peripheral edema).

Because of his breathlessness, I would like to take a full history to establish his symptomatic status and investigate him further with:

- Complete blood count, ESR, and CRP, as well as three sets of blood cultures to exclude associated infective endocarditis.
- Chest X-ray, ECG, color Doppler echocardiography, as well as renal and liver function tests.

If these tests do not reveal any cause of breathlessness, I would like to assess his respiratory system clinically and do further tests to see any evidence of respiratory illness, such as spirometry and HRCT of the chest.

Examiner: You carefully identified two mid-sternotomy scars of this patient. Now tell me, what would be the explanation for these scars?

Candidate: As there is no scar on his legs, therefore, two mid-sternotomy scars mean the patient had redo or reoperative heart surgery. Possibly it was done due to replacing a degenerative (bioprosthetic valve) or dysfunctional prosthetic valve sometimes complicated with infective endocarditis.

Examiner: Okay, let us see the patient had a vein graft harvesting scar along with one mid-sternotomy scar. Then what might be the cause for it?

Candidate: Before doing any valve replacement, we usually do CAG to exclude concomitant coronary artery disease (CAD).

With these scars, I think he may have had aortic valve disease requiring AVR with coexistent coronary artery bypass surgery (CABG) due to associated CAD.

Examiner: Okay ... let us think if you are getting click following the carotid pulse (2nd heart sound) and a soft ejection systolic murmur, what does it indicate?

Candidate: A loud prosthetic valve closure clicks synchronized with second heart sound indicates metallic aortic valve prosthesis (on the other hand, if it is synchronized with 1st heart sound, it indicates metallic mitral valve prosthesis) as the biological valve does not produce any click.

A systolic murmur (usually soft) accounts that the prosthetic valve can sometimes be heard and represents innocent turbulent flow as the valve orifice area will never truly match that of the native valve.

Examiner: How will you maintain adequate anticoagulation of a patient with valve replacement?/How will you anticoagulate a patient with valve replacement?

Candidate: We must ensure adequate anticoagulation in a mechanical prosthetic valve to prevent valve thrombosis and thromboembolic risks such as stroke or TIA.

Patients with recently used bilateral tilting disc prosthesis in an aortic position can be anticoagulated to achieve a target INR of 2–3 (2.5). However, a patient with a similar mechanical prosthetic valve in mitral position or concomitant AF or with more than one valve replacement should be anticoagulated to a target INR of 2.5–3.5 (3).

Examiner: Okay, fast forward 3 years, you have seen the patient back into the clinic, and you detect a new early diastolic murmur, decreased prosthetic clicks, and high-volume collapsing pulse. What is the possible significance of this?

Candidate: Here, my key concern would be whether this patient had developed valvular incompetence with his replaced aortic valve. Most importantly, in that case, we must exclude infective endocarditis first.

I would also want to assess this by doing three sets of blood C/S and color Doppler echocardiography to assess:
- The function of the prosthetic valve as well as associated vegetations
- Or any new valvular lesions might be causing the diastolic murmur.

Examiner: Tell me some important complications of the prosthetic valve.

Candidate: Complications are:

Valve thrombosis with thromboembolic events (warfarin reduces but does not abolish the risk of ischemic stroke or TIA):
- Under anticoagulation—increases the risk of ischemic stroke or valve obstruction due to valve thrombosis.
- On the other hand, over anticoagulation—increases the risk of bleeding or hemorrhagic stroke as well as bleeding from other sites. So we have to check PT with INR at a regular interval for dose adjustment of anticoagulant drugs.

Valve leakage: Most notably due to infective endocarditis, other causes may be due to:
- Wear/tear of the valve, which is more common in bioprosthesis.
- Or near-total or even total dehiscence of the valve from its siting.

Anemia: It may be due to subacute bacterial endocarditis or resulting from intravalvular mechanical hemolysis through or around a dysfunctional prosthetic valve.

Jaundice: May be due to intravalvular hemolysis (prehepatic jaundice).

Prosthetic Mitral Valve

Mr Harry, a 65-year-old man, complained of breathlessness. Examine the cardiovascular system.

(After finishing cardiovascular system examination within 6 minutes of time)

Candidate: I would like to complete my examination by measuring blood pressure, checking for the radiofemoral delay, doing urine dipsticks, and looking at the patient's observations chart.

Examiner: Would you like to present your case, please?

Candidate:

I believe this middle-aged gentleman has had signs of mechanical MVR, which appears to be functioning well (in prosthetic mitral valve—a systolic murmur indicates incompetence).

My important positive findings are:

He has a midline sternotomy scar.

Metallic prosthetic click was audible without a stethoscope, which coincides with the 1st heart sound.

Pulse is 76 beats/min, regular with normal in volume and character.

No evidence of PHTN (palpable and loud P2 or left parasternal heave).

No evidence of heart failure (crepitations, raised JVP or peripheral edema).

No stigmata of infective endocarditis.

No evidence of oral anticoagulation (e.g., bruising of skin may suggest over anticoagulation).

Because of his breathlessness, I would like to take a full history to establish his symptomatic status and investigate him further with:
- Complete blood count, ESR and CRP, as well as three sets of blood cultures to exclude associated infective endocarditis.
- Chest X-ray, ECG, color Doppler echocardiography, as well as renal and liver function tests.

If these tests do not reveal any cause of breathlessness, I would like to assess his respiratory system clinically and do further tests to see any evidence of respiratory illnesses, such as spirometry and HRCT of the chest.

Examiner: Would you like to tell me about the possible reasons for MVR in this gentleman?

Candidate: As there is no evidence of PHTN and the patient is on sinus rhythm, mitral stenosis would be the less likely cause for this patient. Other possibilities are mitral regurgitation or infective endocarditis.

Examiner: Tell me about the different types of prosthetic valves.

Candidate: These include:
Mechanical valve:
- Starr-Edwards valve (a ball and cage device; not used nowadays)
- Medtronic-Hall valve
- Björk-Shiley valve
- St Judes valve

Bioprosthetic valve:
- Xenografts: Porcine valve and pericardial valve
- *Homografts*: These are cadaveric aortic or pulmonary valve.

Examiner: Tell me the advantages of mechanical and bioprosthetic valves?

Candidate: Mechanical valves are significantly more durable than bioprosthesis and are, therefore, the valve of choice in those <60 years, where there is no contraindication to long-term anticoagulation.

On the other hand, the principal advantages of bioprosthesis are the lack of need for any long-term anticoagulation. Anticoagulant is usually prescribed for the first 3 months, during which time the bioprosthesis has become fully endothelialized.

Examiner: What are the main disadvantages of a mechanical and bioprosthetic valve?

Candidate: While mechanical valves have the advantage of being durable, there is a significant risk of clotting on those valves (valve thrombosis), which directly affects their function. Despite the necessary time intake of anticoagulation, there is always a risk of thromboembolic stroke.

The main disadvantages of bioprosthesis are a higher incidence of degeneration and structural failure requiring redo or reoperation, which has a higher risk than initial surgery. A total of 30-60% of cases develop failure within 10-15 years.

Examiner: Would you like to tell me how MVR can be done?

Candidate: MVR was an exclusively open-heart procedure requiring cardiopulmonary bypass until recently. However, recently a transcatheter approach has become available in that case; most importantly we will not get a mid-sternotomy scar.

Examiner: What is the usual time until a tissue mitral valve will require replacing again?

Candidate: Typically, it may last around 15 years on average, although this may be less in the younger patient.

Examiner: Now, tell me, how will you follow up a patient with metallic valve replacement?

Candidate: The patient should be kept in a regular follow-up by taking an appropriate history, clinical examination, and further investigations. I would like to perform:
- Serial echocardiography to check that the valve is well functioning or not.
- As he would need to be anticoagulated with warfarin, monitoring his INR is mandatory, and the target INR would be 2.5-3.5 for the mitral valve.

Examiner: Okay, let us think about this patient with MVR complaining of breathlessness. Your examination and further cardiovascular investigations revealed normal findings, including FBC, CRP, blood C/S, ECG, and ECHO. Now tell me, what would be the next step for this patient?

Candidate: As all of these do not reveal any cardiovascular cause (as well as anemia) of breathlessness, then I would like to assess his respiratory system clinically and want to do further investigations to see any evidence of respiratory diseases such as:
- Spirometry
- Chest X-ray
- HRCT of the chest.

Atrial Septal Defect

This 25-year-old gentleman complains of cough and occasional palpitation. Please examine his cardiovascular system.

(After finishing full cardiovascular system examination within 6 minutes of time)

Candidate: I would like to complete my examination by looking at the full sets of clinical observations chart, measuring blood pressure, doing urine dipsticks, and checking for the radiofemoral delay.

Examiner: Would you like to present your case, please?

Candidate:

I believe this gentleman had an atrial septal defect, and the most likely unifying diagnosis, which would explain the phenotypic features and ASD in this instance, is that of Down syndrome.

The findings that I had elicited from the examination are:

He had an irregularly irregular pulse suggestive of atrial fibrillation, which might be the first presentation of ASD.

The second heart sound was widely split, and the two components of the split were not influenced by respiration (fixed splitting).

There was an ejection systolic murmur (due to increased flow across the valve) over the pulmonary area.

I believe that this was hemodynamically little significant ASD because of the absence of a number of clinical findings such as:

He did not have evidence of PHTN such as loud P2, left parasternal heave (right ventricular volume overload), pansystolic murmur of the TR at the left sternal edge, and raised JVP. Moreover, I could not see any evidence of right heart failure (peripheral edema or ascites). He also had no evidence of infective endocarditis or Eisenmenger syndrome, including clubbing or cyanosis.

Down syndrome was suggested by the classical phenotypic features of:
- Typical facies (low set small hypoplastic ears, prominent epicanthic folds, upslanting fissures, brush field spots in the iris, flat nasal bridge, and glossoptosis).
- Simian palmar crease
- Short inward curving of the little finger.
- Wide gap between first and second toes.

Patients with Down syndrome may have mild intellectual disabilities and motor developmental delay; however, I did not assess for these.

I would like to take a full history to establish his symptomatic status, and my investigation of choice would be an echocardiogram to confirm the diagnosis and quantitate the degree of shunting and estimate pulmonary arterial pressure.

Examiner: How will you investigate the case?

Candidate: I would like to do an ECG, which may reveal AF, first-degree heart block, partial RBBB with left axis deviation in primum defect, right axis deviation in secundum defect.

A plain chest X-ray demonstrates increased pulmonary vascular markings, dilated pulmonary artery and cardiomegaly if there is heart failure, as well as pulmonary plethora.

The most important test would be TTE, which can be used to identify types (primum, secundum), assess the size of the shunts and their effects on RV function (PHTN).

Bubble contrast may be needed to reveal these defects. However, diagnosis is confirmed by transesophageal echocardiography to define anatomy in more detail and assess suitability for the deployment of a percutaneous closure device.

Cardiac catheterization is indicated to determine pulmonary arterial pressure, pulmonary vascular resistance and to determine shunt quantification from sequential oxygen saturations.

Moreover, cardiac MRI can provide further structural information, especially in more complex congenital lesions.

Examiner: How will you manage the case?

Candidate: The patient should be referred to a specialist ACHD for follow-up. In many cases, no intervention is required in a patient with ASD. However, closure can be achieved surgically (for ostium primum and sinus venosus defect) or more recently with percutaneous closure device (secundum ASD only, if there is no contraindication such as no LA appendages thrombus or anomalous pulmonary venous drainage, adequate rim to anchor device). This should be offered in the following circumstances:
- After paradoxical embolism causing a stroke
- For symptomatic ASD (breathlessness)
- In an asymptomatic patient who has evidence of a significant shunt (ratio pulmonary or systemic flow >1.5).
- In any patient, if there is evidence of significant PHTN (pressure >2/3rd systemic), the closure should only be offered if this can be shown to be reversible on right heart catheterization with a vasodilatation test and shunt fraction (e.g., the ratio of pulmonary to systemic blood flow) is at least 1.5.

Examiner: Would you like to tell me some of the complications of ASD?

Candidate: The most important complications would be:
- Paradoxical embolism causing a stroke
- RV dilation or right heart failure
- Atrial arrhythmia (AF, atrial flutter)
- Severe PHTN and Eisenmenger syndrome where closure is contraindicated.

Ventricular Septal Defect

This 30-year-old man feels well and is under cardiology follow-up, please examine his CVS.

(After finishing cardiovascular system examination within 6 minutes of time)

Candidate: I would like to complete my examination by looking at the full sets of clinical observations chart, measuring blood pressure, doing urine dipsticks, and checking for the radiofemoral delay.

Examiner: Would you like to present your case, please?

Candidate:

The pulse is regular and venous pressure is not elevated. Apex beat is normal in position and character.

There is a loud pansystolic murmur with an ejection character best heard at the left sternal edge, which is also audible at the apex.

He has no evidence of PHTN, left ventricular failure.

He has no evidence of infective endocarditis as well as concomitant AR due to prolapse of the right coronary cusp that can occur, particularly in perimembranous VSD.

He also has no evidence of morphological features of known disease association such as Down syndrome or Turner syndrome.

I believe this gentleman has evidence of ventricular septal defect, which is likely a small hemodynamically insignificant left to right shunt (Maladie de Roger).

I would like to take a full history to establish his symptomatic status, mainly looking for symptoms of heart failure and PHTN; my investigation of choice would be an echocardiography (2D, M-mode and color Doppler) to confirm the diagnosis, to quantitate the degree of shunting, and to estimate left ventricular function and pulmonary arterial pressure.

Examiner: Well said.... would you please tell me what other investigations can be done for this young gentleman for further evaluation?

Candidate: In that case, I would like to start with an ECG, which may demonstrate electrocardiographic findings of left, right, or combined ventricular hypertrophy depending on the size and direction of the shunt. However, if VSD is small, a normal ECG can be expected.

Then I would like to do a chest X-ray that may demonstrate cardiomegaly due to left ventricular dilatation or enlarged main pulmonary artery with reduced peripheral vascular markings in a patient with PHTN in hemodynamically significant VSD.

Cardiac MRI can be used to evaluate further ventricular volumes, function, and shunt quantification where echocardiography has not been diagnostic. However, cardiac catheterization is not routinely required. It can be used to determine pulmonary vascular resistance if pulmonary arterial pressure is suggested to be raised on echocardiography and for shunt quantification and exclude other associated congenital anomalies such as PDA or aortic coarctation.

Examiner: How will you manage the case?

Candidate: Clinically, this young gentleman has had evidence of hemodynamically insignificant small VSD, and if further investigations suggest it then, the only management that is required is the reassurance of the patient that the condition is entirely harmless.

However, if large defects or those presenting with complications, VSD are most commonly closed surgically, but in case of anatomically suitable muscular VSD-percutaneous catheter-based closure is now an option.

Examiner: That's great! Now tell me the contraindications of VSD closure?

Candidate: Closure is contraindicated at the extremes of the symptomatology spectrum, such as those who have developed Eisenmenger syndrome or asymptomatic patients with small, hemodynamically insignificant lesions with no evidence of left ventricular volume overload. However, severe PHTN is also a contraindication to closure.

Patent Ductus Arteriosus

Please examine the CVS of this asymptomatic 45-year-old gentleman.

(After finishing cardiovascular system examination within 6 minutes of time)

Candidate: I would like to complete my examination by looking at the full sets of clinical observations chart, measuring blood pressure, doing urine dipsticks, and checking for the radiofemoral delay.

Examiner: Would you like to present your case, please?

Candidate:

I believe this patient most likely had a PDA. However, other differentials for this patient could be PS.

The findings that I had elicited from this examination were:

He had continuous machinery murmur heard in the infraclavicular and infrascapular region.

There were no features of left or RVH or PHTN, and he did not have a collapsing pulse, which would be present in a severe patent ductus arteriosus.

Importantly, the patient is presented in adulthood with his PDA, which suggests it is not severe. If it were a large PDA, it would likely have been picked up during childhood resulting in his PDA being closed.

I would like to take a full history to establish his symptomatic status and the diagnostic investigation is likely to be an echocardiogram to confirm the diagnosis, confirm the absence of left or right heart involvement, and estimate pulmonary arterial pressure to establish that this is a nonsevere (small) PDA.

Examiner: Let us go back to your examination, and you did some maneuvers during the examination. You said the murmur was present due to PS or PDA. Tell me about the maneuvers.

Candidate: In this case, the murmur was loudest in expiration instead of in inspiration that would be classical for a PDA compared to a PS, which would be louder in inspiration.

The position of the radiation to the back of being over the left infrascapular is more classical for a patent ductus arteriosus.

In PS, the murmur tends to radiate to the center of the back and the shoulders.

Examiner: You said at the beginning, you would like to do an echocardiography. Now tell me what other investigations would you like to perform?

Candidate: Here, other relevant investigations would be a 12 lead ECG and plain X-ray chest radiography related to complications of the PDA. A normal CXR and ECG would be expected with a small PDA with no cardiac sequelae. RVH and prominent pulmonary vessels could be evident with shunt causing PHTN. Cardiomegaly and pulmonary congestion may be evident with PDA, which gives rise to left ventricular failure in severe PDA.

Cardiac catheterization helps to the quantification of the shunt along with the determination of pulmonary artery pressure and pulmonary vascular resistance.

Another important test would be cardiac MRI that provides structural information, complex congenital heart disease identification, and ventricular function quantification.

Examiner: Well said. Now please tell me how you will manage this asymptomatic PDA case?

Candidate: The patient should be referred to a specialist for adult congenital heart disease for follow-up.

Asymptomatic patient with small hemodynamically insignificant lesion with no clinical evidence of shunt on examination is managed conservatively and requires no closure. Indications of closure by percutaneously or surgically include:

- Signs of LV volume overload
- Or patients with PHTN but with pulmonary arterial pressure less than two-thirds of the systemic pressure or pulmonary vascular resistance less than two-thirds of systemic vascular resistance.

Intracardiac Device

A 50-year-old man previously complained about reduced exercise tolerance and one episode of syncopal attack. Please examine his CVS.

(After finishing cardiovascular system examination within 6 minutes of time)

Candidate: I would like to complete my examination by looking at the full sets of clinical observations chart, measuring blood pressure, doing urine dipsticks, and checking for the radiofemoral delay.

Examiner: Would you like to present your case, please?

Candidate:

> This elderly gentleman has an incisional scar with a subcutaneous mass in the infraclavicular position.
>
> However, he has no evidence of local infection, such as redness or tenderness over that area.
>
> He also has evidence of congestive cardiac failures such as raised JVP, peripheral edema, and bilateral basal crepitations.
>
> But he does not have any evidence of infective endocarditis.
>
> I believe this gentleman has a congestive cardiac failure and a subcutaneously implanted cardiac device in the infraclavicular region. The differential diagnosis would be a conventional bradycardia pacemaker (single/dual), cardiac resynchronization therapy with biventricular pacing with (CRT-D) or without defibrillator (CRT-P) or a standard ICD.
>
> I would like to take a full history from the patient to establish his symptomatic status and the nature of the implanted device.

Examiner: Let us think this patient has had a CRT-D device. Would you like to tell me the indications of the device?

Candidate: CRT-P or biventricular (triple chamber) pacing is considered in the following situations to synchronize all chambers:
- If the patient has LVEF <35%
- NYHA II-IV on optimal medical therapy
- Sinus rhythm and QRS duration >150 milliseconds (ms) (if LBBB morphology may be >120 ms)

Here, extra LV pacemaker leads via coronary sinus improve mortality or symptoms.

On the other hand, ICD, where the "shock box" also delivers antitachycardia pacing (ATP) improves mortality.

It is considered primary prevention in post-MI patients (MI >4 weeks ago) with an NYHA no more than class III.
- LVEF <35% and nonsustained VT and positive EP study or
- LVEF <30% and a QRS duration of ≥120 ms
- *Familial conditions with a high risk of sudden cardiac death (SCD)*: LQTS, ARVD, Brugada, HCOM, complex congenital heart disease

It is also considered as secondary prevention (without treatable cause):
- Sudden cardiac arrest due to VT or VF or hemodynamically compromised VT or VT with LVEF <35% (not NYHA IV) **(Table 1)**

Examiner: How will you investigate the case?

Candidate: In fact, the relevant investigations will depend upon the clinical presentation of the patient; for example, if a patient with an implantable device presents with symptoms and signs of infection, then I would like to do serial blood cultures and inflammatory markers with suspicion of device-related infections or device-related infective endocarditis.

Table 1: Implantable device treatment options for a patient with severe LV dysfunction (EF <35% stratified by NYHA class, QRS duration, and the presence/absence of LBBB).

QRS interval	NYHA I	NYHA II	NYHA III	NYHA IV
QRS <120 ms	ICD if there is a high risk of sudden cardiac death			ICD/CRT not clinically indicated
120–149 ms without LBBB	ICD	ICD	ICD	CRT-P
120–149 ms with LBBB	ICD	CRT-D	CRT-P/D	CRT-P
≥150 ms with or without LBBB	CRT-D	CRT-D	CRT-P/D	CRT-P

Source: The NICE guidelines.

Other general investigations include 12 lead ECG, CXR P/A view, and an echocardiography.

Examiner: What important advice would you like to give a patient with CRT-D or pacemaker device?

Candidate: There has been long-standing concern regarding the safety of MRI scans in a patient with pacemaker and ICD due to direct electrical effects of induced current within the leads. So, most hospitals consider MRI in a patient with such devices to be absolutely contraindicated.

CHAPTER 4

Clinical Examination: Respiratory System

- ❑ Respiratory System Examination
- ❑ Interstitial Lung Disease
- ❑ Rheumatoid Lung
- ❑ Bronchiectasis
- ❑ Cystic Fibrosis
- ❑ Pneumonia
- ❑ Chronic Obstructive Pulmonary Disease
- ❑ Cor-pulmonale
- ❑ Bronchial Asthma
- ❑ Lung Cancer
- ❑ Lobectomy
- ❑ Pneumonectomy
- ❑ Lung Transplant

Respiratory System Examination

1. Meticulously, read the clinical scenario; this shall help you predict what you are going to find and do only what you have been asked.
2. Carefully greet the examiners in a nice, decent, and balanced manner—this will definitely carry a positive impact on them.
3. Sanitize your hands with antiseptic liquid (antiseptic liquid is provided to you in the station).
4. Greet the patient, introduce yourself, confirm your patient identity and take permission (Hello, Mr X…. Good morning, I am Mohammad Ali….One of the working doctors here today….I have been asked to examine you….Is that okay with you?).
5. Explain to the patient in easy yet precise terms about your procedure—this shall help to get required cooperation from the patient (I would like to examine your hands, face, neck, chest, and legs if that is okay with you?).
6. Ask about the pain and discomfort and reassure the patient (Do you have any pain or discomfort?………I would be gentle during the examination, please let me know if you feel any pain or discomfort).
7. Adequately positioned (position the patient 45° in bed).
8. Sufficiently expose the patient appropriate to the examination (please maintain dignity… Expose the patient from head to the mid-abdomen).
   [Explain every subsequent step before doing it so that the patient will be more cooperative and this will help you score better in skill-7 (maintaining patient's welfare)]
9. *General survey*: Stand at the end of the bed, take your time to observe (see the patient as a whole, do not rush to examination, look for bedside clues and other clues in the patient).
   - Bedside clues:
     - Oxygen therapy (O_2-mask, nasal cannula), bilevel positive airway pressure machine (BIPAP)/continuous positive airway pressure (CPAP) machine [interstitial lung disease (ILD), chronic obstructive pulmonary disease (COPD)]
     - Inhaler or nebulizers machine (asthma, COPD, bronchiectasis)
     - Sputum pots (COPD, bronchiectasis, lung abscess)
     - Chest drains (malignant pleural effusion, empyema, pneumothorax)
     - Walking aids which may suggest the patient may have reduced exercise tolerance
   - Ask the patient to breathe in and out and cough……….. (Could you take a deep breath in for me; Could you cough for me please?) and note—whether this is productive or dry?
     - Productive cough (bronchiectasis, cystic fibrosis if young, COPD, lung abscess)
     - Dry: ILD if older, asthma if young.
   - Age:
     - Young patient: Asthma, cystic fibrosis (bronchiectasis), pneumonia, pneumothorax.
     - Old: More likely COPD, ILD, malignancy, lobectomy, pneumonectomy, pneumothorax.
   - Comfortable versus tachypnea…Is the patient short of breath at rest? Is the patient able to speak in a full sentence?
     - Use of accessory muscles (indrawing of the intercostal muscle, use of abdominal muscle, tracheal tug)
     - Pursed lip breathing
     - Nasal flaring (spreading of the nostrils while breathing)
     - Tripod position (leaning forward with arm and elbow supported on over bed table—the inability to lie flat)

- Body built:
  - Overweight: Obstructive sleep apnea (OSA), obesity hypoventilation syndrome (OHA)
  - Cachexia: COPD, bronchogenic carcinoma, bronchiectasis (cystic fibrosis in the young patient)
- Any audible wheeze (expiratory):
  - COPD, bronchial asthma and rarely—cardiac asthma, carcinoid, anaphylaxis
- Any stridor (inspiratory):
  - Upper airway obstruction
- Face neck:
  - Horner's syndrome (Pancoast tumor)
  - Radiation burn suggests underlying lung carcinoma (collapse, fibrosis, cavity, consolidation)
  - Amiodarone pigmentation: May have pulmonary fibrosis
  - Systemic lupus erythematosus (SLE) rash: Lung fibrosis, effusion
  - Microstomia, tight shiny skin, tipped nose, telangiectasia suggests systemic sclerosis: (PHTN), fibrosis.
  - Lupus pernio suggests sarcoidosis (?Fibrosis)
  - The heliotrope rash suggests dermatomyositis [(?Diffuse parenchymal lung disease (DPLD)]
  - Cushingoid face suggests steroid use [(?Sarcoidosis, asthma, COPD, connective tissue disease (CTD)]
- Chest: "Take a deep breath for me, please.":
  - Pectus carinatum, pectus excavatum (chest deformity).
  - Increased anteroposterior (AP) diameter (barrel shape chest) suggests COPD.
  - Restricted movement one side: Collapse, fibrosis, pneumonia, lobectomy, and pneumonectomy.
  - Restricted movement on both sides: DPLD/ILD, bilateral bronchiectasis, COPD.
  - Bulge: Pneumothorax and pleural effusion.
  - Chest wall retraction: Collapse, fibrosis, lobectomy, and pneumonectomy.
  - Radiation tattoos/burn: Lung carcinoma.
  - Dilated veins over chest wall with congested face and congested arm suggest superior vena cava obstruction (SVCO) due to carcinoma of lung or lymphoma.

10. *Close inspection of the hand*:
    - Rheumatoid arthritis (Z-deformity, boutonniere or swan neck deformity, joint pain, and swelling) may have DPLD, effusion, bronchiolitis obliterans, bronchiectasis.
    - Sclerodactyly, thin tight shiny skin suggests systemic sclerosis may have DPLD or PHTN.
    - Bruising and skin purpura suggest steroid use; may have COPD, DPLD, bronchial asthma (BA).

11. *Ask the patient to extend his hand and examine the dorsum of hands for*:
    - Clubbing suggests bronchial carcinoma, DPLD, typically idiopathic pulmonary fibrosis (IPF), suppurative lung disease (bronchiectasis, lung abscess, and empyema).
    - Tar staining on the finger suggest smoker; increase the risk of COPD, lung cancer.
    - Yellow nail syndrome (?bronchiectasis)
    - Peripheral cyanosis (bluish discoloration of the nail) suggests hypoxia (respiratory failure)
    - Fine tremor associated with beta-agonists therapy suggests COPD and BA; Tacrolimus therapy in a post-transplant patient (look for scar mark).
    - Wasting of the small muscle of the hand suggests C8, T1 lesion (Pancoast tumor)

12. Ask the patient to turn his hands up and examine palms for ....
    - Palmar erythema (?CO_2-retention)
    - Feel radial pulse (rate, rhythm), if high volume bounding pulse suggests CO_2 retention (?respiratory failure)
    - Count respiratory rate in 15 seconds × 4 whilst feeling the pulse.

13. Ask the patient to pull his wrist back and examine flapping tremors which suggest hypercapnia (?Type 2 respiratory failure, ?COPD)

14. *Examine both eyes same time for*:
    - Pallor (pull down your lower eyelid for me, please)
    - Horner syndrome (partial ptosis, meiosis, enophthalmos, anhidrosis)
    - Jaundice indicates malignancy
    - Suffused conjunctiva presents in secondary polycythemia (hypoxia-induced)
15. Examine mouth ("Open the mouth for me and lift the tongue, please..") for central cyanosis at the dorsal surface of the tongue and lips (suggests hypoxia—?respiratory failure), fish mouth (narrow mouth opening with skin puckering) and telangiectasia suggest systemic sclerosis–may have PHTN or DPLD.
16. Ask the patient to turn his head ("Please turn your head to the left side and relax..") and examine jugular venous pressure (JVP) and look for raised JVP and hepatojogular reflux [discussed in cardiovascular (CVS)]:
    - Raised JVP suggests PHTN, cor-pulmonale or heart failure, fluid overload, pulmonary embolism (PE).
    - Nonpulsating raised JVP suggests SVCO.
    - JVP waveform: If the "a-wave" is prominent, suggesting right atrial hypertrophy, or large "v-wave" suggests tricuspid valve (TR).
17. *Close inspection of the chest*:
    - Scar:
        - The small (1–2 cm) mid-axillary scar in the intercostal space for the previous chest drain
        - Small (1–2 cm) VAT scar in posterior intercostal space
        - Mediastinoscopy scar (5 cm) in the suprasternal notch
        - Large horizontal posterolateral thoracotomy scar (for lobectomy or pneumonectomy)
    - Chest asymmetry:
        - Pneumonectomy (usually for cancer)
        - Thoracoplasty [rib removed/previously used for tuberculosis (TB)]
    - Skin change:
        - Erythema or thickened skin indicates recent or previous radiotherapy
18. *Palpation*:
    - Tracheal position (palpation of the trachea can be uncomfortable; so, warn the patient and apply gentle pressure—I am going to feel your windpipe, this may be slightly uncomfortable.....)
        - Ensure the neck musculature is relaxed—chin slightly downward.
        - Dip index finger into the thorax beside the trachea.
        - Compare this space to another side of the trachea using the same process.
        - A difference in the amount of space between the sides suggests deviation.
        - The trachea deviated away from pneumothorax and large pleural effusion.
        - The trachea deviates toward the lobar collapse, fibrosis, and pneumonectomy.
    - Check for the cricosternal distance (the distance between the suprasternal notch to the cricoid cartilage; normal should be 3-4 fingers). If the distance is <3 fingers suggest lung hyperinflation (?COPD)
    - Apex beat position (displacement suggests mediastinal shifting or poorly palpable due to hyperinflation of the chest)
    - Right ventricular heave is noted in cor-pulmonale (right heart failure secondary to PHTN due to chronic hypoxic lung diseases such as COPD, ILD, or bronchiectasis)
    - Chest expansion:
        - Place your hands on the patient's chest, inferior to the nipple
        - Wrap your fingers around either side of the chest
        - Bring your thumb in the midline so that they touch each other
        - Ask the patient to take a deep breath.
        - If one side of your thumbs move less, suggest reduced expansion on that side (? lung collapse, pneumonia)
19. *Percussion of the chest*:
    - Percuss the following areas comparing side-to-side:
        - Supraclavicular (lung apical zone), infraclavicular, chest wall (3–4 location), axilla

[Resonant: normal; Hyperresonant: pneumothorax; Dullness: consolidation (woodiness), pleural effusion (stony dull), collapse, and tumor. Loss of cardiac dullness suggest hyperinflated lung]
20. *Auscultation of the chest*:
    - Assess the quality of breath sound:
        - Bronchial breath sound suggests consolidation (?fibrosis)
        - Vesicular breath sound with prolonged expiration suggests asthma, COPD, bronchiectasis.
        - Absent breath sound suggests pleural effusion or pneumothorax or central collapse, or pneumonectomy.
    - Added sound:
        - Rhonchi—asthma, COPD (rarely also in anaphylaxis, sarcoid, cardiac asthma).
        - (End) Late inspiratory fine crackles—pulmonary fibrosis or pulmonary edema.
        - Early-mid inspiratory coarse crackles: Bronchiectasis, resolving pneumonia.
        - If crackles are present, then ask the patient—"Can you cough for me please?"; Crackles that alter with coughing suggests infections or secretions (bronchiectasis); if unaltered (fixed), suggests ILD.
        - Pleural rub—pleurisy due to any cause.
    - Ask the patient to say 99.......Each time you put on your stethoscope and listen for vocal resonance.
        - Increased vocal resonance: Consolidation, cavitation, mass, dense lung fibrosis, lung collapse with mediastinal shift to the side of the lesion, bronchiectasis (if vocal resonance is increased, then examine for whispering pectoriloqy by asking the patient to whisper 99 and determine if this sound is increased that suggests consolidation or fibrosis)
        - Decreased vocal resonance: Pleural effusion, pneumothorax, lobectomy, pneumonectomy, and lung fibrosis.
21. Ask the patient to sit forward and cross their arms, then examine the patient for lymph nodes in the anterior and posterior triangle, supraclavicular, and axillary region:
    - Lymphadenopathy suggests cancer, TB, sarcoidosis, and lymphoma.
22. *Assess the patient's posterior chest*: Inspection, palpation, percussion, and auscultation.
23. Examine the sacrum for edema (fluid overload for cor-pulmonale)
24. *Examination of the leg*:
    - Peripheral edema (?cor-pulmonale)
    - Assess the calves for a sign of deep vein thrombosis (DVT)
    - Erythema nodosum (?sarcoidosis)
    - Erythema multiform (?mycoplasma)
    - Purpuric eruption (?steroid use)
25. *Formulate your comment and diagnosis*:
    - The diagnosis (COPD, DPLD, fibrosis, effusion, bronchiectasis)
    - Causes (smoking, cystic fibrosis, CTD, drugs)
    - Possible complications (PHTN, cor-pulmonale, respiratory failure)
26. Thanks to the patient at the end of the examination and cover him up before turning around to the examiner.
27. Wash hands again.
28. To complete the examination, offer the examiner to look at the patient's observation chart, sputum pots (if any), to perform pulse oximetry, bedside spirometry, and to look at the patient's chest radiograph.

Note: The anterior part of the chest is mainly formed of the upper lobe, and the posterior part of the chest is mainly formed of the lower lobe.

Case Presentation

If you are confident of the diagnosis, it is far more impressive to state the diagnosis and justify it by the presentation of the important relevant positive and negative findings, otherwise present the case in a systemic manner mentioning the important positive and negative findings. Try to give a possible cause of the condition, e.g., pulmonary fibrosis most likely secondary to SLE. It is better to comment on the severity, any complications of the disease (e.g., pulmonary HTN) or of the treatment (e.g., Cushing syndrome secondary to steroid use)

I would like to complete my examination by examining sputum pots, patient's observation charts, doing pulse oximetry and spirometry; examine lymph nodes (if you did not examine the lymph nodes during examination).

I believe this gentleman has evidence of…….(Diagnosis)….(Cause)…..(Complication)

This gentleman is lying comfortably at rest with an average built…He has tar staining of the nail, pulse…..respiratory rate…clubbing…cyanosis…JVP…trachea….chest movement….percussion note…breath sound…added sound…vocal resonance

He has (no) evidence of PHTN, Cor-pulmonale, respiratory failure.

Interstitial Lung Disease

Mr John, 65-year-old presented with progressive breathlessness. Examine the respiratory system.

(After finishing respiratory system examination within 6 minutes of time)

Candidate: I would like to complete my examination by checking the patient's observation chart, examining sputum pots (if any), doing bedside spirometry and pulse oximetry, and examining lymph nodes (if you do not examine the lymph nodes during your examination).

Examiner: Would you like to present your case, please?

Candidate:

I performed a respiratory system examination on Mr John, based on my clinical findings, I believe this patient has a diagnosis of interstitial lung disease.

On inspection, this gentleman was breathless at rest and on ambulatory oxygen requiring relatively high flows.

On general physical examination, he presented with tachypnea, tachycardia and mild finger clubbing in both hands and feet.

On chest inspection, there were no obvious scar marks, deformity or engorged vein. He had a normal chest expansion with a resonant percussion note.

On chest auscultation, he had a vesicular breath sound; there were some fine end-inspiratory crackles at both lung bases that did not alter with cough; vocal resonance was normal.

The important negative findings in this case: There were no obvious stigmata of connective tissue disease specifically,
- Any small joint arthropathy for rheumatoid arthritis or SLE,
- Rashes suggestive of dermatomyositis,
- Any evidence of scleroderma in hands and face (tight shiny skin of face and hands, sclerodactyly, calcinosis)

No evidence of PHTN (right ventricular heave, raised JVP, palpable loud P2) or cor-pulmonale (evidence of PHTN plus peripheral edema) or respiratory failure (central cyanosis or CO_2 retention flap).

Examiner: Tell me some differentials that could be possible with these findings? Or tell me some differentials of bilateral basal crepitations?

Candidate: Keeping in mind bilateral basal crepitations, other possible differentials could be:
- *Bronchiectasis*: Here, I would expect coarse crepitations that alter with coughing and also a productive cough with a bedside sputum pot.
- Next, it could be a case of heart failure; therefore, some inspiratory crepitations, peripheral edema, along with features of PHTN (such as raised JVP) with or without a murmur, would be expected.
- Resolving pneumonia would be another possibility with fever, fine crepitations in the chest and absent clubbing. However, no features suggested these differentials.

Examiner: Okay, as you have mentioned, your diagnosis is an interstitial lung disease. Do you have any ideas of what his underlying cause would be?

Candidate: In terms of his age and the fact that he is clubbed, I think it is most likely to be idiopathic pulmonary fibrosis (IPF).

Examiner: What do you know about Hamman-Rich Syndrome?

Candidate: It is a clinical condition characterized by rapidly progressive cryptogenic lung fibrosis with a very poor prognosis.

Examiner: As this patient is breathless, how would you investigate him?

Candidate: First of all, I would like to do a routine set of blood including complete blood count (CBC) with erythrocyte sedimentation rate (ESR) and C-reactive protein (CRP), urea and electrolytes (U/Es), serum creatinine, liver function tests (LFTs), autoimmune and vasculitis screen such as antinuclear antibody (ANA), anti-cyclic citrullinated peptide antibody testing (anti CCP Ab), rheumatoid arthritis factor to exclude underlying CTD, as well as serum Ca, serum angiotensin converting enzyme (ACE) to exclude sarcoidosis.

A chest X-ray for seeing any appearance of interstitial opacities based on patterns like a reticular, nodular, or reticulonodular shadow.

The next test would be a high-resolution computed tomography (HRCT) scan of the chest which may show bilateral predominantly subpleural and basal reticular opacities with associated traction bronchiectasis, ground-glass opacities, and honeycombing.

Pulmonary function test: Here, I expect a restrictive pattern on spirometry that may include:
- Normal or reduced forced expiratory volume (FEV1)
- Markedly reduced forced vital capacity (FVC), so FEV1/FVC ratio will be normal or increase
- Reduced lung volume and total lung capacity
- Finally, reduced diffusing capacity of the lung for carbon monoxide (DLCO)

An electrocardiogram (ECG) and echocardiogram for any evidence of PHTN or right ventricular failure.

After doing all of these tests, I would like to refer this patient to the interstitial lung disease multidisciplinary team (MDT) to make a decision about diagnosis and understand the possible underlying etiology. Any diagnostic uncertainty should be confirmed by lung biopsy that would be decided by MDT. It can be done by a transbronchial biopsy or an open lung biopsy.

Examiner: How could you manage a patient with a diagnosis of idiopathic pulmonary fibrosis?

Candidate: The management of an IPF patient is a MDT approach. This may include:
- Respiratory specialist nurses (to help the patient with their shortness of breath and improve quality of life).
- Physiotherapist for a pulmonary rehabilitation program (PRP); PRP includes physical training, patient education, and nutritional and psychological support. The physical therapist starts from breath retraining and relaxing postures, increasing chest expansion, and relaxing the inspiratory muscles and increasing patients' exercise capacity.
- Respiratory physicians consider medical therapies that include supportive treatments where necessary, such as oxygen and drugs like nintedanib or pirfenidone.
- Also a surgeon to decide whether they need lung transplantation

Nonpharmacological measures include vaccination, stopping smoking, chest physiotherapy, and avoidance of industrial and occupational exposure, if any, causing DPLD.

Moreover, pharmacological measures if the patient has ground-glass opacities in HRCT suggest inflammation and, therefore, a potential response to corticosteroid and immunosuppressive drugs such as azathioprine and cyclophosphamide.

If there is established fibrosis in HRCT, which suggest end-stage lung disease are less likely to respond to steroid and other immunosuppressive drugs in that case, I will treat them with newer antifibrotics (nintedanib or pirfenidone).

In very advanced cases, patients with no absolute contraindication should be referred for consideration of unilateral lung transplantation.

Rheumatoid Lung

Mrs Convey, a 62-year-old woman, presented with progressive breathlessness. Examine the respiratory system.

(After finishing respiratory system examination within 6 minutes of time)

Candidate: I would like to complete my examination by checking the patient's observation chart, examining sputum pots (If any), doing bedside spirometry, pulse oximetry, and examining lymph nodes (If you do not examine the lymph nodes during your examination).

Examiner: Would you like to present your case, please?

Candidate:

> I performed a respiratory system examination on this elderly lady; she was breathless at rest requiring high flow oxygen with a nasal mask.
>
> On chest examination, there were no obvious scar marks. She had bilateral decreased chest expansion with bi-basal dullness on percussion. She had some fine end-inspiratory crackles at both lung bases, which did not alter with coughing.
>
> Moreover, most importantly, there was a symmetrical deforming arthropathy of the small joints of the hands, keeping with rheumatoid arthritis. Some steroid purpuras over the extremities were also noted.
>
> There were no other peripheral stigmata of chronic lung disease such as clubbing, cyanosis, or CO_2 retention flap.
>
> No evidence of PHTN or Cor-pulmonale or respiratory failure.
>
> With all of these findings, I believe this patient has interstitial lung disease secondary to rheumatoid arthritis.

Examiner: You mentioned rheumatoid arthritis that causes interstitial lung disease. Could you tell me some other respiratory complications of rheumatoid arthritis?

Candidate: Although rheumatoid arthritis-related lung disease nowadays is seen much less frequently due to earlier and more aggressive treatment regimens. However, rather than ILD, there are some other respiratory manifestations of rheumatoid arthritis, such as:

- The most common presentation would be pleural thickening or pleural effusions. Here, I would expect absent breath sounds with diminished vocal resonance.
- Bronchiectasis may present with coarse inspiratory crackles, which alters with coughing and some expiratory wheeze.
- Bronchiolitis obliterans may be associated with reduced cricoid-sternal distance (hyperinflation), high-pitched expiratory wheeze, and late inspiratory squeak.
- Pulmonary nodule usually remains asymptomatic but can become infected, cavitated or bronchopulmonary fistula, and mainly at the upper lobe.
- *Caplan's syndrome*: This is the presence of pneumoconiosis in a patient with rheumatoid arthritis.
- *Organizing pneumonia* can occur with fever, dyspnea, and multifocal consolidation.
- Others may include PHTN, pulmonary arteritis, pneumonitis (this may occur due to rheumatoid arthritis itself or as methotrexate-induced), bronchial carcinoma (very rarely).

Examiner: Okay, that is fine. Please tell me, can rheumatoid interstitial lung disease be present in the absence of arthritis?

Candidate: Interstitial lung disease often occurs in patients with known rheumatoid disease. However, in some cases, it may precede the onset of arthritis by months or even years.

Examiner: You mentioned pleural effusion as a respiratory manifestation. What would be the features of a rheumatoid pleural effusion?

Candidate: The characteristic findings of pleural effusion caused by rheumatoid arthritis include:
- Exudative
- High lactate dehydrogenase (LDH) (>700 IU/L); low glucose (<1.6 mmol/L); low PH (<7.2)
- A high rheumatoid factor titer (>1:320)
- High cholesterol levels

Examiner: How would you investigate this patient?

Candidate: At first, I would want to take a full history from this patient, mainly asking about medications and occupational history. Then, I would want to do some simple bedside tests such as oxygen saturation and arterial blood gas (ABG) if the patient is hypoxic. I would also like to do routine blood tests, specifically full blood count with ESR and CRP, U/Es, serum creatinine and LFTs. Next, I would want to do a chest X-ray; this may show bilateral interstitial shadowing, reticulonodular shadow and loss of lung volume.

The most important test for this patient would be an HRCT of the chest; I would refer the patient for a HRCT scan, which may show subpleural reticulation, traction bronchiectasis, and basal honeycombing with ground-glass opacity. Other things that I also could do would be to send the patient for pulmonary function tests. Here, I would be looking for a restrictive defect with reduced lung volume and impaired gas transfer.

Given my concern about rheumatoid arthritis, I would want to do an autoimmune screen and a full rheumatic disease screen.

Examiner: You have done all of these investigations and confirmed your case as an interstitial lung disease related to rheumatoid arthritis. Now please tell me how would you manage this patient?

Candidate: This patient should have ongoing access to an MDT. This includes rheumatology and respiratory physicians, surgeons, physiotherapists, occupational therapists, and specialist nurses. We would first treat the underlying rheumatic disease with appropriate disease-modifying drugs, which will also help improve lung function and delay progression.

Bronchiectasis

Mr Donald, a 56-year-old man, presented with progressive breathlessness and cough. Examine the respiratory system.

(After finishing respiratory system examination within 6 minutes of time)

Candidate: I would like to complete my examination by checking the patient's observation chart, examining sputum pots (if any), doing bedside spirometry, pulse oximetry, and examining lymph nodes (if you do not examine the lymph nodes during your examination).

Examiner: Would you like to present your case, please?

Candidate:

Respiratory system examination on this gentleman, I believe this patient has left-sided lower lobe bronchiectasis.

The patient was comfortable at rest with average built, and I noticed a sputum pot by the bedside. He had finger clubbing, productive cough, and some inspiratory clicks audible from the end of the bed with the unaided ear.

On chest auscultation, this gentleman also had a vesicular breath sound with prolonged expiration and some end-inspiratory coarse crepitations that alter with coughing at the left lower chest. There was also some expiratory wheeze at the left lower chest.

Otherwise, he had a normal chest expansion, resonant percussion with normally placed trachea and apex beat, and no scars on his chest.

Important negative findings include:
- There was no evidence of pulmonary hypertension, respiratory failure, or cor-pulmonale.
- No evidence of complications such as consolidation, collapse, fibrosis, or effusion.
- In terms of etiology, there was no evidence of lymphadenopathy, tar staining, SVCO, radiation burn (suggests underlying carcinoma) or yellow nails and lymphedema (suggest yellow nail syndrome)
- And also, no evidence of long-term central venous catheter.

Examiner: You diagnosed this case as bronchiectasis based on some important positive findings, so tell me some other differentials with these findings.

Candidate: Presence of a productive cough, clubbing, and coarse crackles has the following differentials:
- Pulmonary fibrosis, here I would expect bilateral symmetrical fine end-inspiratory crackles that do not alter with coughing. The cough would be usually dry, but in some cases, it may be productive due to concomitant infection.
- Bronchogenic carcinoma, here a nicotine stain together with lymphadenopathy, clubbing, and cachexia may be expected.
- Next, it would be a case of lung abscess, the patient of lung abscess, usually may appear with high fever and toxic. However, this patient had no evidence of infection.

Examiner: How would you investigate someone that you suspect to have bronchiectasis?

Candidate: The first investigation step would be a routine blood test including full blood count (FBC) with ESR, CRP, U/Es, and LFTs.

All patients should have sputum samples sent for Gram staining and C/S, acid-fast bacillus (AFB) staining, fungal and mycobacterial culture.

The next step would be a chest X-ray that may often look normal in early disease.

The HRCT of the chest is the gold standard test which may show signet ring sign (bronchial diameter greater than adjacent vessel diameter), tramlines and honeycomb appearance.

Spirometry (should be performed both for diagnosis as well as disease monitoring) and ABG. Other tests to identify the cause include:
- Immunoglobulin level (look for any evidence of immunodeficiency)
- Human immunodeficiency virus (HIV) serology
- Aspergillus serology for allergic bronchopulmonary aspergillosis (ABPA)
- Autoimmune screen for connective tissue disease
- Sweat test and *CFTR* gene for cystic fibrosis
- Nasal biopsy (if suspected mucociliary dyskinesia- refer to a specialist)

Examiner: What would be the spirometry findings in this patient?

Candidate: Most common abnormality is an obstructive pattern with FEV1: FVC <70%.

In advanced disease, there may be a restrictive pattern with FEV1: FVC >70% secondary to scarring, atelectasis and may also be for underlying pulmonary fibrosis. Therefore, the patient may show mixed obstructive and restrictive patterns.

Examiner: You have a patient with a diagnosis of bronchiectasis. Let us say it is a case of idiopathic bronchiectasis. How would you manage that patient?

Candidate: Management of idiopathic bronchiectasis would be guided by an MDT. This would include:
- *Respiratory physician*: To treat any possible infections or complications by using appropriate antibiotics (according to bacterial sensitivity) and other drugs therapy (such as bronchodilators, inhaled corticosteroids, nebulized hypertonic saline-mucolytics, antifungals), and vaccination (commonly influenza and pneumococcal)
- Smoking cessation and nutritional supplementation and long-term oxygen therapy (LTOT) if required
- Chest physiotherapy for postural chest drainage and devices such as a flutter may aid sputum expectoration and mucus drainage.
- Chest surgeons should also be involved for any surgical resection (in case of localized bronchiectasis, which is poorly controlled with medical therapy), bronchial artery embolization for massive hemoptysis and lung transplantation in advanced bilateral disease.
- Specialist nurse and also with an occupational therapist.

Examiner: Tell me some common causes of bronchiectasis.

Candidate: Bronchiectasis can be idiopathic. Other causes apart from idiopathic bronchiectasis include:
- Mucociliary defects, for example:
  - Cystic fibrosis [young patient, short stature, cachexia, and may have a sign of diabetes mellitus (DM)]
  - Kartagener syndrome (dextrocardia, situs inversus; feel the liver if dextrocardia, especially in a young patient)
  - Immotile cilia syndrome
- Respiratory childhood infections such as tuberculosis, measles, and pertussis.
- *Bronchial obstruction*: That may occur by a foreign body, endobronchial tumor, enlarged lymph nodes can also cause obstruction (due to tuberculosis, sarcoidosis, and malignancy)
- Immunodeficiency that may be due to congenital or acquired hypogammaglobulinemia or acquired immunodeficiency syndrome (AIDS)
- *Autoimmune disease* such as rheumatoid arthritis (rheumatoid lung), Sjogren's syndrome or inflammatory bowel disease [here ulcerative colitis (UC) > Crohn's disease (CD)]
- ABPA
- COPD (30% of the COPD patient may have associated bronchiectasis)

Examiner: Tell me some possible complications of bronchiectasis.

Candidate: Most common complications of bronchiectasis are:
- Pneumonia (the patient may show bronchial breath sounds, increased vocal resonance with fever and chills)
- Empyema (with decreased breath sounds and diminished vocal resonance)

- Lung collapse (the position of the trachea will be shifted to the same side and absent breath sounds if it is central collapse)
- Fibrosis (with bronchial breath sounds and shifted trachea to the same side of the lesion)
- Recurrent pneumothorax (there will be reduced chest expansion, hyper-resonance to percussion and absent breath sounds, in case of tension, pneumothorax trachea will be shifted to the opposite side).
- Cor-pulmonale (raised JVP, right ventricular heave, cyanosis, peripheral edema are the possible findings) and respiratory failure (cyanosis with CO_2 retention flaps)
- Amyloidosis (peripheral edema with bedside urinary proteinuria, peripheral neuropathy or carpal tunnel syndrome)
- Hemoptysis

Examiner: A patient with bronchiectasis can be infected with different types of organisms. Can you please tell me about some common pathogens involved in it?

Candidate: Common organisms are the:
- *Hemophilus influenzae* (most common)
- *Pseudomonas aeruginosa* (characterized by the greenish sputum and green coloration of the colonies due to production of the pigment pyocyanin)
- *Staphylococcus aureus*
- *Streptococcus pneumoniae*
- *Klebsiella pneumoniae*
- *Aspergillus* species (cystic fibrosis is most likely associated with it)
- *Mycobacterium tuberculosis* and other mycobacteria
- *Burkholderia cepacia* and *Mycobacterium abscessus* (both have the worst prognosis and are difficult to eradicate. Chronic infection with either of these organisms renders a patient ineligible for lung transplantation)

Cystic Fibrosis

Mr David, a 25-year-old man, presented with progressive breathlessness and cough. Examine the respiratory system.

(After finishing respiratory system examination within 6 minutes of time)

Candidate: I would like to complete my examination by checking the patient's observation chart, examining sputum pots (if any), doing bedside spirometry, pulse oximetry, and examining lymph nodes (if you do not examine the lymph nodes during your examination).

Examiner: Would you like to present your case, please?

Candidate:

I performed a respiratory system examination on Mr David. Based on my clinical findings, I believe this patient has a diagnosis of bronchiectasis secondary to cystic fibrosis.

On inspection, Mr David was cachexic, short stature, and breathless at rest requiring supplemental oxygen therapy by a nasal mask.

He had a productive cough, and I noticed a bedside sputum pot containing copious quantities of purulent sputum. He also had evidence of a port-a-cath in the left axilla and a gastrostomy tube in situ.

On general physical examination, he was tachypneic, tachycardic, clubbed, edematous with raised JVP.

On chest examination, he had vesicular breath sounds with prolonged expiration and coarse inspiratory crackles throughout the lung field. Bilaterally, reduced chest expansion with resonant percussion.

There were no obvious scars, trachea, and apex beat were normally placed. Also, there was no evidence of cyanosis or CO_2 retention flap.

Examiner: You mentioned, this patient has evidence of a port-a-cath in his left axilla. Could you please tell me what do you know about this?

Candidate: Port-a-cath is an implanted device for long-term venous access usually placed at the right side of the chest; this consists of a circular port for needle access that is surgically inserted beneath the skin and is attached to a venous catheter, the tip of which usually lies in the superior vena cava, jugular vein, or subclavian vein.

Given that patients usually require repeated courses of intravenous (IV) antibiotics, they may have evidence of long-term venous access such as a port-a-cath, like this patient. A port-a-cath is used to give IV fluids, chemotherapy, other drugs, blood transfusions, and used to take blood samples as well.

Examiner: You also mention a gastrostomy tube. Please tell me why this patient has a gastrostomy tube?

Candidate: This patient may have pancreatic insufficiency as a complication of cystic fibrosis, which, in combination with a catabolic state due to chronic or recurrent infection, leads to high-calorie requirements and thus, the patient may need supplemental feeding with a gastrostomy tube.

Examiner: How would you confirm the diagnosis of cystic fibrosis?

Candidate: The diagnosis of cystic fibrosis can be made by screening for the most common CFTR mutations on a blood sample and also by performing a sweat test (in cystic fibrosis—the abnormally high chloride content of >60 mmol/L will be found).

All infants in the UK are now screened for cystic fibrosis as part of the Guthrie test at just a few days old. This involves the measurement of immunoreactive trypsin levels via a heel prick blood sample, and a significantly raised level is suspected for cystic fibrosis.

Examiner: Please tell me how you would manage someone with cystic fibrosis?

Candidate: Individuals with cystic fibrosis should have ongoing access to an MDT. This includes respiratory physicians, surgeons, physiotherapists, dieticians, psychologists, occupational therapists, specialist nurses, and social workers.

Treatment of cystic fibrosis with bronchiectasis is:
- Daily chest physiotherapy incorporating postural drainage
- Active cycle of breathing techniques and exercise

Patients are also treated with a combination of nebulized therapies, including mucolytic agents such as recombinant deoxyribonuclease (DNase) and hypertonic saline, as well as oral azithromycin. Patients will usually need regular 2-week courses of IV antibiotics.

In case of pancreatic insufficiency, pancreatic enzymes are taken to aid digestion at every meal. Fat-soluble vitamin supplementations or supplemental feeding either nasogastrically or via a gastrostomy may be needed. Patients who develop cystic fibrosis-related diabetes will usually require insulin therapy.

The *CFTR* modulating therapies such as ivacaftor and Orkambi have marked improvement in lung function and exacerbation frequency in eligible patients who carry specific mutations that respond to these medications.

Examiner: You diagnosed the case as cystic fibrosis. Would you please tell me what the pathogenesis of cystic fibrosis is?

Candidate: It is an autosomal recessive disorder due to a defect in the CFTR gene located on chromosome 7. Delta F508 is the most common one with over 1,250 mutations.

All exocrine tissues contain CFTR protein, and a defective CFTR protein prevents chloride moving out of cells, then Na^+ hyper reabsorption occurring to keep intracellular electrochemical balance, the osmotic pull of water into the cells, dehydration of extracellular surfaces, that produce thick viscous secretions easily amenable to colonization and infection.

Examiner: You mentioned cystic fibrosis is an autosomal recessive disorder. Can you tell me the prevalence of cystic fibrosis in the community?

Candidate: Cystic fibrosis occurs in 1 in 2,500 live births, and the carriers of cystic fibrosis are 1 in 25.

As this is an autosomal recessive disorder, if both parents are carriers of the cystic fibrosis gene:
- The chance of another child being affected (homozygote) is 1 in 4 (25%)
- The chance of their child being free from the cystic fibrosis is also 1 in 4 (25%)
- And the chance of a child being a carrier (heterozygote) is 1 in 2 (50%)

Examiner: Tell me what other systems are affected by cystic fibrosis patients?

Candidate: Cystic fibrosis is a multisystem disease, among them lung disease being the major cause of morbidity and mortality.
- It affects the digestive system:
  - By causing pancreatic insufficiency and malabsorption of fat and protein.
  - Cystic fibrosis-related diabetes (CFRD).
  - In newborns, it can cause meconium ileus and distal intestinal obstruction syndrome.
  - It can also affect the liver and cause focal biliary cirrhosis leading to or with portal hypertension.
  - Cholelithiasis.
- In reproductive system:
  - Male subfertility (>90%, failure of the development of vas deferens) and defective sperm transport, whereas spermatogenesis is normal.
  - Female subfertility is secondary to viscid cervical secretions. However, only 20% will be infertile.
- *On kidneys*: It can cause nephrolithiasis.
- *On the musculoskeletal system*: May cause osteoporosis.
- *On ear, nose, throat (ENT)*: It may cause sinus disease and nasal polyposis. The nasal polyp in children should always raise the suspicion for cystic fibrosis.

Pneumonia

Mr Michel, a 50-year-old man, presented with fever and productive cough for 5 days. Examine the respiratory system.

(After finishing respiratory system examination within 6 minutes of time)

Candidate: I would like to complete my examination by checking the patient's observation chart, examining sputum pots (if any), doing bedside spirometry and pulse oximetry, and examining lymph nodes (if you do not examine the lymph nodes during your examination).

Examiner: Would you like to present your case, please?

Candidate:

I performed a respiratory system examination on Mr Michel. Based on my clinical findings, I believe this patient has a diagnosis of consolidation at the left base, possibly due to S. pneumoniae.

This gentleman was febrile, tachycardic, and dyspneic at rest requiring ambulatory oxygen therapy, and he had a herpetic lesion on the lips that suggested underlying streptococcal pneumoniae.

On chest examination—there were no obvious scars or engorged veins—restricted chest movement with reduced chest expansibility on the left side. There was also dullness to percussion at the left base.

On auscultation, there were bronchial breath sounds and increased vocal resonance with coarse crepitations at the left base.

There was no evidence of clubbing, lymphadenopathy, cachexia, or tar-stain on fingers.

No evidence of pulmonary hypertension, cor-pulmonale, respiratory failure, or venous thrombosis.

Examiner: Tell me some important differential diagnoses with these clinical findings?

Candidate: I have some differentials such as:
- Tubercular consolidation, here I would expect a long history of fever, weight loss and anorexia with commonly an upper lobe consolidation.
- Bronchogenic carcinoma, here cachexia, clubbing, lymphadenopathy, tar staining would be expected.
- Pulmonary embolism, here I expect features of raised venous pressure and venous thrombosis.

Examiner: How would you investigate a patient with consolidation?

Candidate: At first, I would like to take a full history from the patient, such as fever, chest pain, cough, and breathlessness.

My initial investigations would include pulse oximetry and baseline blood test, including FBC, inflammatory markers—ESR, CRP, U/Es, serum creatinine, and LFTs.

Next, most importantly, a chest X-ray; here, I expect dense homogenous opacity with air-bronchogram or its complications such as parapneumonic effusion or abscess or cavitation.

Sputum for Gram staining, AFB staining, culture sensitivity, and cytology (for malignant cells)

Other blood tests, including:
- Blood culture
- Serological testing for *Mycoplasma* and *Legionella*
- Arterial blood gas sampling

Urine analysis for:
- Proteinuria and hematuria
- *Legionella* antigen
- Pneumococcal antigen

To exclude other differentials, I would like to do an ECG, D-dimer, CTPA or V-Q scan if suspecting PE. Finally, a CT scan of the chest to exclude underlying malignancy.

Examiner: So, you have a diagnosis of pyogenic pneumonia. Can you tell me what are the common organisms causing pneumonia in the community?

Candidate: Pneumonia occurs secondary to airborne infection, which includes bacteria, viruses, fungi, parasites, among others. The typical bacterias which cause pneumonia are:
- *S. pneumoniae* (most common, accounting for 60–70% of cases)
- *S. aureus* (following influenza viral illness or in IV drug users)
- *Klebsiella pneumoniae* (debilitated patients, elderly, alcoholics)
- *H. influenzae*

Atypical organisms are *Mycoplasma pneumoniae* (second most common cause, accounting for 15–20% cases), *Legionella* spp, *Chlamydia* spp, *Coxiella* spp.

Viral causes include influenza, *Cytomegalovirus* (CMV), Varicella-Zoster virus, and other respiratory viruses (*Coronavirus*).

Examiner: What do you know about the CURB-65 criteria for managing community-acquired pneumonia?

Candidate: CURB-65 means (one point is given for any of the following):
- Confusion
- Urea >7 mmol/L
- Respiratory rate of ≥30/minutes
- Blood pressure (systolic) <90 mm Hg
- Age ≥65 years

Patients with 1 or less score of the above criteria are regarded as having less severe pneumonia. Score 2 is for moderate severity, and score 3 or more is regarded as having severe pneumonia.

Examiner: How would you manage a patient having pneumonia?

Candidate: The CURB-65 score can be used to decide upon prognosis and management. If patients have a CURB-65 score 1 or less, they can be treated as an outpatient with oral antibiotics such as, oral amoxicillin or flucloxacillin (in case of *S. aureus*)

In case of severe pneumonia where CURB-65 score 3 or more, the patient should be treated with IV antibiotics and require hospitalization. Antibiotics include:
- Co-amoxiclav + clarithromycin or,
- Cefuroxime + clarithromycin or,
- Cefotaxime + clarithromycin

As well as oxygen therapy to maintain an oxygen saturation of 94–98% in the absence of COPD, IV fluids for hypovolemia, low molecular weight heparin for thromboembolic prophylaxis, and adequate nutritional supplementation.

Examiner: Tell me some acute and chronic complications of pneumonia.

Candidate: Acute complications include empyema, fistula, and organizing pneumonia. Patients may develop bronchiectasis as a chronic complication.

Examiner: Are there any preventive measures for pneumonia?

Candidate: All patients aged 65 years or at risk of the invasive pneumococcal disease admitted with CAP and who have not previously received the pneumococcal vaccine should receive the 23-polyvalent pneumococcal vaccine (23-PPV).

Chronic Obstructive Pulmonary Disease

Mr George, a 66-year-old man, presented with progressive breathlessness. Examine the respiratory system.

(After finishing respiratory system examination within 6 minutes of time)

Candidate: I would like to complete my examination by checking the patient's observation chart, examining sputum pots (if any), doing bedside spirometry, pulse oximetry, and examining lymph nodes (if you do not examine the lymph nodes during your examination).

Examiner: Would you like to present your case, please?

Candidate:

I performed a respiratory system examination on Mr George. Based on my clinical findings, I believe this patient has a diagnosis of COPD.

On inspection, this gentleman was breathless at rest, requiring oxygen therapy by nasal mask and had a productive cough.

There was some steroid purpura on his skin and tar staining on his fingers. I also noticed that a blue salbutamol inhaler device was on the table.

On chest examination, he had a tracheal tug and reduced cricoid-sternal distance and the visible indrawing of the lower intercostal muscles. Chest expansion reduced slightly with resonant percussion.

On auscultation, he had vesicular breath sounds with prolonged expiration. There were some scattered crepitations and occasional wheezes.

No evidence of PHTN (raised JVP, left parasternal heave, loud palpable P2) or respiratory failure (a sign of CO_2 retention, collapsing pulse, warm periphery, flapping tremor, palmer erythema, or cyanosis due to hypoxia) or Cor-pulmonale (evidence of PHTN plus peripheral edema). Moreover, he had no evidence of lymphadenopathy or clubbing.

I would like to take a full history from the patient, mainly focusing on dyspnea, cough, wheeze, weight loss, and smoking history for better assessment of the patient.

Examiner: What are the other differential diagnoses with these clinical findings? And how would you differentiate them?

Candidate: My first differential diagnosis would be bronchial asthma; however, the age of onset for BA is quite earlier than COPD, and the cough would be usually dry.

One important differential would be bronchiectasis. Here, I expect finger clubbing along with coarse inspiratory crepitations, which alter with coughing. However, I could not find any of this.

It can be a case of congestive cardiac failure that may be presented with fine crackles on lung bases with peripheral edema and raised JVP with other features of heart disease.

Examiner: You mentioned some important negative findings. Please tell me what you would think if these findings were present in your case?

Candidate: If there were any features of PHTN with evidence of right heart failure, I would think about cor-pulmonale, which may be the long-term complication of COPD.

If there were CO_2 retention flaps with bounding pulse, then I would think about the acute exacerbation of COPD with type-2 respiratory failure.

In case of lymphadenopathy in a COPD patient, I would think about associated bronchogenic carcinoma or infection such as TB.

If clubbing is present in a case of COPD, then I have to exclude underlying lung cancer, lung abscess or bronchiectasis (30% of COPD patients may have associated bronchiectasis, which is usually detected in HRCT).

Examiner: How would you investigate this patient?

Candidate: My initial investigations would include bedside observations specifically with a pulse oximetry and ABG to confirm any respiratory failure (hypoxia with hypercapnia suggests type-2 respiratory failure).

Then, I would like to do a baseline blood test that includes a FBC and inflammatory markers (looking particularly for polycythemia and signs of infection), U/Es, and LFTs.

Moreover, a baseline chest X-ray [that may show enlarged lung, air pockets (bullae) or a low flat diaphragm in advanced COPD].

The most important investigation for this patient is spirometry with a reversibility test to demonstrate airflow obstruction. On this test, I would expect:
- Markedly reduced FEV1
- Normal or reduced FVC, so the FEV1/FVC ratio will also be reduced (<70%), suggests airflow obstruction.
- And also, there will be increased total lung capacity (TLC), functional reserve capacity (FRC), and residual volume (RV)
- Reduced vital capacity (VC) and transfer factor of the lung for carbon monoxide (TLCO).
- The reversibility test will show no significant reversibility.

An HRCT of the chest would be the most sensitive test to rule out alternative diagnoses and presurgical assessment before lung volume reduction surgeries or bullectomy.

Finally, an ECG and echocardiogram to see any evidence of PHTN or associated heart disease.

Examiner: How would you classify the severity of COPD via spirometry?

Candidate: According to NICE guideline, the severity of COPD is categorized using the FEV1. After confirming the postbronchodilator obstructive pattern on spirometry (FEV1/FVC <70%), then I would focus on the patient's FEV1 compared to their predicted value.
- If the FEV1 >80% predicted but an obstructive pattern—mild COPD
- FEV1 50-80% with an obstructive pattern—moderate COPD
- FEV1 30-50% with an obstructive pattern—severe COPD
- And FEV1 <30%—very severe COPD

Examiner: You mentioned some steroid-induced purpura on the patient's skin. Tell me some other steroid-induced complications for this patient.

Candidate: Other complications include Cushingoid appearance, proximal myopathy, diabetes mellitus, hypertension (HTN). Furthermore, the most common complication of steroid inhalers would be oropharyngeal or esophageal candidiasis (that can be prevented by advising him to rinse his mouth after each time he uses it and by using a spacer device).

Examiner: As your patient is a case of stable and advanced COPD and using long-term oxygen therapy, how would you manage him at this stage?

Candidate: At first, I would like to take some general measures that include vaccination for the common respiratory organisms, pulmonary rehabilitation involving chest physiotherapy, and, most importantly, smoking cessation.

At this point, as my patient is breathless and on oxygen therapy and also using a salbutamol inhaler; therefore, I would like to give him triple-drug therapy according to NICE guideline. That is the combination of:
- Long-acting β2 agonists (LABA) (salmeterol, formoterol)
- Inhaled corticosteroid (ICS) (fluticasone, beclomethasone)
- Long-acting muscarinic antagonist (LAMA) (tiotropium, glycopyrronium)

Noninvasive ventilation (NIV) may be appropriate if hypercapnia is on LTOT. Other measures include oral doxofylline, theophylline, mucolytics, and roflumilast.

Surgery may be appropriate in selected patients, such as:
- Lung volume reduction surgery, bullectomy to increase lung compliance.
- Moreover, patients with no absolute contraindications should be referred for consideration of unilateral lung transplantation.

Examiner: What do you know about long-term oxygen therapy? What are the indications for using LTOT?

Candidate: LTOT is supplementary oxygen therapy given for at least 16 hours a day to try and treat a stable COPD patient who is classically hypoxic and to reduce the risk of cor-pulmonale.

Indications include (patient must be a nonsmoker and in a stable condition) Persistently, hypoxic patient with two measurements of PO_2 <7.3 kPa or those with a PO_2 of 7.3–8 kPa and one of the following:
- Nocturnal hypoxemia
- Peripheral edema
- PHTN
- Secondary polycythemia

Cor-pulmonale

Mr Benham, a 65-year-old, presented with progressive breathlessness. Examine the respiratory system.

(After finishing respiratory system examination within 6 minutes of time)

Candidate: I would like to complete my examination by checking the patient's observation chart, examining sputum pots (If any), doing bedside spirometry, pulse oximetry, and examining lymph nodes (If you do not examine the lymph nodes during your examination).

Examiner: Would you like to present your case, please?

Candidate:

I performed a respiratory system examination on Mr Benham. Based on my clinical findings, I believe this patient has cor-pulmonale secondary to COPD.

This gentleman was cyanosed and breathless at rest, requiring oxygen therapy and had an engorged neck vein.

The patient was tachypneic, tachycardic with bounding pulse, edematous and also had evidence of raised JVP with CO_2 retention flap.

On chest examination, he had a tracheal tug with the intercostal recession. He had also reduced chest expansion, resonant percussion, palpable P2 and left parasternal heave.

On auscultation of the chest: There were vesicular breath sounds with prolonged expiration and some scattered crepitations on both lung bases.

A systolic murmur is also audible in the lower left parasternal area, probably due to associated TR.

Examiner: Well, you diagnosed this case as a cor-pulmonale secondary to COPD. Now, this patient is breathless, cyanosed and has a CO_2 retention flap. What does it mean for a COPD patient? How would you manage him now?

Candidate: With these findings, I would think about the acute exacerbation of COPD with respiratory failure and also may have PHTN. Now regarding treatment:

- I would like to treat this patient in an emergency setting and start with nebulized bronchodilators, either salbutamol or ipratropium bromide. In the meantime, I would like to do a bedside ABG and chest X-ray. If SaO_2 <88% or PaO_2 <7.3 kPa, I would manage this with controlled oxygen therapy, start at 24–28%, and my aim would be 88–92% saturation, this will adjust according to ABG.
- The next step would be steroid either IV hydrocortisone 200 mg or oral prednisolone 30 mg once daily for the next 7–14 days.
- If there is any evidence of infection, I would treat this with the appropriate antibiotic, e.g., amoxicillin/clarithromycin/doxycycline.
- Physiotherapy to aid sputum expectoration.
- If no response to nebulizer or steroid, then I will go for NIV or respiratory stimulant drug doxapram (if NIV is contraindicated or not available)
- Moreover, finally, intubation and ventilation if the patient remains unresponsive with pH <7.20 or unconscious or any contraindications of NIV.

Examiner: Tell me some common causes of cor-pulmonale?

Candidate: Around 10–40% of patients with COPD develop cor-pulmonale. Other than COPD, the causes include:
- Interstitial lung disease
- Obstructive sleep apnea

- Hypoventilation disorder, including obesity-related hypoventilation
- Neuromuscular disorders
- Kyphoscoliosis
- Bilateral bronchiectasis

Examiner: You were asked about the management of this patient; you mentioned the NIV. Please tell me when you will give NIV to the patient and tell me some contraindications to using it.

Candidate: I would like to give NIV if there is respiratory acidosis despite immediate maximum standard medical treatment on controlled oxygen for no more than one hour to achieve a pH in the range of 7.25–7.35. If the pH is <7.20, then I will proceed to invasive ventilation.

Contraindications to NIV include:
- Hemodynamically unstable patient
- Confused/agitated patient
- Life-threatening hypoxemia
- Fixed upper airway obstruction
- Vomiting
- Facial burns or trauma/recent facial or upper airway surgery
- Copious respiratory secretion
- Upper gastrointestinal surgery or bowel obstruction
- Undrained pneumothorax
- Patient declines treatment

Examiner: Tell me about the surgical management of a COPD patient.

Candidate: The most common surgical option for a COPD patient is lung volume reduction surgery (this is used to treat people with upper lobe emphysema with CO_2 retention and low exercise capacity). Other options include bullectomy, endobronchial valves and also lung transplantation (specifically for a very advanced stage of COPD like cor-pulmonale).

Examiner: Do you know any measures for symptomatic relief of breathlessness in end-stage COPD?

Candidate: If the patient has end-stage-COPD and if control of symptoms is his priority, in that case, the use of opioid or benzodiazepine medications (lower dose of opioid use, <30 mg daily oral morphine equivalent) for symptomatic relief of breathlessness is appropriate.

Examiner: What are the causes of acute exacerbation of COPD?

Candidate: Respiratory infection is responsible for approximately half of COPD exacerbations. Common bacterial pathogens of acute exacerbations include *H. influenzae*, *S. pneumoniae*, and *Moraxella catarrhalis*. Less commonly involve methicillin-resistant *Staphylococcus aureus* (MRSA) and *Chlamydia pneumoniae*.

Others include some allergens such as pollens, wood or cigarette smoke, toxins, including a variety of different chemicals, air pollutions, pneumothorax, failing to follow a drug therapy program, e.g., improper use of an inhaler.

In one-third of all COPD exacerbation cases, the exact cause cannot be identified.

Bronchial Asthma

Mrs Julia, a 24-year-old lady, presented with dyspnea. Examine the respiratory system.

(After finishing respiratory system examination within 6 minutes of time)

Candidate: I would like to complete my examination by checking the patient's observation chart, examining sputum pots (if any), doing bedside spirometry and pulse oximetry, and examining lymph nodes (if you do not examine the lymph nodes during your examination).

Examiner: Would you like to present your case, please?

Candidate:

I performed a respiratory system examination on Mrs Julia. Based on my clinical findings, I believe this patient has bronchial asthma.

On inspection, this young lady was dyspneic at rest and had a dry cough with an audible wheeze from the end of the bed.

She had a normal chest on inspection without any scar marks or engorged veins.

Trachea and apex beat were normally placed with normal chest expansion and resonant percussion.

On chest auscultation, she had vesicular breath sounds with prolonged expiration and a widespread, polyphonic wheeze.

There were no peripheral stigmata of chronic lung disease (specifically tar staining on fingers, edema, cyanosis, clubbing or CO_2 retention flap).

No evidence of PHTN, respiratory failure, or cor-pulmonale.

Examiner: Tell me some other possible differential diagnoses of these findings, and how would you differentiate them?

Candidate: My first differential would be COPD. In case of COPD, I would expect a relatively older patient with tar staining on fingers and productive cough.

Next, I would think about bronchiectasis; here, I would expect finger clubbing, productive cough with evidence of a bedside sputum pot and some coarse crepitations on chest auscultation.

Other possibilities may include:
- Pulmonary edema
- Large airway obstructions (foreign body/tumor)
- SVCO
- And rarely obliterative bronchiolitis (specifically in the elderly patient)

However, clinical findings are not suggesting any of these findings.

Examiner: How would you investigate a bronchial asthma patient?

Candidate: Initially, I would like to start with:
- A baseline observation particularly looking at pulse oximetry levels and ABG in an acute setting (mainly if the patient is hypoxic).
- Next, a baseline blood test including a full blood count, inflammatory markers, and UEs.
- A baseline chest X-ray (here I would expect normal findings but may show hyperinflation).
- Peak expiratory flow (PEF) monitoring (here, a diurnal variation of >20% over 2 weeks is considered significant).
- Spirometry with reversibility test (this may show an obstructive defect with markedly reduced FEV1, normal or reduced FVC so that FEV1/FVC will also be reduced. Reversibility usually >15% improvement on FEV1 following beta-2 agonist).

- ECG and echocardiogram to exclude any CVS disease.
- Finally, an HRCT to exclude other possible differentials.

Examiner: What do you expect specifically in the full blood count of this patient?

Candidate: I would expect the white cell count may be raised due to infection or if the patient has been on a recent course of steroids. The eosinophil count may also be raised due to asthma.

Examiner: You have a differential of COPD, so tell me, how would you differentiate COPD and BA with spirometry features?

Candidate: Both would show an obstructive picture on spirometry. However, asthma is a reversible obstruction; I would expect there to be an improvement following the use of a bronchodilator—usually 200 mL on a peak flow or an improvement by 15%.

Examiner: How would you treat an asthma patient?

Candidate: I would like to follow NICE guidelines for treating such patients. In the case of newly diagnosed asthma,
- I would start with short-acting beta agonists (SABA).
- The next step would be SABA + low dose ICS.

If symptoms are not controlled on previous steps, future steps would be:
- SABA + low dose ICS + LABA [with or without leukotriene receptor antagonists (LTRA)]

Then we can switch to:
- Maintenance and reliever therapy (MART) with low dose ICS next to medium-dose ICS, or
- We can consider changing back to a fixed dose of moderate to high dose ICS and a separate LABA.

If all measures fail, then we may need to use oral steroids or refer to the respiratory specialist at that point.

Examiner: Think this patient is admitted in emergency department with a respiratory rate >25, PEF 33-50% of predicted and unable to complete a sentence in one breath. What would be your next steps in her management?

Candidate: At first, I would like to assess the severity of this attack with the above features; I think this is a case of an acute severe asthma attack.
- Supplemental oxygen to maintain saturations 94-98% would be my first step of immediate management.
- Nebulized salbutamol 5 mg or terbutaline 10 mg along with ipratropium bromide 0.5 mg/6 hourly will be the next step.
- Hydrocortisone 100 mg IV or prednisolone 40-50 mg PO should also start with a continuous reassessment every 15 minutes along with pulse oximetry, ABG, ECG, and checking vitals.
- If the above measures failed, then a single dose of $MgSO_4$ 1.2-2 g IV over 20 minutes would be my next step.
- At this point, if the patient's condition does not improve, I would refer the patient to ICU for consideration of ventilatory support and intensification of medical therapy.
- If the patient is improving, then nebulized therapy should continue for 4-6 hours and prednisolone 40-50 mg PO for 5-7 days.

Lung Cancer

Mr Bennett, a 62-year-old man, presented with dyspnea and cough. Examine the respiratory system.

(After finishing respiratory system examination within 6 minutes of time)

Candidate: I would like to complete my examination by checking the patient's observation chart, examining sputum pots (if any), doing bedside spirometry, and pulse oximetry.

Examiner: Please present your case findings and tell me your diagnosis.

Candidate:

I performed a respiratory system examination on Mr Bennett; I believe he has a Pancoast syndrome due to left apical lung carcinoma with associated collapse-consolidation.

Positive findings include:

The patient was cachexic with reduced triceps fat fold thickness, breathless at rest and had a productive cough, clubbing, and tar staining of the fingers.

There were some palpable lymph nodes in the left axilla and supraclavicular fossa.

There was wasting of small muscles of the left hand with reduced sensation in the C8-T1 dermatomes due to left brachial plexus involvement. Also, I noticed left partial ptosis, miosis, and enophthalmos, suggesting left Horner's syndrome.

On chest examination, the position of the trachea shifted to the left with normal cricoid-notch distance. There was reduced chest expansion of the left upper chest with a dull percussion note and increased vocal fremitus.

On auscultation, there was bronchial breathing over the left upper chest.

I would like to ask about the history of progressive weight loss, chronic cough, hemoptysis, pain and weakness of the hand, hemifacial anhidrosis, as well as risk factors of lung malignancy, particularly smoking history.

Examiner: As you are suspecting, the patient has lung cancer, so how would you proceed with investigations?

Candidate: Initial investigations would include routine blood tests:
- FBC, ESR, CRP looking for signs of anemia and infection.
- LFTs [maybe deranged with hepatic metastases; raised alkaline phosphatase (ALP) with bony metastasis].
- Kidney function may help guide future treatment.
- U/Es looking for hyponatremia [syndrome of inappropriate antidiuretic hormone secretion (SIADH)] and hypokalemia [ectopic adrenocorticotropic hormone (ACTH); Cushing] associated with small cell lung cancer.
- Clotting profile for disseminated intravascular coagulation (DIC).
- Serum calcium [hypercalcemia may present due to bony metastasis or parathyroid hormone-related protein (PTHrP) production]

Chest radiograph (may identify the location and size of the tumor as well as collapse, consolidation, and pleural effusion).

Spirometry to guide fitness for surgery as well as overall lung function.

Sputum analysis for malignant cells and to exclude associated infections.

If the patient has evidence of pleural effusion, then I would like to proceed with pleural fluid aspiration and study. Here, I would usually expect hemorrhagic, exudative effusion (LDH >2/3 of normal; >0.6 of serum; pleural fluid protein >0.5 of serum) with low pH <7.3, low glucose and raised amylase.

If the patient's history were suspicious enough, I would go onto a staging CT. Positron emission tomography (PET) scan to look for evidence of malignancy and metastasis.

Finally, the most important step would be trying to identify a tissue diagnosis. This can be done by bronchoscopy [transbronchial lung biopsy, sometimes ultrasonography (USG) guided] or percutaneously CT scan guided with the help of a radiologist.

Examiner: Okay, let us go back to the examination; you carefully noted the case as a Pancoast syndrome with associated collapse and consolidation. Now please tell me some other features that might present someone with lung cancer?

Candidate: Other features include:
- *Pleural effusion*: Here, I would expect reduced chest expansion with dull percussion notes and diminished breath sounds over the affected area.
- *SVCO*: I would expect here some signs such as facial swelling, arm swelling, as well as a distended vein in the neck and chest.
- *Recurrent laryngeal nerve palsy*: This may cause hoarseness of voice.
- *Metastatic features*: Lung cancer often metastasis to other parts of the body, such as the brain, bones, adrenal gland, and liver. Cancer those spreads can cause pain, headaches, nausea, or other signs and symptoms depending on what organ is affected.
- It can be present with also paraneoplastic features.

Examiner: That is great. Would you like to tell me some paraneoplastic features of lung cancer?

Candidate:
- In case of squamous cell cancer, may present with hypercalcemia due to release of PTHrP, or clubbing or hypertrophic pulmonary osteoarthropathy (HPOA).
- In case of adenocarcinoma—there may be gynecomastia.
- Small cell carcinoma may present with hyponatremia due to SIADH, ectopic Cushing due to ACTH, Lambert-Eaton myasthenic syndrome.
- Other paraneoplastic features include peripheral neuropathy, inflammatory myopathy, cerebellar syndrome.

Examiner: Let us say your patient has lung cancer confirmed by histological diagnosis. Can you tell me about the different types of lung cancer you may see?

Candidate: Lung cancer can be divided into:
Small cell carcinoma (oat cell carcinoma), usually central, arise from Kulchitsky cells and secretes many polypeptides. Typically presents with a short history, and 60–70% of patients have disseminated disease at presentation.

Nonsmall cell carcinoma, they are predominately:
- Adenocarcinoma [a most common type in nonsmokers, commonly causing peripheral lesion, and accounting for 50% of non-small cell lung cancer (NSCLC)]
- Squamous cell carcinoma (accounting 30% of NSCLC, typically causing central and cavitating lesions)
- Bronchoalveolar carcinoma (A subtype of adenocarcinoma that develops at multiple sites and spread along the pre-existing alveolar walls)
- Large cell carcinoma (this is the least common type, also known as undifferentiated carcinoma)

Examiner: Well said. How would you manage a patient with lung carcinoma?

Candidate: Treatment of lung cancer will depend on lung cancer stage and histology in conjunction with a patient's wishes, comorbidities, and performance status; and will be decided by a specialist MDT.

Nonsmall cell lung cancers are often treated with surgery and radical radiotherapy, depending on the location and stage. In advanced non-small cell lung cancer, patients are generally treated palliatively, and this may include chemotherapy.

The presence of specific molecular abnormalities such as epidermal growth factor receptor (EGFR), anaplastic large-cell lymphoma kinase (ALK) or PDL1 means that specific targeted therapies such as tyrosine kinase inhibitors, ALK inhibitors, or immunotherapy can be used to improve prognosis.

Small cell lung cancers often are not amenable to surgery; here, chemotherapy is the mainstay of treatment, and if the disease is limited, it is combined with radiotherapy.

Examiner: You told me about different treatment options for lung carcinoma. Tell me the functional criteria for pneumonectomy and some contraindications of it?

Candidate: Functional criteria for pneumonectomy include:
- FEV1 of >1.5 liters
- FEV1 >50% of the observed FVC, and
- Normal $PaCO_2$ with the patient at rest

Contraindications to surgery where palliative treatment is given:
- Patient refusal
- FEV1 <1.5 liters for lobectomy; <2 liters for pneumonectomy
- SVCO where stenting and radiotherapy are suitable options
- Malignant pleural effusion (chest tube drain with pleurodesis for recurrent effusion)
- Pancoast tumor
- Vocal cord paralysis

Lobectomy

Mr Ashok, a 63-year-old man, presented with dyspnea. Examine the respiratory system.

(After finishing respiratory system examination within 6 minutes of time)

Candidate: I would like to complete my examination by checking the patient's observation chart, examining sputum pots (if any), doing bedside spirometry, pulse oximetry, and examining lymph nodes (if you do not examine the lymph nodes during your examination).

Examiner: Would you like to present your case, please?

Candidate:

Mr Ashok has had a right-sided upper lobectomy.

The positive findings include:

He was comfortable at rest and had nicotine staining on his fingers, and I noticed a salbutamol inhaler on the table.

On inspection of the chest, there was a well-healed scar of right lateral thoracotomy with underlying chest wall deformity (the right upper ribs are pulled in—depressed chest wall)

The trachea and apex beat deviated to the right side of the chest.

Chest expansion was reduced on the right upper zone with dull percussion in that area anteriorly but resonant posteriorly.

On chest auscultation, there was bronchial breathing in the right upper zone over the deviated trachea; breath sounds, and vocal resonance were also reduced anteriorly but were normal posteriorly.

There was no evidence of clubbing, lymphadenopathy, or peripheral edema and JVP was not raised.

I would like to ask the patient about the underlying respiratory disease that leads to lobectomy, any complications following the surgery and any current symptoms, particularly the shortness of breath and exercise tolerance.

This gentleman is a smoker, and as he is using an inhaler which suggests COPD and I suspect his lobectomy was done due to previous primary lung cancer, most probably non-small cell carcinoma (squamous cell carcinoma strongly associated with smoking). However, other possibilities include:
- Solitary pulmonary nodule of unknown cause
- Pulmonary adenoma causing hemoptysis
- Localized bronchiectasis or pulmonary tuberculosis resistant to medical management.

Examiner: How would you differentiate pneumonectomy and lobectomy clinically?

Candidate: In a lobectomy:
- The trachea may be deviated (toward the side of the lobectomy).
- Breath sounds may be normal or may be reduced.
- The percussion note is likely to be normal.

In a pneumonectomy:
- The trachea definitely will be deviated to the opposite side.
- Breath sounds will be absent throughout the lung field, apart from the apex where there is bronchial breathing (this correspond with airflow through the deviated trachea).
- The percussion notes would be dull throughout the lung field, although not stony dull.

Examiner: How would you investigate the case?

Candidate: As the patient is symptomatic, I would like to start with some baseline blood tests, including CBC, ESR, CRP, U/Es, serum creatinine, and urine R/E.

Then, I would like to do a chest X-ray where I would expect an absence of resected lobe with volume loss, altered rib anatomy, and trachea shifts toward the resection side.

In terms of breathlessness, a further test would be spirometry with reversibility test, ECG and echocardiography to exclude CVS disease, as a cause of breathlessness.

Examiner: What are the possible indications for a lobectomy?

Candidate: Indications for a lobectomy would be lung cancer, aspergilloma, TB, lung abscess, and COPD.

Examiner: Well said. Would you like to comment on operative mortality of lobectomy and pneumonectomy? Is there any difference between the right and left-sided procedures?

Candidate: Operative mortality for lobectomy is approximately 2–4%, and for pneumonectomy, this rises to 6%.

There is a marked difference in mortality risks between the right and left side following a pneumonectomy; right-sided pneumonectomy is associated with higher overall mortality (10–12%) as compared to left-sided (1–1.3%).

Although reasons are uncertain for this difference, however, the most likely cause may be due to life-threatening complications that are encountered at higher frequency following right-sided procedures such as postpneumonectomy space empyema, pulmonary edema, and bronchopleural fistula.

Pneumonectomy

Mrs Gupta, a 65-year-old lady, is undergoing follow-up from the respiratory physicians. Examine her respiratory system and present your findings to the examiner.

(After finishing respiratory system examination within 6 minutes of time)

Candidate: I would like to complete my examination by checking the patient's observation chart, examining sputum pots (if any), doing bedside spirometry and pulse oximetry, and examining lymph nodes (if you do not examine the lymph nodes during your examination).

Examiner: Would you like to present your case, please?

Candidate:

Mrs Gupta has had a left pneumonectomy.

The positive findings include she was comfortable at rest, had finger clubbing, and nicotine stains on general inspection.

On inspection of the chest, there was a posterolateral thoracotomy scar on the left with flattening of the left chest wall.

The trachea and apex beat deviated to the left side of the chest. Chest expansion was reduced on the left side with dull percussion throughout the whole left lung field.

On chest auscultation, there was bronchial breathing in the left upper zone over the grossly deviated trachea, and breath sounds were absent in rest of the left lung field. There was no evidence of lymphadenopathy, peripheral edema, or raised JVP.

I would like to ask the patient about the initial symptoms and diagnosis that led to the initial surgery, any complications following surgery, and any current symptoms, particularly about the shortness of breath or exercise tolerance.

However, as she had finger clubbing along with tar staining, therefore, I suspect this pneumonectomy may be due to NSCLC.

Examiner: Well, you have carefully noticed the patient's thoracotomy scar and other significant findings, and you mentioned that this is a case of pneumonectomy. Now would you please tell me about some other possible indications for a pneumonectomy?

Candidate: Other possible indications for a pneumonectomy include:
- Localized bronchiectasis with uncontrolled symptoms such as recurrent hemoptysis.
- Old TB [before the establishment of anti-TB therapy or resistance to treatment— extensively drug-resistant (XDR)-TB/multidrug-resistant (MDR)-TB].
- Bronchial obstruction with destroyed lung.
- Traumatic lung injury.

Examiner: How would you work up a patient for surgery, or how would you assess their potential fitness for surgery?

Candidate: I would like to take a full history and also want to examine the patient adequately. Moreover, I would like to go for lung function tests, including gas transfer factor assessment as well as cardiopulmonary exercise testing.

Examiner: Before performing lobectomy, what FEV1 would you want the patient to have?

Candidate: I would expect the patient has an FEV1 of at least 1.5.

Examiner: And for a pneumonectomy?

Candidate: I would expect the patient to have an FEV1 of at least 2.

Examiner: Let us think she had pneumonectomy due to lung cancer 2 years ago. Now, she presented with supraclavicular lymphadenopathy. What may be the cause of it?

Candidate: I would think either this patient's lung cancer is recurring back, causing lymph node metastasis, or she may have been suffering from lymphoma or infection (such as TB).

Examiner: What are the complications of pneumonectomy?

Candidate: Pulmonary complications include pulmonary edema, postpneumonectomy syndrome. Pleural space complications include postpneumonectomy empyema, bronchopleural fistula, esophagopleural fistula, chylothorax, acute hemothorax, contralateral pneumothorax.

Cardiac complications include arrhythmia, myocardial infarction (MI), PE, intracardiac shunting, and cardiac herniation.

Others are esophageal motility disorders, gastric volvulus, acute kidney injury, pneumopericardium, and postpneumonectomy paralysis.

Examiner: You mentioned postpneumonectomy syndrome as a complication of pneumonectomy. Please tell me, what do you know about this?

Candidate: This syndrome results from the extensive compression of the distal trachea and main bronchus due to mediastinal shifting and compensatory hyperinflation of the remaining lung. Postpneumonectomy syndrome occurs almost exclusively in patients with right-sided pneumonectomy, approximately 6 months after surgery, but can occur years after the procedures.

The syndrome is characterized by progressive breathlessness, cough, inspiratory stridor, and pneumonia. Treatment includes surgical repositioning of mediastinum and filling of postpneumonectomy space with nonabsorbable material with or without stenting of bronchi. It can be fatal if left untreated.

Lung Transplant

Mr Jimmy, a 49-year-old man, presented with breathlessness. Examine the respiratory system.

(After finishing respiratory system examination within 6 minutes of time)

Candidate: I would like to complete my examination by checking the patient's observation chart, examining sputum pots (if any), doing bedside spirometry and pulse oximetry, and examining lymph nodes (if you do not examine the lymph nodes during your examination).

Examiner: Would you like to present your case, please?

Candidate:

I performed a respiratory system examination on Mr Jimmy; he has had the right lung transplant associated with chronic lung transplant rejection.

This gentleman was breathless at rest, tachypneic, tachycardic, and bilaterally clubbed. He was taking oxygen therapy via nasal cannula. He had a Cushingoid appearance with some skin purpura.

On chest examination, there was a right thoracotomy scar.

There was reduced chest expansion in both lungs with a dull percussion note over the left base.

On auscultation, there were fine inspiratory crackles to the mid-zone in the left lung and a few scattered inspiratory squeaks in the right lung.

There was no evidence of infection or drug reaction.

I would like to ask the patient about the underlying respiratory disease that leads to transplant, any complications following transplant and any current symptoms, particularly about the shortness of breath and exercise tolerance.

However, there were fine inspiratory crackles in the left lung, and a thoracotomy scar on the right lung along with finger clubbing suggest that the lung transplant was for interstitial lung disease.

Examiner: Well, you mention he has transplant rejection, and if it is established, what may be the cause for this rejection?

Candidate: The patient was dyspneic and had some scattered inspiratory squeaks in his transplant lung and also some features of steroid-induced side effects.

With all of these findings, I would suspect this is a chronic transplant rejection case possibly due to bronchiolitis obliterans syndrome, for which he takes high doses of steroids and is on continuous oxygen therapy.

Examiner: Okay.... Now tell me, how will you investigate the case?

Candidate: In the post-transplant patient, routine investigations may include baseline blood tests CBC, ESR, CRP looking for active infections and drug levels of relevant immunosuppressants.

Then, I would like to do spirometry with a reversibility test looking for the obstructive deficit, which may suggest bronchiolitis obliterans syndrome.

Examiner: Would you like to tell me some of the indications for a lung transplant?

Candidate: The most common conditions for which lung transplants are performed are interstitial lung disease, cystic fibrosis, bilateral bronchiectasis, COPD, pulmonary vascular diseases-idiopathic pulmonary HTN, and alpha-1 antitrypsin deficiency.

The rare disease may include Langerhans cell granulomatosis and lymphangioleiomyomatosis.

Examiner: To be eligible for a lung transplant, what are the criteria that should be fulfilled?

Candidate: Lung transplantation should be considered for adults with chronic, end-stage lung disease who meets three criteria:
1. He should have >50% risk of death from lung disease within 2 years if the transplant is not performed.
2. He should have >80% likelihood of surviving at least 90-days post-transplant.
3. He should have >80% likelihood of a 5-year post-transplant survival from a general medical perspective, provided adequate graft function.

Moreover, finally, they have no contraindications, such as:
- *From history*:
  - Bloodborne viral infections [HIV, hepatitis B virus (HBV), hepatitis C virus (HCV), etc.]
  - Current smoker
  - Unsuitable psychological profile
- *From investigation*:
  - Organ dysfunction other than respiratory disease
  - Concomitant unresolved malignant disease
  - Active pulmonary infections

Examiner: As you mention, the patient has been suffering from chronic lung transplant rejection due to bronchiolitis obliterans. What are the other complications of a lung transplant?

Candidate: Early complications of lung transplant include:
- Acute rejection or primary graft dysfunction is common, and most patients will experience at least one episode in the first 6 months post-transplant.
- Chronic rejection is usually due to bronchiolitis obliterans syndrome, which is the leading cause of death after the first year of transplant, and the incidence approaches 50% by 5 years.
- Other significant complications include infections such as bacterial, mycobacterial, fungal, and viral (commonly CMV and herpes simplex)

Patients are also at increased risk of malignancy:
- Post-transplant lymphoproliferative disease (PTLD) is the most common malignancy in the first year after transplant.
- Skin malignancies are also common and should be regularly screened for.

Complications of immune suppression may include:
- Typical steroid side effects from glucocorticoids include a Cushingoid appearance, decreased bone density, skin thinning, and diabetes.
- Patients on tacrolimus may also develop diabetes or may have a tremor, mainly if levels are high.
- Patients on cyclosporine may develop gum hypertrophy.
- Renal and hearing impairments may occur in long-term use of antirejection medications and frequent antibiotic courses, including aminoglycosides.

Examiner: This patient has a lung transplant due to interstitial lung disease. Can you please tell me when you plan for a lung transplant in a patient with interstitial lung disease?

Candidate: The timing of referral to the lung transplant team depends on the lung condition. However, ideally, referrals should be made early in suitable patients.

In case of interstitial lung disease, which carries the worst prognosis of all diseases, is the indications for lung transplantation. All patients with usual interstitial pneumonia or fibrotic nonspecific usual interstitial pneumonia (NSIP) who have no contraindications should be considered for referral for lung transplant regardless of their lung function.

Patients with other types of interstitial lung disease, such as nonfibrotic/cellular NSIP:
- Should be referred to if their FVC <80% or
- Their transfer factor is <40%, or
- Any oxygen requirement or symptomatic dyspnea

This does not mean that these patients will be immediately listed; however, they can complete a full and timely transplant assessment and be listed if shown to be rapidly deteriorating, e.g., >10% drop in FVC within 6 months.

CHAPTER 5

Clinical Examination: Gastrointestinal System

- Gastrointestinal Tract Examination
- Chronic Liver Disease
- Cirrhosis with Portal Hypertension
- Hepatomegaly with No Stigmata of Chronic Liver Disease
- Hereditary Hemochromatosis
- Primary Biliary Cholangitis/Cirrhosis
- Ascites
- Hepatosplenomegaly
- Isolated Splenomegaly
- Hemolytic Anemia (Hereditary Spherocytosis)
- Autosomal Dominant Polycystic Kidney Disease
- Renal Transplant
- Liver Transplantation
- Renal-pancreas Transplant
- Chronic Pancreatitis
- Crohn's Disease
- Percutaneous Endoscopic Gastrostomy

Gastrointestinal Tract Examination

1. Meticulously, read the clinical scenario; this shall help you predict what you are going to find and do only what you have been asked.
2. Carefully greet the examiners in a nice, decent, and balanced manner—this will definitely carry a positive impact on them.
3. Sanitize your hands with antiseptic liquid (antiseptic liquid is provided to you in the station)
4. Greet the patient, introduce yourself, confirm your patient identity, and take permission (Hello, Mr X.... Good morning, I am Mohammad Ali....One of the working doctors here today....I have been asked to examine you....Is that okay with you?).
5. Explain to the patient in easy yet precise terms about your procedure—this shall help to get required cooperation from the patient (I would like to examine your hands, face, neck, tummy and, legs if that are okay with you?).
6. Ask about the pain and discomfort and reassure the patient (Do you have any pain or discomfort?.........I would be gentle during the examination, please let me know if you feel any pain or discomfort).
7. Adequately positioned (initially, position the patient 45° in bed).
8. Sufficiently expose the patient appropriate to the examination (Please maintain dignity... Expose the patient from mid-chest to inguinal area). "Please sit up and take off your shirt and undo the top button of your trouser, just notched them down a little but not below the level of your underwear, if that's okay with you."
   [*Explain every subsequent step before doing it so that the patient will be more cooperative and this will help you score better in skill-7 (maintaining patient's welfare)*]
9. *General survey*: Stand at the end of the bed, take your time to observe (see the patient as a whole, do not rush to examination, look for bedside clues and other clues in the patient).
   - Bedside clues: Look for environmental clues behind the chair, bedside table or under the bed, such as special shoes for a patient with diabetic feet, walking aids required for osteoporotic fractures from prolonged under-nourishment or steroid therapy, medic-alert bracelet, glucometer, artificial tears for Sjögren's syndrome, insulin pump or inhaler (which look like an asthma inhaler).
   - Age
   - Body built: Obese, low body mass index (BMI), cachectic.
   - Comfortable or not (?pain, agitation, and confusion)
   - Face and neck:
     - Parotid enlargement: Chronic liver disease (CLD) and sarcoidosis
     - Temporalis wasting: CLD and malignancy
     - Cushingoid face: Steroid use for autoimmune hepatitis, inflammatory bowel disease (IBD), sarcoidosis, renal/liver/pancreas transplantation or Cushing syndrome
     - Lipoatrophy/hearing aid: Mesangiocapillary glumerolunephritis (MCGN)
     - SLE rash: Autoimmune hepatitis, renal failure, renal transplant
     - Jaundice: CLD, obstructive jaundice, chronic hemolytic anemia
     - Spider nevi: CLD
     - Tattoo: CLD due to viral hepatitis
     - Purpura: Steroid use, myelofibrosis
     - Central lines for hemodialysis catheter: Renal failure

- Xanthelasma: Primary biliary cholangitis (PBC), nephrotic syndrome
- Muddy complexion: Chronic hemolytic anemia
- Thalassemic facies
- Facial plethora + Conjunctival injection: PRV
- Lupus pernio (chronic raised indurated hardened lesion on the skin often purplish in color usually seen on the nose, ear, cheeks, lips, and forehead): Sarcoidosis
- Systemic sclerosis facies (taught skin with microstomia): ?Malabsorption (bacterial overgrowth?)
○ Chest:
- Gynecomastia, sparse hair, Spider nevi: CLD
- Purpura: Steroid use (?)
○ Abdomen:
- Distension (ascites, large mass, bowel distension)
- Flank fullness: Ascites
- Umbilicus shifted down: Ascites/organomegaly.
- Dilated vein (IVCO, Caput medusa)
- Scars

10. Ask him to extend his hands and examine the dorsum of hands for:
    ○ Clubbing (IBD, CLD, celiac disease, familial adenomatous polyposis coli)
    ○ Leukonychia (whitened nail bed) suggests hypoalbuminemia due to CLD, nephrotic syndrome, malabsorption
    ○ A-V fistula [thrill (felt), bruit (heard) suggests functioning fistula; recent needling suggests the patient is on hemodialysis for end-stage renal disease (ESRD) or renal replacement therapy (RRT) in a post-transplant failure]
    ○ Rheumatoid arthritis (RA) change in the hands; splenomegaly (?Felty's syndrome) or hepatosplenomegaly (?Amyloidosis)
    ○ Tattoos, needle track marks: HBV, HCV, HIV infection.
    ○ Koilonychia (spooning of the nails) suggests IDA: Chronic Blood loss (?malignancy), malabsorption.
    ○ Sclerodactyly, thin tight shiny skin suggests systemic sclerosis—may have small bowel bacterial overgrowth (malabsorption), renal failure, autoimmune hepatitis.
    ○ Bruising (purpura), thinning of the skin suggests steroid use: ?Autoimmune hepatitis, IBD, sarcoidosis.
    ○ Splinter hemorrhage suggests infective endocarditis (?Splenomegaly).

11. Ask him to turn his hands up and examine palms for:
    ○ Palmar erythema (reddening of the palm) suggests liver disease.
    ○ Dupuytren's contracture (thickening of the palmer fascia suggests alcoholic liver disease/familial).
    ○ Carpal tunnel scar suggests ?amyloidosis.
    ○ Janeway lesion, Osler nodes suggest infective endocarditis (?Splenomegaly).

12. Ask him to pull his wrist with the patient arm unsupported in that position for 15 seconds and examine for flapping tremor ("Keep your arms nice and straight for me and cock your wrist right back...")—hepatic encephalopathy, uremia or CO_2 retention (respiratory failure).

13. Inspect the patient's arm:
    ○ Purpura, ecchymosis (?Thrombocytopenia due to idiopathic thrombocytopenic purpura (ITP) or other hematological disorders and look for organomegaly or chronic steroid use or coagulopathy due to any cause (?Liver disease/drugs)
    ○ Spider nevi
    ○ A-V fistula
    ○ Needle track marks (HBV, HCV, HIV)
    ○ Excoriations (Cholestasis due to PBC)

14. Examine the axilla (Please keep your hands to hip):
    ○ Lymphadenopathy suggests malignancy, TB, lymphoma, sarcoidosis.
    ○ Scars of lymph node biopsy
    ○ Hair loss (CLD, IDA, malnutrition)
    ○ Acanthosis nigricans (brown to black velvety hyperpigmentation of the skin suggest underlining carcinoma or obesity due to any cause or insulin resistance)

15. Examine eye ("pull down your lower eyelid for me please"):
    ○ Anemia can be a feature of many abdominal diseases other than blood loss,

such as malabsorption, chronic IBD, chronic kidney disease (CKD), abdominal malignancy, or it may be the features of hematological malignancy (so, look for lymphadenopathy and hepatosplenomegaly)
- Jaundice suggest CLD, acute viral hepatitis, hemolysis (usually associated with anemia), obstructive jaundice (? pancreatic carcinoma) or PBC
- Xanthelasma: PBC, nephrotic syndrome

16. *Examination of mouth ("open your mouth widely for me please.... And lift up your tongue to the roof")*:
    - Hyperpigmentation suggests Addison's disease
    - Pigmented macules on the lips suggest Peutz-Jeghers syndrome
    - Ulcer suggests Crohn's disease, celiac disease
    - Oral candidiasis (?Immune deficiency due to HIV or post-transplant patient)
    - Tongue (glossitis)—smooth swelling of the tongue with associated erythema suggest Iron, vitamin B12, folate deficiency
    - Angular stomatitis (inflamed, red areas at the corners of the mouth suggest iron, vitamin B1/B12, folate deficiency)
    - Lip hyperplasia suggests chronic disease, acromegaly
    - Telangiectasia on the lip and tongue suggests Osler-Weber-Rendu syndrome (?HHT)
    - Gum hypertrophy: Cyclosporine therapy (?organ transplant), phenytoin, calcium channel blocker (CCB) and AML
    - Large tongue: Amyloidosis, acromegaly

17. *Examination of the neck*: Ask the patient to turn his head and examine the neck for JVP
    - Raised JVP with prominent V wave, enlarged tender liver + peripheral edema suggest TR (?Carcinoid syndrome)
    - Raised JVP with edema suggests volume overload: ?renal transplant failure (if there is renal transplant scar) or ESRD

18. *Ask him to sit forward and examine for lymphadenopathy*:
    - Virchow's node—left supraclavicular fossa to suggest gastric malignancy
    - Cervical lymphadenopathy suggests infection (?TB) or malignancy or lymphoma or CLL (look for ?hepatosplenomegaly)

19. *Chest*:
    - Spider nevi (a central red spot with a reddish extension; >5 significant) suggest CLD
    - Gynecomastia (over the development of male mammary glands) suggests liver disease, digoxin and spironolactone therapy
    - Sparse hair suggests CLD
    - Lung biopsy scars could be ?sarcoidosis
    - Permcath or its scar (?hemodialysis)

20. Inspect the back for scar or spider nevi.

21. Ask him if he has any pain in this back and examines for sacral edema.

22. Take permission to lower the bed flat and lay the patient flat on the bed (you may ask the patient to bend his knees to relax the abdominal muscle).

23. *On your knees, closely inspect the abdomen and ask him to take a deep breath*:
    - Scar (stretch the abdomen skin if the patient is obese to see the scar):
        - Rooftop incision scar suggests upper GIT surgery (gastrectomy)
        - The Mercedes Benz scar (vertical extension of the rooftop incision suggests liver transplantation)
        - Left subcostal scar suggests splenectomy (?chronic hemolytic anemia)
        - Right subcostal scar (Kocher's incision) due to cholecystectomy due to chronic HA.
        - Laparotomy scar suggests cholecystectomy due to chronic hemolytic anemia; Crohn's disease
        - Peritoneal dialysis (Tenckhoff catheter)
        - Right iliac fossa (RIF) scar renal transplant or appendicectomy
        - Left iliac fossa scar (Rutherford Morrison's scar) suggests renal transplantv
        - Paramedian scar suggests general abdominal surgery (?colectomy)
        - Midline scar/Multiple scars (?Crohn's disease)
        - Loin incision suggests an open renal procedure.

- Groin incision: Vertical (vascular surgery), oblique (repair of hernia)
- Ascites tapping scar
- *Percutaneous endoscopic gastrostomy (PEG) tube*: If you find a PEG tube, look for a neurological problem affecting swallowing or head neck malignancy.
- Dilated vein:
  - Engorged periumbilical vein: Caput medusa suggests portal HTN due to ?CLD (filling away from the umbilicus), IVCO (filling toward the umbilicus)
  - Do milking test on the dilated veins below the umbilicus, feel for a thrill, auscultation for venous hum
- Cullen's sign (Bruising surrounding umbilicus) suggests retroperitoneal bleed (? Pancreatitis/raptured AAA)
- Grey turner sign (Bruising in the flanks) suggests retroperitoneal bleed (Pancreatitis/raptured AAA)
- Striae (reddish/pink suggests chronic steroid use or Cushing syndrome)
- Stomas:
  - Left iliac fossa (colostomy)
  - RIF (ileostomy)
  - RIF and contains urine (urostomy)

24. Ask if he has any pain in the abdomen (Do you have any pain in your tummy?).
(If the patient has pain in an area, start palpating away from the site of the pain)
- Light palpation: Palpate each of the quadrants and asses for any of the below:
  - Tenderness
  - Rebound tenderness: Peritonitis
  - Muscle guarding: Localized or generalized
  - Masses
- Deep palpation: If any masses are identified, then assess
  - Location, size, shape, consistency, mobility, pulsating—a pulsatile mass suggests vascular etiology.

25. Palpate for the liver lower border from RIF upwards, asking the patient to breathe in during palpation, and percuss for it and feel its edge and measure how many centimeters...... below the costal margin and note...
- Consistency:
  - Soft [nonalcoholic steatohepatitis (NASH), heart failure, TR]; firm (CLD, CHA, sarcoidosis) hard; malignancy
- Edge:
  - Sharp (CLD, malignancy, CHA, sarcoidosis)
  - Rounded (NASH, heart failure, PRV, sarcoidosis)
- Tenderness:
  - Acute viral hepatitis, congestive liver, liver abscess, Budd–Chiari syndrome
- Surface:
  - Nodular (cirrhosis, metastasis) or smooth

26. Palpate for the spleen from RIF diagonally toward the left hypochondrium
27. If you cannot find the spleen ask the patient to roll on his right side and support the left costal area with your left hand and feel for the spleen with your right-hand fingers.
28. *Percuss the Traube's area for dullness or percuss left 9th intercostal space (ICS) anterior axillary line on deep inspiration*:
- If note changes from resonance on deep expiration to dull on deep inspiration. Then positive Castell's sign.
- Splenomegaly:
  - If you find splenomegaly, then measure how many centimeters below the costal margin, and comment on edge, consistency, surface, and tenderness.
- For massive ascites, do the dipping method for palpating organs.

29. *Palpate for kidneys and do ballottement*: Kidney will be ballotable anterior and posteriorly
30. *Percuss for ascites*:
- Percuss from the center of the abdomen to the flank until dullness is noted.
- Keep your finger on the spot at which the percussion note became dull.
- Ask the patient to roll onto the opposite side to which you have detected the dullness and keep the patient on his side for 30 seconds
- Repeat your percussion in the same spot
- If the fluid was present (ascites), then the area that was previously dull now be resonant

- If the flank is now resonant, percuss back to the midline, which if ascites is present will now be dull (the dullness has shifted).
31. *Auscultation*:
    - Bowel sound:
        - Normal—gurgling
        - Abnormal—if tinkling (bowel obstruction: ?Crohn's disease)
        - Absent—ileus/peritonitis
    - Aortic bruit—auscultate just above the umbilicus—AAA
    - Renal bruits—auscultate just above the umbilicus slightly lateral to the midline.
32. *Examine the legs for*:
    - Edema (CLD, renal failure, NS)
    - Clubbing
    - Necrobiosis lipoidica: DM, RF
    - Pyoderma gangrenosum: IBD, RA
    - Erythema nodosum: IBD, sarcoidosis
    - Purpura
    - Vitiligo: ?Autoimmune hepatitis, PBC
33. *Formulate the diagnosis*:
    - Diagnosis (hepatosplenomegaly, renal transplant, CLD)
    - Possible cause (viral hepatitis, alcohol, CHA, myelofibrosis)
    - Complication (?Decompensated CLD, choledocholithiasis, nephrolithiasis)
34. Thank to the patient at the end of the examination and cover him up before turning around to the examiner.
35. Wash hand again.

Abdominal Case Presentation

I believe this gentleman has evidence of .....(diagnosis) ....(cause) .....complication

This gentleman is lying comfortably in bed with average built

Positive findings ...

No evidence of CLD or hepatic encephalopathy

I would like to complete my examination by examining hernia orifices, external genitalia, doing P/R, urine dipstick, and looking at the patient observation chart.

Chronic Liver Disease

Mr Bowman, a 55-year-old man, presented with abdominal fullness. Examine the abdomen and present your findings (After finishing GIT examination within 6 minutes of time).

Candidate: I would like to complete my examination by looking at the patient's observation chart, examining hernia orifices, external genitalia, doing PR, and urine dipsticks.

Examiner: Would you like to present your case, please?

Candidate:

I have performed an abdominal examination on this middle-aged gentleman. Based on my clinical findings, I believe this patient has CLD.

Positive findings include:

On inspection, this gentleman is cachectic, jaundiced with paper money skin, diffuse multiple superficial capillaries visible (telangiectasia) in the upper arm.

He has multiple spider nevi in the location of the SVC distribution, bruising, and gynecomastia.

He also has tattoos and needle track marks on his arms.

On abdominal palpation, the patient has evidence of hepatomegaly, which is 3 cm below the costal margin, firm in consistency and nontender.

There is no sign of portal hypertension (splenomegaly, caput medusa, and ascites).

There is no ascites, asterixis, encephalopathy or any other evidence of hepatic decompensation.

In terms of etiology, this patient has evidence of tattoos and needle marks on his arms along with other stigmata of CLD. I would suspect this patient may have chronic viral hepatitis (hepatitis B/HCV likely) with all of these findings.

Examiner: Okay. Tell me some causes of CLD?

Candidate: In the UK, the commonest causes of CLD are alcoholic liver disease or nonalcoholic fatty liver disease.

Globally probably the commonest cause is viral hepatitis (hepatitis B and C). Other important causes include:
- Autoimmune disorders, such as autoimmune hepatitis
- PBC or PSC
- Hemochromatosis
- Wilson's disease
- Alpha-1 antitrypsin deficiency
- Budd–Chiari syndrome
- Constrictive pericarditis and cardiac failure
- Liver disease may also be associated with various drugs.

Examiner: What investigations would you do on this gentleman if this was the first consultation you have had with him?

Candidate: I would start by taking a full history, including:
- Alcohol history
- Drug history such as methyldopa, methotrexate, amiodarone, etc.
- I/V drug abuse or blood transfusion
- Travel history
- Family history
- High risk of sexual history
- History of all other comorbidities

In terms of investigations, I would like to perform baseline blood tests such as full blood count (FBC), urea and electrolytes (U & E's), LFTs, and a coagulation screen.

To identify the etiology, I would like to do the following tests:
- Serological tests to identify viral infections such as HCV, HBV, CMV, and EBV.
- Serum ferritin as a screen for hemochromatosis
- Serum ceruloplasmin for Wilson's disease
- Serum immunoglobulins and autoantibody screen (ANA, AMA, smooth muscle antibody, and LKM antibody) for PBC, PSC and autoimmune hepatitis.

To identify the complications, I would consider progressing to imaging with:
- An ultrasound (to see the evidence of liver architecture, hepatomegaly, SOL, splenomegaly, and ascites), a CT, and possibly arrange a biopsy.
- A noninvasive test of liver fibrosis may also be appropriate, e.g., a fibrotest or fibroscan.
- An upper GIT endoscopy for esophageal varices

It would be worth considering sending tumor markers for hepatocellular carcinoma (HCC) [AFP (alpha-fetoprotein)].

Examiner: Please tell me what findings you may have found from blood tests in a CLD patient?

Candidate: In a patient with CLD, the synthetic function of the liver will be impaired that including low albumin, low platelet, prolonged prothrombin time (PT) with INR.

Examiner: You mentioned, this patient has hepatomegaly on the background of chronic viral hepatitis. What do you expect here?

Candidate: In the advanced stage of chronic viral hepatitis, I would expect nonpalpable small liver. However, if hepatomegaly is present in a patient with chronic viral hepatitis induced CLD; we must exclude the possible hepatoma. Otherwise, I would think this is the early stage of chronic viral hepatitis.

Examiner: Then how would you proceed with hepatoma?

Candidate: There is a high incidence of hepatoma with HBV or HCV infection, and patients should be screened for these with alpha-fetoprotein and USG of the abdomen.

Examiner: How would you treat a patient with hepatitis C virus-induced CLD?

Candidate: In terms of management of a hepatitis C virus patient:
- Alcohol intake should be reduced as it hastens disease progression.
- Antiviral therapy with ribavirin and peginterferon can be tried if the patient is viremic with abnormal liver histology. Novel oral anti-HCV medication includes two drugs combination with sofosbuvir and daclatasvir.

Examiner: Tell me some complications of CLD.

Candidate: It includes:
- Portal hypertension
- Ascites with splenomegaly with hypersplenism
- Hemorrhage, usually upper GI (gastric ulcers and erosions still occur more frequently than variceal bleeding)
- Spontaneous bacterial peritonitis
- Hepatic encephalopathy
- Hepatorenal syndrome
- Hepatopulmonary syndrome

Examiner: What is decompensated CLD? What are the precipitating factors which can lead to decompensated CLD?

Candidate: Clinically decompensated CLD will present with a combination of jaundice, ascites, asterixis, encephalopathy, hepatorenal or hepatopulmonary syndrome in the acute setting.

The liver can compensate for a significant amount of hepatocyte injury. However, it can decompensate as a result of ongoing liver injury and additional stress. The precipitating factors include:
- Continued alcohol intake or sedative or electrolyte imbalance
- Untreated chronic active viral hepatitis, GI bleeding, large salt intake, dehydration, constipation

Examiner: You mentioned hepatic encephalopathy as a feature of decompensated CLD. What do you know about encephalopathy?

Candidate: Hepatic encephalopathy or portal-systemic encephalopathy is a neuropsychiatric syndrome caused by hepatic failure associated with acute or CLD.

Hepatic encephalopathy is caused by the body's inability to remove ammonia from the bloodstream, and the collection of neurotoxins in the blood affects brain activity.

Hepatic encephalopathy can be classified by as:
- *Type A*: Acute liver failure
- *Type B*: The presence of portosystemic "shunt" that allows blood to bypass the liver without intrinsic liver disease
- *Type C*: Chronic liver failure (cirrhosis of the liver)

Hepatic encephalopathy may present with intellectual impairment, personality changes, and reduced level of consciousness.

It is associated with diminished quality of life, impaired daily function, decreased work productivity, and frequent hospitalization for the treatment of acute episodes.

Examiner: You mentioned encephalopathy. How would you examine for encephalopathy specifically?

Candidate: So, we have mentioned the presence of asterixis; also, assess for constructional apraxia, for example, and ask the gentleman to draw a five-pointed star.

Examiner: How do you grade the severity of hepatic encephalopathy?

Candidate: Hepatic encephalopathy can be graded using the Conn score, which is also called West Haven classification, where higher scores indicate a higher severity, as follows:
- *Grade 0*: No personality or behavioral abnormality detected.
- *Grade 1*: Lack of awareness, anxiety and euphoria, shortened attention span.
- *Grade 2*: Apathy or lethargy, minimal disorientation for time or place, inappropriate behavior, subtle personality change, impaired performance of subtraction.
- *Grade 3*: Somnolence to semi stupor but responsive to verbal stimuli, confusion, gross disorientation.
- *Grade 4*: Coma-unresponsive to verbal or noxious stimuli.

Examiner: Let us think you have a patient with CLD presented with obesity, diabetes mellitus, hypertension, and hyperlipidemia. What might be the cause of liver disease?

Candidate: I wound think about the NASH.

Examiner: What will you think if a CLD patient presented with tender liver, ascites, and no hepatojugular reflux?

Candidate: I would think about Budd–Chiari syndrome, which may involve inferior vena cava as there is no hepatojugular reflux.

Examiner: Well, please tell me about the severity of cirrhosis; how do you grade the severity of cirrhosis?

Candidate: The most commonly used grading system for the severity of cirrhosis is the modified Child–Pugh system, which scores clinical and biochemical parameters out of three to obtain a score.

The parameters include encephalopathy, bilirubin, INR, ascites, and albumin. Severity is classified according to the Child–Pugh score into:
- Class A (5–6 points) where 1-year survivals of 100%
- Class B (7–9 points) with 1-year survivals of 80%
- Class C (10–15 points) with 1-year survivals of 50%

There are other scores, such as the model for end-stage liver disease (MELD) score, also available.

Examiner: Would you like to tell me some about hepatorenal syndrome?

Candidate: Hepatorenal syndrome (HRS) is a functional and reversible form of acute kidney injury in a patient with acute or chronic severe liver disease in the absence of any other identifiable causes of renal pathology.

Two types of HRS are described as:

Type 1: It is characterized by rapid deterioration of renal function that usually occurs within 2 weeks.

Type 2: It has a more insidious onset; it is characterized by a steady and progressive decline in

Table 1: Classification of jaundice.		
Prehepatic *(due to excessive breakdown of red blood cells)*	**Hepatocellular** *(due to hepatocyte injury)*	**Posthepatic** *(due to obstruction to the normal flow of bile)*
• Hemolytic anemia • Gilbert's syndrome • Crigler–Najjar syndrome	• Alcoholic liver disease • Viral hepatitis • Iatrogenic, e.g., medication • Autoimmune hepatitis • Hereditary hemochromatosis • Primary biliary cirrhosis • Hepatocellular carcinoma	• Intraluminal causes, such as gallstones • Mural causes, such as cholangiocarcinoma, strictures, or drug-induced cholestasis • Extra-mural causes, such as pancreatic cancer or abdominal masses (e.g., lymphomas)

renal function over weeks and sometimes months, as well as recurrent, diuretic-resistant ascites.

Hepatorenal syndrome is difficult to reverse without hepatic transplantation unless the patient has a spontaneous recovery of liver function (e.g., postalcoholic hepatitis).

Medical therapy, mainly vasoconstrictor therapy, is used as a temporizing measure to improve renal function while the patient with HRS awaits liver transplantation if the patient is an appropriate candidate.

Surgical options for patients with hepatorenal syndrome include the transjugular intrahepatic portosystemic shunt (TIPS) procedure and liver transplantation.

Examiner: In this case, your patient has jaundice. Would you please tell me what are the types of jaundice and some causes of it?

Candidate: Jaundice can be classified as **(Table 1)**:

Examiner: Let us think a CLD patient presented with ascites. How would you manage such a case?

Candidate: We should start with:
- A low sodium diet (90 mmol or 5.2 g salt/day)
- Fluid restriction (if hyponatremia <120 mmol/L)
- Beta-blockers (propranolol) to reduce portal HTN.
- Spironolactone from 100–400 mg/day, in all patients able to tolerate the drug without excessive hyperkalemia.
- Loop-diuretics should be initiated next, usually furosemide from 40–160 mg/day.

If these measures fail or if the patient has significant symptoms related to the ascites, therapeutic paracentesis with albumin replacement should be carried out.

Radiological procedures such as TIPS may help relieve portal hypertension, but the risk of encephalopathy is increased as nitrogen waste effectively bypasses the liver with a resultant increased concentration in the systemic circulation.

Surgical measures such as portosystemic and Porto-venous shunts are much less likely done these days but still play a role in recurrent ascites.

Ultimately, definitive treatment is liver transplantation for end-stage liver disease when medical management fails.

Examiner: You noticed some stigmata of CLD are present in this patient. Tell me other stigmata of CLD that you can find in the limbs.

Candidate: There are many findings, such as
- *In nails*: I would find leukonychia, clubbing, and tarry nails.
- *In hands*: Palmar erythema, Dupuytren's contracture
- *In arms*: Jaundice, bruising, excoriation from pruritis, spider nevi, tattoos, needle track marks, cutaneous abscess at the site of I/V drug injection, asterixis, skin bronzing (hemochromatosis).

Cirrhosis with Portal Hypertension

Mrs Polin, a 59-year-old woman, presented with abdominal swelling. Examine the abdomen and present your findings.

(After finishing abdominal system examination within 6 minutes of time)

Candidate: I would like to complete my examination by looking at the patient's observation chart, examining hernia orifices, external genitalia, doing PR, and urine dipsticks.

Examiner: Would you like to present your case, please?

Candidate:

On examination of this elderly lady, I believe she has signs and symptoms consistent with decompensated liver cirrhosis with portal hypertension, possibly due to alcoholic cirrhosis or NASH.

Positive findings include on inspection, Mrs Polin is obese and icteric; she has abdominal distension with peripheral edema.

She also has evidence of finger clubbing, palmar erythema, gynecomastia with bilateral parotid swelling, and corneal arcus possibly related to hyperlipidemia or age.

She has multiple spider nevi on the trunk and face, multiple petechiae and ecchymoses.

On abdominal examination, the patient has evidence of two small scars suggesting paracentesis or liver biopsies; caput medusa; nontender Hepatosplenomegaly and ascites with positive shifting dullness. Also, a hepatic venous hum is present.

She has no signs of hepatic encephalopathy or hepatic bruits.

There are no features of hemochromatosis, such as bronzing of the skin. No evidence of tattoos and needle track marks on her arms.

Examiner: You have a diagnosis of liver cirrhosis, and you suspect this is due to alcoholic liver disease or NASH. Please tell me what the points are in favor of it.

Candidate: This patient is obese, has features consistent with cirrhotic liver disease, and has nontender hepatomegaly. In most cases, a cirrhotic liver is small and shrunken. However, hepatomegaly may be present due to fat deposition in cases where it is due to alcohol or nonalcoholic fatty liver disease (NAFLD).

The most common cause of cirrhosis in the UK is alcohol and NASH.

She is obese; this may be in keeping with steatohepatitis (NASH).

She has parotid swelling, which is classically associated with an alcoholic cause.

Examiner: What is hepatic venous hum? Moreover, let me know some conditions where you can find a hepatic bruit.

Candidate: The hepatic venous hum is a murmur that is audible in portal hypertension or HCC. It results from collateral formation between the portal system and remnants of the umbilical vein. It is best heard over the epigastrium.

A hepatic bruit over the liver can be heard with:
- Alcoholic hepatitis or
- Hepatic carcinoma (primary or secondary)

Other rare causes include:
- Hepatic arteriovenous malformations
- Intestinal arteriovenous malformations
- Hepatic hemangioma
- TIPS

Examiner: You have carefully noted that this patient has finger clubbing. Tell me some other GIT causes of clubbing.

Candidate: Other GIT causes of clubbing include:
- Inflammatory bowel disease
- Celiac disease
- GI lymphoma
- Rarely tropical sprue and Whipple's disease

Examiner: As we know, a cirrhotic patient may present with anemia. Can you please tell me some causes of it in a patient with liver cirrhosis?

Candidate: The principal causes of anemia in a cirrhotic patient are:
- Blood loss from portal hypertensive gastropathy or anemia of chronic disease
- Alcohol excess causes bone marrow suppression and poor nutrition.

Examiner: If a patient with CLD is still drinking alcohol, what will be your approach to stop this? Furthermore, tell me the treatment options for alcohol misuse.

Candidate: Any patient with liver disease should stop alcohol intake immediately. I would advise this patient for abstinence.

The treatment options for alcohol misuse depend on the extent of your drinking and whether you are trying to drink less (moderation) or give up drinking completely (abstinence).

He may be offered a short counseling session known as a brief intervention.

Other approaches include:
- Alcoholics anonymous
- Cognitive-behavioral therapy
- Family therapy
- Maintain drinking diary or
- Drug therapy: Several medications are recommended by the National Institute for Health and Care Excellence (NICE) to treat alcohol misuse. These include acamprosate, disulfiram, naltrexone, and nalmefene.

Examiner: Tell me some of the circumstances where alcohol abstinence is strongly recommended.

Candidate: There are several situations where abstinence is strongly recommended, including if:
- Liver damage, such as liver disease or cirrhosis
- Other medical problems, such as heart disease, which can be made worse by drinking
- Taking medication that can react badly with alcohol, such as antipsychotics
- Pregnant or planning to become pregnant
- Abstinence may also be recommended if you have previously been unsuccessful with moderation.

Examiner: Tell me, what do you know about alcohol withdrawal syndrome?

Candidate: Chronic alcohol consumption enhances gamma-aminobutyric acid (GABA) mediated inhibition in the CNS and inhibits NMDA-type glutamate receptors. Alcohol withdrawal can lead to the opposite effects that mean decreased inhibitory GABA and increased N-methyl-D-aspartate (NMDA) glutamate transmission.

Mild symptoms usually start within 6–12 hours of the alcohol-free period, such as anxiety, shaky hands, headache, nausea, vomiting, insomnia, and sweating.

More serious problems range from hallucinations usually starting within 12–24 hours and seizures within the first 2 days after the cessation.

Delirium tremens usually start within 48–72 hours after you put down the glass. These are severe symptoms that include vivid hallucinations and delusions. Only about 5% of people with alcohol withdrawal have them; this may be associated with confusion, racing heart, high blood pressure, fever, and heavy sweating.

Management includes: Benzodiazepine (chlordiazepoxide) is the 1st line treatment along with I/V vitamin B and C.

Examiner: What are the systemic consequences of alcohol in a patient with chronic alcoholism?

Candidate: Alcohol abuse has multi-system consequences, including:
- Cardiac problems include dilated cardiomyopathy and hypertension.

- Gastrointestinal problems include pancreatitis, peptic ulceration, and upper GI cancers.
- Neurologically there may be cerebellar atrophy, polyneuropathy, Wernicke's encephalopathy, and Korsakoff's syndrome.

Many of these clinical problems have specific clinical features, so I would like to examine some of them.

Examiner: How would you manage a case of cirrhosis?

Candidate: Treatment depends on the underlying disease.
- In case of alcoholic liver disease, abstinence is mandatory, as well as dietary and lifestyle advice with vitamin B supplementation in a patient with chronic alcohol consumption.
- In viral hepatitis—antiviral therapy
- In autoimmune hepatitis—immunosuppression (prednisolone, azathioprine)

For the prevention of complications, all patients:
- Should stop consuming alcohol
- Should be immunized against hepatitis, pneumococcal, and yearly influenza vaccines.
- Should keep surveillance for hepatoma, which involves 6-monthly abdominal ultrasound and AFP
- Should undergo endoscopy as surveillance for esophageal varices. If varices present, non-selective beta-blockers can be used as primary prophylaxis.
- Prophylactic antibiotics (e.g., norfloxacin) are indicated following an episode of spontaneous bacterial peritonitis.

Finally, liver transplantation: A decision can be made by MDT.

Hepatomegaly with No Stigmata of Chronic Liver Disease

Mr Bowman, a 55-year-old man, complained of abdominal fullness. Examine the abdomen and present your findings.

(After finishing GIT examination within 6 minutes of time)

Candidate: I would like to complete my examination by looking at the patient's observation chart, examining hernia orifices, external genitalia, doing PR, and urine dipsticks.

Examiner: Would you like to present your case, please?

Candidate:

This patient has hepatomegaly with a non-tender palpable liver edge 4 cm from the costal margin in the mid-clavicular line, which is firm in consistency.

This patient is well-nourished and has no evidence of anemia, jaundice, or other stigmata of CLD.

There is no evidence of splenomegaly or lymphadenopathy.

No audible bruits or hepatic venous hum or no signs of hepatic encephalopathy.

This patient has isolated hepatomegaly with no stigmata of CLD; at this point, my differential diagnosis would be broad that include liver disease due to:

Alcoholic liver disease/alcoholic hepatitis, NAFLD, HCC or secondaries to the liver, or viral hepatitis.

Other causes include congestive heart failure, chronic constrictive pericarditis (raised JVP, peripheral edema, and breathlessness are important clinical clues), carcinoid syndrome (nodular liver, facial flushing, telangiectasia, wheezing, and TR murmur are important clinical clues), hydatid cyst.

Examiner: If this patient presents with tender hepatomegaly, what would be the possibilities?

Candidate: Possibilities of tender hepatomegaly include:
- Acute viral hepatitis
- Liver abscess
- Congestive liver
- Budd–Chiari syndrome
- Hepatoma also can cause tender liver.

Examiner: How will you differentiate them clinically?

Candidate: I would like to take a full history and examine the other systems also.

In case of acute viral hepatitis: Clinically, I would expect jaundice along with tender liver and absence of other stigmata of CLD.

In case of the congestive liver due to congestive cardiac failure (CCF) or chronic constrictive pericarditis or cor pulmonale: The patient may present with dyspnea, raised JVP, and peripheral edema.

In liver abscess: High fever and toxic patient, usually non-icteric and tender liver.

In Budd–Chiari syndrome: Acute onset, abdominal pain, and tender liver with ascites

In hepatoma: Usually, it appears on the background of liver cirrhosis with portal hypertension, but very rarely, it can appear without evidence of cirrhosis.

Examiner: If I allow you to take some history from this patient, what is the important history you will take from him?

Candidate: I would like to ask the patient regarding:
- Is there any history of nausea, vomiting or abdominal discomfort?
- Any history of anorexia or weight loss.

- Any history of fever.
- Family history of liver disease.
- Other comorbidities such as metabolic syndrome, cardiac failure, and emphysema.
- Any joint pain or swelling.
- I/V drug abuse
- Medications including over-the-counter and herbal medicines or any hepatotoxic drugs.
- Alcohol and drinking habits.
- Moreover, I would ask for any recent travel history.

Examiner: How would you investigate this patient?

Candidate: At first, I would like to do a baseline blood test including CBC, ESR, and CRP, U/E's, serum creatinine, and blood sugar.

The most important test would be:
- Liver function tests that include: AST, ALT, serum alkaline phosphatase, serum bilirubin, PT, and serum albumin

To identify the etiology of hepatitis, I would like to do:
- Viral screening for especially hepatitis B and C
- Iron profile for hemochromatosis
- Serum copper and ceruloplasmin for Willson's disease

Autoimmune screening for:
- *Autoimmune hepatitis*: IgG, ANA, anti-smooth muscle antibody, and anti-liver-kidney microsomal type 1 Ab, soluble liver-kidney antigen.
- *Primary biliary cirrhosis*: IgM, anti-mitochondrial AB (M2)
- *Primary sclerosing cholangitis*: IgM, ANA, and ANCA
- *Alcoholic liver disease*: IgA

Then I would like to proceed with further tests with imaging include:
- Chest X-ray
- A USG of the hepatobiliary system
- CT scan of the abdomen
- Fibroscan of the liver

Finally, for definitive diagnosis, an invasive test includes a liver biopsy (gold standard test) that may be required.

Examiner: You mentioned about fibroscan of the liver. Please tell me some more about it.

Candidate: Transient elastography or fibroscan is a novel, noninvasive, and rapid bedside method for assessing liver fibrosis by measuring liver stiffness as well as steatosis (fatty change). It is commonly used to determine fibrosis in CLD, particularly:
- *Viral hepatitis*: Hepatitis B, hepatitis C
- HIV/HCV co-infection
- NAFLD or NASH
- Alcoholic liver disease

The fibrosis result is measured in kilopascals (kPa). It is normally between 2–6 kPa. The highest possible result is 75 kPa.

Fibroscan fibrosis results and the patient's medical history are used to determine fibrosis scores.
- *Fibrosis score F0–F1*: No liver scarring or mild liver scarring
- *Fibrosis score F2*: Moderate liver scarring
- *Fibrosis score F3*: Severe liver scarring
- *Fibrosis score F4*: Advanced liver scarring (indicates cirrhosis)

Examiner: Okay, let us think you have a patient with anasarca and massive proteinuria. Now presented with acute abdominal pain and tender hepatomegaly, what is your diagnosis?

Candidate: I think this is a case of nephrotic syndrome, which causes Budd–Chiari syndrome. As the nephrotic syndrome is a hypercoagulable state, and it can lead to venous thrombosis.

Examiner: A patient presented with cachexia, anemia, jaundice, supraclavicular lymphadenopathy, and nontender hepatomegaly, along with a palpable umbilical nodule. What is your diagnosis with these findings?

Candidate: Putting all of these findings together, I believe this patient has malignancy, either HCC or secondaries with lymph node metastasis.

Hereditary Hemochromatosis

A 40-year-old man presented with arthralgia, fatigue, and sexual dysfunction; please examine the abdomen.

(After finishing GIT examination within 6 minutes of time)

Candidate: I would like to complete my examination by looking at the patient's observation chart, examining hernia orifices, external genitalia, doing PR, and urine dipsticks.

Examiner: Would you present your case?

Candidate:

I believe this gentleman has hereditary hemochromatosis (HH).

He has slate gray (bronze) pigmentation with reduced body hair with gynecomastia.

The liver is enlarged 3 cm from the costal margin, firm in consistency, and nontender.

There is synovitis in the 2nd and 3rd metacarpophalangeal (MCP) joint and has evidence of scaring in the right antecubital fossa that I suspect may be due to regular venesection here.

Furthermore, the bedside blood glucose meter and BM Stix mark on his finger suggest the presence of DM.

He has no other stigma of CLD.

No signs of portal HTN such as ascites, caput medusa, or splenomegaly.

No evidence of hepatic decompensation such as jaundice, asterixis, encephalopathy, or ascites.

In terms of etiology for this presentation, There is no evidence of tattoo or Dupuytren's contracture or parotid enlargement or evidence of metabolic syndrome other than DM to say the common cause of liver diseases such as:
- Alcoholic liver disease
- NASH
- Or chronic viral hepatitis.

However, taken together with the history of arthralgia, DM, hypogonadism with evidence of venesection, and characteristic skin color changes, my most likely diagnosis would be HH.

I would like to complete my assessment by performing fundoscopic examination for diabetic retinopathy, urine dipstick for glucose or protein, neurological examination for neuropathy, examining for joint involvement, and cardiovascular examination to exclude cardiomyopathy.

Examiner: How would you investigate the case?

Candidate: I would like to do baseline blood tests that include CBC, U/E's, serum creatinine, blood sugar, HbA1C, and LFT including transaminases, alkaline phosphatase, serum bilirubin, as well as serum albumin and PT with INR to see the synthetic liver function.

Meanwhile, serum ferritin and transferrin saturation are useful for diagnosis and monitoring of response to treatment.

Alfa fetoprotein—as it is a strong risk factor (>200 fold) for HCC.

Finally, I would like to do a genetic test (HFE genotyping) to confirm the diagnosis.

Examiner: How would you treat someone with HH?

Candidate: As the HH has multi-system involvement, an MDT approach with input from other specialties is strongly recommended.

The most important general measures would be to avoid alcohol (alcoholism may accelerate iron accumulation in a patient with HH due to unknown mechanism) and iron supplementation in this diet.

Weekly venesection (500 mL) until the serum ferritin is (0–20 µg/dL); and transferrin saturation <50%. Maintenance phlebotomy is to keep the serum ferritin and iron in the lower limit of the normal range, usually once every 3 months.

Desferrioxamine, an iron chelator, can be used as an injection to reduce iron storage, particularly those patients if anemia and hypoproteinemia preclude phlebotomy.

In those with advanced liver cirrhosis or HCC, liver transplantation is indicated if the patient is fit enough to undergo the procedure.

Examiner: Okay, that's fine. Now tell me, how does hemochromatosis typically present?

Candidate: There may include an asymptomatic presentation with abnormal blood tests such as a raised ferritin. Sometimes it can be presented via screening programs of first degree relatives of HH patients.

The symptomatic patient usually presents with the classical triad of fatigue, arthralgia, and gonadal or sexual dysfunction; later presentation would be a complication of hemochromatosis such as:
- Liver cirrhosis
- Type 1 diabetes mellitus (T1DM)
- Skin discoloration
- Dilated cardiomyopathy with or without arrhythmia

Examiner: How is HH inherited?

Candidate: HH is inherited in an autosomal recessive fashion. It is usually due to mutation in the HFE gene (coded for iron absorption), located on chromosome 6, leading to impaired absorption of iron with resultant iron overload. The most commonly affected organs are the liver (leading to CLD), pancreas (leading to DM), heart (leading to cardiomyopathy or arrhythmia), anterior pituitary and glands (leading to hypo or hypergonadotropic hypogonadism or rarely panhypopituitarism) and joints (causing pseudogout with chondrocalcinosis).

Examiner: What are your recommendations for the screening program?

Candidate: A screening program should be undertaken in first degree relatives of the patient with hemochromatosis by doing an iron profile.

In case of a male, if baseline ferritin >300 and transferrin saturation >50%, however, in case of females, if ferritin >200 and transferrin saturation >40%, then we should go for HFE genotyping to confirm our cases of iron overload.

However, we should keep in mind that the presence of an identifiable HFE gene does not necessarily mean the disease will be expressed as the disease is of variable penetrance.

On the other hand, HH is very common in Caucasian mainly Celtic and Northern European populations—so all adult people of Northern European ancestry with unexplained raised serum ferritin (>300 µg/L male; >200 µg/L female) and random transferrin saturation (>50% male, >40% female) and normal FBC should be checked for *HFE* gene.

Examiner: Could you tell me the prognosis of the HH patient?

Candidate: If cirrhosis has not been established and venesection is introduced, then survival will be equivalent to the general population.

Primary Biliary Cholangitis/Cirrhosis

Mrs Sarah Kaur, a 40-year-old woman, presented with pruritus. Examine her abdomen and present your findings.

(After finishing GIT examination within 6 minutes of time)

Candidate: I would like to complete my examination by looking at the patient's observation chart, examining hernial orifices, external genitalia, digital rectal examination, and urine dipstick.

Examiner: Would you like to present your case, please?

Candidate:

> *This middle-aged lady appears to be suffering from CLD. She is lying comfortably at rest with an average built. She has signs of CLD in the form of:*
>
> *Gynecomastia, multiple spider nevi in the location of superior vena cava (face, upper limb, and trunk), fragile skin, which bruises easily and evidence of recent weight loss.*
>
> *Most importantly she has evidence of hepatomegaly. A palpable liver edge 3 cm below the costal margin, which is non-tender, firm in consistency, sharp margin, smooth surface, nonpulsatile with no bruit over it.*
>
> *She is jaundiced but has no other clinical signs of decompensation such as ascites or flapping tremor (encephalopathy).*
>
> *She has no clinical signs of portal hypertension such as splenomegaly, ascites or caput medusa.*

Examiner: Keeping that in mind, what do you think the cause of CLD could be here?

Candidate: In terms of etiology for this, she had generalized pigmentation, excoriation (due to scratching) and xanthelasma that strongly suggest the underlying cause could be primary biliary cholangitis, previously termed primary biliary cirrhosis.

She lacks parotid swelling or Dupuytren's contracture, which would classically be associated with alcoholic liver disease.

She is not overweight and has no clinical evidence of DM (such as needle mark for glucose monitoring), so she is less likely to have NASH as a cause of CLD.

There is no needle marks or tattoo that place her at high risk for viral hepatitis.

There are no features of hemochromatosis such as bronzing/tanning of the skin or evidence of arthropathy (MCP joint or knee) as a cause of CLD.

Or, she has no evidence of Wilson diseases such as Kayser–Fleischer (KF) rings or neurological manifestation (extrapyramidal or cerebellar sign), or she has no clinical evidence of emphysema that suggest alpha-1 antitrypsin deficiency as a cause of CLD.

At this point, I would like to take a full history from the patient, particularly alcohol history, drug history, family h/o liver disease or h/o comorbidity such as DM, HTN, and travel history.

So, if the patient is nonalcoholic and has no features suggestive of NASH, then my most likely clinical diagnosis would be a CLD due to primary biliary cholangitis.

Examiner: What investigations would you do on this lady if this was the first consultation you held with her?

Candidate: At this point, in terms of the investigation, I would like to perform a basic blood test that includes FBC with ESR, urea, serum creatinine, LFTs such as serum glutamic pyruvic transaminase (SGPT), serum glutamic oxaloacetic transaminase (SGOT), gamma-glutamyl transferase (GGT), alkaline phosphatase and serum albumin and coagulation screen such as PT, and also perform blood-borne viral screening such as HBsAg, anti-HCV Ab, and anti-HBc total.

Check for iron profile such as serum ferritin, percentage saturation, immunoglobulin and ceruloplasmin, and other autoantibody screens.

I would consider progressing to imaging with an ultrasonography of the hepatobiliary system, possibly CT scan, and possibly arrange a liver biopsy.

Noninvasive tests of liver fibrosis may also be appropriate such as fibroscan (liver elastography) to see the evidence of fibrosis and steatosis of the liver.

It would be worth considering sending tumor markers which, in case of HCC that would be AFP and des-gamma-carboxy prothrombin (DCP).

Examiner: You mentioned autoantibodies here. Which specific autoantibodies would you request?

Candidate: I would like to do ANA, AMA, ASMA (smooth muscle Ab), and anti-LKM-Ab.

Examiner: Okay! Now let us think this young lady had a positive AMA and evidence of obstructive jaundice such as increased serum bilirubin, GGT, and alkaline phosphatase. What diagnosis would you perform to know the suspect?

Candidate: I would think that the most likely diagnosis is primary biliary cholangitis, which was previously termed primary biliary cirrhosis.

Examiner: So, if I was to tell you, this lady has strongly suspected PBC clinically, and you are getting biochemical evidence of obstructive jaundice, but autoantibody screen revealed AMA negative, then what would you think?

Candidate: In that case, I would think about AMA-negative PBC.

As we know, in PBC, AMA will be positive almost 95% cases. A total of 5% of cases, it can be negative and termed as an AMA-negative PBC. In that case, other autoantibodies such as ASMA and ANA may be positive. These patients may require a liver biopsy to establish our diagnosis.

The guidelines of American Association for the study of liver disease for PBC diagnosis are—two of the three following criteria:
1. AMA positive
2. Elevated alkaline phosphatase
3. Histological evidence of PBC was seen on liver biopsy.

Examiner: Now tell me, how does it typically present?

Candidate: Fatigue (78% cases) and intense itching are the commonest presenting symptoms; pruritus usually develops several months or years ago before the development of jaundice; here, the jaundice is the last manifestation of PBC.

Hypothyroidism should be excluded first in case of unusual fatigability. Around 20% of cases of PBC may have associated hypothyroidism or rarely thyrotoxicosis.

There is a strong association of other autoimmune diseases in PBC patients, such as:
- Scleroderma (Raynaud's disease, tight skin, sclerodactyly, dysphagia)
- RA (deformity polyarthritis)
- Sjögren's syndrome (dry eye and dry mouth)
- Myasthenia gravis or
- Vitiligo

Primary biliary cholangitis can progress to CLD, cirrhosis with portal HTN, and rarely HCC.

Some patients may have features of complications such as deficiency of fat-soluble vitamins lead to:
- Osteomalacia (due to vitamin D deficiency)
- Osteopenia or osteoporosis (so, BMD should be done 2–3 yearly)
- Bleeding risk (due to vitamin K deficiency)

Examiner: What are the available treatment options for a patient with PBC?

Candidate: Ursodeoxycholic acid (13–15 mg/day) is the treatment of choice for the PBC patient that improves biochemical indices, delays histological progress, decreases variceal formation as well as improves liver transplantation. Moreover, with ursodeoxycholic acid, liver transplantation has free survival 85% at 10 years, 65% at 20 years.

Pruritus is generally assumed to be caused by circulating bile acid and be helped by anion exchange resin cholestyramine. Besides, rifampicin, phenobarbitone, naltrexone may also help in pruritus.

General measures include:
- Avoidance of smoking
- Reduce alcohol intake and
- Supplementation of the diet with the fat-soluble vitamin (ADEK) if biochemical evidence of deficiency then may require injectable correction as well.

Examiner: But, if the condition deteriorates despite medical management, then what will be your approaches for such a patient?

Candidate: Then, the only other option would be listing her for liver transplantation.

Ascites

Mr Ismail, a 79-year-old man, presented with abdominal fullness. Examine his abdomen and present your findings.

(After finishing GIT examination within 6 minutes of time)

Candidate: I would like to complete my examination by looking at the patient's observation chart, examining hernia orifices, external genitalia, doing PR, and urine dipsticks.

Examiner: Would you like to present your case, please?

Candidate:

I believe this patient had ascites due to intra-abdominal malignancy with peritoneal and lymph node metastasis.

Positive findings include:

This gentleman was cachexic, anemic, and had left-sided supraclavicular lymphadenopathy.

On abdominal examination:

His abdomen was distended, soft, and non-tender with the everted umbilicus.

The abdomen was dull to percussion in the flanks, with shifting dullness.

There was no evidence of visible collateral vessels, hepatosplenomegaly, lymph node enlargement or no palpable mass in the abdomen.

There was no evidence of stigmata of CLD or hepatic encephalopathy. No evidence of elevated venous pressure, no peripheral edema.

Examiner: You mentioned the cause of ascites here is an intra-abdominal malignancy with metastasis. Why and what are the other possibilities here?

Candidate: This patient was of elderly age with anemia, ascites, and supraclavicular lymphadenopathy. With all of these features, I suspect this is a case of intra-abdominal malignancy with peritoneal and lymph node metastasis.

However, on the background of ascites and lymphadenopathy, my strong differential diagnoses would be TB and lymphoma.

Although CLD is the most common cause of ascites, almost 80%, however, this patient had no stigmata of CLD.

There was no evidence of engorged neck vein or peripheral edema, so less likely to have a CCF.

No evidence of anasarca; that may also exclude nephrotic syndrome.

Other possibilities are:
- Budd–Chiari syndrome (tender hepatomegaly with features of portal HTN, usually no stigmata of CLD)
- Myxedema (myxedematous facies, delayed relaxation of the ankle jerks)

Examiner: What important history would you want to take from this gentleman?

Candidate: I would like to take the history of particular symptoms that may help to find some causes of ascites, such as:
- Either he has any history of fever that may indicate TB or lymphoma.
- Any history of hematemesis or melena; ruptured esophageal varices, or esophageal malignancy.
- Alteration of bowel habit with or without per rectal bleeding; that may indicate lower GIT malignancy

- Any urinary symptoms such as urgency, hesitancy, incontinence; may indicate renal pathology.
- History of loss of appetite or unintended weight loss.
- Personal or family history of malignancy or liver disease.
- Alcohol history
- Any travel history or suggestive history of HBV or HCV infection (previous blood transfusion or I/V drug abuser)

Examiner: How would you like to investigate this case?

Candidate: I would like to perform baseline blood tests, which include FBC looking for any evidence of:
- Anemia (due to chronic blood loss from underlying malignancy or esophageal varices or due to as a part of anemia of chronic disease)
- Low platelet count (as a consequence of portal hypertension)
- High ESR and CRP (due to chronic infection or malignancy)

Synthetic liver function, in particular (to see any evidence of liver disease)
- Abnormal LFTs with low albumin levels and raised PT

Renal function:
- Urine R/E
- Creatinine and electrolytes (looking for any renal disease or coexistent renal impairment)

Imaging tests include:
- A chest X-ray to see any evidence of pleural effusion, mediastinal lymphadenopathy, or any mass lesion.
- Importantly an abdominal ultrasound (to see any evidence of CLD, particularly hepatosplenomegaly, confirmation of ascites or intra-abdominal mass or lymphadenopathy, or evidence of portal hypertension by Doppler study)
- CT scan
- An endoscopy to exclude underlying malignancy or esophageal varices.
- If history suggests, I will go for colonoscopy (to exclude the lower GIT malignancy)

The most important test would be ascitic fluid analysis with:
- Ascitic fluid albumin, total protein, ADA, amylase, triglyceride, glucose, and LDH
- Ascitic fluid total and differential white cell count
- Ascitic fluid gram stain and culture (for conventional microbes and acid-fast bacilli) and gene expert test for TB
- Ascitic fluid malignant cell.

As this patient has supraclavicular lymphadenopathy, another important test would be supraclavicular lymph node FNAC (less invasive) or biopsy (invasive and best test).

CT scan of the chest and abdomen: If the above measures fail to detect the cause of ascites, I would like to proceed with a more invasive test—diagnostic laparoscopic laparotomy and peritoneal biopsy.

Examiner: Would you like to tell me some characteristics of ascitic fluid in different clinical situations?

Candidate: I would expect:

In case of malignancy: Lymphocyte predominant exudative ascites, usually hemorrhagic or bloody with low glucose and with or without malignant cell.

Tubercular ascites: Lymphocyte predominant exudative ascites, usually transparent or serous fluid with low glucose and high ADA.

Liver cirrhosis: Transudative ascites with few cells and serous appearance.

In case of spontaneous bacterial peritonitis: Caused by a single organism with transudative ascites with WBC >500 cells/mm^3 (>50% neutrophil or >250 cell/UL neutrophil).

In secondary bacterial peritonitis: Neutrophil predominant polymicrobial, exudative ascites with high LDH (>225 mU/L), low glucose (<50 mg/dL), and high amylase.

In pancreatic ascites (due to acute pancreatitis): Exudative ascites with high amylase, low LDH (<225 mU/L), low glucose (<50 mg/dL).

In case of chylous ascites (due to lymphatic obstruction): Exudative ascites with the characteristic milky-white appearance and a high triglyceride level (> 1.1 g/L or 110 mg/dL) confirm it.

Examiner: How do you classify transudative and exudative ascites in patients with low serum albumin?

Candidate: This can be done by calculation of Serum Ascitic Albumin Gradient (SAAG);

The SAAG indirectly measures portal pressure and can be used to determine if ascites are due to portal hypertension.

SAAG calculation: SAAG = (serum albumin) − (ascitic fluid albumin)
- A high SAAG (>1.1 g/dL) suggests the ascitic fluid is a transudate.
- A low SAAG (<1.1 g/dL) suggests the ascitic fluid is an exudate.

A high SAAG (i.e., transudate) suggests the presence of portal hypertension:
- Cirrhosis, hepatic failure, hepatic venous occlusion—e.g., Budd–Chiari syndrome, sinusoidal obstruction syndrome (veno-occlusive disease), fulminant hepatic failure, alcoholic hepatitis, kwashiorkor malnutrition, and cardiac failure.

Causes of a low SAAG (i.e., exudate) include:
- Malignancy (hepatic/peritoneal), infection (TB), acute pancreatitis, nephrotic syndrome, and hypothyroidism (rarely)

Examiner: Let us think a patient presented to you with ascites where ascitic protein is 30 g/L, and SAAG is >11 g/L. What will be the cause of these findings?

Candidate: On this patient, the most likely cause of high SAAG and high protein would be:

Portal hypertension, due to extrahepatic, causes Budd–Chiari syndrome or veno-occlusive disease.

Very rarely, around 30% of cases, a cirrhotic patient may present with high SAAG and high protein, although a cirrhotic patient typically presented with a low protein <25 g/L and a high SAAG > 11 g/L.

Examiner: Is there any alternative way that can differentiate it?

Candidate: An alternative way of differentiating between exudate and transudate is using lactate dehydrogenase activity (LDH), which is also measured from ascitic fluid.
- LDH <225 U/L = transudate
- LDH > 225U/L = exudate

The use of SAAG has mostly replaced this.

Hepatosplenomegaly

Mr Harry, a 50-year-old man, presented with fever and abdominal fullness. Examine his abdomen and present your findings.

(After finishing GIT examination within 6 minutes of time)

Candidate: I would like to complete my examination by looking at the patient's observation chart, examining hernia orifices, external genitalia, doing PR, and urine dipsticks.

Examiner: Would you like to present your case, please?

Candidate:

This patient has hepatosplenomegaly; the liver is enlarged 4 cm from the costal margin, which is nontender and firm in consistency; the spleen is enlarged up to 3 fingers breadth from the costal margin along its long axis, which is also nontender and firm in consistency.

The patient is anemic, and there are bilateral cervical and supraclavicular lymphadenopathy, which are firm, nontender, discrete, and freely mobile.

The patient is non-icteric, and there is no other evidence of stigmata of CLD.

No evidence of rheumatoid hand or butterfly rash.

I would like to take a full history from the patient to reach my diagnosis. As the patient has fever, hepatosplenomegaly, anemia, and lymphadenopathy, the most likely possibilities are:

Lymphoproliferative disease including CLL or ALL or lymphoma and rarely CMV, EBV, TB, or sarcoidosis.

Examiner: Let us think this patient has no lymphadenopathy. Then what would be your differential diagnosis?

Candidate: Then, I would like to think about the myeloproliferative disorder and tropical infections such as malaria or kala-azar.

Examiner: Okay! However, if this patient is presented with anemia, jaundice, spider nevi, venous hum, an engorged vein in addition to hepatosplenomegaly, what do these indicate?

Candidate: It indicates CLD with portal hypertension. The cirrhotic liver is often small and impalpable. However, some exceptions are alcoholic liver disease, NASH or PBC, as well as cirrhosis complicated by hepatoma.

Examiner: That's fine. Imagine a patient of pancreatic malignancy presented with anemia, jaundice, ascites, supraclavicular lymphadenopathy, and hepatosplenomegaly. Now how will you explain these signs to me?

Candidate: There are lots of signs that have developed in this case; I would like to explain this, respectively.

- In case of anemia—this is due to multiple causes such as chronic blood loss, nutritional deficiency, or bone marrow infiltration.
- Jaundice may be due to CBD obstruction (due to head of pancreas malignancy) or liver metastasis.
- Ascites may be due to peritoneal dissemination or hepatic vein thrombosis (e.g., Budd–Chiari syndrome) as malignancy is a hypercoagulable state that increases the risk of venous thrombosis.
- Hepatomegaly due to liver metastasis or hepatic vein thrombosis leading to Budd–Chiari syndrome.
- Splenomegaly due to portal or hepatic vein thrombosis, as malignancy is a hyper-

coagulable state that increases the risk of thrombosis.
- Lymphadenopathy is mainly due to lymph node metastasis.

Examiner: If you have a patient with a hard, knobbly enlarged liver, what will be the possible causes for it?

Candidate: The likely possibilities are:
- Malignancy (either primary or secondary)
- Polycystic liver disease
- Macronodular cirrhosis (following hepatitis B with widespread necrosis)
- Hydatid cysts (may be eosinophilia; rupture may cause by anaphylaxis)
- Syphilitic gummas (late benign syphilis; rapid response to penicillin)

Examiner: How would you differentiate between a splenic and renal mass?

Candidate: The four characteristics of a splenic mass are as follows:
1. Dull to percussion
2. Not ballotable
3. Palpable splenic notch
4. The palpating finger cannot get above a splenic mass.

Isolated Splenomegaly

Mr Steven, a 55-year-old man, presented with abdominal fullness. Examine his abdomen and present your findings.

(After finishing GIT examination within 6 minutes of time)

Candidate: I would like to complete my examination by looking at the patient's observation chart, examining hernia orifices, external genitalia, doing PR, and urine dipsticks.

Examiner: Would you like to present your case, please?

Candidate:

This patient has an enlarged spleen up to 6 fingers breadth from the costal margin along its long axis, which is nontender and firm in consistency.

The patient is anemic, but there are no stigmata of CLD.

No evidence of lymphadenopathy or hepatomegaly.

No evidence of rheumatoid hand or butterfly rash.

No bony deformity, hypotonia, or short stature.

This patient has isolated massive splenomegaly with anemia; at this point, my differential diagnosis would be chronic myeloid leukemia, myelofibrosis, malaria, and kala-azar.

Examiner: Tell me some causes of splenomegaly.

Candidate: In case of massive splenomegaly (>8 cm): The causes are—
- Myeloproliferative disorder (CML, myelofibrosis)
- Tropical infections such as kala-azar, malaria
- AIDS with myocardium avium complex

In case of moderate splenomegaly (4–8 cm):
- Lymphoproliferative disorders (CLL, lymphoma) are usually associated with lymphadenopathy.
- Portal hypertension
- Thalassemia
- Glycogen and lipid storage diseases (e.g., Gaucher's disease) and other causes of massive splenomegaly.

In case of mild splenomegaly:
- Other myeloproliferative disorders (e.g., polycythemia rubra vera)
- Hemolysis
- Infections (e.g., EBV, infective endocarditis)
- Autoimmune disease (e.g., RA, SLE)
- Infiltrative conditions (e.g., amyloid, sarcoid)

Examiner: What important history would you want to take from this patient to proceed with a diagnosis?

Candidate: I would like to ask about constitutional symptoms first, such as:

Is there any fever, night sweats, malaise, or any weight loss?—these may suggest an underlying infective, malignant or autoimmune condition, or represented as B-symptoms in NHL.

Is there any fatigue, malaise or bleeding manifestations?—that indicates pancytopenia.

Any history of bones or joint pain?—that may indicate myeloproliferative diseases or secondary hyperuricemia-induced gout.

Is any history suggestive of autoimmune diseases such as RA or Felty's syndrome? Is any history suggestive of liver disease, malignancy, or lymphoma?

Is any history of using radiation therapy, chemotherapy, immunosuppressive therapy, or organ transplantation?

Are any risk factors for HIV infection?

Is any recent travel history specifically to malaria and kala-azar endemic zone?

Examiner: Can you please tell me how would you investigate a patient with splenomegaly?

Candidate: I would like to start with routine blood tests such as FBC with ESR with peripheral blood film, thick and thin film for malaria, LFT's, and U&E's.

Other blood tests include serum LDH, Beta-2 microglobulin, autoimmune profile, and HIV testing.

The next important tests would be imaging that includes:
- Chest X-ray
- USG (initially to evaluate splenomegaly) as well as evidence of CLD.
- CT scan of the chest, abdomen, and pelvis will be required to evaluate lymphadenopathy or disseminated malignancy.
- PET scan is highly sensitive for NHL (although not specific, and may also be positive in infection or metastatic malignancy)

Another important test would be:
- Lymph node excision biopsy rather than FNAC (intact tissue is required for histological assessment) if associated lymphadenopathy.
- Furthermore, bone marrow biopsy (this will diagnose conditions such as lipid storage diseases, mycobacterial infection, kala-azar, granulomatous diseases, lymphoid or myeloid disorders and also required to evaluate for extranodal disease during the staging of NHL's).

Examiner: Let us think you have a patient with splenomegaly, anemia, and lymphadenopathy. Now tell me, what will be the possible causes for these findings?

Candidate: The patient has splenomegaly, anemia, and lymphadenopathy; I think the most likely cause would be lymphoproliferative disorders (usually associated with hepatomegaly):
- Leukemia (ALL, CLL) or lymphoma
  Next, I would like to think about malignancy.
- Here splenic vein thrombosis may cause splenomegaly and may have hepatomegaly due to liver metastasis.

And also, Felty's syndrome (look for rheumatoid hand and nodules).

Examiner: If splenomegaly is associated with anemia and jaundice without any stigmata of CLD, what would be the reasons for it?

Candidate: Most likely, this would be a case of hereditary (e.g., hereditary spherocytosis, thalassemia) or acquired hemolytic anemia (e.g., AHA).

Rarely this would be a case of SLE, pernicious anemia, or infective endocarditis.

Examiner: Well said. Now would you like to tell me, if splenomegaly is present with facial plethora and conjunctival injection, what might be the cause?

Candidate: This would be a case of polycythemia rubra vera.

Examiner: Let us think you have a patient with short stature and yellow-brown skin pigmentation. On examination, you have found splenomegaly, bony deformity, and hypotonia. Now tell me, what do you think the diagnosis is here?

Candidate: Putting all of these together, my possible diagnosis would be lysosomal storage disease (Gaucher's disease).

Hemolytic Anemia (Hereditary Spherocytosis)

Mrs Jenifer, a 25-year-old North European lady, presented with weakness. Examine her abdomen and present your findings.

(After finishing GIT examination within 6 minutes of time)

Candidate: I would like to complete my examination by examining hernial orifices, external genitalia, digital rectal examination, and urine dipstick and looking at the patient observation chart.

Examiner: Would you present your case, please?

Candidate:

I believe this lady has had hemolytic anemia.

Positive findings include:

She is moderately anemic and mildly icteric but has no stigmata of CLD. She has splenomegaly which is 5 cm from the costal margin and along its long axis.

The underlying cause of this triad of anemia, jaundice, and splenomegaly would be hemolytic anemia.

Here the causes of hemolytic anemia would be hereditary, such as hereditary spherocytosis, hereditary elliptocytosis, thalassemia, sickle cell anemia (but in case of sickle cell anemia, auto splenectomy is an expected finding).

It may be acquired autoimmune hemolytic anemia. Or, it may be secondary hemolytic anemia due to SLE, infective endocarditis, other infections such as infectious mononucleosis or lymphoproliferative disorder.

In this case, secondary hemolytic anemia would be unlikely due to the absence of other stigmata of these disorders.

Examiner: Let us think—the patient has a strong family history of hematological disorder—such as her mother had a history of severe anemia during her childhood, and she was treated by combined splenectomy and cholecystectomy; then what would be your diagnosis?

Candidate: In this clinical scenario of the young European leady—my diagnosis would be hereditary spherocytosis. Half of the affected adults have gallstone, mainly when the hemolysis is severe. However, in a severe case of hereditary spherocytosis, a combined splenectomy and cholecystectomy is not uncommon.

Examiner: She does indeed have hereditary spherocytosis; how is it inherited?

Candidate: It is usually inherited in autosomal dominant fashion and mainly due to defect in one of the five different genes that encode for protein (beta-spectrin protein) of RBC membrane in chromosome 8 that causes the characteristic spherical structure of RBC, which are rapidly cleared in the spleen leading to extravascular hemolysis and splenomegaly.

Examine: How does the patient with HH usually present?

Candidate: Most of the patients usually presents with a classical triad as in this lady include anemia, jaundice, and splenomegaly.

Sometimes it could be an asymptomatic presentation, particularly through the screening program of first degree relatives with hereditary spherocytosis.

Examiner: Okay.... now tell me, how will you investigate the case?

Candidate: The initial test would be a complete blood count with peripheral blood film with the typical appearance of spherocytes.

Unconjugated bilirubin, serum LDH, and reticulocyte count would be high, and serum haptoglobin will be low or absent.

I would like to do a Coombs test to exclude the differential diagnosis of an immune-mediated hemolysis that may give rise to spherocytosis in the blood film.

The more specific test for hereditary spherocytosis (HS) would be EMA binding, an eosin-based fluorescent dye that binds RBC membrane protein. The mean fluorescence is lower with HS detected using flow cytometry.

If EMA binding test is not always available, I would do an osmotic fragility test, although the sensitivity and specificity of this test are low. This test measures the RBC resistance to hemolysis while being exposed to varying levels of dilution of a solid solution.

Examiner: Tell me about the complications of HS.

Candidate: The most concerning complication is that of aplastic crisis and usually precipitated by infections such as parvovirus infection-causing BM suppression; in that case, a high rate of destruction of RBC can no longer be compensated for increased production.

Anemia is the principal concern in HS and may require a serial blood transfusion.

Biliary colic and obstruction are frequent complications as gallstones are found in 50% of cases (right upper abdominal pain may be the presenting problem due to acute cholecystitis leading to the diagnosis of HS in many patients).

Examiner: What treatment is available for a patient with HS?

Candidate: In fact, no therapy is available to target the faulty membrane protein. However, folic acid supplementation is essential—as the requirement is increased with the increased RBC production, particularly during pregnancy.

After this, we have to treat the complications such as a patient with anemia being treated with serial blood transfusion.

Splenectomy is indicated in moderate to severe symptomatic hereditary spherocytosis. However, it is associated with a 200 fold increase in mortality risk from infections. The spleen contains macrophages, which filter and phagocytose bacteria. Postsplenectomy infection is caused most commonly by encapsulated organisms; *Neisseria meningitis*, *Streptococcus pneumonia*, and *Haemophilus influenzae*. So a patient who undergoes splenectomy will require prior vaccination to be administered, and after this, they will need to keep up to date with his/her vaccination status, particularly his/her meningococcal and pneumococcal vaccines and his/her influenza vaccines need to keep up to date.

The patient should also receive prophylactic penicillin to reduce the risk of infection.

Another important step would be a bracelet or patient holding the alert card to the next medical staff, and she should advise seeking urgent medical attention, may require admission for broad-spectrum intravenous antibiotics if an infection develops.

If she travels abroad—I would like to warn him regarding the risk of severe malaria and advise adequate prophylaxis with medication (antimalarial), repellent, and nets.

Autosomal Dominant Polycystic Kidney Disease

Mrs Ann, a 54-year-old lady, complained of abdominal fullness. Examine her abdomen and present your findings.

(After finishing GIT examination within 6 minutes of time)

Candidate: I would like to complete my examination by looking at the patient's observation chart, examining hernia orifices, external genitalia, doing PR, and urine dipsticks.

Examiner: Would you like to present your case, please?

Candidate:

I believe this patient has autosomal dominant polycystic kidney disease with ESRD.

On examination:

She has a distended abdomen with bilateral ballotable flank masses that do not move with respiration, resonant percussion note, and I can get above these masses.

There are also scars from previous vascular access sites (A-V shunt) for hemodialysis with evidence of recent needling in AV-fistulae.

No evidence of hepatosplenomegaly.

She is euvolemic (normal JVP, no peripheral edema) and not anemic.

(Please mention if other evidence of ESRD such as half and half nail, scratch mark, and parathyroidectomy scar if present).

Examiner: What are the extrarenal manifestations of autosomal dominant polycystic kidney disease (ADPKD)?

Candidate:
- Hypertension due to excess renin release
- Polycythemia due to excess erythropoietin release
- Cerebral aneurysms—subarachnoid hemorrhage as a consequence of a ruptured cerebral aneurysm, which is the most serious complication of ADPKD. Aneurysms occur in 4% of younger patients and up to 10% of older patients.
- Other extrarenal cysts, such as liver cysts, are present in up to 70% of cases and rarely cause symptoms—pancreatic cysts in 9% of cases and splenic cysts in 5% of patients. The cyst has also been reported in the thyroid, parathyroid, lung, pituitary gland, ovary, uterus, testes, seminal vesicles, epididymis, bladder, and peritoneum.
- Valvular heart diseases—aortic regurgitation and mitral valve prolapse causing MR are more common in these populations.

Examiner: Tell me, how would you evaluate extrarenal features in a patient with ADPKD?

Candidate: As ADPKD is a multi-system disorder, I would like to look for other features and associations of the disease and proceed as follows:
- Blood pressure measurement—to look for hypertension that predates the onset of renal failure.
- Cardiovascular system examination—for any evidence of mitral valve prolapse, aortic regurgitation, and left ventricular heave.
- Neurological system examination—for evidence of old stroke due to ruptured berry aneurysm or 3rd nerve palsy due to compression by the posterior communicating artery aneurysm.

Examiner: What are the usual presentations of a patient with autosomal dominant polycystic kidney disease?

Candidate: They may present with:
- Hypertension
- Signs and symptoms of renal failure (which usually starts in the fourth decade of life)
- Proteinuria
- Hematuria
- Symptoms associated with the extrarenal manifestations of polycystic kidney disease include cysts in the liver, pancreas, spleen, epididymis, or thyroid.
- Loin pain may occur due to a hemorrhage or infection in the cysts or renal stone.

Examiner: Tell me, what do you know about the genetics of adult polycystic kidney disease?

Candidate: This is typically an autosomal dominant disease. A variety of genetic defects have been described.
- Autosomal recessive polycystic kidney disease 1 accounts for 85% of cases and has been associated with a mutation in chromosome 16. Moreover, ADPKD2 has been associated with a mutation in chromosome 4.
- Autosomal recessive polycystic kidney disease is a rare disease, presenting in infancy and frequently causing severe renal and liver diseases.

Examiner: As we know, ADPKD is an autosomal dominant disease; how would you screen a patient with positive family history?

Candidate: In case of adults (age 20 or more), screening can be done by imaging, such as:

USG: Diagnostic criteria in patients with positive family history:
- Two unilateral or bilateral cysts for; age <30 years
- Two cysts in each kidney for; age 30–59 years
- Four cysts in each kidney for; age >60 years

Contrast-enhanced CT or MRI: More sensitive than USG—

In case of a younger patient (age <20 years): Genetic testing is the most appropriate strategy to investigate younger with a family history of ADPKD. The major indication for genetic screening in ADPKD is for subjects who are considering donating a kidney to a relative affected by the disease.

Examiner: Now tell me, how would you treat someone with PKD?

Candidate:
- Control of blood pressure is the primary step of management, ideally with ACE inhibitors or ARB. There should also be aggressive control of hyperlipidemia as CKD is a major risk factor for ischemic heart disease.
- Adequate nutritional supplementation—patients should be on a high fluid, low salt diet. Phosphate binders if high serum phosphate.
- Anemia should be corrected by adequate iron replacement and erythropoietin if needed.
- In CKD stage I-III, vasopressin receptor antagonist, e.g., tolvaptan, may be of use.
- If the serum PTH is elevated, Vitamin D supplementation should be considered.
- For persistent hyperparathyroidism, I would consider calcimimetics or parathyroidectomy.
- In case of ESRD, the patient may require RRT and/or renal transplant.

Examiner: Tell me some indications of MRA in an ADPKD patient.

Candidate: Indications for MRA are as follows:
- Family history of stroke or intracranial aneurysms.
- Development of symptoms suggesting an intracranial aneurysm (complete or surgical 3rd nerve palsy).
- Job or hobby in which a loss of consciousness may be lethal.
- Previous history of intracranial aneurysms.

Examiner: Do you know of the indications for a nephrectomy polycystic kidney?

Candidate: Nephrectomy should be avoided; however, at times, it may be required. One indication is to make room for a transplanted kidney if massively enlarged. Other indications would be:
- Progression to renal cell carcinoma,
- Persistent pain,

- Recurrent pyelonephritis
- Large and significant hematuria
- Recurrent stone formation

Examiner: Tell me, what do you know about end-stage renal failure in ADPKD?

Candidate: ESRD occurs in 50% of ADPKD patients by 60 years of age.

Mean age of onset is 56 years (truncating PKD1 mutations), 68 years (nontruncating PKD1 mutations), or 78 years (PKD2 mutations).

Patients with ADPKD who progress to end-stage renal disease may require the following procedures—hemodialysis, peritoneal dialysis, or renal transplantation.

Kidney transplantation is the optimal kidney replacement treatment, and the results in ADPKD patients are better than in the general ESRD population.

Although ADPKD is not a contraindication for peritoneal dialysis, it is less commonly used than hemodialysis given the challenge of accommodating a large volume of peritoneal dialysate and an increased risk of abdominal wall hernias. In hemodialysis treatment, patients with ADPKD may have an increased risk of aneurysmal dilatation of arteriovenous fistulas.

Examiner: Would you always need to perform a nephrectomy before transplantation?

Candidate: It does not always need to perform a nephrectomy. Ideally, the new kidney will be transplanted with both of the old kidneys left in place. However, on occasion, it may be necessary simply to make room for the new kidney if the existing kidney is massively enlarged.

Examiner: Let us think you are a doctor in A&E's, and a patient presented with left loin pain. On examination, the patient has a left-sided palpable kidney. Now tell me, what would be the differentials for a single palpable kidney?

Candidate: My important differential diagnosis for a single palpable kidney would be:
- Polycystic kidney disease (with only one palpable kidney)
- Hydronephrosis—rarely palpable; can be due to ureteric obstruction.
- Hypertrophy of a single functioning kidney
- Or renal cell carcinoma.

Examiner: You mentioned bilateral renal cysts in ADPKD. Do you know of any other conditions that cause bilateral renal cysts?

Candidate: Although the most common cause of bilateral renal cysts is ADPKD, there are some other diseases also, such as:
- Multiple simple cysts
- Tuberous sclerosis
- Von Hippel–Lindau syndrome
- Meckel–Gruber syndrome
- Laurence–Moon–Bardet–Biedl syndrome
- Trisomies: 13 (Patau syndrome), 18 (Edward syndrome), 21 (Down syndrome)

Examiner: Can you please tell me how will you identify hepatomegaly along with a cystic kidney?

Candidate: In patients with hepatomegaly and right renal mass, it may be difficult to palpate above the renal mass. This may falsely indicate the presence of a single large renal mass. However, detecting the presence of a descending liver edge in inspiration, the resonant percussion over the mass below the liver edge and the ballotable nature of the mass will help diagnose both hepatomegaly and a renal mass.

Examiner: Okay! Now tell me some causes of bilateral palpable kidneys.

Candidate: It would include bilateral renal cysts (e.g., ADPKD), bilateral hydronephrosis, amyloidosis, bilateral renal cell carcinoma (occurs in von Hippel–Lindau syndrome).

Renal Transplant

Mrs Salena, a 63-year-old woman, complained of abdominal tenderness. Examine her abdomen and present your findings.

(After finishing GIT examination within 6 minutes of time)

Candidate: I would like to complete my examination by looking at the patient's observation chart, examining hernial orifices, external genitalia, digital rectal examination, and urine dipstick.

Examiner: Would you like to present your case, please?

Candidate:

I examined this elderly lady. Based on my clinical findings, I believe this patient has had a functioning renal transplant for renal failure due to adult polycystic kidney disease.

This lady is lying comfortably in bed with an average body built.

On inspection, there is a large 'J' shaped scar with fullness in the right flank and an impression of swelling under the scar in the RIF.

On palpation, there is an easily palpable rounded mass under the scar, which feels like a kidney in the RIF, that is not tender (tenderness suggests graft rejection or graft infection) and has no bruit.

She has bilateral ballotable masses in her loins that I can get above and that does not move with respiration, suggesting polycystic kidneys.

She does have a palpable AV fistula with a palpable thrill in the left arm. However, there was no evidence of recent needling.

No other organomegaly was detected.

There is no evidence of ongoing RRT or transplant failure (evidence of volume overloads such as raised JVP and edema).

There is no evidence of other access points for hemodialysis.

No evidence of toxicity from immunosuppression, e.g., gum hypertrophy (cyclosporine), tremor, hirsutism, evidence of skin malignancies, or thinning of the skin or other symptoms that may be associated with steroid use (truncal obesity, rounded plethoric face, petechiae, striae rubra, and ecchymosis).

Examiner: Let us think, you have a patient with nonpalpable kidneys. What may be the other clinical signs you look for the causes of renal transplant here?

Candidate: In the absence of evidence indicating the underlying pathology of the native kidney, such as ballotable renal masses in ADPKD, the likely underlying cause for ESRF is chronic glomerulonephritis.

Most importantly, I would search for diabetic nephropathy; here, I would expect:
- BM stick marks on fingertips, necrobiosis lipoidica, diabetic dermopathy, Charcot joint for DM.
- Lipodystrophy at sites of insulin injection.

In the case of Alport's disease—hearing aids and other features of nephrotoxicity and ototoxicity.

In the case of mesangiocapillary glomerulonephritis, type 2 is usually associated with facial lipodystrophy.

Examiner: You carefully identified the palpable transplanted mass in the RIF. Can you offer some differential diagnoses for that mass in the RIF?

Candidate: Commonly, it may be a case of cecal carcinoma, Crohn's disease, or ileocecal tuberculosis. Rare possibilities are—ileocecal abscess (e.g., Ameobiasis or *Yersinia* spp.), lymphoma, ovarian tumor (in a female), appendicular lump or abscess.

Examiner: This patient has a functioning renal transplant. So, if you have had a kidney transplant that is not working properly, what are the findings you may expect clinically?

Candidate: I would expect this patient may have evidence of:
- Volume overload (raised JVP, sacral/peripheral edema, and fine crepitations at lung base for pulmonary edema without evidence of heart failure)
- Graft tenderness
- Fever or any evidence of infection
- Any evidence of actively used means of vascular excess, e.g., evidence of recent needling in the arteriovenous (AV) fistula, a current central line for hemodialysis, and Tenckhoff catheter in situ for peritoneal dialysis.
- Signs of uremia (excoriation of the skin in response to pruritus, fetor, distal sensory-motor neuropathy, signs of uremic pericarditis).
- And finally, I would like to take a history of oliguria (urine output checking).

Examiner: When would you start discussing with the patient and working the patient up for transplantation?

Candidate: Patients should be worked up for transplantation as they approach end-stage renal failure (eGFR <15 mL/minute) but before they require dialysis (peritoneal or hemodialysis).

When they receive transplantation is based on the availability of donors. It is known that transplanting patients before they end up on mainly hemodialysis carries a better prognosis.

Examiner: You mentioned immunosuppression and how this patient does not have any obvious side effects or toxicity from immunosuppression. Tell me, what are the possible side effects or complications of long-term immunosuppression?

Candidate: Most drugs can predispose to infection and malignancy, which may be detected on clinical examination, particularly:

- Skin malignancies such as squamous cell carcinoma, basal cell carcinoma or post-transplant lymphoproliferative disease or lymphoma (previous biopsy or resection scar mark for SCC/BCC).
- Steroids can lead to thinning of the skin, purpura with characteristic easy bruising, and fat redistribution with a cushingoid appearance.
- Cyclosporine can lead to tremors, hirsutism and gingival hyperplasia and cause renal impairment itself.
- Tacrolimus can lead to neurotoxicity (tremor, seizure, blurred vision, encephalopathy), Q-T prolongation and can also cause diabetes (new-onset diabetes after transplant/NODAT).

Examiner: If a renal transplant patient has a surgical scar on the neck, what will be the cause for it?

Candidate: I would think that the scar may be a parathyroidectomy scar as a consequence of tertiary hyperparathyroidism, which may develop in a patient with end-stage renal failure.

Examiner: Tell me some contraindications to renal transplant.

Candidate: The contraindications include:
- Recent or active malignancy.
- Active infection (e.g., TB).
- Active vasculitis such as ANCA-positive vasculitis.
- A severe respiratory condition such as severe COPD or pulmonary fibrosis, uncontrolled asthma.
- Severe ischemic heart disease.
- Severe peripheral vascular disease such as a large uncontrollable abdominal aneurysm.
- Severe obesity (BMI >40) due to the technical difficulty.
- Donor matching.

Examiner: As we know, commonly, a kidney transplant is placed in the pelvis. Can you tell me why it is done here?

Candidate: Because of:
- Good blood supply
- There is sufficient space for the kidney.

- Proximity to the bladder for ureteric anastomosis
- Easy access to perform renal biopsies or nephrostomies (in the event of a ureteric stricture) without puncturing the peritoneum or risk abdominal viscera.

(A kidney can be transplanted on either side of the pelvis, depending on the quality of the vascular supply, and venous drainage. As many patients with ESRD have diabetes, vasculopathy is expected; therefore, an assessment of the arterial supply during transplant workup is important).

Examiner: What is the commonest cause of death in a patient with a renal transplant?

Candidate: The commonest cause of death in all patients with renal disease is vascular (MI or CVD). After this, the commonest causes of death are infections and malignancy. Both are related to chronic immunosuppression.

Liver Transplantation

Mr John, a 62-year-old man, presented with abdominal discomfort. Examine his abdomen and present your findings.

(After finishing GIT examination within 6 minutes of time)

Candidate: I would like to complete my examination by looking at the patient's observation chart, examining hernial orifices, external genitalia, digital rectal examination, and urine dipstick.

Examiner: Would you like to present your case, please?

Candidate:

I believe this patient has a functioning liver transplant due to alcoholic liver disease.

Positive findings include:

He has a classic bilateral rooftop with a sternal extension scar (Mercedes–Benz scar). Two further scars are inferior to this, suggestive of postoperative drain sites.

No palpable liver edge

In terms of the etiology of liver transplantation, he had evidence of gynecomastia, Dupuytren's contracture, and also evidence of enlarged parotid bilaterally.

I think his graft is functioning well as there are no other stigmata of CLD such as jaundice, leukonychia. There are no signs of portal hypertension (splenomegaly, ascites, caput medusa), as well as no signs of encephalopathy (flapping tremors, confusion).

He has also no evidence of complications from immunosuppression such as gum hypertrophy, tremor, or cushingoid appearance.

Examiner: So, you have a diagnosis of post-liver transplant, and you also carefully noted all-important physical findings. Now tell me how you will investigate the case?

Candidate: At first, I would like to take a full history from the patient, mainly focusing on the underlying cause of the liver transplant, recent symptoms of liver disease, recent drug and alcohol history.

In terms of investigations, I would like to start with an assessment of the function of the graft. Then, I would like to do routine liver function tests, including synthetic function with serum albumin and clotting profile (e.g., PT).

Then I would like to do a FBC, including inflammatory markers, particularly in view of immunosuppression.

Moreover, I would like to emphasize the potential for renal insufficiency with the need for routine renal function testing, including U/E's, serum creatinine, and urine R/M/E.

Finally, where there is a doubt regarding the diagnosis, a CT would better evaluate the abdominal anatomy and where there is a suspicion of postoperative complications such as infection, collection, anastomotic leak or stricture, the threshold for performing such imaging would be low.

Examiner: Ok. So, how will you manage this case?

Candidate: This may involve discussing the current treatment options prior to transplantation and the underlying cause. In transplant patients, there is a need for immunosuppression, and current immunosuppressive regimens are corticosteroids in combination with a calcineurin inhibitor such as tacrolimus or ciclosporin and an antiproliferative agent such as mycophenolate mofetil.

Then there should be regular review and surveillance for rejection with tapering of immunosuppression when possible.

Examiner: You mentioned this patient has a Mercedes–Benz Scar due to liver transplantation. Tell me some other differentials of this scar.

Candidate: A Mercedes–Benz Scar should indicate a large upper abdominal operation. The differential diagnosis for these operations would include:
- A liver transplant
- Radical gastrectomy
- Whipple's procedure
- Bilateral adrenalectomies can also be carried out through a Mercedes–Benz scar.

Examiner: Let us think this patient has another scar mark in the left iliac fossa and a mass directly underneath it. What do you think about it? What are the possibilities?

Candidate: If there are a scar and a mass in the left iliac fossa, it is more likely to be the renal allograft of simultaneous kidney-liver transplantation, which can be done in the following situations:
- Paracetamol overdose
- Cirrhosis and hepatorenal syndrome
- Polycystic kidney and liver disease (ADPKD)
- Glomerulopathy associated with alcoholic cirrhosis or with chronic hepatitis B or C infections
- Metabolic diseases, such as primary hyperoxaluria.

Examiner: You have a diagnosis of a liver transplant due to alcoholic liver disease. So, tell me, what positive aspects do you have for this? Moreover, what are the other indications of liver transplants?

Candidate: If there is no evidence of the underlying cause of native liver failure, then I am aware of the commonest indication for liver transplantation in alcoholic liver disease. However, he has evidence of Dupuytren's contracture and enlarged parotid bilaterally, so I suspect this is a case of a liver transplant due to alcoholic liver disease.

Other possible indications are:
- Cirrhosis (this may be due to a large number of conditions including but not limited to alcoholic liver disease, nonalcoholic fatty liver disease, chronic viral hepatitis, autoimmune liver diseases, hemochromatosis, Wilson's disease, or alpha-1-antitrypsin deficiency)
- HCC, and
- Acute fulminant liver failure (the most common cause in the UK being paracetamol overdose)

Examiner: Is there any way that you will be able to detect the underlying liver disease from examining a transplant patient?

Candidate: It is difficult always that I will be able to detect the underlying liver disease from examining the patient only. In that case, I would like to take a detailed history from the patient. However, I would expect some clues during my examination, such as:
- The presence of a scar from venesection usually in the cubital fossa, bonze pigmentation, evidence of arthropathy, fingertip pinprick for diabetes, and associated clinical signs of cardiomyopathy, which may indicate an underlying diagnosis of hemochromatosis.
- Tattoos and evidence of I/V drug abusers could suggest chronic viral hepatitis. Hepatitis C is also associated with porphyria cutanea tarda and cryoglobulinemia, and here we can find purpura and livedo reticularis.
- Significant xanthelasma, tendon xanthoma, excoriation marks, and generalized pigmentation could suggest primary biliary cirrhosis (now known as primary biliary cholangitis).
- Signs of lower zone emphysema in the chest may suggest alpha-1-antitrypsin deficiency.
- Loss of hepatic jugular reflux indicates Budd–Chiari syndrome.
- Kayser–Fleischer ring and Akinetic-rigid syndrome indicate Wilson's disease.
- Raised JVP, third heart sound indicate CCF.

Examiner: Please tell me, what do you know about acute fulminant liver failure?

Candidate: Acute liver failure is defined as a multi-system disorder in which severe acute impairment of liver function with encephalopathy occurs within 8 weeks of the onset of symptoms and no recognized underlying CLD.

Examiner: Let us think you have a liver transplant patient, now presented with ascites, asterixis, and jaundice. What does it indicate for this patient?

Candidate: With all of these findings, I would think this patient is now in hepatic decompensation. The presence of asterixis or ascites is strongly suggestive of inadequate graft function. Jaundice may also be an indicator of graft dysfunction, particularly if other signs of decompensation are noted.

Examiner: If a patient presented with jaundice but has no evidence of CLD, portal hypertension, ascites, or encephalopathy related to his/her transplant, then what will be the cause of his/her jaundice?

Candidate: It seems that the patient's liver transplant is working very well, I would consider the case may be extrahepatic (may be due to hemolysis) in nature and would want to investigate for this by doing direct and indirect bilirubin, including other tests.

Examiner: The transplant itself may or may not be palpable. If a transplanted liver is easily palpable, then what does it mean?

Candidate: If a transplanted liver is easily palpable, it does not necessarily mean there is a problem with the graft and could simply reflect a size mismatch between donor and recipient. Usually, no mass is palpable in the right upper quadrant as the new liver is placed in the same place as the old one. Occasionally, a liver edge may be palpable, although hepatomegaly is uncommon in a healthy liver transplant.

Examiner: What are the criteria for referral to a liver unit for transplantation?

Candidate: In the context of liver failure, the KCH (King's College Hospital) criteria identify patients at particularly high risk of death who should be discussed with a liver transplant unit. The KCH criteria divide patients into paracetamol-induced acute liver failure and non-paracetamol-induced liver failure.

In case of paracetamol-induced acute liver failure:
- Arterial lactate >3.5 (4 hours after resuscitation)
- Or PH <7.3 or arterial lactate >3.0 (12 hours after resuscitation)
- Or any 3 of: INR >6.5, Creatinine >300, encephalopathy grade III, or IV

And in case of non-paracetamol-induced acute liver failure:
- Arterial lactate >3.5 (4 hours after resuscitation)
- Or, INR >6.5
- Or any 3 of: INR >3.5, age <10 or >40 years, serum bilirubin >300 mmol/L, time from onset of jaundice to development of coma >7 days, etiology being a drug reaction.

On the other hand, liver transplantation in CLD is generally considered where there is evidence of end-stage cirrhosis.

Renal-pancreas Transplant

Mr Samir, a 58-year-old man, complained of abdominal tenderness. Examine his abdomen and present your findings.

(After finishing GIT examination within 6 minutes of time)

Candidate: I would like to complete my examination by looking at the patient's observations chart, examining hernial orifices, external genitalia, digital rectal examination, urine analysis for proteinuria and glycosuria, and also fundoscopy.

Examiner: Would you like to present your case, please?

Candidate:

On examination of this gentleman, I believe this patient has a combined kidney-pancreas transplant, possibly due to type-1 diabetes mellitus with ESRF, and both are well functioning.

Positive findings include:

There were two scars, one in each iliac fossa. Moreover, typically each of the two scars has a palpable mass directly underneath it.

She does have a palpable AV fistula with a palpable thrill in the left arm. However, there was no evidence of recent needling.

No evidence of bruising from insulin injection or fingertip pinprick marks of glucose monitoring.

No evidence of ongoing RRT or transplant failure and also no evidence of other access points for hemodialysis.

No evidence of toxicity from immunosuppression, e.g., gum hypertrophy, evidence of skin malignancies, thinning of the skin, or other symptoms that may be associated with steroid use.

Examiner: Why has this patient undergone both a kidney-pancreas transplant? What are the benefits of doing it combinedly?

Candidate: A combined kidney-pancreas transplant intends to cure both the patient's diabetes and end-stage renal failure. With the potential that the patient could then be free of hemodialysis and insulin therapy also reduce the risk of vascular complications of diabetes.

Examiner: Can a pancreas transplant reduce all the complications of diabetes?

Candidate: Simultaneous pancreas and kidney transplantation lead to decreased mortality and improved quality of life, avoiding frequent blood sugar monitoring, insulin injections, and dialysis.

It is unclear at this stage whether or not successfully transplanted patients avoid all the long-term complications of diabetes. However, glucose and lipid metabolism are improved, and new diabetic nephropathy is prevented by successful pancreatic transplantation.

Diabetic neuropathy either remains static or else improves, but the effect on retinopathy is not yet clear.

Examiner: Who should receive a combined transplant?

Candidate: Simultaneous pancreas and kidney transplantation are effective for selected patients with poorly controlled diabetes with related end-stage renal disease.

Generally, patients undergoing simultaneous pancreas and kidney transplantation have type 1 diabetes mellitus (T1DM), although it is sometimes performed for type 2 diabetes mellitus (T2DM) if they meet specific criteria.

The decision for selection is made from a combination of outcomes from an MDT meeting and the patient's choice.

Examiner: You mentioned that this patient's transplants are functioning well. Please tell me, what are the points you want to note with a functioning transplant?

Candidate: In the case of functioning pancreas transplant, I would expect the absence of:
- Bruising from insulin injections.
- Fingertip pinprick marks of glucose monitoring.
- Glycosuria on dipstick testing.
- Peripancreatic collection and pancreatitis (mostly seen in the early postoperative period)

In case of functioning renal transplant:
- No evidence of volume overload and
- No tenderness over the transplanted area.

Most importantly, I would check for urinary output. Normal urine output suggests a well-functioning kidney.

Examiner: What type of renal transplantations do you know?

Candidate: Kidney transplant can either be from a life or a deceased donor. Live donors can be related to the patient or can be altruistic donors. Cadaveric donors can be donated after circulatory death or neurological death.

Examiner: Which do you think is better, a live kidney donation or cadaveric combined transplantation?

Candidate: A live kidney has several advantages over a cadaveric kidney in that the donor and the recipient can be brought together in the same hospital, minimizing handling time for the kidney, and it minimizes both warm and cold ischemic time for the donated kidney, hopefully leading to a better graft function.

However, if a patient's diabetes (or his/her underlying cause for renal failure) has not been treated, that disease will likely recur in a kidney. In contrast, a cadaveric kidney and pancreas combined transplant can cure the patient's diabetes and has the potential for a longer-lasting surviving graft over and above an isolated live kidney.

Examiner: How is the pancreas drained? Do you know any complications of this route?

Candidate: Traditionally, pancreatic transplants were bladder drained (the pancreatic duct was anastomosed to the bladder). In this way, urinary amylase could be monitored and acts as an early sign of graft pancreatitis or pancreatic rejection. The complications of this route of drainage are:
- Reflux pancreatitis
- Persistent hematuria
- Recurrent UTIs and
- Metabolic acidosis (pancreatic bicarbonate loss, particularly during episodes of dehydration)

More recently, to avoid these complications, pancreatic transplants perform with primary enteric drainage (transplanted pancreases are attached to the small bowel and drained through the bowel).

Chronic Pancreatitis

A 35-year-old lady presented with abdominal pain that radiates to the back; please examine her abdomen.

(After GIT examination within 6 minutes)

Candidate: I would like to complete my examination by looking at the patient's observation chart, examining hernia orifices, external genitalia, doing PR, and urine dipsticks.

Examiner: Would you present your case, please?

Candidate:

I believe this lady has had chronic pancreatitis that would keep her presentation of abdominal pain, which radiates to the back.

She is extremely tender in the epigastric region.

She has multiple fentanyl patches that suggest she has had chronic pain.

She also has a tracheostomy, and central line scar suggests recent ICU admission possibly due to the development of acute pancreatitis with complications such as ARDS or renal failure.

In terms of the etiology of this pancreatitis, she does not have evidence of CLD or parotid swelling or Dupuytren's contracture, which would be in keeping with chronic alcohol use.

There is no evidence of cholecystectomy scar, so it is unlikely to have gallstone.

Examiner: How does chronic pancreatitis typically present?

Candidate: Most commonly, patients present with chronic upper abdominal pain that radiates to the back, usually aggravated after taking a meal, particularly fatty meal-classically grumbling in nature. The intensity of the pain may be variable mild-to-severe intensity with intermittent or regular flare-ups that are typically better when sitting up and leaning forward.

Some patients may present with pancreatic insufficiency such as fat absorption causes steatorrhea with a loose, greasy, pale, and foul-smelling stool that is difficult to flush away, weight loss, and many of them may develop DM (classically type-3 DM that are prone to develop recurrent hypoglycemia) and features of fat-soluble vitamin (A, D, E, K) deficiency such as weak bones, proximal myopathy, easy bruising. In some cases, the patient may remain asymptomatic.

Examiner: What are the causes of pancreatitis?

Candidate: The two most common causes are already mentioned:
- Chronic alcohol abuse
- Gallstone related

Other causes are:
- Hypertriglyceridemia
- Hypercalcemia
- Drugs such as steroid and azathioprine, thiazide diuretics, etc.
- Smoking
- Secondary to ERCP
- Trauma or autoimmune pancreatitis
- Sometimes may be idiopathic

Examiner: Are there any causes of pancreatitis which perhaps run in families?

Candidate: These are the genetic causes of pancreatitis:
- *Cystic fibrosis*: It is an autosomal recessive disorder usually associated with a respiratory problem related to bronchiectasis (CFTR gene will be detected in blood)
- PRSSI (AD hereditary pancreatitis)

- SPINK-1 (which has more complex genetics)

Blood tests for genetic causes should be done where the most common causes are excluded, such as alcohol and gallstone disease or any younger patient with unexplained chronic pancreatitis particularly.

Examiner: Ok, now tell me how will you investigate the case?

Candidate: At first, I would like to take a full history from the patient that includes:
- Alcohol or smoking history
- Drug history
- Family history
- Weight loss
- Diarrhea/steatorrhea
- History of DM
- As well as other symptoms, particularly pain in the abdomen

Then I would like to do a baseline blood test that includes FBC, U/E's, serum creatinine, serum calcium, and lipid profile.

To see the evidence of pancreatic insufficiency, I would like to do blood sugar and HbA1C, coagulation screen (vitamin-K deficiency), vitamin D level, serum magnesium (magnesium level is probably the most useful test for insufficiency), serum albumin, and measurement of fecal elastase, which may be normal in mild pancreatitis, and also do a plain X-ray abdomen to see the evidence of pancreatic calcification.

Here, the most important test would be a CT scan of the hepatobiliary system, including pancreas, to see the evidence of size, shape, contours of the pancreas or evidence of pancreatic calcification or dilatation of the main pancreatic duct as well as stone in CBD, pancreatic duct or GB.

Serum amylase and lipase will be normal, usually in chronic pancreatitis.

Examiner: How will you manage the patient?

Candidate: The mainstay of treatment in pancreatitis would include:
- Avoidance of cause of pancreatic inflammation.
- Aiming to reduce pain by using painkillers.
- As well as pancreatic enzyme replacement therapy (amylase, lipase, protease)

The most important lifestyle modification would be completely eliminating smoking and alcohol and being advised to take a healthy balanced diet.

If there is any evidence of malabsorption, I would like to consider an adequate dose of Creon, typically 75,000–1,25,000 units given during each meal and 50,000 units presnacks. Concomitant use of a proton pump inhibitor (PPI) is essential to prevent the acid breakdown of Creon in the stomach.

ERCP with stenting may be required in a patient with pancreatic duct stricture.

Examiner: What complications of pancreatitis do you know?

Candidate: Complications can be divided into acute or chronic.

Acute pancreatitis is a multi-system disorder that can lead to some local and systemic complications.

Local complications include:
- Necrotizing pancreatitis
- Pancreatic abscess
- Hemorrhage from a pseudoaneurysm of the splenic artery (hemosuccus pancreatitis)
- As well most importantly, pancreatic pseudocyst (with a defined nonepithelial wall) can be infected or have a compressive effect on the pancreas, causing a duodenal, biliary and pancreatic obstruction.

The systemic feature includes:
- ARDS, pleural effusions, atelectasis, renal failure, stroke, disseminated intravascular coagulation (DIC), etc.

Over the long-term, pancreatitis can lead to:
- Portal or splenic vein thrombus
- Exocrine and endocrine pancreas insufficiency
- As well as pancreatic pseudocyst that is more common in chronic pancreatitis than acute.

Examiner: You mentioned pseudocyst formation. How that is the best drained?

Candidate: Typically, it is performed 6 weeks after the presentation of pancreatitis, as in many cases, it resolves spontaneously within the period. It is usually done USG-guided (trans-gastrically) endoscopic approach by using AXIOS stent.

Crohn's Disease

A 35-year-old lady presented with abdominal pain. Examine her abdomen.
  (After finishing gastrointestinal examination within 6 minutes of time)

Candidate: I would like to complete my examination by looking at the patient's observation chart, examining hernia orifices, external genitalia, doing PR, and urine dipstick.

Examiner: Would you present your case, please?

Candidate:

I believe this patient has IBD. The positive findings on the clinical examination, which has to lead me to this diagnosis, are that:

First of all, this is a young patient who has no evidence of gastrointestinal disease peripherally. However, on examination of the abdomen, she has evidence of previous multiple abdominal surgeries suggesting a chronic, relapsing abdominal condition, which has led to a crisis requiring surgical intervention on several occasions such as fissure, fistula or emergency operation for perforation, hemorrhage or toxic megacolon.

Also, she has a stoma in the region of the RIF—the content of the stoma is semiliquid; on closer inspection, I also noticed the ileostomy is not flushed to the skin but has a spout protruding from the abdominal wall to prevent skin excoriation from the irritative small bowel content.

She also has a scar consistent with a previous stoma site in the left iliac fossa, possibly due to an end-ileostomy with a mucous fistula at the time of previous emergency surgery to avoid leakage from the retrosigmoid stump.

I asked the patient to cough to look for a parastomal hernia that is absent here.

Examiner: Can you tell me why this is not colostomy?

Candidate: In a colostomy, stoma positioned in the left iliac fossa. In contrast, the colostomy will flush the skin as fecal contents coming from the large bowel do not cause skin irritation.

Examiner: Could you tell me the other presentation of IBD?

Candidate: Clinically, the patient with IBD usually presents with recurrent abdominal pain and diarrhea with or without blood—classically have a relapse, remission illness.
  Other abdominal symptoms could be vomiting, weight loss, or anemia.
  There may be oral ulceration and a palpable mass in the RIF in acute exacerbation of Crohn's disease.
  Some patients may present with acute exacerbation, usually characterized by diarrhea worsening over several days, which is bloody in both ulcerative and Crohn's colitis. In that case, we have to assess the severity by Truelove–Witts' criteria.
- *Mild*: <4 stools per day (with or without blood), no systemic disturbance, normal ESR
- *Moderate*: >4 stools per day with minimal systemic disturbance
- *Severe*: >6 stools per day with blood with evidence of systemic disturbance by fever, tachycardia, anemia, and an ESR >30

Some patients may have extraintestinal manifestations such as:
- Finger clubbing
- Uveitis (painful red eye, decreased visual acuity)

- Large and small joint arthropathy, sacroiliitis (often unilateral)
- *Skin lesion*: Pyoderma gangrenosum; Erythema nodosum
- Peripheral edema from hypoalbuminemia
- Sclerosing cholangitis usually presents with obstructive jaundice.

Some patients may have cushingoid change due to complications of steroid therapy.

Examiner: Can you describe some differences between Crohn's disease and ulcerative colitis?

Candidate: There are several differences between Crohn's disease and ulcerative colitis. The main differentiating factors are the site of inflammation and the extent of the inflammation across the bowel wall.

CD can affect any part of the intestinal tract from mouth to the anus and is characterized by skip lesion, whereas UC affects only the large bowel and affects the sigmoid colon, rectum more than any part of the large bowel.

UC does not normally cause any problem with the anus though CD can cause a number of problems with anal fissure and fistula.

CD characteristically causes the full thickness of the bowel (transmural) inflammation, which can cause fistulae, whereas UC mainly causes superficial inflammation in the mucosa. Histologically CD causes noncaseating granuloma, whereas UC is more likely to cause crypt abscesses.

During an endoscopic procedure in CD, I would expect cobblestoning, creeping fat and fistulae, whereas, in UC, we would expect deep ulceration with pseudopolyps.

In the X-ray abdomen in CD, we would expect a string sign due to bowel wall thickening, while UC is more likely to have a lead pipe sign due to loss of haustra.

On autoimmune screening, the CD is ASCA (anti-saccharomyces cerevisiae antibody) positive, where UC is associated with p-ANCA positive and commonly associated with primary sclerosing cholangitis.

Examiner: What are the investigations you would like to do?

Candidate: I would like to do some baseline blood tests that include CBC, ESR, CRP, U/E's, serum Creatinine, LFTs, and fecal calprotectin.

Moreover, here, the most important test would be colonoscopy with biopsy for histopathology.

Examiner: What are the treatments for Crohn's disease?

Candidate: During acute attack:
- Steroids
- Cytotoxic medications; azathioprine, cyclosporine
- Biological therapy; infliximab, adalimumab
- Metronidazole
- Enteral nutrition
- 5-ASA treatment

Between attack—to maintain remission:
- Azathioprine
- 5 ASA
- Smoking cessation

Percutaneous Endoscopic Gastrostomy

A 65-year-old man has a weakness of the limbs. Examine his limbs.

(After finishing GIT examination within 6 minutes of time)

Candidate: To complete my examination, I would like to complete my examination by looking at the patient observation chart, examining hernia orifices, external genitalia, doing PR, and urine dipstick.

Examiner: Would you please present your case?

Candidate:

This elderly gentleman was in a wheelchair.

During my examination, I noticed he had a tube in the epigastrium for feeding—widespread wasting and fasciculation in his hands and forearm and also in the tongue.

I also noticed bulbar dysarthria while examining him.

His abdominal examination was entirely normal.

I believe this patient has had evidence of motor neuron disease (MND) requiring a PEG tube.

In case of MND, the patient may develop dysphagia—in that case, the normal feeling is impossible, so to maintain normal enteral nutrition and prevent aspiration pneumonia, a PEG tube was done.

Examiner: Could you please tell me the other indications of PEG tube insertion?

Candidate: Gastrostomy may be indicated in numerous situations, usually those in which normal (or nasogastric) feeding is impossible, so to establish the enteral access of feeding, a PEG tube is done.

The causes of these situations may be neurological disorders such as stroke, cerebral palsy, brain injury, Parkinson's disease, or multiple sclerosis.

Moreover, PEG is use in case of head and neck malignancy to prevent malnutrition. The underlying mechanism of this malnutrition includes the obstructive effect of the tumor, oropharyngeal mucositis due to aggressive treatment with high dose radiotherapy and/or chemotherapy and reduced appetite.

Examiner: Tell me some contraindications to the PEG tube?

Candidate: There are some absolute contraindications to the PEG tube:
- Serious coagulation disorder (INR >1.5, APTT >50 sec, platelet <50,000/mm^3)
- Sepsis
- Severe ascites
- Peritonitis
- Gastric outlet obstruction
- Abdominal wall infection at the site of placement
- Inability to perform esophagogastroduodenoscopy

Examiner: If you have a patient with a stroke when you consider PEG?

Candidate: In case of stroke, if a permanent neurological deficit causes difficulty in swallowing, then usually PEG is done. In stroke patients, the initial 14 days of enteral feeding are maintained by the NG tube then consider PEG.

Examiner: Now, please tell me some complications of PEG insertion.

Candidate: There are some procedure-related complications such as:
- Visceral perforation
- Intra-abdominal hemorrhage
- Peritonitis

- Stomal sepsis
- Colonic perforation
- Pneumonia

And subsequent complications would be:
- Occlusion
- Displacement

- Buried bumper syndrome (gastric part of the tube migrates into the gastric wall)
- Pneumonia
- Kissing ulcer—gastric ulcer either at the site of the button or on the opposite wall of the stomach.

CHAPTER 6

Clinical Examination: Nervous System

- Examination of Upper Limb
- Examination of Lower Limb
- Examination of Cranial Nerves
- Examination for Disequilibrium
- Examination of Eye
- Peripheral Neuropathy
- Peripheral Neuropathy: Atypical Features
- Chronic Inflammatory Demyelinating Polyneuropathy
- Sensory Ataxia
- Charcot–Marie–Tooth Disease
- Claw Hand
- Spastic Paraparesis
- Cord Compression
- Cervical Myelopathy
- Stroke/Cerebrovascular Disease
- Cerebellar Disorder (Upper Limb)
- Cerebellar Ataxia
- Multiple Sclerosis
- Motor Neuron Disease (Kennedy's Disease)
- Bulbar Palsy (Motor Neuron Disease)
- Myotonic Dystrophy
- Myasthenia Gravis (Ocular)
- Parkinson's Disease
- Tardive Dyskinesia
- Involuntary Movement (Chorea)

Examination of Upper Limb

- Meticulously, read the clinical scenario; this shall help you predict what you are going to find and do what you have been asked.
- Carefully greet the examiners in a nice, decent, and balanced manner—this will positively impact them.
- Sanitize your hands with antiseptic liquid (antiseptic liquid is provided to you in the station).
- Greet the patient, introduce yourself, confirm your patient identity and take permission *(Hello, Mr X.... Good morning, I am Mohammad Ali.... one of the working doctors here today.... I have been asked to examine you.... Is that okay?)*.
- Explain to the patient in easy yet precise terms about your procedure—this shall help to get required cooperation from the patient *(I would like to examine your nerves that supply your arms and hands if that is okay with you)*.
- Ask about the pain and discomfort and reassure the patient *(Do you have any pain or discomfort? I would be gentle during the examination, please let me know if you feel any pain or discomfort)*.
- Adequately positioned (position the patient either sitting or lying).
- Sufficiently expose the patient appropriate to the examination.

Explain every subsequent step before doing it so that the patient will be more cooperative and this will help you score better in skill-7 (maintaining patient's welfare).

- A general survey of the patient (see the patient as a whole, do not rush to examination, look for bedside clues and other clues in the patient).
- *During greeting the patient*: Shake the hand, note if any myotonia (myotonic dystrophy) and note his speech:
  - *Slurred speech* (loss of some letters): Suggest upper motor neuron lesions (UMNL), (e.g., stroke), bulbar, pseudobulbar palsy (look for crossed hemiplegia)
  - *Staccato speech* (pauses between words): Suggest cerebellar disorder.
  - Scanning speech (it is a type of ataxic dysarthria in which spoken words are broken up into separate syllables, often separated by a noticeable pause, and spoken with varying force) suggests UMNL + cerebellar lesion.
- *Bedside clues*:
  - Mobility or walking aids (canes or walking sticks, crutches, walker, rollator, wheelchair, mobility scooter), ankle-foot orthosis (foot drop), urinary catheter, spirometer (suggest respiratory compromise), medications, steroid card (bracelet or necklace).
  - State of the muscles of both upper and lower limbs, and face.
  - *Tremor*: Resting/static–parkinsonism; intentional–cerebellar disorder.
  - *Fasciculation*: Anterior horn cell diseases-motor neuron disease (MND), multifocal motor neuropathy, and syringomyelia.
  - *Nystagmus*: Cerebellar disorder.
  - Myotonia, triangular facies, partial ptosis with frontal baldness–myotonic dystrophy.
  - *Facial nerve palsy*:
    - If lower motor neuron facial palsy with crossed hemiplegia–Pons lesion [cardiovascular disease (CVD), multiple sclerosis, tumor].
    - If upper motor neuron facial palsy (lower face involvement) with same sided hemiplegia with flexed arm—Internal capsule lesion (CVD).
  - Bilateral ptosis, unlined face, loss of nasolabial fold, and wrinkle with jaw support sign—Myasthenia gravis.
  - Expressionless face with resting tremor—Parkinsonism.
  - Wasted muscle of the face, neck and arm ± ptosis-Facioscapulohumeral myopathy.

- Pes cavus and hammer toe suggest long-standing neurological disability—Charcot–Marie–Tooth disease (CMTD), Friedreich's ataxia.
- *Flexion of the upper limb*: Hemiplegia and dystonia.
- *Involuntary movement*: Dystonia/chorea/myoclonus/choreoathetosis/pseudoathetosis.

- *Examine the muscle state*:
  - Inspect for wasting/disuse atrophy, hypertrophy, fasciculation, tremor, scars (?CTS, muscle biopsy scar over the triceps and deltoid, sternotomy scar in chest indicate thymectomy for myasthenia gravis, scar over the anterior and posterior aspects of the neck suggest previous cervical decompression).
  - Palpate for fasciculation and tenderness by tapping on muscle.
- *Pronator drift*: Ask the patient to close their eyes and place arms outstretched forward with the palm facing up—observe the hands and arms for a sign of pronation as well as look for pseudoathetosis (?sensory ataxia: central/peripheral). If pronator drift occurs in one of the arms, it indicates upper motor neuron pathology of the contralateral side. Now, assess for rebound phenomenon to identify a cerebellar syndrome.
- *Examine the tone*:
  - Ask the patient to let their arm go floppy (*please relax and let your arm be nice and floppy*) while moving each major joint.
  - Support the patient's arm by holding their hand and elbow.
  - Move the wrist through its full range of motion (flexion, extension, rotational).
  - Pronate and supinate the forearm–feel for any spasticity.
  - Flex and extend the elbow joint.
  - Flex/extend/abduct/adduct the shoulder joint.
- *Interpretation*:
  - Spasticity is velocity-dependent, i.e., the faster you move the limb, the worse it is. This is why you get the spastic catch (clasp knife-resistance to initial movement then sudden release)—it indicates pyramidal lesion (corticospinal tract).
  - Rigidity is not velocity dependent, i.e., it feels the same if you move the limb fast or slowly—it suggests extrapyramidal disease such as parkinsonism—cogwheel rigidity (best assessed in the wrist, when extrapyramidal rigidity with superimposed tremor) and lead-pipe rigidity (when rigidity is detectable throughout the range of motions, best assessed at elbow joint)
  - *Hypotonia*: Lower motor neuron lesions (LMNL), cerebellum.
- *Examine the power*:
  - *Shoulder*: "Put your arms up like that for me and stop me pushing you down and now pull down to my arms."
    - Abduction (C5)
    - Adduction (C6/C7)
  - *Elbow*: "Bend your elbow and now pull me toward you and push me away."
    - Flexion (C5/6)
    - Extension (C7)
  - *Wrist*: "Cock your wrist back and stop me pushing you down; point your wrist downward and stop me pushing it up."
    - Extension (C6)
    - Flexion (C6/7)
  - *Finger*:
    - Finger extension (C7): "Put your fingers out straight and close together and stop me push them down."
    - Finger abduction (T1): "Spread your fingers and do not let me push them together."

    Check for first dorsal interosseous (FDI), abductor digiti minimi (ADM)
    - Thumb abduction (C8/T1): "Point your thumbs to the ceiling and stop me push them down."
    - Power drip (C5-T1): "Squeeze my fingers nice and tightly............then relax."
    - Pincer grip (ulnar nerve C8-T1)
- *Interpretation*:
  - Weakness of extension > flexion, abduction > adduction, distal > proximal: UMNL.
  - Distal > proximal, extension > flexion, adduction > abduction: LMNL.

- Proximal > distal, adduction > abduction: Proximal myopathy, look for facial muscles and neck: facioscapulohumeral.
- *Abduct thumb* (toward the ceiling): Median nerve (abductor pollicis brevis).
- *Then adduct with card test*: Ulnar nerve (adductor pollicis).
- *Then extend thumb*: Radial nerve (extensor pollicis brevis).

- *Examine the reflexes*: Make sure the limb is properly relaxed and that the tendon you are percussing is under some tension but not fully stretched. Percuss the tendon at least twice to ensure that the reflex that you have elicited (or not) is reproducible.
  - Biceps reflex (C5/6)
  - Triceps reflex (C7)
  - Supinator reflex (C6)
  - Do not assume the reflex is absent without doing Jendrassik maneuver—ask the patient to clench their teeth.
  - *Hoffman's sign* (UMNL): Hold the middle finger, flick the middle finger distal phalanx by thumb; flexion of distal phalanx of the thumb, and index fingers indicates UMNL.
  - Mid-cervical reflex (inverted supinator jerk—where the biceps jerk is absent but generates a supinator jerks with reflex flexion of the fingers (or when tapping biceps, triceps will contract) it suggests cervical myelopathy with cervical C5/6 nerve root damage.

- *Examine coordination*:
  - *Finger-to-nose test*:
    - Ask the patient to touch their nose with the tip of their index finger, then touch their fingertips.
    - Position your finger so that the patient has to fully outstretched their arm to reach it.
    - Ask them to continue doing this finger to nose motion as fast as they can do it and look for past pointing, intention tremor (tremor that increases in amplitude the closer to the target the finger is) suggest cerebellar disorder.
    - If you suspect peripheral neuropathy or dorsal column lesion-(you can ask him to do this with closing eyes: impaired coordination—sensory ataxia).
  - *Dysdiadochokinesia*:
    - "Can you tap over your hands faster?" An inability to perform (very slowly/irregular) suggests cerebellar ataxia (can also be impaired in sensory ataxia or parkinsonism due to bradykinesia).

- *Examine for sensation*:
  - *Pinprick sensation*: Touch the patient's sternum with a neurotip (pinprick sensation) to confirm they can feel it. Now ask the patient to close their eyes and to say "Yes" when they are touched.
    - *Assess* each of the dermatomes (C5: deltoid and lateral arm, C6: lateral forearm and hand, C7: middle two ring fingers, C8: medial hand, T1: medial forearm, T2: medial arm) of the upper limbs and compare right to the left by asking the patient if it feels the same on both sides or same as on your chest (*is it sharp as like in your chest?*).
    - *Then*, look for nerve lesions (if lateral 3 and a half fingers + lateral two-thirds of palm, then it is median nerve palsy; if medial one and a half fingers + medial one-third palm sensory loss, then it is ulnar nerve palsy; radial fossa (anatomical snuffbox) radial nerve palsy).
    - If the sensation is reduced peripherally, assess from a distal point and move proximally and circumferentially to identify "glove pattern" sensory loss suggest peripheral neuropathy, usually bilateral.
    - If necessary, keep going all the way up the arm, trunk, and neck until the normal sensation is felt. This may reveal a sensory level, which is suggestive of a spinal lesion.
    - If *he* does not feel the whole arm, then it is hemianesthetic sensory loss that suggests cerebral hemisphere lesion.
  - *Light touch sensation*: Use a cotton wool wisp (for light touch) and do the same as a pinprick.

- *Joint position sense*: Show him first—*"that is your finger is up and down; now close your eyes, and tell me where it is?"* Move finger while supporting up and down and ask him where it is? If joint position is impaired in the distal interphalangeal (DIP), move to the proximal interphalangeal (PIP), metacarpophalangeal (MCP), wrist, elbow, and shoulder joint.
- *Vibration sense*: First, tap a 128 Hz tuning fork, then place it onto the patient's sternum or on the head and establish that the patient can feel it buzzing. Now ask the patient to close their eyes and place it on the DIP joint of the forefinger and ask him if he can feel it buzzing and when it stops buzzing. If vibration sensation is impaired, continue to assess the bony prominence of more proximal joints—the carpometacarpal joint of the thumb, wrist, elbow, and then shoulder.

- Formulate the diagnosis, possible causes, and complications.
- Thanks to the patient at the end of the examination.
- Wash hands.
- To complete the examination, offer the examiner that you would do full neurological examinations of lower limbs and cranial nerve.

Examination of Lower Limb

- Meticulously, read the clinical scenario, this shall help you predict what you are going to find and do what you have been asked.
- Carefully greet the examiners in a nice, decent, and balanced manner—this will definitely carry a positive impact on them.
- Sanitize your hands with antiseptic liquid (antiseptic liquid is provided to you in the station).
- Greet the patient, introduce yourself, confirm your patient identity and take permission (*Hello, Mr X..... Good morning, I am Mohammad Ali....one of the working doctors here today....I have been asked to examine you....Is that okay with you?*)
- Explain to the patient in easy yet precise terms about your procedure—this shall help to get required cooperation from the patient (*I would like to examine your nerves that supply your legs and feet if that is okay with you?*).
- Ask about the pain and discomfort and reassure the patient (*Do you have any pain or discomfort?.........I would be gentle during the examination, please let me know if you feel any pain or discomfort, then I will stop*).
- Adequately positioned (position the patient either sitting or lying).
- Sufficiently expose the patient appropriate to the examination.

Explain every subsequent step before doing it so that the patient will be more cooperative and this will help you score better in skill-7 (maintaining patient's welfare)

- A general survey of the patient (see the patient as a whole, do not rush to examination, look for bedside clues and other clues in the patient). During greeting patient—shake hand, note if any myotonia and any abnormality in his speech.
  - *Speech*:
    - Slurred speech (loss of some letters) suggest UMNL, (e.g., stroke) bulbar, pseudobulbar palsy (look for crossed hemiplegia)
    - Staccato speech (pauses between words) suggests cerebellar disorder.
    - Scanning speech (it is a type of ataxic dysarthria in which spoken words are broken up into separate syllables, often separated by a noticeable pause, and spoken with varying force) suggests combined UMNL and cerebellar lesion.
  - *Bedside clues*:
    - Walking aids (walking sticks), wheelchair, and urinary catheter.
    - State of the muscles of both upper and lower limbs.
    - *Facies*: Myasthenia gravis, myotonic dystrophy, polymyositis, parkinsonism, facial nerve palsy (UMNL/LMNL).
    - Fasciculation and wasting—anterior horn cell disease (MND, multifocal motor neuropathy).
    - *Nystagmus*: Cerebellar disorder
    - *Scars*: Frequent fall
    - *Flexed upper limb posture*: Hemiplegia
    - Externally rotated hips and flexed knee (frog sign) suggest hypotonia: LMNL or cerebellum.
    - Deformity of the foot (Pes cavus and hammer toe) suggests long-standing neurological diseases such as Friedreich's ataxia, hereditary motor and sensory neuropathy (HSMN) (CMTD).
    - Ankle foot orthosis suggests foot drop (common peroneal nerve palsy).
- *Examine the muscle state*:
  - Wasting (LMNL)
  - Disuse atrophy (UMNL)
  - Fasciculation
  - Palpate for tenderness, fasciculation (by tapping)
- *Examine for tone:* Ask the patient to relax/go floppy like a rag-doll and ask about the pain.

- Leg roll (hold the patient's knee and roll it from side to side; watch the foot, it should flap independently)
- Leg lift (place your hands behind the knee, then briskly flip the knee joint up from the below)—if the tone is normal, the heel will stay on the bed, but if it is increased, the heel will flip up off the bed then repeat it on another side.
- Knee flexion and extension
- Ankle clonus (At first ensure the knee and ankle are in slightly flexed position and support the leg with your hand under their knee, then move the foot up and down and from side to side to encourage relaxation, now rapidly dorsiflex and partly evert the feet; hold it there with reasonably firm pressure; clonus is felt as rhythmical beats of dorsiflexion/plantar flexion, more than 3 is abnormal).

- *Interpretation*:
  - *Hypotonia*: LMNL
  - *Hypertonia*: Spasticity (clasp knife); rigidity (lead pipe/cogwheel)

For scoring muscle strength, use the Medical Research Council (MRC) muscle power assessment scale. *"I would like to examine your muscle strength to check how strong you are."*

- *Hip*:
  - Flexion (L1/2): *"Raise your leg straight up of the bed and keep it there; stop me from pushing it down."*
  - Extension (L5/S1): *"Now, using your legs to push my hand into the bed."*
  - Adduction (L2/3): Position hands-on inner thigh; *"Push your legs together."*
  - Abduction (L4/5): Position hands-on outer thigh; *"Push your legs out."*
- *Knee*:
  - Flexion (S1)—*"Bend your knee and bring your heel to your bottom, and do not let me pull it away."*
  - Extension (L3/4)—*"Kick out your legs and push me away."*
- *Ankle*:
  - Dorsiflexion (L4)—*"Keep your legs flat on the bed–cock your foot up toward your face and stop me push it down."*
  - Plantar flexion (S1/2)—Keep your hand on the undersurface of the patient's foot and ask them, *"Bend your foot down and push my hand away."*
  - Inversion (L4)—*"Push your foot in against my hand."*
  - Eversion (L5/S1)—*"Push your foot out against my hand."*
- *Big toe*:
  - Extension (L5)—*"Point your big toe toward your face and stop me push it down."*
- *Interpretation*:
  - Weakness: Proximal > Distal = Proximal myopathy
  - Weakness: Distal > Proximal; Extension > Flexion; Adduction > Abduction = LMNL
  - Weakness: Distal > Proximal; Flexion > Extension; Abduction > Adduction = UMNL
  - Weakness of foot plantar flexion and eversion = Tibial nerve
  - Weakness of knee extension = Femoral nerve.
  - Weakness of foot dorsiflexion, inversion, and eversion = Common peroneal.
- *Examine for reflex:* Ensure the patient's lower limb is completely relaxed; test the knee and ankle jerk using reinforcement (*clench your teeth*) if required.
  - Knee jerk: (L3/4)
  - Ankle jerk: (L5/S1)
  - Plantar reflex: (S1)

Run a blunt object (orange stick) along the lateral edge of the sole, moving toward the little toe, then medially under the toes, and observe the response of the great toe.
  - *Normal*: Flexion of the great toe and flexion of the other toes.
  - *Abnormal* (Babinski sign): Extension of the great toe and spread of the other toes—UMNL.
- *Coordination*: Heel-shin test—using your finger on the patient's shin and instruct patient—*"Put your heel on your knee, run it down your shin, lift it up, and repeat."*
  - An inability to perform this test (very slowly or irregular) may suggest cerebellar ataxia (can also be impaired in sensory ataxia,

loss of motor strength, parkinsonism due to bradykinesia).
- If you suspect sensory ataxia, ask the patient to do this with closing eyes—if impaired, then suggest sensory ataxia (central/peripheral).
- *Examine for sensation*:
  - *Pinprick sensation*: Touch the patient's sternum with neurotip (pinprick sensation) to confirm they can feel it. Now ask the patient to close their eyes and to say "Yes" when they are touched.
    - Assess each of the dermatomes (upper thigh-L2, lower thigh-L3, medial leg-L4, dorsum of the foot-L5, behind the medial malleolus-S1) of the lower limbs and compare right to the left by asking the patient if it feels the same on both sides or same as on your chest (*is it sharp as like in your chest?*).
    - Then, look for nerve lesions (sensory deficit of sole of the foot-tibial nerve, sensory deficit of anterior thigh and medial knee-femoral nerve, a sensory deficit of lateral aspects of the lower leg and dorsum of the foot-peroneal nerve).
    - If the sensation is reduced peripherally, assess from a distal point and move proximally to identify "stocking" sensory loss suggest peripheral neuropathy, which is usually bilateral.
    - If necessary, keep going all the way up the leg and trunk until the normal sensation is felt. This may reveal a sensory level, which is suggestive of a spinal lesion, if there is abnormal sensation up to the level of the umbilicus, this suggests spinal lesion at around T-10, Nipple-T4, Xiphisternum-T6.
    - If he does not feel the sensation of one whole limb then, it is hemiplegic sensory loss suggests cerebral hemisphere lesion.
  - *Light touch sensation*: Use cotton wool wisp (for light touch) and do the same as pinprick.
  - *Joint position sense*: Ask the patient to close their eyes; grasp the distal phalanx of the great toe at the sides and stabilize the rest of the toe. Now move the joint up and inform the patient (*"This is "up" and this is "down"; now close your eyes and tell me where it is?"*). Then flex and extend the joint and stop at intervals to ask the patient about the position of the toe, whether is it "up" or "down". If joint position is impaired in the great toe, then move to ankle-knee-hip.
  - *Vibration sense*: At first tap, a 128 Hz tuning fork which is then placed onto the patient's sternum and establish patient can feel it buzzing. Now ask the patient to close their eyes and tell you when they can feel it on their feet and when it stops buzzing. At first, test the vibration sense at the distal phalanx of the great toe. If it is not perceived, proceed proximally to the medial malleolus, patella, and ileac crest as appropriate.
- Formulate the diagnosis, possible causes, and complications.
- Thanks to the patient at the end of the examination.
- Wash hands.
- To complete the examination, offer the examiner that you would do full neurological examinations of upper limbs and cranial nerves.

Examination of Cranial Nerves

- Meticulously, read the clinical scenario, this shall help you to predict what you are going to find and do what you have been asked.
- Carefully greet the examiners in a nice, decent, and balanced manner—this will definitely carry a positive impact on them.
- Sanitize your hands with antiseptic liquid (antiseptic liquid is provided to you in the station).
- Greet the patient, introduce yourself, confirm your patient identity and take permission (*Hello, Mr X…..Good morning, I am Mohammad Ali….one of the working doctors here today….I have been asked to examine you….Is that okay with you?*).
- Explain to the patient in easy yet precise terms about your procedure—this shall help to get required cooperation from the patient (*I would like to examine your nerves that supply your face and neck if that is okay with you?*)
- Ask about the pain and discomfort and reassure the patient (*Do you have any pain or discomfort?………I would be gentle during the examination, please let me know if you feel any pain or discomfort*).
- Adequately positioned (position the patient on a chair at eye level—approximately one arm's length away).
- Sufficiently expose the patient appropriate to the examination.

Explain every subsequent step before doing it so that the patient will be more cooperative and this will help you score better in skill-7 (maintaining patient's welfare).

- A general survey of the patient (see the patient as a whole, do not rush to examination, look for bedside clues and other clues in the patient).
  - Comfortable at rest
  - Obvious facial asymmetries (?facial nerve palsy)
  - Position of the eye:
    - Normal alignment/strabismus
    - *Ptosis*: Is it unilateral/bilateral?
  - *Abnormality of speech or voice*: Slurred speech, staccato speech, scanning speech.
  - *Signs around the bed*: Walking aid, wheelchair, hearing aid/glasses.
  - *Myopathic face*: Unlined face, loss of nasolabial folds and wrinkle—facioscapulohumeral, myasthenia gravis, inflammatory myopathy.
  - *Parotid enlargement*: Look for facial nerve palsy
  - *Herpes Zoster rash in-ears*: Facial nerve palsy (Ramsay hunt syndrome)
  - *Cushingoid face + bilateral facial nerve palsy*: Sarcoidosis (look for basal crepitation or lymphadenopathy?)
  - *Nystagmus*: Cerebellar disorder
  - *Intention tremor*: Cerebellar disorder
  - *Flexed upper limb*: Hemiplegia
- *Individual cranial nerve examination*:
  - Olfactory nerve: (I)

  Have you noticed any recent change in your sense of smell?
  - Optic nerve: (CN: II)
- *Inspect pupil*:
  - Size and shape
  - *Symmetry*: Large and fixed in a CN-III palsy, small and reactive in Horner's syndrome.
- *Visual acuity*: Decreased visual acuity has many causes—refractive error, amblyopia, ocular media opacities such as cataract or corneal scarring, retinal disease such as retinitis pigmentosa, age-related macular degeneration, optic nerve pathology such as optic atrophy or optic neuritis, lesion higher in the visual pathway.
- Optic nerve (CN-II) pathology (ON, OA) usually causes a decrease in visual acuity in that eye. In contrast, optic disc swelling from raised increased intracranial pressure (ICP) (papilledema) usually does not affect visual acuity until it is at a late stage.

- The patient who normally uses distance glasses; ensure these are worn for assessment—ask the patient to cover their one eye and read the lowest line they are able to—(Snellen's chart from 6 meters, if cannot read 6/60, move 1 meter closer until he cannot 1/60, then counting finger from 30 cm, then a perception of light).
- *Visual field*: Do not go for field examination without acuity testing before it. No field examination if there is a defect in acuity.
  - *At first, assess for visual inattention*: Ask the patient to look at the bridge of your nose with both eyes open while you place your index finger just inside the outer limit of your temporal field, now move your fingers (wiggling) in turn and then both at the same time and ask the patient to point to the finger that moves. The patient will only point one finger when you move both at the same time if there is visual inattention. The condition may be found in people with visual field loss (hemianopia) following a stroke or brain injury on the opposite side.
  - Then look for central visual field with red hat pin (central scotoma in optic neuritis). *Finally, check for the mono-ocular visual field*: Ask the patient to cover their left eye with left hand—meanwhile, cover your right eye and should be staring directly at the patient—then ask the patient to look into your eye and not to move their head or eyes during the assessment—ask the patient to tell you when they are able to see your fingertip wiggling (better to use red hat pin)—outstretch your arms and ensure they are situated at an equal distance between your fingertips (red hat pin) at the outer border of one of the quadrants of your visual field—slowly bring your fingertip of your visual field until the patient sees—repeat this process for each quadrant at 10 o'/2 o'/4 o'/8 o'. If you can see your fingertip but the patient cannot, this would suggest a visual field defect, map out any visual field defects you detect. Repeat the same assessment procedure on the other eye.
- *Pupillary reflex*: The room should be dimly lit to see the pupillary reflexes properly (ask the examiner, *"is it possible to dim the light?"*)
  - *Direct light reflex*: (Afferent CN-II, efferent CN-III) shine a light into the pupil and observe constriction of the pupil. Lack of constriction or sluggish reaction may suggest pathology—optic nerve/brainstem/drugs.
  - *Consensual pupillary reflex*: Shine a light again into the pupil but this time observe the contralateral pupil—a normal consensual response involves the contralateral pupil constriction. Lack of a normal consensual response may suggest damage to one or both optic nerves or damage to the Edinger-Westphal nucleus.
- *Swinging light test*: Rapidly move the pen-torch between the two pupils, shining the light for 3 seconds in each eye.
  - This test may detect a relative afferent pupillary defect (RAPD)—caused by damage to the tract between the optic nerve and optic chiasma (e.g., optic neuritis in multiple sclerosis). It is also known as a Marcus-Gunn pupil. A relative afferent pupillary defect can be detected by paradoxical dilatation of the affected pupil (normally, it should constrict when light is shining into it). It points to pathology in the afferent pathway (optic nerve) on this site. This test is important to compare the function of the two optic nerves, so when the light is shone into the eye in which the optic nerve is not functioning well, it dilates.
- *Accommodation reflex*:
  - Ask the patient to focus their vision on a distant object (light site/clock on the wall).
  - Place your finger/object approximately 15 cm in front of the eyes.
  - Ask the patient to switch from focusing on the distant object to the nearby finger or object.
  - Observe the pupils; normally, they should be constricted and convergence bilaterally.

- *Fundoscopy*: Darker the room (ask the examiner, "*is it possible to dim the light*"). Warn the patient that you will need to get close to their faces. The patient should ideally have their pupils dilated with a short-acting mydriatic eye drop. Ask the patient to focus on a distant object.
  - Assess for red reflex.
  - Position yourself at a distance of around 30 cm from the patient's eye.
  - Look through the ophthalmoscope and ensure the light is directed into the pupil.
  - Observe for a reddish/orange reflection in the pupil.
  - Move-in closer and examine the eyes with the ophthalmoscope.
  - Find a vessel on the fundus and focus on it using the dial on the ophthalmoscope.
  - Follow the vessel along with the optic disc; if you cannot find the optic disc, stay on the same vessel and follow it the other way.
  - *Assess the optic disc*: Color (pale color indicates optic atrophy), margin (blurred margin indicates papilledema or optic neuritis), cupping (glaucoma).
  - *Assess the retinal vessel*: Cotton wool spots, arteriovenous (AV) nipping, neovascularization.
  - *Finally, assess the macula*: Ask the patient to look directly into the light—Drusen noted in macular degeneration.

Examine III, IV, VI Cranial Nerve

Look for ptosis (*causes*: oculomotor nerve palsy, Horner's syndrome, myopathy—myasthenia gravis, myotonic dystrophy, congenital, senile or age-related)

Eye Movement

Pursuit movement: Hold your finger about 30 cm directly in front of the patient's eye and ask them to look at it. Look at the eyes in primary position for any deviation (squint/strabismus) or abnormal movement. Now check each extra-ocular muscle individually by asking the patient to track movement in the shape of an "H", lateral movement is assessed followed by elevation and depression to about 30° of lateral gaze. Observe for restriction of the eye movement and note any double vision and nystagmus (*"Keep your head still, move with your eyes and follow my finger, if you see double or feel any pain then tell me"*).

- Note that double vision (eye cannot move) suggests cranial nerve palsy. All muscles of the eye movements are supplied by 3rd cranial nerve (oculomotor) except superior oblique (moves eye down medially), which is supplied by the 4th cranial nerve (trochanter); lateral rectus (moves laterally) supplied by 6th cranial nerve (abducens).
- Note nystagmus for cerebellar lesion.
- Internuclear ophthalmoplegia (INO) suggests multiple sclerosis (one of the eyes is not adducting; the other abducting eyes have nystagmus; by covering the eye with nystagmus, the nonadducting eye adducts normally suggest a lesion in the MLF of the nonadducting eye).

Saccadic eye movement: Hold your hand about 30 cm to the side of your head, ask the patient to look at your palm, then back to your nose when you ask them to do this on both sides. The movement should be quick and accurate; if there is an overshot (the eyes will go too far past the target, then correct themselves back to the target) suggests cerebellar disease.

Trigeminal Nerve (V)

Sensory

- Assess light touch and pinprick sensation in the forehead (V1), check (V2), and jaw (V3) branch of the trigeminal nerve.
- If you find the loss of sensation in the face, examine sensation behind the ear (C2) and neck, if lost suggests hemianesthetic sensory loss (cerebral hemisphere lesion) where corneal reflex will be intact.
- If the sensation is intact behind the ear and neck, which suggests CN-V lesion (midbrain lesion; internal capsule) where corneal reflex will be absent.
- Now ask the examiner… *"I would like to check for corneal reflex."*

Motor
- Ask the patient to clench their teeth then feel the bulk of masseter and temporalis bilaterally.
- Ask the patient to open their mouth and apply resistance under the jaw—note any deviation—here Jaw will deviate to the affected side.

Jaw Jerk
- Ask the patient to open mouth loosely—place your finger horizontally over the chin, now tap on your finger with a tendon hammer.
- *Normal*: Slight closure of the jaw.
- *Abnormal*: Brisk complete closure of the jaw suggests UMNL.

Facial Nerve (VII)
Inspect the patient face at rest for asymmetry (forehead wrinkles, angle of the mouth, nasolabial folds). Ask the patient to perform the specific facial movement:
- Raise your eyebrows as like you are surprised—note any asymmetry.
- Close your eyes tightly and do not let me open them—note the power.
- Blow out your checks, and do not let me deflate them—note the power.
- Can you do a wide smile for me?— note any asymmetry.
- Can you try to whistle for me?
- Close your lips tight and do not let me open them—note the power.

Other Things to Check
- Inspect external auditory meatus for herpes zoster rash (Ramsey Hunt syndrome)
- Have you noticed any change in hearing (hyperacusis)?
- Have you noticed any change in taste sensation to the front part (anterior two-thirds) of your tongue?

Vestibulocochlear Nerve (VIII)
- *Gross hearing testing*: Explain to the patient that you are going to say a number or word (name, age), and you would like to take them to repeat it back to you. Mask the ear not being tested by pressing the tragus. If the patient repeats the correct word or number, repeat the test at 15 and 60 cm.
- *Rinne's test and weber's test*: Usually not done in the exam.

IX and X Nerve
- *Assess soft palate and uvula*: Look for any obvious deviation of the uvula?
- Ask the patient to say "Ahhhh", then observe uvula moving upward and note any deviation? (deviation away from the side of the lesion—uvula supplied by vagus nerve deviates to the unaffected side).
- Ask the patient to cough; damage to nerve IX and X can result in a bovine cough.
- Ask the patient to take a sip of water—note any delayed swallowing or coughing?

XI–Accessory Nerve
- Ask the patient to shrug shoulders and resist pushing it down; assess the power of the trapezius muscle.
- Ask the patient to turn head to one side and resist you pushing it to the other; assess the power of sternocleidomastoid muscle.

XII–Hypoglossal Nerves
- Inspect tongue for wasting and fasciculation at rest.
- Ask the patient to protrude the tongue and look for any deviation (deviates toward the side of the lesion).
- Place your finger on the patient's cheek and ask to push their tongue against it—assess the power.
  - Formulate the diagnosis, possible cause, and complications.
  - Thanks to the patient at the end of the examination.
  - Wash hands
  - To complete the examination, offer the examiner that you would do full neurological examinations of both upper and lower limbs.

Examination for Disequilibrium

- Meticulously, read the clinical scenario (e.g., the patient has difficulty walking or the patient has had frequent falls, please examine gait and proceed), this shall help you predict what you are going to find and do what you have been asked.
- Carefully greet the examiners in a nice, decent, and balanced manner—this will definitely carry a positive impact on them.
- Sanitize your hands with antiseptic liquid (antiseptic liquid is provided to you in the station).
- Greet the patient, introduce yourself, confirm your patient identity and take permission (*Hello, Mr X.....Good morning, I am Mohammad Ali....one of the working doctors here today....I have been asked to examine you....Is that okay with you?*).
- Explain to the patient in easy yet precise terms about your procedure—this shall help to get required cooperation from the patient (*I would like to examine your nerves that supply your face and neck, upper and lower limbs if that is okay with you?*).
- Ask about the pain and discomfort and reassure the patient (*Do you have any pain or discomfort?.........I would be gentle during the examination, please let me know if you feel any pain or discomfort*).
- Adequately positioned (position either sitting or lying on the bed).
- Sufficiently expose the patient appropriate to the examination.

Explain every subsequent step before doing it so that the patient will be more cooperative and this will help you score better in skill-7 (maintaining patient's welfare).

- *General survey*: Stand at the end of the bed, take your time to observe (see the patient as a whole, do not rush to examination, look for bedside clues and other clues in the patient).
  - Walking aids, wheelchair, ankle-foot orthosis suggests foot drop; Glucometer suggests diabetic peripheral neuropathy; medications (antiparkinsonism drugs).
  - Look for wasting, fasciculations, pes cavus, or foot drop.
  - Observe the patient for vital clues as they stand up from the chair (use of arms in proximal myopathy).
- *Examine patient's gait*:
  - Initially, stand the patient and ensure stability on standing, assess the base—is it narrow or broad, broad base suggests a cerebellar disorder.
  - Ask the patient to walk to the end of the room, turn, and walk back (taking a few steps with them first)—assess posture, arm swing, stride length base, symmetry, balance, and for abnormal movement (resting tremor).

  Common abnormalities are:
  - *Ataxic gait*: Broad-based, unsteady gait suggests cerebellar pathology or sensory ataxia.
  - *Parkinsonian*: Small, shuffling steps, festinant (hurrying) stooped posture, and reduced arm swing suggests parkinsonism (usually unilateral first, in some cases with freezing and slow turning).
  - *High steeping gait*: Usually caused by foot drop suggests the weakness of the ankle dorsiflexion (common peroneal nerve palsy).
  - A stamping gait in proprioceptive sensory loss (dorsal column or peripheral neuropathy).
  - *Waddling gait*: Pelvic girdle sway from side to side, legs lifted off the ground with the aid of tilting the trunk suggests proximal myopathy.
  - *Circumduction or hemiplegic gait*: One leg held stiffly (extended knee) and swing round in an arc with each stride.

- Scissor gait (spastic paraparesis) is similar to hemiparetic gait, but it is bilateral—both are stiff and circumducting—feet may be inverted and scissor.
- If gait appears to be normal, then look for tandem (heal to toe) gait.
  - Ask the patient to walk in a straight line heel to toe *(Could you walk heel to toe as if on a tight rope?)*, this may bring out subtle gait ataxia—an abnormal heel to toe test suggests impaired proprioception and cerebellar disorder (can be impaired in weakness also).
- Ask him to walk on heels for L5 weakness (assess ankle dorsiflexion power)
- Ask him to walk on toes for S1 weakness (gastrocnemius lesion)
- *Do the Romberg test*:
  - Ask the patient to stand unaided with their feet together and eyes closed (be ready to support them). The test is positive if there is a loss of balance (swaying on closing the eyes indicates sensory ataxia due to dorsal column lesion or peripheral neuropathy)
- Ask him to sit on the bed and stand with a crossed arm to see the evidence of proximal myopathy.
- Examine eyes for nystagmus suggests cerebellar disorder or INO in multiple sclerosis patients.
- Test for coordination in the upper limb (finger nose test and dysdiadochokinesia) and lower limb (heel-shin test).
- Complete neurological examination of the lower limb (particularly for a joint position and vibration sense for a dorsal column or sensory ataxia for peripheral neuropathy).
- Formulate the diagnosis, possible causes, and complications.
- Thank the patient and cover him.
- Wash hands

Examination of Eye

- Meticulously, read the clinical scenario, this shall help you predict what you are going to find and do what you have been asked.
- Carefully greet the examiners in a nice, decent, and balanced manner—this will definitely carry a positive impact on them.
- Sanitize your hands with antiseptic liquid (antiseptic liquid is provided to you in the station).
- Greet the patient, introduce yourself, confirm your patient identity and take permission *(Hello, Mr X.....Good morning, I am Mohammad Ali....one of the working doctors here today....I have been asked to examine you....Is that okay with you?).*
- Explain to the patient in easy yet precise terms about your procedure—this shall help get required cooperation from the patient *(I would like to examine your nerves that supply your eyes if that is okay with you?)*
- Ask about the pain and discomfort and reassure the patient *(Do you have any pain or discomfort?.........I would be gentle during the examination, please let me know if you feel any pain or discomfort).*
- Adequately positioned (position the patient on a chair at eye level—approximately one arm's length away).
- Sufficiently expose the patient appropriate to the examination.

Explain every subsequent step before doing it so that the patient will be more cooperative and this will help you score better in skill-7 (maintaining patient's welfare).

- A general survey of the patient (see the patient as a whole, do not rush to examination, look for bedside clues and other clues in the patient).
- Initial examination/inspection (in the primary position of the eye)
- Ptosis (unilateral/bilateral; complete/partial)
- Strabismus/squint
- Nystagmus in primary position
    - Lateral nystagmus suggests a unilateral vestibular lesion
    - Vertical downbeat nystagmus suggests craniocervical junction lesion at the level of the foramen magnum (Arnold-Chiari malformation or syringobulbia, vertebrobasilar infarction)
    - Vertical upbeat nystagmus suggests a cerebellar lesion or brainstem lesion.
      - *Size of the pupil*: Constricted, dilated
      - Visual acuity
      - Field of vision (both central and peripheral)
      - Light reflex (separately in both eyes, then do the swinging light reflex for relative afferent pupillary defect (RAPD)]
      - Fundoscopy (papilledema, optic neuritis, or atrophy)
      - *Eye movement* (pursuit and saccade movement): This may bring out nystagmus not seen in the primary position.
- *During pursuit movement*: Ask for diplopia and do the cover test if diplopia is present or nystagmus in lateral/up/downgaze.
- *During saccade movement*: (Ask the patient to look from one object to another, e.g., hand and examiner's nose) Look for nystagmus at that time (horizontal or vertical) and look for hypermetric or hypometric saccades.

Approach to a Patient with Ptosis

If the ptosis is present, then...is it unilateral or bilateral?

- Unilateral usually suggests 3rd nerve palsy, which causes complete ptosis or Horner's syndrome, which generally causes partial ptosis.
- But myopathy (oculopharyngeal muscular dystrophy or myotonic dystrophy) and neuromuscular disorder such as myasthenia gravis usually cause bilateral ptosis, but in

some cases, it may be unilateral presentation; if myasthenia gravis is suspected, then look for eyelid fatigability on upgaze.

Then assess for the pupil:
- Dilated and fixed pupil suggest compressive 3rd nerve palsy, but a medical cause of 3rd nerve palsy due to mononeuritis multiplex [diabetes mellitus (DM), PAN, rheumatoid arthritis (RA), connective tissue disease (CTD), sarcoidosis] may cause pupil sparing 3rd nerve palsy where other features of 3rd nerve palsy will be present.
- If constricted, then think Horner syndrome—look for other features of Horner syndrome (enophthalmos, anhidrosis).
- Normal pupil may suggest myasthenia gravis or myopathy (oculopharyngeal/myotonic dystrophy/mitochondrial myopathy).
- Ask for old portrait photography of the patient if it is long-lasting (congenital) or consider senile ptosis.

Approach to a Patient with Ophthalmoplegia

Usually present with diplopia:
- *Left VI nerve palsy*:
  ○ The patient has left convergent strabismus at rest (in the primary position).
  ○ There is impaired abduction of the left eye (during pursuit eye movement).
  ○ There is diplopia which is maximal on the left lateral gaze.
  ○ Cover testing reveals that the outermost image comes from the left eye.
  Causes are:
  ○ Raised ICP due to any cause (look for papilledema or complaining of early morning headache).
  ○ Brainstem infarction, hemorrhage or tumor, or demyelinating lesion in the pons (usually associated with long tract sign).
  ○ *Subacute meningitis*: Tuberculosis (TB), fungal, carcinoma.
  ○ Mononeuritis multiplex due to DM, PAN, antineutrophil cytoplasmic antibody (ANCA) positive vasculitis, RA, systemic lupus erythematosus (SLE), Sjögren's syndrome, lymphoma, cancer, and amyloidosis.
- *Right III nerve palsy*:
  ○ The patient has complete ptosis on the right; there is right divergent strabismus at rest (primary position).
  ○ The right eye movement is impaired, and the eye is fixed in a down and out position.
  ○ The pupil is fixed and dilated.
  ○ There is diplopia which is maximal on the left superior gaze (angulated diplopia).
  Causes are:
  ○ *Compressive lesion (brainstem sign will be absent here)*: Posterior cerebral artery (PCA) aneurysm, internal carotid artery aneurysm, and meningioma.
  ○ *Brainstem infarction (if sudden onset)*: Weber's (contralateral hemiparesis) and Benedikt syndrome (if contralateral ataxia indicates paramedian midbrain lesion).
  ○ *Brainstem demyelination*: Multiple sclerosis.
- *Right IV nerve palsy*:
  ○ The right eye is higher than the left eye in the primary position (primary gaze)
  ○ During pursuit movement adducted right eye cannot look down.
  ○ There is vertical diplopia that is maximal on looking down and away from the affected eye side, cover testing reveals that the outer image comes from the right eye.
  Causes are:
  ○ Trauma (most common)
  ○ *Brainstem lesion*: Infarction, hemorrhage, demyelination, and tumors.
  ○ Cavernous sinus thrombosis
  ○ Mononeuritis multiplex
  ○ Congenital
- *Complex ophthalmoplegia* (describe the clinical picture in which the eye sign cannot be attributed to just one cranial nerve, which is usually caused by multiple cranial nerve palsy or myopathy or neuromuscular disorder or INO):
  (Left-sided complex ophthalmoplegia)
  ○ The patient has diplopia on looking to the right. The eye movement appears to be grossly intact. Cover testing reveals that the outermost image comes from the left eye.

- This would suggest impairment of the left medial rectus and does not fit with a specific cranial neuropathy (that means other muscles supplied by 3rd cranial nerve is not affected as well as pupil is reacting to the light–so 3rd nerve palsy is not the cause here).
- On the other hand, there is no evidence of nystagmus in the abducted right eye that excludes INO of the left MLF involvement, usually caused by MS, infarction, or trauma.
  The differential diagnosis would be:
  - Mitochondrial myopathy, e.g., Graves ophthalmopathy (look for the evidence of thyroid disease) or Kearns–Sayre syndrome.
  - Oculopharyngeal muscular dystrophy.
  - Myasthenia gravis (look for fatigability by maintaining upgaze; the patient may complain of diplopia, and ptosis will appear).
  - Miller Fisher syndrome (look for dorsal column sign-sensory ataxia and areflexia).
  - Orbital myositis
  - Trauma
  - Chronic progressive external ophthalmoplegia

Approach to a Patient with Nystagmus

Ataxic Nystagmus

- The patient has dissociation of conjugate eye movement. Abduction is normal in both eyes, but adduction is impaired in the left eye. Nystagmus is present in the right abducted eye (best assessed in saccadic eye movement, this may bring out subtle INO).
- When the abducted right eye is covered, adduction of the left eye becomes normal.
- So, my diagnosis is left-sided INO due to a left medial longitudinal fasciculus lesion.
- As it is unilateral INO, so most likely diagnosis would be stroke (infarction or hemorrhage in the brain).
  Other causes would be multiple sclerosis (usually bilateral, but rarely it may be unilateral), tumor, trauma, vasculitis, Wernicke's encephalopathy, and Arnold Chiari malformation.

Cerebellar Nystagmus

Case-1
- This patient has horizontal nystagmus with a fast component to the right.
- There is a loss of smooth pursuit (broken pursuit).
- The saccadic eye movement is abnormal with hypermetric saccades (ocular dysmetria).
- This is cerebellar nystagmus with a right-sided cerebellar lesion.

Case-2
- This patient has vertical nystagmus that beats upward in the primary position (primary gaze).
- The nystagmus increased on an upward gaze.
- So, it is upbeat nystagmus suggestive of the lesion in the anterior vermis of the cerebellum.

Other less likely possibilities are drugs (phenytoin, carbamazepine, and OCP); Wernicke's encephalopathy.

Approach to a Patient with Visual Field Defect

Case-1

This patient has bitemporal hemianopia; this suggests a lesion at the optic chiasma.
Differential diagnoses would be:
- Pituitary tumor
- Craniopharyngioma
- Suprasellar meningioma
- Granulomatous disease (sarcoidosis, tuberculosis)

Pituitary tumor compresses the optic chiasma from below whilst craniopharyngioma compresses the optic chiasma from above. So, pituitary tumors result in temporal hemianopia that progress from the upper to lower field and craniopharyngioma progresses temporal hemianopia from lower to upper field. Importantly look for evidence of pituitary tumors such as acromegaly, gynecomastia (hyperprolactinemia), hypopituitarism, and Cushing syndrome.

Case-2

This patient has a right (complete) congruous homonymous hemianopia. This suggests a lesion behind optic chiasma but more specifically behind the lateral geniculate ganglion (optic tract and lateral geniculate ganglion cause incongruous or incomplete homonymous hemianopia) affecting the left optic radiation.

The differential diagnoses would be CVD (infarct or hemorrhage), intracranial tumor, and trauma.

Look for evidence of:
- Right hemiparesis
- Dysphasia (left dominant hemisphere involvement)
- Left craniotomy scar (previous trauma or surgery)

Case-3

The patient has a right homonymous upper quadrantanopia. This suggests a lesion in the left temporal cortex.

Differential diagnoses would be CVA (infarction/hemorrhage), trauma, tumor, and surgery.

So look for evidence of:
- Left craniotomy scar (for previous trauma or surgery)
- Right-sided hemiparesis
- Dysphasia

Case-4

The patient has a right homonymous lower quadrantanopia. This suggests a lesion in the left (anterior) parietal cortex.

Diagnosis would be cerebral vascular accident (CVA), tumor, and trauma.

Case-5

There is a central scotoma.
- The disc may be pale, and a distinct margin suggests optic atrophy.
- Swollen (blurred margin) and pink suggests optic neuritis/papillitis.
- The normal disc may suggest retrobulbar neuritis.
- The most important causes would be multiple sclerosis (look for ataxic nystagmus, cerebellar signs).

Other causes would be toxins (alcohol), Leber's hereditary optic atrophy, and nutritional (vitamin B12 deficiency/DM).

Peripheral Neuropathy

Mr Tamim, 65-year-old, presented with weakness. Examine the lower limb.

(After finishing full neurological examination within 6 minutes of time)

Candidate: To complete my examination, I would like to examine the cranial nerves and upper limb chronologically.

Examiner: Would you like to present your case, please?

Candidate:

I believe this gentleman has had evidence of predominantly sensory polyneuropathy with some motor signs.

On examination of the lower limb:

He had trophic changes in his legs with a shiny and dry appearance and loss of hair up to midcalves. He also had callus formation in the region of the metatarsal head. He had reduced tone with evidence of distal weakness. Reflexes of the knee were maintained, but ankle jerks were absent, including reinforcement. Coordination was intact.

On sensory testing:

His sensation to soft touch and pinprick was reduced bilaterally in a stoking distribution up to the knees. Vibration sense was reduced to the patella on both sides. Proprioception was reduced to the ankle.

During gait examination, I noticed he had slight ataxia on tandem walking.

Examiner: Would you like me to tell a bit more specific about what type of neuropathy you think this is?

Candidate: At first, I would like to take a full history, cranial nerves examination, and upper limbs examination.

Same time, I would like to look for other signs to detect underlying causes such as alcohol [stigmata of chronic liver disease (CLD), parotid enlargement, palmar erythema], DM (necrobiosis lipoidica, dermopathy, insulin injection site), HSMN (long-standing neuropathy such as pes cavus, hammer toe), subacute combined degeneration of spinal cord (anemia, optic atrophy, UMNL, central sensory ataxia), Friedreich's ataxia (UMNL, pes cavus, cerebellar syndrome, central sensory ataxia), CTD (rash, joint pain, proteinuria), Guillain-Barré syndrome (GBS) (tracheostomy and central line for plasmapheresis).

Moreover, I believe this patient has predominantly sensory polyneuropathy with some motor signs.

Examiner: What important history you would like to take from this patient?

Candidate: I would like to take some relevant history that includes:
- *Mode of onset*: If predominantly motor polyneuropathy develops over hours to days, then we have to think about—most commonly GBS.

Other possibilities include:
- Acute intermittent porphyria
- Toxins such as diphtheria or botulinum
- Heavy metal poisoning, e.g., lead

Duration and disease course—(acute <6 months, chronic >6 months)
- Waxing and waning course suggest chronic inflammatory demyelinating polyneuropathy (CIDP), inherited neuropathy may develop over the year.
- History of (H/O) DM in most polyneuropathies as it is the leading cause of peripheral neuropathy.

- H/O alcohol intake or drinking habits
- Any suggestive history of malignancy (features such as loss of appetite, weight loss, or other systemic manifestations)
- Suggestive history of RA or CTD with vasculitis (such as arthritis, rash, dry eye, and dry mouth)
- Drugs:
  - Anticancer drugs such as vinblastine and cisplatin.
  - Antibiotic such as fluoroquinolones, nitrofurantoin, isoniazid and metronidazole.
  - Other drugs are chloroquine and amiodarone.

Examiner: Now tell me, what sort of causes would you think for that type of neuropathy?

Candidate: My differentials in this case—
I would like it split into the metabolic cause of diabetes is at the top of the list. Other metabolic causes would include:
- Vitamin deficiencies such as vitamin B1, vitamin B6, and vitamin B12.
- Hyperthyroidism
- Uremia

Other causes of sensory peripheral neuropathy could be split into toxic causes, of which alcohol would be at the top of the list, which would cause predominantly sensory polyneuropathy as well. Furthermore, there could be some other causes, such as:
- Antibiotics
- Chemotherapy agents
- Other medications can be prescribed, such as amiodarone.

Some inflammatory conditions may also consider:
- Connective tissue disease (ANCA positive vasculitis or RA)
- Chronic inflammatory demyelinating polyneuropathy
- Sarcoidosis
- Paraneoplastic neuropathy is either due to a solid organ malignancy (lung cancer) or those associated with paraproteinemia.

Examiner: Based on the multiple causes of the neuropathy you mentioned, are there any simple bedside tests or measures you could do to try and work out the cause of this patient's problem?

Candidate: I would like to do—
- Fundoscopy looking for any evidence of diabetic retinopathy.
- Bedside urine test looking for glucose and protein and bedside blood sugar measurement.

Examiner: Let us for a moment assume he does not have diabetes and you are looking for an alternative cause for peripheral neuropathy. How would you go about investigating him?

Candidate: I would like to start with some basic blood tests such as full blood count (FBC), erythrocyte sedimentation rate (ESR), and C-reactive protein (CRP).
- Here macrocytic anemia suggests vitamin B12 deficiency or alcohol use.
- High ESR and CRP suggest autoimmune inflammatory disorder or paraneoplastic cause.
- Urine routine/examination (R/E), serum creatinine, blood urea and electrolytes (U&Es).
- Liver function tests

Other tests include:
- Thyroid function
- As well as vitamin levels, particularly vitamin B12.

Common causes of neuropathy can be identified from the history, examination, and these simple blood tests.

If the cause of neuropathy is not clear from these simple investigations, the following can be done, and he should be referred to a neurologist.
- Immunological tests including antinuclear antibody (ANA), ANCA, or extractable nuclear antigen (ENA) profile.
- Serum and protein electrophoresis
- Serum angiotensin converting enzyme (ACE) level and chest X-ray (CXR)

Finally, and most importantly, I would like to do—the electrophysiological study, including electromyography (EMG) and nerve conduction study (NCS).

Examiner: What actually are you looking for in the nerve conduction studies of this patient?

Candidate: To determine whether this is demyelinating in nature or whether this is axonal.

Demyelination is shown by slowed conduction velocity with prolonged latency.

On the other hand, an axonal loss is shown by the reduced amplitude of the compound muscle action potential (CMAPs) and sensory nerve action potential (SNAPs) while nerve conduction velocity (NCV) will remain unchanged.

In the case of symmetrical peripheral neuropathies, usually, 80% of cases are axonal. So, it also helps to determine whether the involvement is symmetrical or asymmetrical, small or large fiber or both are involved, which can also help identify the etiology such as with the demyelinating conditions more likely to be associated with an underlying inflammatory condition such as CIDP, rarely monoclonal gammopathy of undetermined significance (MGUS), motor sensory neuropathy (MSN), hereditary motor and sensory neuropathies (HMSN), multifocal motor neuropathy, hereditary neuropathy with pressure palsy, polyneuropathy, organomegaly, endocrinopathy, monoclonal gammopathy, and skin changes (POEMS) syndrome.

Examiner: What do you mean by length-dependent peripheral neuropathy?

Candidate: In case of length-dependent peripheral neuropathy, symptoms usually begin in the most distal segment of the lower limb, especially in the lower extremities and progress in an ascending pattern. As a general rule, sensory symptoms begin in the hands when sensory symptoms in the leg have progressed up to the knee.

These neuropathies are nonlength dependent and are more likely to be the CIDP/acute inflammatory demyelinating polyneuropathy (AIDP) or other inflammatory origins (e.g., CTD)

Examiner: Tell me, what do you mean by small and large fiber neuropathy?

Candidate: Small fiber neuropathy is characterized by impairment of small caliber sensory nerve fiber usually presented with severe pins and needles sensation or feeling as though the feet are ice cold, and difficulty in determining whether both water is hot or cold with the foot (dysesthesia). In small fiber neuropathy, pinprick sensation and a light touch will be markedly affected, but joint position and vibration sensation are relatively preserved. Important causes include DM, alcohol, hypothyroidism, amyloidosis, leprosy, and drugs (isoniazid, cisplatin, and metronidazole).

Large fiber sensory loss usually presents with impairment of balance, which may be assessed in the dark or when vision cannot overcome the loss of proprioception.

Examiner: How will you manage a patient with neuropathic pain?

Candidate: At first, I would be looking at a tricyclic agent which is licensed for the treatment of neuropathic pain, such as amitriptyline or nortriptyline.

If the patient develops any of the side effects of tricyclic agents such as dry mouth, drowsiness, and constipation, in that case, we will use an antiepileptic drug, such as gabapentin or pregabalin, which also is licensed for the management of neuropathic pain.

A serotonin-noradrenaline reuptake inhibitor (SNRI) called duloxetine is another alternative option if sedation is the main problem.

We can also consider topical therapies such as capsaicin if tablets are not being tolerated.

Peripheral Neuropathy: Atypical Features

Mr Kayle, a 45-year-old man, is having a problem with hand function. Examine the upper limb neurologically.

(After finishing full neurological examination within 6 minutes of time)

Candidate: To complete my examination, I would like to examine the cranial nerves and lower limb chronologically.

Examiner: Would you like to present your case, please?

Candidate:

I performed an upper limb neurological examination of this middle-aged gentleman. Based on my clinical finding, I believe he has evidence of peripheral neuropathy with atypical features.

Positive findings include:

When I asked the patient to close his eyes and placed arms outstretched forward with the palm facing up, I noticed that he had an involuntary writhing type of movement when his eyes were closed (pseudoathetosis).

Motor system examination revealed, his tone was normal and symmetrical with reduced power more marked in proximal muscle groups.

Regarding jerks, biceps reflexes were absent. However, the rest of the reflexes were present with reinforcement.

Coordination was impaired in keeping with sensory ataxia.

The soft-touch sensation was intact throughout, but pinprick as well as joint position sense were impaired distally.

Most importantly, vibration sensation was absent throughout the right arm but was present more proximally on the left-hand side.

So, in summary, these findings are consistent with a lower motor neuron syndrome.

As the patient has nonlength dependent proximal muscle weakness with preserved hand strength and asymmetric sensory change with prominent sensory ataxia, which is more marked on the right side, the common causes of peripheral neuropathy are diabetes, hypothyroidism, and chronic alcoholism are much less likely in this case. I believe these are more in keeping with an inflammatory cause of neuropathy.

Depending on the onset of the presentation, if it is coming acutely with the context of areflexia, I would consider something such as GBS [acute motor sensory axonal neuropathy (AMSAN) and Miller Fisher syndrome (MFS)].

If with a chronic presentation, we could consider CIDP or paraneoplastic or other multisystem disorders, (e.g., Sjögren's syndrome, vasculitis).

Examiner: How will you investigate this case?

Candidate: At first, I would like to take a full history from the patient. Then in terms of the investigation, we should start with routine blood tests, such as FBC with ESR with CRP, urea and electrolytes, and liver function tests.

Further, blood tests should be done in peripheral neuropathies such as HbA1c, thyroid function tests, and checking for things such as vitamin B12 and virology.

If there is clinical suspicion, you could also check for things such as:
- Paraneoplastic syndrome with a paraneoplastic screen such as antineuronal-Ab (e.g., Hu, Yo).

- Neurophysiological tests such as nerve conduction studies and EMG can be used to look at whether this is an axonal or a demyelinating process, which can help guide diagnosis.

Other tests that can be used include: Examining the cerebrospinal fluid (CSF) in the form of a lumbar puncture:
- In case of CIDP or GBS, I would expect albuminocytological dissociation (the protein to be raised, but the cell count to be relatively normal).

Examiner: Let us say this was an acute presentation, and you had diagnosed Guillain-Barré syndrome; how would you manage this patient on the ward?

Candidate: In an acute setting, it would be important to approach the patient in an airway, breathing, circulation, disability, exposure (ABCDE) manner and resuscitate them as necessary.

The vast majority of patients with GBS can be managed supportively on the ward; however, you would need to monitor their FVC to look for any involvement of the respiratory muscles.

If the FVC were less than 1.5, you would need to consider whether there was evidence of ventilatory failure present.

You may need to do an arterial blood gas and discuss with higher levels of care, such as intensive care, whether it would require a ventilator in this patient.

Patients who have severe symptoms, such as those who cannot walk, may require other therapies such as plasma exchange or intravenous immunoglobulin.

Examiner: Let us think it from another point of view; if this was a chronic situation and you diagnosed CIDP, how might you go about managing that?

Candidate: So, in the chronic presentation, such as CIDP, it would require an MDT approach.

It would require regular review from a neurology team to consider whether any symptomatic therapies such as neuropathic pain agents required or any disease-modifying therapies such as plasma exchange, intravenous immunoglobulin (IVIG), steroids or other immunosuppression therapies could be required.

Other members of the MDT would include physiotherapy, occupational therapy, and the orthotics team.

Examiner: Would you please tell me the subtypes of GBS?

Candidate: GBS subtypes are:
- *Demyelinating*: AIDP
  - Sensory symptoms and muscle weakness, often with cranial nerve weakness and autonomic involvement.
- *Axonal*:
  - Acute motor axonal neuropathy (AMAN)
  - Isolated muscle weakness without sensory symptoms in <10%; cranial nerve involvement uncommon
  - Acute motor and sensory axonal neuropathy
  - Severe muscle weakness similar to AMAN but with sensory loss
- *Miller Fisher variant*:
  - Sensory ataxia, eye muscle weakness (ophthalmoplegia), areflexia but usually no limb weakness.

Chronic Inflammatory Demyelinating Polyneuropathy

Mr Thomas, 35-year-old, presented with weakness in the upper limb. Examine the upper limb neurologically.

(After finishing full neurological examination within 6 minutes of time)

Candidate: To complete my examination, I would like to examine the cranial nerves and lower limb chronologically.

Examiner: Would you like to present your case, please?

Candidate:

On examination of the upper limb:

There are no trophic changes with no evidence of ulcer and callosities.

There are distal wasting and weakness.

I was unable to elicit any reflexes.

However, the sensation of all four modalities (light touch, pinprick, joint position, vibration senses) is entirely normal.

Coordination cannot be performed due to marked weakness.

The diagnosis is pure motor peripheral neuropathy.

To complete my examination, I would like to examine the cranial nerves and lower limb chronologically.

Examiner: Okay, that is great. What will be the important differential diagnosis of this typical pure motor neuropathy?

Candidate: Most important differential diagnosis would be a case of MND (particularly progressive muscular atrophy variety—its pure form is characterized by minimal signs of the pyramidal sign, but here fasciculation is expected findings as anterior horn cells are involved).
Other possibilities are:
- If wasting and fasciculation are not prominent, weakness is the prominent feature with fatigability then – Myasthenia Gravis (complex ophthalmoplegia, ptosis would be expected).
- Distal myopathy such as—myotonic dystrophy (look for myotonia during the handshake, frontal balding, fascial muscle wasting, ptosis)
- Inclusion body myositis (wasting and weakness of fingers and wrist flexors. Here, weakness of the wrist and finger flexors are often disproportionate to that of the extensor compartment.)

Examiner: Okay. Now tell me some causes of pure motor neuropathy.

Candidate: In the case of acute onset, I would like to think most commonly:
- GBS (AIDP/AMAN variety) or rarely acute intermittent porphyria, lead poisoning, and diphtheria. However, in the case of acute neuropathy, wasting is an uncommon feature.

In case of chronic presentation (where wasting is a common feature), I would think:
- CIDP usually has a symmetrical presentation, but if it is an asymmetrical presentation, I would like to think of multifocal motor neuron (MMN) variety or drugs such as Dapsone.

Examiner: What is the likely cause of this gentleman's symptoms?

Candidate: CIDP classically distal acquired demyelination syndrome (DADS) variety.

Examiner: Tell me the difference between CIDP and multifocal motor neuropathy.

Candidate: Multifocal motor neuropathy is an acquired, autoimmune, demyelinating neuropathy that causes progressive distal weakness and atrophy. There is often asymmetrical limb wasting and weakness (arms > legs). It is very slowly progressive, up to a period of 30 years. Fasciculations occur in 50% of cases. Immunoglobulin M (IgM) anti GM1 ganglioside antibodies are frequently positive. Respond to treatment with IV immunoglobulin.

The CIDP features that would differentiate this from multifocal motor neuropathy disease would be an asymmetrical distribution with raised CSF protein, autonomic dysfunction, and possible sensory involvement.

Sensory Ataxia

Mrs Karen, 35-year-old, presented with difficulty in walking. Examine the lower limb neurologically.

(After finishing full neurological examination within 6 minutes of time)

Candidate: To complete my examination, I would like to examine the cranial nerves and upper limb chronologically.

Examiner: Would you like to present your case, please?

Candidate:

Mrs Karen has lower motor neuron syndrome, which is symmetrical, nonlength dependent and predominantly sensory; sensory-motor neuropathy.

On motor system examination, she had reduced tone, areflexia, power was reduced throughout the lower limb (both proximal and distal weakness was found). She only had antigravity movement in hip flexion (nonlength dependent). She was hesitant on coordination (heel-shin test) testing because of her weakness.

On sensory testing, her sensation was impaired of all four modalities of sensation to the mid-shin.

On checking her gait, she was unsteady when standing, walked with a broad-based gait.

As she was clearly unsteady when standing still, so I did not perform Romberg's test. However, here I expect Romberg's to be positive, given the degree of sensory impairment (sensory ataxia).

During walking, I noted she was wearing a steroid wrist band (medic Alert bracelet).

Although features are atypical (patient has significant sensory ataxia and nonlength dependent weakness—both proximal and distal muscles are involved), we would need to consider the common causes of peripheral neuropathy first, these would include:
- Diabetes
- Alcohol excess
- Vitamin B12 deficiency
- Hypothyroidism

As the signs are atypical, and I noticed she was wearing a wrist band (getting steroid), I would like to consider immune-mediated neuropathy.

Most importantly, I would like to take a full history from the patient, and if this was an acute onset, we need to consider GBS (AMSAN or Miller Fisher variant where ophthalmoplegia is expected along with sensory ataxia and areflexia).

If the onset is gradual or slowly progressive or waxing and waning (increase and decrease) courses—I would like to think CIDP—symmetrical proximal and distal weakness with sensory loss variety of CIDP (usually demyelination).

In this presentation, we should also consider systemic inflammatory conditions such as Sjögren's syndrome, SLE, and RA.

Examiner: Well said. You brilliantly noticed atypical features of peripheral neuropathy here include nonlength dependent weakness with significant sensory ataxia that guide you about immune-mediated neuropathy. Could you tell me the other features of atypical presentation of immune-mediated neuropathy?

Candidate: Most notably, if it is an asymmetrical motor and sensory presentation such as a history of symptoms starting in the hands, trunk, or face (ophthalmoplegia, facial weakness, or sensory loss), would be clear evidence of non-length dependency or features of multisystem autoimmune disease like inflammatory arthropathy, rashes, or Sicca syndrome.

Alternatively, neurophysiological study shows demyelinating polyneuropathy and or signs of dorsal root ganglionopathy.

Examiner: You have suggested a possible immune-mediated cause. What features in the history might help support the diagnosis?

Candidate: I would be looking at the onset of the symptoms and progression of the illness.

If the onset was acute and rapidly progressive, e.g., if she noticed weakness in the lower limbs first then rapidly progressed to involve upper limbs (an ascending type of weakness) over days, I would consider a diagnosis GBS.

If the onset is chronic and slowly progressive over a longer period, I would like to consider CIDP.

If the patient has a waxing and waning course of illness, I would suspect inflammatory or immune-mediated neuropathies. Therefore, I would like to ask if it has gotten better and worse over time or is it static?

In addition, I would like to ask him where did the symptoms start? If the symptoms started in the hands or face, that would be unusual, except it is immune-mediated similarly if they have any truncal symptoms as well.

If the patient is presenting with predominantly ataxic syndromes, this would be likely due to immune-mediated cause.

It is essential to look for any symptoms or signs suggestive of systemic inflammatory conditions such as the suggestive history of inflammatory arthropathy, photosensitive rash, and oral ulceration.

I would also like to ask about dry eyes and dry mouth (sicca syndrome), which would be more suggestive of Sjögren's syndrome.

I would also need to explore the patient's previous and current medications like any biologic or chemotherapy agents, which could explain these symptoms as well.

Examiner: Okay. This patient presented with dry mouth and dry eye. How will you investigate the case to establish your diagnosis?

Candidate: At first, I would like to do basic blood tests, including CBC with ESR, CRP, U&Es, renal function tests as well.

Then I would do, importantly, a neurophysiological study (NCS and EMG).

Finally, to establish my diagnosis, I usually like to do autoantibody screening that includes RA, ANA, and ENA profiles for anti-Ro, anti-LA antibody.

Other tests for Sjögren's syndrome are Schirmer's test, Rose Bengal test, and Labial gland biopsy.

Examiner: Well. Let us think this patient has electrophysiological evidence of demyelinating polyneuropathy and positive RA factor, ANA factor, anti-Ro and anti-LA. How will you treat the case?

Candidate: So my diagnosis would be immune-mediated demyelinating polyneuropathy due to Sjögren's syndrome.

A most important part of management includes increasing the production of saliva and tears so that we can use pilocarpine or cevimeline.

Immune suppression by steroids and disease-modifying antirheumatic drugs (DMARDS) include, most importantly, hydroxychloroquine with or without methotrexate.

Examiner: Tell me, what are the subtypes of CIDP?

Candidate: Chronic inflammatory demyelinating polyneuropathy is an acquired immune-mediated polyradiculoneuropathy characterized by heterogeneous clinical manifestations. In addition to typical CIDP, some atypical forms are considered to be CIDP subtypes, such as:
- Multifocal acquired demyelinating sensory and motor (MADSAM)
- Distal acquired demyelinating symmetric
- Multifocal motor neuropathy
- Multifocal acquired demyelinating sensory and motor neuropathy (Lewis-Sumner syndrome)
- Anti-myelin-associated glycoprotein (MAG) polyneuropathy
- Pure sensory
- Pure motor and focal
- Complicated with other neurological disorders, such as multiple sclerosis, myasthenia gravis, CMTD, Churg–Strauss syndrome, and cerebral palsy.

Charcot–Marie–Tooth Disease

Mr Leo, 45-year-old presented with progressive weakness and a change in the appearance of his legs. Examine the lower limb neurologically.

(After finishing full neurological examination within 6 minutes of time)

Candidate: To complete my examination, I would like to examine the cranial nerves and upper limb chronologically.

Examiner: Would you like to present your case, please?

Candidate:

Mr Leo had generalized wasting of his muscle groups, particularly in the distal muscles. Given the appearance of an inverted champagne bottle and he has gross pes cavus with high arched feet.

His tone was flaccid bilaterally throughout the lower limbs.

Power was reduced, particularly in the distal muscle groups, and I could not elicit any reflexes even with potentiation.

His coordination did appear to be intact, but his pinprick and light touch sensation was reduced up to the knee, and his joint position was impaired in the distal phalanx. His vibration was also reduced up to the medial malleolus.

When I examined his gait, he had a high step stamping gait with bilateral foot drop consistent with sensory ataxia.

He found it very difficult to stand still with his feet together due to unsteadiness.

During my examination, I noticed the patient had ankle-foot orthoses at the side of his bed—these devices are used may be due to correct his foot drop. I also noticed wasting of the muscle groups of the upper limb, which was more marked distally.

I would like to take a full history from the patient, and I also want to examine upper limbs and cranial nerves.

Given the presence (in CMT, it will present in 70% case) of pes cavus, the signs show that the neuropathy is long-standing and mostly consistent with Charcot-Marie-Tooth.

Examiner: You mentioned there, you want to take a history from the patient. What other aspects of history would be particularly important?

Candidate: I would like to take the history of onset and progression of the disease, and I would pay particular attention to the family history by expecting someone such as a parent or sibling, or maybe an aunt or uncle to be affected by Charcot-Marie-Tooth.

Examiner: If we want to investigate the patient for Charcot-Marie-Tooth, how should we proceed?

Candidate: Testing for this sort of genetic neuropathy is quite different from the investigation plan for most acquired polyneuropathies.

In this scenario, basic blood tests are unlikely to be helpful. However, the neurophysiological study can be very useful and are an appropriate first stage.
- This test will demonstrate severe and uniform slowing of conduction velocity or reduced amplitude in both the motor and sensory nerves, keeping with a genetic neuropathy.
- Besides, it may be possible to determine if the neuropathy is axonal or demyelinating, which would help you to target genetic testing appropriately.

This is a genetic condition, so a blood test looking for Charcot-Marie-Tooth genetic studies would be essential.

Many different mutations can cause a Charcot-Marie-Tooth phenotype, and this stage of the investigation is best managed by a specialist in neuromuscular disease.

Examiner: Why is the distinction between demyelinating and axonal neuropathy's helpful or important in the investigation of Charcot-Marie-Tooth?

Candidate: There are multiple types of Charcot-Marie-Tooth (mainly AD but rarely AR or X-linked dominant or recessive).

Type 1: Demyelination type approximately affects 30% of Charcot-Marie-Tooth patients and causes severe demyelination, thereby impairing NCV.

Type 2: Axonal type approximately affects 20–40% of Charcot-Marie-Tooth patients. As it is an axonopathy, average NCV is usually not affected.

Other types are:
- CMT3—Dejerine–Sottas disease, very rare, and severely impaired NCV
- CMT4—Spinal type
- CMT5—Pyramidal type
- CMT6—with optic atrophy
- CMTDI—Dominant intermediate type
- CMTRI—Recessive intermediate type
- CMTX—X-linked type

Examiner: You mentioned pes cavus. Would you please tell me the importance of pes cavus here and tell me some other causes of it?

Candidate: Pes cavus is a high arch of the foot that does not flatten when the patient weight bears. It is seen in only 70% of patients with CMTD. It is an important clinical sign, and if present, indicates that the neuropathy is long-standing and therefore likely to be hereditary. This is the main clue for the diagnosis. Other causes of pes cavus include:
- *Unilateral*: Malunion of calcaneal or talar fracture, burns, sequelae of compartment syndrome, poliomyelitis, spinal trauma, and spinal cord tumors.
- *Bilateral*: Friedreich's ataxia, muscular dystrophies, spinal muscular atrophy, cerebral palsy, syringomyelia, hereditary spastic paraparesis, and spinal cord tumor.

Examiner: Is there any other deformity of the foot that can possible in a Charcot-Marie-Tooth patient?

Candidate: Other foot deformities can also happen, including high arched foot, hammertoes, and contractures of the Achilles tendon.

Examiner: Why are pain and temperature sensations usually unaffected in patients with Charcot-Marie-Tooth disease?

Candidate: Pain and temperature sensations are carried by unmyelinated nerve fibers, and therefore not affected.

Examiner: What does forme fruste of the disease present?

Candidate: This is seen in family members of patients with CMTD, displaying only minor signs, e.g., pes cavus and absent ankle jerks.

Examiner: So, now tell me, how will you treat this gentleman?

Candidate: I am not aware of any disease-modifying treatments that are currently available. However, PXT3003 is in phase 2 clinical trials to treat people with CMT type 1A, the most common form of the disease. It works by blocking PMP22, a protein whose over-production in some CMT1A patients causes nerve damage.

The principles of management include supportive care in the context of an MDT with appropriate genetic counseling. In addition, early implementation of physiotherapy, foot orthosis, or splint can improve functions and significantly delay ankle contracture.

Surgical treatment may be required later in the disease for foot deformity.

Confirming the diagnosis is important by genetic testing as it would help to detect family members who may also be affected and also allow the patient to understand what is affecting them.

Claw Hand

Mrs Ahmed, 38-year-old, has difficulty in hand function. Examine the upper limb neurologically.
(After finishing full neurological examination within 6 minutes of time)

Candidate: To complete my examination, I would like to examine the cranial nerves and lower limb chronologically.

Examiner: Would you present your case?

Candidate:

There is wasting and weakness of the thenar and hypothenar eminence and small muscle of the hand with dorsal guttering.

There is hyperextension of the MCP joint and flexion of the interphalangeal joint resulting in claw hands.

As there is generalized wasting of small muscles of the hand that suggests a lesion is affecting the anterior horn cells, nerve roots, or lower motor neurons that originate from the C8, T1.

Examiner: Now tell me what the cause is and how you will differentiate them?

Candidate: If there is no sensory loss, hyporeflexia, and bilateral involvement, then I would like to think:
- Motor neuron disease if only lower motor sign in both upper and lower limb as well as cranial nerve examination (progressive muscular atrophy), but if hyperreflexia with bilateral plantar extensor in the lower limb then we have to think amyotrophic lateral sclerosis (ALS). Fasciculation in the tongue and limbs is a strong clue to diagnose MND.
- Peripheral motor neuropathy such as multifocal motor neuropathy (50% case may have fasciculation) or CIDP.

If there are bilateral involvement and sensory loss, then I have to think:
- Syringomyelia—here dissociated (loss of pain and temperature sensation with preserved joint position and vibration sense), suspended, cape distribution (upper limb and chest) sensory loss is expected with associated lower limb spastic paraparesis.
- Cervical spondyloradiculopathy or myelopathy usually affects C6, C7; therefore, significant wasting is uncommon but rarely can affect C8, T1. A cervical collar or scar in the neck for previous surgery is a strong clue to the diagnosis. If there is cervical myeloradiculopathy, then the lower limb spastic paraparesis and dorsal column sign are expected.
- Bilateral cervical ribs involving brachial plexus, especially lower trunk and medial cord; and here classical C8 and T1 distribution sensory loss are prominent and symptoms provoked by particular posture and movement such as sleeping in the limbs and cleaning windows.
- Charcot-Marie-tooth disease......there distal wasting of the lower limb and pes cavus and or hammer toe is a strong clue with positive family history for CMT.
- Combined ulnar and median nerve lesion due to any cause.
- Arthritis leading to disuse atrophy—here, wasting out of proportion to weakness associated with joint deformity, the rheumatoid nodule is a clue to the diagnosis.

If it is unilateral and associated with sensory loss in the C8 and T1 distribution, then we have to think:
- Pancoast tumor involving brachial plexus and sympathetic chain (where Horner syndrome is an expected finding) is usually associated with tar staining, clubbing, and lymphadenopathy.
- Cervical rib involving brachial plexus.
- Tumors at the C8-T1 level (neurofibroma).

- Combined median and ulnar nerve palsy (characteristic sensory loss is the strong clinical clue).

Examiner: How will you investigate the case?

Candidate: At first, I would like to take a full history from the patient and examine the cranial nerves and lower limbs thoroughly.

Investigations will depend on further assessment and clues from history.

Here, the most important investigations would be neurophysiological study and magnetic resonance imaging (MRI) of the cervical spine to reach my diagnosis.

Other tests include baseline blood tests, X-ray cervical spine, CXR—posteroanterior (P/A) view and genetic test if required.

Examiner: How will you treat such a case?

Candidate: Here, management will depend on the underlying etiology.

I would like to manage the patient under an MDT involving a neurologist, physiotherapist, occupational therapist, specialist nurse, and if required, rheumatologist as well as a neurosurgeon.

As a part of relieving symptoms, I would give the patient amitriptyline or gabapentin for neuropathic pain.

Spastic Paraparesis

Mr Tylor, 35-year-old, presented with progressive difficulty in walking. Examine the lower limb neurologically.

(After finishing full neurological examination within 6 minutes of time)

Candidate: To complete my examination, I would like to examine the cranial nerves and upper limb chronologically.

Examiner: Would you like to present your case, please?

Candidate:

This patient presented with evidence of spastic paraparesis.

The patient has wasting of the lower limb.

The tone was increased bilaterally with evidence of nonsustained clonus at the ankles.

Power was reduced in both lower limbs, more marked in the proximal distribution.

There was hyperreflexia with bilateral upgoing plantars.

The sensation is impaired in all four modalities, including pinprick, light touch, joint position, and vibration senses.

He had a broad-based ataxic scissor gait and was Romberg positive. There was no spinal deformity, tenderness, or scar.

To further assess this gentleman, I would want to perform upper limb and cranial nerve examination as well as check for sensory level.

These features suggest a myelopathic cause of spastic paraparesis.

Here, the differential diagnosis would be broad, and I would like to take history, particularly looking at the onset and progression of the symptoms.

If this has come on very suddenly within seconds to minutes, then a vascular cause such as a spinal stroke due to anterior spinal artery occlusion or thrombosis is the possibility; however, I would not expect the patient to present with such spasticity in the acute phase.

If this has come acutely in the context of back pain or red flags associated with back pain, then I would think cord compression due to an intervertebral disk herniation (above the L1/2 vertebrae), trauma, collapsed vertebrae most commonly metastatic malignancy such as colon, pancreas, or thyroid; multiple myeloma or tuberculosis (pott's disease). However, I would expect a definite sensory level with the absence of signs above the lesion and early bowel-bladder involvement.

If this has come on subacutely (over days) then an inflammatory or infective pathology could be the cause. In inflammatory condition, I would like to think about multiple sclerosis presenting as a transverse myelitis syndrome. If it were infective, then classically, Varicella zoster virus (VZV) would be the culprit. Other infective causes of myelitis would be human immunodeficiency virus (HIV), human T-lymphotropic virus type 1 (HTLV1), Herpes virus, cytomegalovirus (CMV), etc.

If the presentation is chronic (over a period of time), then metabolic causes such as vitamin B12 deficiency or rarely copper or vitamin E deficiency can also be the cause.

If the patient's symptoms came on very gradually and progressive, we need to consider slowly growing tumors (meningioma), neurodegenerative conditions like Friedreich's ataxia, spinobulbar ataxia, or hereditary spastic paraparesis. Where positive family history is the clue to the diagnosis and most importantly, in case of hereditary spastic paraparesis, sensory signs will be absent.

Examiner: Let us think this is a case of chronic progressive myelopathy; what would be your investigation strategy?

Candidate: MRI of the spine is vital in this patient but would not necessarily need to be urgent, given the chronic nature of the symptoms.

We need to consider any reversible nature, so things such as vitamin B12, copper, and vitamin E levels would need to be measured. These can be reversed with supplementation.

If there is a positive family history, genetic screens for hereditary spastic paraparesis can be arranged, and the patient can be referred to the genetic counseling team.

Examiner: Well said. You already mentioned you want to examine the cranial nerves and upper limb to complete your examination. Now let uss think about a patient presented with spastic paraparesis. What other clinical evidence can help to identify the underlying etiology along with history?

Candidate: In fact, it is very important to take a full history from the patient as well as a thorough neurological examination to reach my diagnosis, such as:

I want to examine the eye—if I get the evidence of optic neuritis (pale optic disc, relative afferent pupillary defect) and INO, then I would think—multiple sclerosis.

If I get the evidence of optic neuritis, then I would think B12 deficiency, Friedreich's ataxia, spinocerebellar ataxia, taboparesis as well.

I would like to see the evidence of cerebellar dysfunction, such as scanning speech, nystagmus, cerebellar ataxia, dysdiadochokinesia then I would like to think multiple sclerosis, Friedreich's ataxia, B12 Deficiency, and spinocerebellar ataxia.

If I get the evidence of a definite sensory level with no signs above the lesion, then I would like to think of cord compression first or transverse myelitis (due to multiple sclerosis/sarcoidosis/SLE).

If I get dysarthria, then I like to think about demyelination (multiple sclerosis) or MND (where an absence of sensory sign is the expected finding).

If I get the evidence of dissociated sensory loss (preserved posterior column but the loss of spinothalamic) then,

- If it is a sudden onset, I would think anterior spinal artery occlusion, where evidence of atrial fibrillation (AF) is an expected finding. Then I want to examine the CVS to identify the cause of it.
- If it is slowly progressive, then I would think syringomyelia where lower motor neuron sign (wasting of the small hand muscles, fasciculation, and loss of reflex) in the upper limb is the expected finding.

If I get evidence of a surgical scar in the spine, then I would like to think of previous surgery for trauma or spinal cord pathology such as a tumor.

If I get the evidence of dorsal column sign with spastic paraparesis, then I would like to think most importantly:
- Cervical myelopathy
- B12 deficiency (anemia with other expected findings)
- Friedreich's ataxia (where pes cavus is an expected finding)
- Taboparesis (Argyll Robertson pupil is an expected finding)
- Tropical spastic paraparesis

If I get spastic paraparesis with no sensory sign, then I would like to think most importantly:
- MND (where wasting with fasciculation are expected findings) or
- Hereditary spastic paraparesis (very rarely, it may have a dorsal column sign).

If I get dorsal column sign with evidence of peripheral neuropathy (stocking pattern sensory loss with loss of ankle jerks), then I would like to think about vitamin B12 deficiency and tropical spastic paraparesis (more commonly in an Afro-Caribbean patient, where proximal > a distal weakness).

Cord Compression

Mr Harry, 55-year-old complaining of back pain. Examine the lower limb neurologically.

(After finishing neurological examination within 6 minutes of time)

Candidate: To complete my examination, I would like to examine the cranial nerves and upper limb chronologically.

Examiner: Would you like to present your case, please?

Candidate:

This middle-aged gentleman has evidence of spastic paraparesis.

There is a muscular weakness in both lower limbs, more marked distally.

The tone is increased bilaterally with ankle clonus on the left side. There is hyperreflexia with bilateral upgoing planters.

Soft-touch and pinprick sensations are diminished in both legs extending upward up to the hip.

Joint position and vibration senses are intact.

The patient has evidence of bladder involvement as a catheter in situ.

To further assess this gentleman, I would want to perform upper limb, cranial nerve examination and, most importantly, want to check for a definite sensory level as well as I would like to take a full history from the patient particularly, onset, and progression of the disease course.

Examiner: That is great. Okay, let us think the patient is complaining of recent onset of back pain, and you have examined the cranial nerves and upper limb, which is completely normal, and he has definite sensory loss at the level of T8, then what will be your differential diagnosis?

Candidate: At this point, it suggests:

Spinal cord compression (compressive myelopathy) possibly from trauma, tumor, or intervertebral disk prolapse at T7-8 level, then we will need to be urgently investigated by MRI of the thoracic spine.

As the patient is elderly, cachectic, most likely, it would be secondary to the spine with collapsed vertebrae. The primary malignancy could be Ca-lung, prostate, kidney, GIT, etc., or it could be multiple myeloma, lymphoma, or infective spondylitis such as Pott's disease or brucellosis.

Moreover, most importantly, I want to examine for anemia and lymphadenopathy and take a full history from the patient to identify an underlying cause.

Other less likely possibilities in the clinical scenario would contribute to inflammatory or infective (noncompressive myelopathy) such as transverse myelitis (it could be the first presentation of MS), lupus, sarcoid, other viral infections—VZV, herpes simplex virus (HSV), HIV infections.

Other possibilities are intradural or extramedullary tumors such as neurofibroma, meningioma, sarcoma, or intramedullary tumors (ependymoma, astrocytoma)

Examiner: How will you investigate the case?

Candidate: If it is an acute onset or rapidly progressive symptoms, then the most important test would be a same-day MRI of the thoracic spine particularly, looking to exclude acute compression that may need urgent surgical decompression or metastatic disease that could require same day radiotherapy as well as I want to consider for steroid.

Other important investigation that would be for this gentleman:

- CBC with ESR with peripheral blood film (PBF), urine R/E, blood urea, serum electrolytes, and serum creatinine.
- CXR P/A view, ultrasonography (USG) of whole abdomen (W/A)
- Protein and immunoelectrophoresis
- Skeletal surveys for multiple myeloma or secondaries

Second line investigations would be:
- Computed tomography (CT) scan of the chest and abdomen
- Bone marrow study

Cervical Myelopathy

Mr Wilson, 65-year-old, presented with difficulty in hand function. Examine the upper limb neurologically.

(After finishing full neurological examination within 6 minutes of time)

Candidate: To complete my examination, I would like to examine the cranial nerves and lower limb chronologically.

Examiner: Would you like to present your case, please?

Candidate:

On examination of the upper limb of this elderly patient showed, the patient was wearing a neck collar (?scar in the neck for previous surgery)

There were segmental wasting and weakness with fasciculation corresponding to C5-C6 nerve roots (biceps and supinator muscles) with normal hand muscle (C8-T1) and triceps muscle (C7).

Biceps and supinator jerks (C5-C6) were absent with inversion of the reflexes (a contraction of the triceps with biceps reflex testing and finger flexion with supinator testing with hyperreflexia at the lower level of the lesion), but triceps jerks are brisk.

There is a segmental sensory loss in C5 (lateral upper arm) and C6 (lateral forearm and thumb) with normal sensation in the C7 (middle finger) and C8 (ring and little finger) to all four modalities of examinations.

There is myelopathy hand sign (when eyes are closed and the hands outstretched and supinated—there is the abduction of the little finger), and there is pseudoathetosis (involuntary writhing of the fingers due to dorsal column involvement)

Dynamic Hoffman sign was positive.

So, my diagnosis is cervical myelopathy. To complete my examination, I would like to examine the cranial nerves and lower limb as well.

Examiner: Okay, this is a case of cervical myeloradiculopathy, so what do you expect in cranial nerve and lower limb examination?

Candidate: So, firstly, I would expect to find a completely normal cranial nerve examination. However, I expect pyramidal weakness in the lower limb with hypertonia, hyperreflexia, ankle clonus, and bilateral plantar extension.

Sensory system examination, I expect impaired joint position and vibration sense. But other modalities of sensation will be intact in that case (may rarely involve in advanced cases).

In gait examination, I expect wide-based scissor gait and Romberg test will be positive.

So, in my lower limb examination, I would get spastic paraparesis with dorsal column signs.

Examiner: Okay. That is fine, so you are getting a mixed picture of lower motor neuron signs in the upper limb and upper motor signs in the lower limb in a patient with cervical myelopathy. In that case, what will be your differential diagnosis, and how will you differentiate them?

Candidate: In that case, MND will be a strong differential diagnosis, but segmental sensory loss and dorsal column signs help differentiate it from MND. Or, the presence of bulbar or pseudobulbar dysarthria, an important feature of MND, is an unexpected finding in cervical myelopathy.

In very few cases of cervical myelopathy patients, sensory signs will be absent. In that case, it is very difficult to differentiate it from MND. However, the presence of tongue wasting, fasciculation, and dysarthria are important clues for MND.

Further investigations, particularly MRI of the cervical spine and evidence of denervation with fasciculation in electrophysiological study (EMG and NCS), will help to establish my diagnosis.

Examiner: Okay, can you tell me the other conditions where mixed upper and lower motor neuron signs may be expected?

Candidate: In fact, in our clinical practice, mixed upper and lower motor neuron signs are very common, usually caused by dual pathology.

Such as in this case, thus, the elderly patient may have diabetes where joint position and vibration sense may be absent along with glove and stocking pattern of sensory loss as a result of diabetic peripheral neuropathy or vitamin B12 deficiency.

Another important clinical condition may have mixed LMN (upper limb) and UMN (lower limb) signs that are syringomyelia, but in that case, dissociated and suspended (cape-like) sensory loss will help to reach our diagnosis.

Examiner: So, in case of cervical myelopathy, you have already mentioned you are expecting spastic paraparesis with dorsal column signs in the lower limb. Can you tell me the other clinical conditions that may have similar clinical features?

Candidate: In that case, a differential diagnosis other than cervical myelopathy would be:
With absent ankle jerk with extensor plantar response:
- Friedreich's ataxia
- Subacute combined degeneration of the spinal cord due to B12 deficiency
- Taboparesis

Moreover, another cause can be multiple sclerosis (but in this case, ankle jerk will be increased with other features of multiple sclerosis like cerebellar signs or optic atrophy).

Examiner: Now, tell me, how will you treat a case of cervical myelopathy?

Candidate: The patient should be treated under an MDT. Treatment options for cervical myelopathy may include:
- Nonsurgical treatment such as simple analgesics for relieving pain, cervical intra-articular steroid injections and physiotherapy.
- Surgical procedures include decompressive discectomy/foraminotomy/laminoplasty/hemilaminectomy.

Stroke/Cerebrovascular Disease

Mr Parker, 49-year-old, presented with difficulty in walking. Examine the lower limb neurologically.

(After finishing full neurological examination within 6 minutes of time)

Candidate: To complete my examination, I would like to examine the cranial nerves and upper limb chronologically.

Examiner: Would you like to present your case, please?

Candidate:

This patient presented with evidence of right-sided hemiparesis.

On general inspection, I noticed a flexor posturing of the right upper limb with dystonic posturing of the right hand (the shoulder is held adducted with internal rotation whilst the wrist is flexed and fingers are held extended).

I also noticed he has ankle-foot orthosis as well as a walking aid.

The patient has extensor posturing of the right lower limb.

There are hypertonia and spasticity in the knee and ankle joint.

Hyperreflexia with weakness in a pyramidal distribution (that means flexor muscles are weaker than extensors).

The right plantar response is an extensor.

There is reduced sensation to pinprick and fine touch in the right lower limb.

There is a left hemiplegic gait.

When I asked some more complex questions and gave him more complex instructions, I noticed there was hesitancy in his speech and hesitancy when responding to verbal commands.

To complete my assessment, I would like to assess the speech, visual field and examine the upper limb and cranial nerves.

I would also like to take a full history from the patient regarding the onset and progression of the symptoms, particularly weakness, headache, loss of consciousness, as well as the risk factor assessment for stroke, such as HTN, DM, dyslipidemia, smoking, and family history, and also I want to ask him whether he is a right-handed or left-handed person.

If these symptoms suddenly come on, we need to think about stroke, either ischemic or hemorrhagic. In that case, I would like to examine the pulse to see the evidence of AF, measure the blood pressure (BP) and carotid pulse (to see the evidence of carotid artery stenosis-bruit), which is the most common cause of ischemic stroke, particularly the anterior circulation stroke for this patient as he has evidence of right-sided hemiparesis with dysphasia.

If it is the insidious onset with slow progression and having a headache, convulsion or evidence of papilledema, then brain tumor or other space-occupying lesions due to any cause would be my strong differential diagnosis.

If it is the subacute onset and having a relapse and remitting episodes with evidence of other neurological deficits such as optic neuritis, INO, cerebellar, and dorsal column signs, then I would like to think demyelinating cause such as multiple sclerosis.

Examiner: If the patient had evidence of expressive dysphasia and other signs and your diagnosis is a stroke, how would you classify a stroke like this?

Candidate: These are consistent with an anterior circulation stroke. We would need to identify any visual field defect (homonymous hemianopia or quadrantanopia) on examination of the eyes.

If this were present in the context of the other features, that would be consistent with a total anterior circulation stroke (anterior and middle cerebral artery both supplied by the internal carotid artery).

If it were not present, it would be a partial anterior circulation stroke.

If a patient with cerebral stroke and an anterior circulation is affected, he is most likely to have carotid artery stenosis. In that case, we have to exclude carotid artery stenosis by doing a carotid Doppler study or carotid angiogram. If the stenosis is >70% of the ipsilateral carotid artery, it is termed symptomatic carotid artery stenosis and requires urgent carotid endarterectomy.

Examiner: How would you assess speech in a patient with stroke?

Candidate: There are multiple points of speech such as frequency, comprehension, repetition, naming that should be assessed.

At first, I would like to assess comprehension by asking some simple commands such as *"Close and open your eyes."*

If they are able to understand these, I would like to move to more complex commands such as *"Touch your right ear with your left hand."*

It is then important to check for any evidence of expressive dysphasia or dysarthria. I can ask them to repeat phrases such as *"Baby hippopotamus"* or *"42 West Register Street"*.

Speech production (fluency) can be tested by asking them the question that requires a long answer *"Please tell me what did you have for breakfast this morning."*

We can also test for naming, e.g., holding up a pen and asking them to name it and asking *"what you would use that for."*

If the patient's speech is fluent but is incomprehensible, repetition and naming are impaired, then he had sensory aphasia (Wernicke's dysphasia) due to impairment of the dominant posterior perisylvian area.

If the patient is not fluent, comprehension is normal, but repetition is impaired, then it is Broca's (expressive) dysphasia due to involvement of the dominant precentral area—posterior part of the inferior frontal gyrus.

But, if the patient is not fluent, both comprehension and repetition are impaired, then he has global aphasia. The causative lesion affects both sensory and expressive elements commonly caused by dominant middle cerebral artery (MCA) territory infarct.

Examiner: Okay, now, if the patient presents within the thrombolysis window, how would you manage that situation?

Candidate: With any acutely unwell patient, it is important to approach them in an ABCDE manner and resuscitate them as necessary.

Once the patient is stabilized, it is important to take the history and identify things such as the onset of symptoms.

At first, I would like to exclude some stroke mimics conditions (hypoglycemia, migraine may present with aphasia and hemiparesis, Todd's paresis following a focal seizure, central nervous system (CNS) infections such as fever with neurological symptoms, functional hemiparesis—weakness unlikely to be a pyramidal pattern) with a rapid assessment of the patient and by doing some investigations such as:
- CBC, ESR, CRP, blood C/S, RBS, LFTs and RFTs
- CXR P/A view to see the evidence of cardiomegaly and aspiration
- Electrocardiogram (ECG) to see the evidence of AF or previous infarction

Then I will do an urgent CT scan of the brain; it is often normal in the acute phase in case of embolic stroke or may see thrombus on the proximal, middle cerebral artery, or hyperdynamic signal of blood in hemorrhagic stroke.

I would like to consider thrombolysis with a tissue plasminogen activator because the patient presented with ischemic stroke within the thrombolysis window period (3-4.5 hours) and no contraindication for it. It is given intravenously peripherally and regular (15 minutes) neurological observation to look for any drop in Glasgow Coma Scale (GCS), which may indicate hemorrhagic transformation or edema, causing raised ICP.

We have to perform a post-thrombolysis CT scan within 24 hours or sooner if GCS score drops, and also we have to avoid catheterization, venipuncture, or other invasive procedure for 24 hours.

Then I would like to refer the patient to a specialist stroke unit for an MDT approach involving a neurologist, specialist stroke rehabilitation nurse, physiotherapist, speech and language therapist, and occupational therapist. At the same time, I would like to add antiplatelet clopidogrel (or aspirin and dipyridamole). I would also want to consider deep venous thrombosis (DVT) prophylaxis.

Examiner: Okay, that is good; would you like me to tell the chronic management of a stroke patient?

Candidate: Here, the most important to address the cardiovascular risk factors such as DM, HTN, dyslipidemia, and treat these conditions appropriately.

I also want to consider anticoagulation for cardiac thromboembolism.

Finally, carotid endarterectomy in a patient who has made a good recovery (if >70% stenosis of the ipsilateral internal carotid artery (ICA)] as well as nursing and social care.

Examiner: Now, would you please tell me some complications of stroke?

Candidate: Acute complications are raised ICP due to hemorrhagic transformation or perilesional edema. Another acute complication would be aspiration pneumonia.

Complications due to immobility include pneumonia, contractures, DVT, pressure sores, urinary tract infections, constipation, and disuse atrophy from immobility.

Later complications include depression and reduced social interaction, seizure, and thalamic pain syndrome.

Cerebellar Disorder (Upper Limb)

Mrs Lily, 45-year-old, has difficulty walking. Examine the upper limb neurologically.

(After finishing full neurological examination within 6 minutes of time)

Candidate: To complete my examination, I would like to examine the cranial nerves and lower limb chronologically.

Examiner: Would you like to present your case, please?

Candidate:

I performed the upper limb neurological examination of this middle-aged lady. Based on my clinical finding, I believe she has the right cerebellar syndrome.

This patient is ataxic on the right side.

On upper limb neurological examination, there is dysdiadochokinesia, impaired finger nose testing with past pointing (dysmetria) and an intention tremor (that worsens as the finger approaches the target) on the right side.

There is a failure of the displaced right arm to find its original posture with the eyes closed (Rebound phenomenon).

During my examination, I noticed the patient has scanning dysarthria. However, her muscle power, reflex, and all four modalities of sensation are intact.

To complete my assessment, I would like to examine the cranial nerves, lower limbs, and most importantly, gait.

At first, I would like to take a full history from the patient, particularly cadence of onset as well as the progression of the symptoms.

If the symptoms came on suddenly, I would be thinking about stroke, either ischemic or hemorrhagic or if there is relapse and remitting disease course and other signs such as INO or optic atrophy, then I would like to think—multiple sclerosis.

If it is slowly progressive, then we have to think of a space-occupying lesion in the cerebellum—the primary (medulloblastoma, astrocytoma), secondary or abscess.

As there is a unilateral or asymmetrical sign—degenerative [multiple system atrophy (MSA)], nutritional (vitamin B12 and E) or toxic causes (drugs, alcohol), hypothyroidism, paraneoplastic, hereditary (Friedreich's ataxia, spinocerebellar ataxia) is unlikely here because in these cases, global dysfunction is an expected finding.

Examiner: How will you investigate this case?

Candidate: In this case, brain imaging is the most important investigation. MRI is the gold standard imaging for looking at the posterior fossa. However, CT has a vital role in a hyperacute presentation when hemorrhages are needed to be rapidly excluded.

Examiner: Okay, let us assume you have examined a patient where you are getting evidence of unsteadiness when sitting down and broad-based ataxic gait; however, no other abnormalities in the limbs when tested separately. Now tell me, what is the cause of these types of features?

Candidate: So, the patient has only truncal ataxia, which suggests a lesion of the cerebellar vermis, mostly found in cerebellar degeneration related to alcohol.

Cerebellar Ataxia

Mrs Jane, a 50-year-old, has difficulty walking. Examine the cranial nerves.

(After finishing full neurological examination within 6 minutes of time)

Candidate: To complete my examination, I would like to examine the upper and lower limb chronologically.

Examiner: Would you like to present your case, please?

Candidate:

This lady has evidence of cerebellar ataxia with bilateral signs.

During my cranial nerve examination, I noticed that she has truncal ataxia, evidence of intermittent head tremor, and nystagmus in all directions of gaze. I also noticed scanning/staccato speech during my examination.

She has evidence of reduced visual acuity in the right eye; however, there was no evidence of a relative afferent pupillary defect or pale optic disease suggestive of optic nerve lesion.

She complained of jumpy vision or oscillopsia.

To complete my examination, I would like to see gag reflex, corneal reflex, and examine upper and lower limbs (limb ataxia suggest lobe involvement).

So in terms of the cause of this syndrome, I would like to take a full history from the patient, mainly focusing on the onset and progression of the symptoms and looking for other signs (upper and lower limb).

If these symptoms had come on suddenly, we need to think about stroke; either ischemic or hemorrhagic. In addition, I would expect CVD to be unilateral, whereas this examination showed bilateral signs.

I would then want to screen for other associated neurological signs and symptoms (pyramidal and sensory symptoms) that might suggest certain conditions such as multiple sclerosis; there might be a history of relapse and remitting disease course. However, in that case, INO or features of optic neuritis or atrophy is an expected finding but notably absent here.

A detailed social history would be required to look for risk factors such as alcohol consumption which commonly present with these symptoms. In that case, I would expect evidence of alcoholic liver disease, bilateral parotid enlargement, and peripheral neuropathy as well.

I would also like to take drug history, particularly some drugs that can cause this type of syndrome, such as anticonvulsants (phenytoin, lithium, carbamazepine, phenobarbitone) and also chemotherapy drugs.

I would like to take a suggestive history of systemic illness like hypothyroidism or nutritional deficiency, like B12, copper, or vitamin E deficiency as a cause of the cerebellar syndrome.

I would like to take a family history of the rare genetic cause of cerebellar syndromes such as spinocerebellar ataxia and Friedreich's ataxia, where other features such as pyramidal and a sensory sign can help to reach my diagnosis.

Finally, I would like to think paraneoplastic causes of the cerebellar syndrome as well, and here I expect the evidence of malignancy such as cachexia, anemia, lymphadenopathy, or clubbing.

Examiner: You have presented to me as this is a case of cerebellar ataxia, so how do you confidently say this is not sensory ataxia?

Candidate: There is evidence of nystagmus with scanning or staccato speech in this case, which is unexpected in the sensory ataxia.

However, if I examine the patient's limb, we will get evidence of impaired sensation, particularly joint position and vibration sense in sensory ataxia. In sensory ataxia, we can get the involuntary writhing movements of the fingers and hands with arms outstretched and eyes closed (pseudoathetosis).

If I examine the gait, I would expect broad-based gait in both sensory and cerebellar ataxia. However, if I do the Romberg test in sensory ataxia, the patient sways whilst the eyes are shut. On the other hand, in cerebellar ataxia, usually, the patient will be unable to stand with both feet together—but if possible, then rombergism is more or less the same with eyes open or closed.

Besides, the patient with sensory ataxia will be able to perform heel-shin, and finger nose tests with eyes open but could struggle with eyes closed (in fact, in sensory ataxia, all problems are made worse by removing the patient's visual input).

Examiner: How will you investigate this case?

Candidate: Investigations will be guided by history. However, all patients with cerebellar ataxia will require brain imaging—MRI is the gold standard imaging for cerebellar dysfunction, but CT plays a vital role in a hyperacute presentation when hemorrhage needs to be rapidly excluded.

Other tests include CBC, LFTs, TFTs, bone profile (Ca, PTH), vitamin E, B12, and thiamine levels, serum ceruloplasmin level (to exclude Wilson's), serum phytanic acid level (for suspected Refsum disease), screening for implicated drugs level, autoantibody screen (for paraneoplastic cerebellar degeneration).

Examiner: How will you manage a patient with an ataxic syndrome like this?

Candidate: Given the significant functional impairment due to cerebellar dysfunction, management would take place in an MDT setting with input from physiotherapy, occupational therapy, neurologist, and specialist nurse as appropriate.

The exact management depends on the underlying cause of the cerebellar syndrome, such as avoidance of drugs causing cerebellar dysfunction.

In general, an MDT approach to helping a patient retain their function and independence is useful, e.g., we could:
- Review the patient regularly under a physiotherapist to help with their mobility and give them exercises to preserve their strength.
- Involve the occupational therapists to see what adaptation we would need to make at their home and provide them with any mobility aids to help them with their independence.

Examiner: What types of lifestyle advice would you like to give the patient?

Candidate: I think the first thing we could do is look at the patient's occupation and assess whether they are at any risk whilst they are at work. We could see if there are any adaptation we could make to their workplace to help them continue with their occupation.

The second thing to do is look more broadly at their medical history, particularly their medications. Are there any medications they are taking that could affect the cerebellum or exacerbate any causes of dizziness or unsteadiness?

I would like to advise importantly to reduce their amount of alcohol consumption or stop this altogether. Although alcohol might not cause the cerebellar syndrome, it is known to exacerbate cerebellar symptoms.

Multiple Sclerosis

Mrs Kate, 45-year-old, presented with difficulty in walking. Examine the lower limb neurologically.

(After finishing full neurological examination within 6 minutes of time)

Candidate: To complete my examination, I would like to examine the upper limb and cranial nerves.

Examiner: Would you like to present your case, please?

Candidate:

Mrs Kate had evidence of an asymmetrical spastic paraparesis.

On examination, she had a broad-based ataxic gait, and she used a stick to support her walk. Romberg test was also positive.

She had increased tone bilaterally more on the left compared to the right with sustained clonus in the left leg. Reflexes were brisk bilaterally, more so on the left compared to the right and upgoing plantar on the left side.

Power was reduced on both legs at hip flexion and knee flexion but otherwise well-preserved.

Coordination was impaired probably due to weakness more than true incoordination.

Sensation showed hyperesthesia in the right leg to pinprick, but joint position and vibration sense was impaired distally on both sides.

These findings were in keeping with partial Brown-Séquard syndrome because in complete Brown-Séquard syndrome, I would expect weakness and posterior column signs will be restricted to one side and loss of spinothalamic signs will be on the opposite side.

To complete my examination and further assessment, I would want to perform an upper limb and cranial nerve examination and check for sensory level.

As there is an asymmetry in presentation, I would like to think of myelitis or compressive lesion first rather than a degenerative, hereditary, or nutritional deficiency.

- Firstly, I would think about the compressive causes—probably the most common cause of these signs would be disc prolapse or tumor that may be primary or secondary in terms of metastasis.
- Next, I would like to consider autoimmune processes such as multiple sclerosis or lupus or sarcoid or myelitis due to infections, most importantly, VZV infection or rarely HIV, HSV, CMV, TB.
- After that, I would think about a nutritional deficiency such as B12 or copper or other vitamin deficiency that usually presents symmetrical involvement, which is less likely in this clinical scenario.
- Lastly, I would like to consider hereditary spastic paraparesis, where symmetrical involvement is usual but less likely to have a sensory sign (dorsal column).

In terms of investigations, as the patient has predominant upper motor neuron signs, so the most appropriate investigation would be an MRI scan of the cervicothoracic cord.

Examiner: As your diagnosis is multiple sclerosis and also you want to look for some other signs. So, what sort of signs are you talking about?

Candidate: In that case, the most important part would be examining the eyes, where I want to look for evidence of optic neuritis or neuropathy such as a relative afferent pupillary defect and a pale optic disc.

I want to look for the evidence of INO (one of the eyes is not adducting, and the other abducted eye has nystagmus. By covering the eye with nystagmus, the nonadducting eye normally adducts. It suggests a lesion in the medial longitudinal fasciculus of the nonadducting eye).

Examiner: Other than an MRI scan of the cervico-thoracic spine, are there any other investigations that you think would be helpful?

Candidate: If we consider a diagnosis of multiple sclerosis, we have to look for evidence of the demyelinating plaques in other parts of the CNS, particularly in the periventricular regions as well as in the cerebellum.

The other thing we could do is a lumbar puncture, where we expect a predominantly normal cell count with typical oligoclonal bands. Another test would be visual evoked potential to get evidence of optic neuropathy (delayed latency).

If they were present, that would be very indicative of multiple sclerosis.

Examiner: How would you like to manage this case?

Candidate: I would like to manage him by an MDT approach involving physiotherapist, occupational therapist, social worker, MS specialist nurse, as well as a neurologist to boost the quality of life. At the same time, I would like to give some drugs for symptomatic improvements, such as baclofen for his spasm, gabapentin for neuropathic pain, antimuscarinic (oxybutynin) for urinary symptoms.

I would like to take a full history from the patient; if she has a history of frequent relapse (at least 2 attacks of neurological dysfunction over 2/3 years) followed by reasonable recovery or secondary progression, then I would like to consider disease-modifying agents such as:
- Beta-interferon
- Glatiramer acetate
- Natalizumab is useful in severe relapsing-remitting multiple sclerosis, which is unresponsive to other therapies. However, it is associated with the risk of progressive multifocal leukoencephalopathy, so close monitoring of the patient is required.

Examiner: If this lady has a confirmed diagnosis of multiple sclerosis, and she is now presenting to you with an acute deterioration in her neurological function, such as difficulty in walking. How are you going to manage this acute situation?

Candidate: In that case, I would think that this is likely to be a relapse of her multiple sclerosis.

During the acute situation, we have to treat the case with high dose intravenous corticosteroids such as methylprednisolone (1 g/day for 3 days) to shorten acute relapse and reduce severity but do not influence long-term outcomes.

Before starting steroids, we need to make sure that there are no signs of infection (e.g., negative urine dip) as well as we need to warn the patient about the possible side effects such as insomnia, personality change and even mania, drug-induced gastritis, and very rarely, can cause avascular necrosis of the hip. It is also important to monitor the patient's blood sugar regularly during the treatment period as steroids can cause higher glucose levels.

Motor Neuron Disease (Kennedy's Disease)

Mr Kelvin, 53-year-old, presented with progressive weakness. Examine the upper limb neurologically.

(After finishing full neurological examination within 6 minutes of time)

Candidate: To complete my examination, I would like to examine the cranial nerves and lower limb chronologically.

Examiner: Would you like to present your case, please?

Candidate:

I performed an upper limb neurological examination of this middle-aged gentleman. Based on my clinical findings, I believe this patient had a possible MND.

On examination, there was global wasting which was most prominent distally, especially in the FDI muscles accompanied by a quite prominent fasciculation, particularly in the triceps muscle distribution bilaterally.

Tone and power were reduced globally throughout the upper limb.

I was not able to elicit any reflex even after potentiation.

Most importantly, coordination and sensation of all four modalities were entirely normal.

Therefore, I believe this is a case of lower motor neuron syndrome. The differential diagnosis would be either anterior horn cell disease such as MND or affecting the nerve itself, like multifocal motor neuropathy.

During the assessment period, I noted there was prominent fasciculation in the perioral region and the neck. Given the signs, I would suspect a type of hereditary motor neuron condition called Kennedy's disease.

I would like to assess this patient completely by taking a full history from him, particularly the onset of symptoms progression as well as family history and by further examination of the lower limb and cranial nerve.

Examiner: Well, you carefully identified the specific signs for Kennedy's disease. So, what are the features in history that might help you differentiate that from other anterior horn cell disorders?

Candidate: In sporadic anterior horn cell disorders, e.g., ALS or progressive muscular atrophy (variety of MND), I would expect that to be a rapidly progressing condition affecting the motor nerves.

In Kennedy's disease, which is an X-linked recessive condition affecting the androgen receptors, by taking a history, I would expect insidious onset with slowly progressive symptoms affecting only lower motor nerves.

Another key element of the history would be looking at the family history, particularly expecting someone such as parents or sibling or an aunt or uncle to be affected by Kennedy's disease or unexplained neurological disorders in the past.

Examiner: Let us back to the examination again. What key features help differentiate Kennedy's from sporadic ALS?

Candidate: While I examine a patient with ALS, I would expect to find evidence of both upper and lower motor neuron involvement, such as, if I get evidence of wasting and fasciculation in the lower limb with exaggerated reflex and upgoing plantars, then it is ALS variety of MND which is the most common variety of MND. However, if only anterior horn cells are affected involving both upper and lower limbs, it is called progressive muscular atrophy (a variety of MND).

In this patient, as there is clear evidence of fasciculations around the mouth with predominantly lower motor neuron signs in the limbs would point us toward Kennedy's disease where only lower motor neurons are affected.

Examiner: How will you investigate this case?

Candidate: Here, the most important test would be a neurophysiological study that includes EMG and NCS, where we will get evidence of denervation, particularly fibrillation and fasciculation with an absence of sensory signs.

In terms of multifocal motor neuropathy, which is less likely in this clinical scenario, I may expect to find demyelination (prolonged latency with slowed conduction velocity) in the motor nerve.

Another important test would be an MRI of the brain and spine to exclude main differentials that are cervical cord compression, myelopathy, and brainstem lesions.

Kennedy's disease can be confirmed by genetic testing.

Examiner: How would you like to manage this patient?

Candidate: Given the significant functional impairment due to MND, management would take place in an MDT setting with input from a neurologist, physiotherapist, occupational therapist, neuropsychologist, speech, and language therapist as well as a specialist nurse.

In general, a multidisciplinary team approach to helping a patient retain their function and independence is useful, e.g., we could regularly review the patient under a neurologist looking for symptomatic management and a physiotherapist to help with their mobility and give them exercises to preserve their muscle strength.

Involve the occupational therapists to see what adaptations we would need to make at their home and provide them with any mobility aids to help them with their independence.

Input from the speech and language therapist would help ensure that the patient's diet is appropriate to help reduce the risk of aspiration in these patients.

To support the patient mentally, neuropsychological assessment and counseling can often be arranged with the help of the MND specialist nurses.

Some patients may develop neuromuscular ventilation weakness, and an early morning blood gas analysis can help identify these patients. In such cases, it would be important to make a referral to the respiratory team, and the ventilation specialist nurses, as well as they may need additional support [noninvasive ventilation (NIV)], particularly nocturnally.

Bulbar Palsy (Motor Neuron Disease)

Mr Edward, 43-year-old, presented with progressive weakness. Examine the cranial nerves.

(After finishing full neurological examination within 6 minutes of time)

Candidate: To complete my examination, I would like to examine the upper and lower limb chronologically.

Examiner: Would you like to present your case, please?

Candidate:

This middle-aged gentleman had evidence of bulbar palsy due to MND.

On examination, there were obvious wasting and weakness of the tongue with prominent fasciculation. In addition, the patient had dysarthria with a nasal quality speech ("Donald duck" speech due to palatal weakness).

There was palatal paralysis. However, importantly sensation and eye movement were intact; and the jaw jerk was normal.

On general inspection, he was in a wheelchair. There were wasting and fasciculation in his hands and forearms.

I would like to examine the patient by looking at the evidence of nasal regurgitation or dysphagia. Moreover, most importantly, I would like to examine the upper and lower limb; also cognitive function and respiratory function as well.

Examiner: Well said. You mentioned that you could examine both upper and lower limbs neurologically, so what other signs would you be particularly looking for here?

Candidate: In this case, I have only detected lower motor neuron features that suggest progressive bulbar palsy, a variety of MND. However, if it is ALS, a most common form of MND, I would expect a combination of upper and lower motor neuron signs that means spastic weakness with an exaggerated reflex in combination with characteristic wasting and fasciculation in the limbs with an absence of a sensory sign.

Examiner: Let us move to a step forward to investigating this patient. What kind of tests would you like to perform?

Candidate: I would like to perform EMG and NCS as a part of the neurophysiological study at the peripheral nerve looking for evidence of denervation (fibrillation and fasciculation) and lack of sensory changes.

Other tests would be routine blood tests and, most importantly, the lung function test (FVC) to see the evidence of respiratory involvement.

Examiner: Now, move to the management plan and tell me the important things to consider in managing such degenerative disorders involving the motor system?

Candidate: So, the only drug treatment that I am aware of is riluzole (glutamate antagonist), licensed in MND that slows disease progression by an average of 3 months. However, it does not improve function and quality of life, and it is costly.

In fact, management is mostly supportive and would take place in an MDT setting where the primary team members would be a consultant neurologist and an MND nurse specialist.

In this patient, importantly, I would like to involve the speech and language therapist to assess their swallowing ability in case they need any changes to their diet or fluids and consider if they need nonoral feeding such as a percutaneous endoscopic gastrostomy (PEG) tube.

I would also like to involve the occupational therapist and physiotherapist who can work to support the patient at home and establish any other circumstances that need to be looked at home.

Lastly, I would want this patient's respiratory function assessed regularly as some patients may develop neuromuscular ventilation weakness. In such cases, it would be important to make a referral to the respiratory team and to the ventilation specialist nurses, as well as they may need additional support (NIV), particularly nocturnally.

Examiner: Okay, now tell me some other causes of bulbar palsy.

Candidate: Other causes are:
- Myasthenia gravis where the myopathic face, ophthalmoplegia, bilateral ptosis with fatigability is the expected findings.
- Neuropathy, particularly GBS or multifocal motor neuropathy.
- Myopathy; here, I would not expect tongue wasting and fasciculation.

Examiner: Would you please tell me the pathological basis of fasciculation in MND?

Candidate: In MND, there is progressive axonal degeneration of the upper and lower motor neurons; axonal loss results in the surviving axons recruiting and innervating more myofibrils than usual, resulting in large motor units. So, fasciculation results from the spontaneous firing of the large motor units.

Myotonic Dystrophy

Mr Patel, 35-year-old, has difficulty in fine activity with the hands. Examine the upper limb neurologically.

(After finishing full neurological examination within 6 minutes of time)

Candidate: To complete my examination, I would like to examine the cranial nerves and lower limb chronologically.

Examiner: Would you like to present your case, please?

Candidate:

> I believe this patient has evidence of myotonic dystrophy.
>
> He had a symmetrical distal weakness with wasting, but the power of the proximal muscles was preserved. The tone was normal. Deep tendon reflexes were reduced, only elicited after reenforcement.
>
> Importantly, the sensation of all four modalities was intact.
>
> Coordination was normal within the limbs.
>
> During my examination, I noticed he had a long thin expressionless face (lifeless face) with bilateral partial ptosis with frontal baldness and wasting of the facial muscles.
>
> I also noticed a walking aid with ankle-foot orthosis, possibly due to bilateral foot drop with a high steppage gait.

So I looked for evidence of myotonia:
- I asked the patient to grip my hand tightly for 5 seconds, then release. He was unable to open it quickly.
- When I asked him to do repeated handgrip exercises, the myotonia phenomenon gradually reduced in intensity (warm-up effect in myotonic dystrophy)
- I asked the patient to close the eyes as tightly as he could, then I noticed there was difficulty opening the eyes after tight closure.
- Finally, after gentle percussion of the thenar eminence with tendon hammer, I noticed dimpling and adduction of the thumb with slow relaxation.

To complete my examination, I would like to examine the cranial nerves and lower limb as well as gait.

Examiner: If I give you some more time to further assess the patient, what other findings do you want to look for?

Candidate: I would like to examine the cranial nerves where I expect weakness and wasting of the bilateral temporalis, masseter, fascial, and sternocleidomastoid muscle groups.

There may be evidence of bilateral cataracts (loss of red reflex).

Slurred and nasal voice due to combined tongue and pharyngeal myotonia.

I would examine the CVS for evidence of cardiomyopathy and arrhythmia like irregular pulse, low blood pressure, or presence of a pacemaker.

Also, I would like to check for evidence of DM (finger prick marks), bilateral gynecomastia with testicular atrophy.

Examiner: How will you investigate this case?

Candidate: As this is an autosomal dominant disease and has a 50% chance of transmitting the disease to the next generation, there is a high possibility of having a positive family history. So,

I would like to take a full history from the patient, most importantly, a positive family history of this type of illness.

I would like to do the basic blood tests, most importantly blood sugar level with HbA1c.

I would like to do a full cardiac assessment by doing an ECG, echocardiography, and, if required, a 24-hour Holter monitoring.

In ECG, I would expect a low voltage QRS complex, prolonged PR interval and prolonged QTc, or often arrhythmias [AF, supraventricular tachycardia (SVT), ventricular tachycardia (VT)].

Echocardiography will give evidence of cardiomyopathy.

The neurophysiological study may show myotonic discharge (dive-bomber potentials), which presents in EMG and help to exclude other differential diagnoses.

Here the most important test would be to confirm our diagnosis—blood test for genetic study to demonstrate trinucleotide repeat expansion (>50 *CTG* gene) in chromosome 19 (type 1 myotonic dystrophy) or tetranucleotide repeat expansion (>75 *CCTG* gene) in chromosome 3 (type 2 myotonic dystrophy).

Examiner: What do you know about anticipation?

Candidate: Early-onset and progressively worsening signs and symptoms in successive generations are called anticipation.

In type 1 myotonic dystrophy, a genetic mutation occurs in the dystrophia myotonica protein kinase (DMPK) on chromosome 19. Here, the mutation is an expansion of a CTG trinucleotide repeat sequence above its maximal upper limit of 35. Here, dynamic mutation causes an increase in several repeats with successive generations and hence causes earlier onset and disease severity.
- If it is 50–150 repeats, then it produces mild disease (present at age 20–40 years with mild myotonia and cataract with normal life span).
- If it is 150–1,500 repeats, then it produces classic myotonic dystrophy (present at the age 10–30 years with life expectancy 45–55 years).
- If it is >2,000 repeats, then it presents as congenital myotonic dystrophy. Present at birth with myotonia, respiratory deficits, and intellectual impairment with a 30–40 years life expectancy.

On the other hand, in myotonic dystrophy type 2, it is also an autosomal dominant condition, causing proximal myotonic myopathy, involving tetranucleotide (CCTG) repeat sequence on chromosome 3, which is usually milder. Proximal muscles (thigh, hip, shoulder) affect first. The patient typically has no cognitive involvement and does not have a congenital form.

Examiner: Let us say this is a case of myotonic dystrophy. How will you manage this case?

Candidate: In fact, there is no cure; however, the principles of management include supportive care in the context of an MDT with appropriate genetic counseling. The patient should be signposted to patient groups, such as the myotonic dystrophy support group.

Muscle weakness can be managed with physiotherapy and orthosis such as a foot or wrist splint, so need the involvement of the physiotherapist and occupational therapist.

Speech and language therapy can help with any communication and swallowing difficulties.

Myotonia, if symptomatic, may be helped by procainamide or phenytoin.

Pain management will often require gabapentin or amitriptyline.

Cardiology referral—there may be a need for pacemaker insertion or ophthalmology referral for cataracts.

A medic alert bracelet should be provided, and we have to avoid statins which may worsen myopathy, and particular care should be taken with anesthesia which may increase the chance of respiratory failure precipitated by sedatives and neuromuscular blocking agents.

Examiner: Now tell me some other causes of myotonia?

Candidate: Most important differentials would be:
- *Myotonia congenita (Thomsen's disease)*: Autosomal dominant disorder. Usually present in the first few years of life due to a chloride

ion channelopathy affecting skeletal muscle. It is a nonprogressive illness that presents with muscle stiffness and hypertrophy. There is difficulty in muscle relaxation after forceful contraction without having other features of myotonic dystrophy such as weakness, cataract, and frontal balding.

- *Paramyotonia congenita*: Autosomal dominant disorder due to a sodium ion channelopathy that presents in the first decade of life. In comparison to the myotonic dystrophy, patients usually complain of paradoxical myotonia that is worse after exercise and triggered by cold.

Myasthenia Gravis (Ocular)

Mrs Bunch, 30-year-old, has difficulty in dressing. Examine the cranial nerves.

(After finishing full neurological examination within 6 minutes of time)

Candidate: To complete my examination, I would like to examine the upper and lower limb chronologically.

Examiner: Would you like to present your case, please?

Candidate:

While I started examination, I noticed she had an expressionless face with flat affect (lifeless face) and partial ptosis in the left eye, and when I was examining this patient's eye movements, she complained of some diplopia. However, I could not see any evidence of ocular cranial nerve palsy (complex ophthalmoplegia).

I, therefore, checked for the sustained elevation of the eyelids for 20-30 seconds; this actually unmasked asymmetric bilateral partial ptosis that also improves following eye closure for a short period. It suggests that the patient had variable ptosis with fatigability of the eyelids.

The pupil was normal in character with reacting to the light. Other cranial nerves examination was entirely normal.

However, interestingly at the end of the examination, I noticed she had a jaw supporting sign (the patient sits with the hands under the chin to support the weak jaw and neck) which was absent initially. At the same time, I noticed nasal speech due to weakness of the pharyngeal and tongue muscles.

These findings would be entirely in keeping with a diagnosis of myasthenia gravis.

Given the fatigability of the ptosis, I would also like to examine the patient's upper and lower limbs looking for fatigability (determine fatigability at the deltoid muscle by first testing shoulder abduction, then asking the patient to repeatedly abduct and adduct the shoulder usually 10-15 times in one side, comparing the strength with the opposite nonexercised side, there will be marked increase of deltoid weakness in the exercised muscle to characterize whether this is ocular or generalized myasthenia gravis.

Examiner: Now tell me, how will you proceed to reach your diagnosis?

Candidate: Firstly, I would like to take a full history of the patient, mainly looking at the symptom onset and progression of the illness.

Asking specifically about whether the symptoms are worse at the beginning or the end of the day or whether they are worse after a sustained period of exercise. Has she noticed any difficulty in swallowing, mastication, speech, or breathing?

I would also like to take a suggestive history of proximal myopathy—has she noticed any difficulty in walking upstairs or rising out of a chair unaided?

In terms of investigations, I would send antibodies for acetylcholine receptors, and I would also arrange for neurophysiological testing, including EMG with repetitive stimulation test or single fiber EMG (most sensitive). In myasthenia gravis, I would expect to see a decremental effect on the action potentials in EMG or "jitter" in single fiber EMG.

Examiner: What other bedside tests can be done in myasthenia gravis?

Candidate: We can do a bedside ceiling test. Here, I will ask the patient to keep the eyes in sustained upward gaze and keep the hands outstretched and supinated; ask to count loudly 1–50, then fatigable ptosis will be evident in one or both eyes and the patient can no longer hold the arm up and hence dysarthria (nasal, lingual, labial) and result in dysphonia.

We can also look for a "peek sign" of orbicularis fatigability (eyelid begins to separate after manual opposition to sustained closure).

Another important test would be the bedside tensilon (edrophonium) test, which involves injecting a short-acting acetylcholinesterase inhibitor to see the improvement of the symptoms and signs. It is now rarely performed as the high incidence of false-positive and false-negative and the possibility of precipitating heart block.

Or, Ice pack test that can also be performed bedside. An ice pack is applied to the ptotic eyelid for 2–5 minutes, and improvement of ptosis is noted. This test has high sensitivity and specificity but may be difficult for patients to tolerate.

Examiner: Let us say the patient's antibodies were sent off, but they came back as negative. Is there anything else you could do to help confirm the diagnosis of myasthenia?

Candidate: In fact, acetylcholine receptor antibody (Ach-Receptor-Ab) is positive in 90% of generalized and 75% in ocular myasthenia. If ach-receptor-Ab is negative, then I would like to do anti-muscle-specific kinase (anti-Musk) Ab which can be positive in 50% of cases of generalized myasthenia gravis patients who are Ach-Receptor-Ab negative. Patient with anti-musk Ab is usually female with prominent neck, bulbar, and respiratory weakness.

However, in seronegative (if both antibody tests are negative) myasthenia gravis, a diagnosis would be based on EMG with repetitive stimulation test or single fiber EMG. If characteristic findings were present in the absence of antibodies, this would be diagnostic for seronegative myasthenia gravis.

Examiner: Let us say that you have completed your examination as described and, in fact, all the signs were limited to the eyes. Would you, therefore, be confident diagnosing this patient with ocular myasthenia?

Candidate: If the symptoms are confined just to the eyes, we should follow-up the patient for 2 years after onset.

This is because if we expect generalization to happen, it will likely happen within those first 2 years. So, therefore, having followed up with the patient for that period, if they still do not have any signs in their limbs, then I would be more comfortable with diagnosing ocular myasthenia.

Examiner: Let us say this patient is diagnosed with generalized myasthenia gravis; how would you go about managing that?

Candidate: This initial therapy should be in the form of pyridostigmine which works by preventing the breakdown of acetylcholine at the neuromuscular junction. This helps with symptom management but does not affect the underlying condition.

A CT chest or MRI should be arranged looking for any evidence in particular of thymic hyperplasia or thymoma, and if this is identified, we should consider thymectomy.

Immunosuppression in the form of steroid initially. Then steroid-sparing agents (methotrexate, azathioprine, or cyclosporine) should be started—this helps to affect the underlying disease.

Patients who are quite resistant to therapy and are on maximum oral therapy should be discussed with seniors to consider whether or not they require intravenous immunoglobulin.

Examiner: Do you know what sort of issues arises when we use steroids to treat patients with myasthenia?

Candidate: In myasthenia gravis, there are both short-term and long-term effects of the steroids.

There is a paradoxical phenomenon called the "steroid dip"—where the patients with myasthenia may get paradoxically worse with the initiation of steroid therapy—this is more likely to happen if large doses are started too soon. Hence, any patient with significant symptoms, especially bulbar problems or respiratory involvement, will usually be admitted to the hospital for close observation during this phase. This is whereby the weakness gets worse as the treatment is started.

Where the symptoms are less severe, and we will be starting this treatment as an outpatient, we should start it as a low dose and slowly titrate the dose upward with regular monitoring.

Examiner: What do you know about the myasthenic crisis?

Candidate: Myasthenic crisis (MC) is a complication of myasthenia gravis, characterized by worsening muscle weakness resulting in respiratory failure that often requires intubation and ventilation. It affects 20–30% of myasthenic patients, usually within the first year of illness, and it is a severe and reversible neurological emergency.

Most patients may have a predisposing factor that triggers the crisis,
- Often an infection, particularly, respiratory tract infection.
- It may present as a postsurgical patient in whom exacerbation of muscle weakness from myasthenia gravis causes delayed extubation.
- Certain drugs can aggravate the condition, such as beta-blockers, calcium channel blockers, propafenone, lithium, penicillamine, quinidine and procainamide, phenytoin, antibiotics—gentamicin, quinolones, macrolides, and tetracyclines.

When a patient with known myasthenia gravis presents with rapidly increasing muscular weakness, with or without respiratory difficulty, it is tough to distinguish between the worsening of myasthenia (MC) or excessive anticholinesterase drugs (cholinergic crisis).

Features suggestive of a cholinergic crisis (overtreatment, but it is rare and usually occur in a dose of pyridostigmine >960 mg/day) include muscle fasciculation, pallor, sweating, hypersalivation, and small pupils. If there is any doubt, perform an edrophonium test. The improvement suggests too little medication (MC); however, aggravation suggests overtreatment (cholinergic crisis). In that case, we should stop all medications, ventilate, and possibly arrange plasmapheresis. This test should only be performed with all the necessary skills and equipment ready for intubation and ventilation.

Treatment of MC includes:
- Intravenous immunoglobulin and plasmapheresis (remove AChR-Ab from the circulation, and it usually works quicker but involves more expensive equipment).
- Most importantly, intubation and ventilation—elective intubation should be considered if the vital capacity show values which are <20 mL/kg.
- Identify and treat the trigger for the relapse (infection, medication).

Parkinson's Disease

Mrs Gomez, 55-year-old, presented with a history of recurrent falls. Examine the upper limb neurologically.

(After finishing full neurological examination within 6 minutes of time)

Candidate: To complete my examination, I would like to examine the cranial nerves and lower limb chronologically.

Examiner: Would you like to present your case, please?

Candidate:

This patient presented with parkinsonian syndrome.

She had hypomimia (expressionless face) with hypophonia (low volume, monotonous, soft speech).

On assessment, I noticed the power was preserved, sensation and coordination were intact. But she had evidence of resting tremor, rigidity and bradykinesia.

The tremor was classically resting tremor with pill-rolling in nature, that classically enhanced by mental activity by asking the patient to count backward from 20 (bradykinesia) with the arms in a semiprone position and resting on her lap.

She had lead-pipe rigidity at the elbow and cogwheel rigidity at the wrist. The rigidity in one arm was enhanced by voluntary movement of the opposite side (tap opposite hand on the knee or wave arms up and down-synkinesis).

Bradykinesia was noted by hypomimia and hypophonia and asked the patient to make repetitive pincer grip movements with the thumb and index finger.

Moreover, she had also difficulty performing two different motor acts simultaneously.

Most importantly, these signs demonstrated asymmetry with classical tremor, rigidity, and bradykinesia are being more marked on the right side.

I was unable to identify features consistent with gaze palsy, suggestive of progressive supranuclear palsy, or multiple systemic atrophy.

To complete my examination, I would like to examine the lower limb, cranial nerves, assess cognitive function (mini-mental state examination), handwriting (micrographia) as well as gait.

I would also like to measure postural blood pressure to see autonomic dysfunction (suggestive of shy dragger syndrome) and look for any other pyramidal or cerebellar signs (suggestive of multiple systemic atrophy).

I believe this lady is most likely to have a diagnosis of idiopathic Parkinson's disease. The features that support this include asymmetric, predominantly upper limb tremor, rigidity, and bradykinesia; and the absence of vertical gaze palsy (limitation of conjugate bilateral eye movement in up gaze and or downgaze, later is more common in progressive supranuclear palsy, which is best assessed during saccadic eye movement), cerebellar features (nystagmus or jumpy vision) and pyramidal signs help me to make progressive supranuclear palsy (PSP) and MSA less likely.

Examiner: Okay, that is great. Would you tell me what you mean by parkinsonism and Parkinson's disease, and how will you differentiate them?

Candidate: Parkinsonism is a movement disorder characterized by bradykinesia and at least one of the following:
- Rest tremor
- Rigidity
- Postural instability

Idiopathic parkinsonism is called Parkinson's disease, where the following features are expected:
- Asymmetrical onset
- Slowly progressive
- Good response to levodopa
- *Furthermore, Parkinson plus signs will be absent here, such as*:
  - Poor response to levodopa
  - Marked symmetry
  - Early-onset of dementia, hallucination, postural instability, history of fall, and autonomic dysfunction (postural hypotension, history of urinary incontinence, impotence)
- *As well as the absence of*:
  - Pyramidal signs (plantar extensors, hyperreflexia)
  - Cerebellar signs (nystagmus or broad-based ataxic gait), or
  - Ocular sign (gaze palsy)

Examiner: Thank you so much. Now would you please tell me the cause of parkinsonism?

Candidate: The most important cause would be drugs, such as:
- Chlorpromazine, metoclopramide, prochlorperazine, sodium valproate, and methyldopa.

Other causes would be:
- Lewy body dementia
- Normal-pressure hydrocephalus
- Postencephalitis (encephalitis lethargica)
- Wilson's disease
- Toxins, such as CO, MPTP, manganese

And Parkinson plus syndromes:
- Multiple system atrophy
- Progressive supranuclear palsy
- Corticobasal degeneration

Examiner: Okay, let us go back to history; if this lady presented with early cognitive dysfunction with the visual hallucination that aggravates after taking levodopa, then what would you think?

Candidate: In that case, I would like to consider an alternative diagnosis, such as Lewy body dementia.

Examiner: Okay, now tell me, if a young patient presented with parkinsonism, then how will you proceed with the case?

Candidate: In that case, I would like to take a full history from the patient. Most importantly, drugs causing parkinsonism or H/O encephalitis in childhood to exclude postencephalitis parkinsonism as well as I want to exclude Wilson's disease where associated liver disease and Kayser-Fleischer (KF) ring is a strong clinical clue to the diagnosis.

Examiner: You have talked to me about the motor side of Parkinson's. What would you ask the patient about nonmotor symptoms of Parkinson's?

Candidate: Parkinson's disease can present with several nonmotor manifestations. One of them is anosmia which can be the earlier sign. Other important nonmotor manifestations are:
- Cognitive impairment
- Mood disorders
- The patient may present with pain
- Also, different sleep disorders such as insomnia, daytime sleepiness with sleep attacks, restless legs syndrome (RLS), rapid eye movement (REM)-sleep behavior disorder.

Examiner: How will manage a patient with Parkinson's disease?

Candidate: The patient should be managed with an MDT approach. A specialist from many areas to coordinate and manage the symptoms and outcome of the patient.

The mainstay of medical management is dopamine replacement. Here, levodopa is given with a peripheral Dopa-decarboxylase antagonist (carbidopa) to reduce the peripheral adverse effect (nausea and hypotension). Dopamine agonist (non-ergot DAs-ropinirole or pramipexole) may be used in combination with levodopa. However, it can be used as a monotherapy in a young patient (below age 65-70 years) with mild-to-moderate impairment.

As the disease progresses, medical therapy for Parkinson's disease becomes more difficult as higher doses of dopamine replacement are required. So, to maintain a long-term response to treatment, we can use increased dose frequency or slow-release formulation and the addition of the catechol-O-methyltransferase (COMT) inhibitors (entacapone 200 mg with each levodopa dose) to prolong the duration of action.

Other drugs include:
- Amantadine is mainly used in advanced diseases to improve dyskinesia.
- Apomorphine is used subcutaneously by an autoinjector as an intermittent rescue injection for off period or by a continuous infusion pump in advanced Parkinson disease.

Tardive Dyskinesia

Mr Jay, 25-year-old, has involuntary movement. Examine the cranial nerves.

(After finishing full neurological examination within 6 minutes of time)

Candidate: To complete my examination, I would like to examine the upper and lower limb chronologically.

Examiner: Would you like to present your case, please?

Candidate:

I noticed the patient had tardive dyskinesia.

This patient has an uncontrolled, jerky, and repetitive movement of the lips, tongue, and jaw; these include:

Facial grimacing, excessive eye blinking

Sticking out of the tongue with tongue-twisting

Lip-smacking and puckering

Jaw opening and closing

Sucking or chewing

There is a slow and writhing movement of extremities (athetosis); these movements are present at rest, diminish with activity. When I asked the patient to squeeze the finger— the finger dyskinesia was diminished.

When I asked the patient to pat the thigh with both hands using the palmar and dorsal surface of the hand alternatively— it accentuated the orofacial dyskinesia (distracting the patient attention from the movement).

I would like to take a full history from the patient, particularly drug history, because it is commonly a result of long-term treatment of dopamine antagonists such as neuroleptics for schizophrenia, bipolar disorder, or other brain conditions or antiemetics (metoclopramide).

Other important differentials can cause movement disorders such as cerebral palsy, Huntington's disease, Parkinson's disease, and Tourette's syndrome. So, to rule out these conditions, I would like to do blood tests (genetic test) as well as brain imaging (CT/MRI).

Examiner: So, how will you manage the case?

Candidate: Here, the main treatment step is to stop the offending drugs and switch to newer antipsychotics (e.g., clozapine) that may be less likely to cause tardive dyskinesia. If not possible, then try to reduce the dose of offending drugs. There are two FDA approved medications to treat tardive dyskinesia that include deutetrabenazine and valbenazine.

Involuntary Movement (Chorea)

Please observe this 45-year-old man who presents with difficulty holding objects (telephone receiver or crockery). Examine the upper limb neurologically.

(After finishing full neurological examination within 6 minutes of time)

Candidate: To complete my examination, I would like to examine the cranial nerves and lower limb chronologically.

Examiner: Would you please present your case?

Candidate:

While I asked the patient to sit still, I noticed he had difficulty doing that, and he had hyperkinetic movement disorder, which was unpredictable, brief, irregular, nonrepetitive, jerky large volume movement that was difficult to control. These were more pronounced with outstretched limbs but importantly the same if his eyes were open or closed.

On closer inspection and examination, I could not find any change in his power, reflex, or sensation.

Coordination was intact with a finger—nose testing, but there was some difficulty with pronation and supination. No evidence of intention tremor or past pointing.

There was abnormal posturing of hands where the wrist was flexed, and fingers were hyperextended. The patient was unable to maintain a sustained posture, tongue protrusion, or eyelid closure (motor impersistence) and showed involuntary tongue movements (bag of worms). Attempting to make a handgrip results in alternate squeezing-relaxing motions (milkmaid grip).

Testing for "finger snap movement" also showed some difficulty but no evidence of bradykinesia.

Examining his eye showed no difficulty with pursuit or saccadic movement, and no nystagmus was present (cerebellar sign).

I would like to complete my examination by examining his gait, dementia screening by doing MMSE, functional impacts of the disorders by asking the patient to tie a shoelace, button, and unbuttoning, and cranial and lower limb neurological examination.

If we consider the differential diagnosis, in this case, we need to think about an immune-mediated inflammatory cause such as SLE and Sydenham's chorea that is rare in the UK now. We also need to consider acute cases.

- Hyperglycemia, and
- CVD involving basal ganglia

If the onset were more chronic, a genetic cause, particularly in the context of positive family history, would need to be considered. The most common of these would be Huntington's disease.

Other less likely possibilities would be Wilson's disease or drugs or polycythemia (Rubra) Vera.

Examiner: How would you investigate such a case like that?

Candidate: It would be very important to take a thorough history to help delineate the cause of the involuntary movement, e.g., if this has come on acutely blood glucose measurement to rule out hyperglycemia or, if it is sudden onset, then the vascular cause should be considered. Urgent imaging of the brain is required, classically, we would be thinking about a lesion in the subthalamic nucleus causing hemiballismus.

If the symptoms suggest SLE/Sjögren's syndrome, such as rash, arthropathy, kerato-conjunctivitis sicca, then I would ask to do ANA, double-stranded deoxyribonucleic acid (dsDNA), antiphospholipid antibody, or ENA profile.

If any suggestive H/O liver disease or KF ring is present, then I would like to exclude Wilson disease by doing copper study such as serum ceruloplasmin level (<300 mg/dL), 24-hour urinary copper (>100 mmol/day).

If we consider that this could be a genetic cause, particularly those who have chronic, insidious onset or any unexplained neurological syndrome in other family members or previous generation or any diagnosis of Huntington's disease in the families, then I will arrange a blood test for Huntington genetic test.

Examiner: Let us think this is a case of Huntington's disease; how will you manage this case.

Candidate: There is still no treatment to slow or stop the disease. Here, the treatment is supportive and symptomatic, and he should be managed with an MDT approach involving a neurologist, specialist nurse, physiotherapist, and occupational therapist.

For symptomatic improvement of involuntary movements, we can use tetrabenazine or deutetrabenazine.

Genetic counseling for the patient who had family members is the key part of the management.

CHAPTER 7

Clinical Communication Skills and Ethics

- Brief Discussion on Communication and Ethics
- Lifestyle Modification of a Rheumatoid Arthritis Patient
- Rheumatoid Arthritis
- Transient Ischemic Attack
- Addison's Disease
- Ulcerative Colitis with the Refusal to Admit Hospital
- Celiac Disease
- Patient with the First Fit
- Emphysema with Smoking Cessation
- Counseling of an Alcohol Drinker
- Discussion on Breaking Bad News
- Pancreatic Carcinoma
- Multiple Sclerosis
- Delayed Diagnosis of Cancer
- Dementia
- Renal Biopsy
- Percutaneous Endoscopic Gastrostomy Tube Insertion
- Intercostal Chest Drain
- Hickman Line
- Lumbar Puncture
- Oesophago-gastro-duodenoscopy Procedure
- Offer a Blood Transfusion
- Needle Stick Injury
- Newly Diagnosed Human Immunodeficiency Virus
- Hospital Superbug-1
- Hospital Superbug-2
- Genetic Counseling
- Counseling for Anticoagulation
- Patient with Poor Compliance
- Nonorganic Disease
- Medical Error-1
- Medical Error-2
- Medical Trial
- Cancer Withhold
- Live Organ Donation
- Advance Care Decision
- Decision about Do-not-resuscitate
- End of Life Decision
- Brainstem Death Testing
- Brainstem Death and Organ Donation
- Hospital Postmortem
- Coroner's Postmortem

Brief Discussion on Communication and Ethics

A clinical interview's main objectives are 4E's that stand for *e*ngaging, *e*mpathy, *e*ducating, *e*nlisting and *e*liciting the patient's expectation. The basic structure of the clinical interview is the C-L-A-S-S strategy. The C-L-A-S-S stands for *c*ontext, *l*istening skills, *a*cknowledgment, *s*trategy, and *s*ummary.

4E

E—It stands for engaging the patient, and engaging really means making contact between the clinician and the patient. This task is considered under three headings—join the patient, elicit the story's agenda, and then set the agenda. Joining the patient has to do with warmth and welcome, introductions, and adapting your language to meet the patient. *"I understand that you wanted to speak to me about ..., is that right?/I wanted to speak to you about ..."* One of the most important issues in eliciting the agenda and the story is allowing the patient to talk uninterrupted. Ideally, leave the patient to speak uninterruptedly. He/She will speak for a maximum of about two minutes; hence the first two minutes are really crucial, and not interrupting is a key technique in facilitating the interview. Now develop a dialogue—*"Would you like to know exactly what is been going on? Or have you got any questions about that or any concerns?"*

E—empathy: The most important part of being an effective communicator and an effective listener is empathy. Acknowledgment is the main issue to show the empathetic response. *"I know that must have felt horrible when ..."*

E—educate the patient: The first issue is assessing the patient's understanding, then assuming questions and ensuring understanding. *"How much do you know about the situations (idea)? Or have any other doctors had a chance to speak to you about things?"* In almost 50% of cases, the patient will not follow medical recommendations or treatments and part of the reason is that the patient may have a particular view of his or her situation, including the possibility that he/she may not recognize the fact that anything is wrong, hence educating the patient is very important and to do that you have to get a feeling of the patient's expectations and to use several techniques. Do not give a long speech and do not be hurry, use a short phrase and allow the information to sink in. Give the information gradually—*"The chest X-ray showed a shadow on the lung ... This was confirmed on the CT scan"*. Be honest, do not promise things that cannot be delivered, such as in a patient with rheumatoid arthritis (RA) we can say—*"We cannot cure this and make it go away completely"*. Do not destroy hope but do not be unrealistic *"Symptoms can be relived or the outlook is uncertain, but there are treatments that can help this condition"*.

E—enlisting and eliciting the patient's expectations: Try to know the patient's expectations or feelings and respond with proper explanation and reassurance.

The technique to perform this 4E task is the **C-L-A-S-S** strategy.

C—context: The meaning of "C" is physical context or the setting of the interview. There are three major components to getting the setting:

Physical space:
- Ensure privacy. Sit down.
- Keep eyes on the same level as the patient's eyes.
- Maintain about 2 feet distance and no physical barriers between you and the patient (e.g., across the corner of the table or chair beside the bed).
- Having a box of tissues nearby is likely to be needed.

Relatives or friends: Make sure the patient is seated nearest to you, and any friend or relative is close to him/her (allow to seat relative/friend next to the patient; not between you and the patient).
Body language and eye contact:
- Try to look relaxed and unhurried.
- Maintain eye contact (unless during the patient's distress)

L—listening skills: Active and uninterrupted listening is the key part of communication.

Asking open-ended questions:
- *How have you been feeling?*
- *Would you like to tell me more about your concerns?*
- *How did you manage with the new treatment?*

Facilitating by:
- Allow the patient to speak uninterrupted.
- Nod to let the patient know you are following him/her.
- And try to repeat a keyword from the patient's last sentence in your first sentence.

Clarifying the issues by saying like:
- *"Please tell me more about that."*
- Or, *"So, if I understand you correctly, you are saying ..."*

Interruptions:
- Try to switch off your phone and phone calls—do not answer, but if you must, apologize to the patient before answering.
- If you know you will be interrupted, try to prepare the patient about it.

A—acknowledgment: The empathetic response validates and legitimizes the patient's feelings.
- As patient's reaction or response to what is happening
- As an item on the agenda between the two of you as that you are going to discuss.

Identify the emotion, identify the reason for the emotion—respond by showing you have made the connection between the emotion and the reason, such as:
- *"Most people would be upset about this."*

In addition to the empathic response, another communication skill is most often used as an acknowledgment technique or as a facilitation technique but can be used at almost any significant point during the interview, and that is touch.

Touching the patient can be an important part of your nonverbal communication skills and may help the patient feel supported and less isolated. However, not all clinicians are comfortable doing it and also not all patients appreciate being touched or liked. So it is important to follow two simple rules:
- Firstly, touch the patient briefly on a neutral area of the body (e.g., the hand or the forearm)
- Secondly, touch the patient briefly and see if the patient appreciates it or withdraws it. If he/she withdraws, then do not try it again. However, many patients appreciate being touched, and if they do, in those cases, touch is a valuable part of your communication skills.

Three more general points about the empathetic response:
1. Normalizing is often useful afterwards.
2. It does not mean you agree with the patient—correct misunderstanding and be firm when necessary. *"No, I don't think that's right, my understanding is that ..."* or *"I am afraid that it is a legal obligation that you are not able to drive for 1 year after having a fit ... I have to advise you that you must tell the DVLA and your insurance company ... and I have to write in your notes that I have told you this."*
3. You can use an empathetic response to your own emotions. *"I can see why you think that ... I can see why you are concerned about that."*

After acknowledging and validating what the patient is feeling, you may want to normalize. This is helpful after you have shown that you have heard what the patient is worried about. It is often unhelpful if you do it before or instead.

S-S—summary and strategy: Check the patient's understanding and summarize the discussion clearly and concisely. Ask about any further queries or questions. If you do not have time for further questions, suggest that they can be addressed at the next appointment and make a clear contact for a follow-up visit. *"I can meet you again to talk over things some more if that would* be helpful." "Do you think it would be helpful if we meet together with your husband/wife (as appropriate) to talk things over?" "If you would like to meet my consultant to discuss the issue then I can help make the arrangement."

The candidate should be kept in mind the ethical and legal issues raised in the clinical scenario during communication skills. Candidates are not expected to have detailed knowledge of the legal issues. For overseas candidates in the UK, detailed knowledge of UK law is not required. However, he/she should be aware of general legal and ethical principles that may affect the case in question.

Ethical Issues

Principles of ethical issues:
1. **Patient autonomy**: It is all about a patient's right to accept or refuse medical advice, the right to know the truth, and share the decision of his/her own management plan. Physicians should always respect the patient's autonomy. After explaining the disease or any medical condition, inform the patient with a full, complete, and right information about the management plan and options and let him/her decide. Do not take decisions on his or her behalf or force him/her to take any decision, just explain the options and let him/her choose as long as he/she has the capacity to understand all the information. Be nice and friendly and maximize patient's abilities to make decisions for himself/herself and respect his/her decision. If the patient refuses the medical advice, which is in his/her best interest, try to explore the reason for that.
2. **Justice**: This is the patient's right to take management without any discrimination. Every patient should be offered the best medical care regardless of his/her origin, religion, or beliefs.
3. **Beneficence**: Every physician must try to do good for the patient, and patient's care would be the priority.
4. **Nonmaleficence**: Never do or induce any harm to the patient.

Example: Percutaneous endoscopic gastrostomy (PEG) feeding of a semi-conscious patient with stroke.

Autonomy: The patient's wishes to be fed or not.

Beneficence and nonmaleficence: PEG feeding may improve the nutritional status of the patient and aid rapid recovery but with the risk of complications from the insertion of the PEG tube and subsequent aspiration pneumonia.

Justice: Heavy resource burden looking after PEG feed patient in a nursing home.

Legal Issues

1. **Patient competence or capacity**: For understanding information and making a decision, in the UK, a person >16 years of age is considered competent until proven otherwise, and no one else can make a healthcare decision on behalf of a competent patient. For any incompetent patient or a patient who lacks capacity (e.g., confusion, coma, dementia, people who committed suicide or with other psychiatric problems, patient <16 years who is not Gillick competent), a physician can decide in the best interest of the patients unless they left an advance directive (living will) or nominated anyone (power of attorney) to make decisions on their behalf.
2. **Signing a consent form**: Every patient has to sign an informed consent form agreement (means that he/she accepts to have the procedure done after explaining the steps of the procedure) containing all the pieces of information before any invasive procedure, and the patient can withdraw any time he/she change his/her mind.
3. **Confidentiality and breaking confidentiality**: Physicians should keep the patient's all medical information and records confidential and respect the patient's privacy by all means. Some special situations where confidentiality can be breached like:
    a. If the patient has given consent.
    b. In the patient's best interest, where a patient lacks capacity or needs another specialist or knows from family about a living will or a power of attorney.

c. In public interest where a patient is harmful to others (e.g., notifiable disease, a patient refuses to inform DVLA, court orders, birth, and death cases).
4. **Driving issue**: It is the legal responsibility of any patient to inform the DVLA if he/she has a condition that bans him/her from driving. Explain to the patient politely about the potential outcome to continue driving. If he/she refuses to do this, the medical team has the responsibility to inform the DVLA and may break his/her confidentiality.
5. **Admission under general or mental health act**: Any patient with suicidal attempts or psychological instability should be admitted to the hospital with or without his/her consent and should be assessed by a psychiatrist to evaluate his/her condition. Moreover, any patient with active infectious disease (active TB) and there is a chance to infect others, he/she is not allowed to discharge.
6. **Illegal drugs (e.g., cocaine)**: Does he/she not legally licensed for a prescription?
7. **Seeking compensation**: Any patient with an occupational disease has the right to claim for compensation (e.g., needle-stick injury of any healthcare worker, patient with mesothelioma or asbestosis).

Lifestyle Modification of a Rheumatoid Arthritis Patient

Your role: You are the doctor in the general medical clinic.

Problem: Discuss the need for lifestyle changes for a patient with rheumatoid arthritis (RA).

Patient's name: Mrs Karen Murphy, a 32-year-old lady.

Please read the scenario printed below. Then, when the bell sounds, enter the room.

You have 14 minutes for your consultation with the patient or relative. Give 1 minute to collect your thoughts and the last 5 minutes for discussion with examiner. If you wish, you may make notes. Where applicable, assume you have the patient's consent to discuss her condition with the relative or surrogate.

Scenario: This patient is a known case of RA. The symptoms started 6 months ago. She has been treated with methotrexate 20 mg weekly but is not responding well to treatment. She still has symptoms of joint pain and morning stiffness. Her liver function tests revealed an abnormal serum glutamic pyruvic transaminase (SGPT) of 69 U/L (normal range: 5–35), although the serum alkaline phosphatase was normal. She is a smoker, obese, and drinks two glasses of wine almost every day. Please discuss lifestyle changes with the patient, which could help to control her RA more effectively.

Your task: You have to discuss to the patient regarding lifestyle modification mainly to stop smoking, reduce alcohol intake, and lose weight.

Do not take a history; Do not examine the patient.

At the end of the station, any notes you make must be handed to the examiners.

[*Note:* Once you get the scenario, you will get 5 minutes to start the station. It is crucial to think and plan HOW TO DEAL WITH THE SCENARIO. As we know, RA is a strong risk factor for cardiovascular morbidity and mortality, and on the other hand, it will increase the risk of liver and kidney disease because of drugs to manage the disease, such as nonsteroidal anti-inflammatory drugs (NSAIDs) and disease-modifying antirheumatic drugs (DMARDs). Lifestyle modification, as a whole, decreases all of the risks and helps reduce symptoms. So, key issue here is to establish the importance of lifestyle change. Therefore, for successful communication, important steps would be:

- Introduction, permission and confirmation of the patient's identity.
- Let the patient speak more (**golden minutes**) to elicit the patient's ideas, concerns, and expectations (**ICE**) to identify the patient's agenda.
- Then explore the appropriate social history to create an appropriate management plan.
- Then explain to the patient the importance of the lifestyle changes as well as an appropriate management plan. During the conversation, you must:
  - Avoid using the medical term (jargon) and use a simple term to understand the patient better.
  - Ensure your patient understands your conversation (Does it make sense for you, Mrs Murphy? Or, is it okay with you?).
  - Be confident, adopt a holistic approach, demonstrate knowledge of MDT working, and consider the potential psychological impact on daily living activities, family life, relationship, employment, and any relevant hobbies.
  - Do not be judgmental; be empathetic, and make sure she does not feel pressured. So, reassure and appreciate her.

- Allow regular pause for clarification and questions as well as to digest the information, raise her concern.
- Remember, nonverbal communications such as smiling (where appropriate), eye contact, nodding, and open body posture to communicate openness or interest to the patient and readiness to listen.
- Provide written information, including follow-up and access to supportive information (website address, leaflet, and brochure) and contact number of the multidisciplinary team (MDT) appropriate member.
- Finally, summarize the key features of the counseling and recheck understanding without spending >1 minute on that at the end of the consultation.

Approach to the Clinical Scenario

Introduction, Permission, and Confirmation of the Agenda

Candidate: Good morning, Mrs Murphy! I am Mohammad Ali, one of the working doctors in this general medical clinic. Today I am here to talk with you, is that okay?

Patient: Good morning, doctor, it's all right.

Candidate: Do you want to invite anyone else to our discussion today?

Patient: No.

Check Understanding

Candidate: I am here to talk with you regarding your arthritis and address your all concerns; before that, would you please tell me more about your condition, like how you are feeling now?

Patient: I have had pain and stiffness in multiple joints involving hands, feet, knees, and shoulders for the last 6 months. My joint pain and stiffness are worse in the morning. Five months ago, I attended the rheumatology clinic, and the doctor told me that I have had RA and would need regular medication to treat it. I have been taking methotrexate for 4 months. I take eight tablets each week and have regular blood tests. I am also taking regular painkillers, although I still have pain and stiffness in my joints. It is not as severe as before but is still affecting my life as well as my job. I am a software engineer and work in computing in an office most of the time. I had a few weeks off sick when the symptoms first started; I have now returned to work, and it is crucial for my career that I do not have more time off sick. So, doctor … is there anything I can do to help treat my arthritis?

Establish the Importance of Lifestyle Change

Candidate: Okay, Mrs Murphy, I am sorry to hear about your condition. In terms of other treatment options, yes … there are lots of available treatment options for RA, including medications, physiotherapy, occupational therapy, and surgery, depending on the severity of the disease and other factors.

The most important factor in improving your condition is lifestyle modification and medications, and I want to talk with you about it. Is that okay with you?

Patient: Yes.

Candidate: Well. As I know from your note that you are overweight, smoke cigarettes, and also drink alcohol. Do you mind if I ask you some questions for a better understanding of your lifestyle?

Patient: Please ask what you want to know, Doctor.

Candidate: How many sticks do you smoke a day? For how long ? Have you ever tried to stop before?

Patient: I have smoked 20 sticks a day for the last 20 years. I never tried to stop it.

Candidate: Do you drink alcohol regularly? For how many years? What is the amount? What types of it?

Patient: I have been taking two glasses of wine every evening for the last 15 years.

Candidate: What about your physical activity? Do you exercise?

Patient: I used to exercise, but now I have to stop it because of my joint pain.

Candidate: As we know, RA is a long-lasting disease, and it can cause damage to your various parts of the body, including joints, heart, lung, liver, eyes, etc. … and people with RA tend to have more chances to develop the disease in such parts of the body. A healthy lifestyle can lower your chance of having these types of bad outcomes and improve your symptoms. You can reduce these bad outcomes by ensuring your arthritis is well controlled and by:
- Stopping smoking
- Reducing alcohol intake
- Eating a healthy, balanced diet; and
- Exercising regularly

As you are a heavy smoker and have smoked 20 sticks a day for 20 years, I believe the 1st step of your lifestyle modification should be to stop smoking as we all know smoking is harmful to our body from every point of view. In addition to increasing the risk of cancer, heart disease, and stroke, smoking may also make RA symptoms worse. Therefore, I strongly advise you to stop smoking, and I can help you to do it.

Address the Patient's Concerns and Questions

Candidate: So, how does that sound? Do you have any concerns or questions?

Patient: I understand that smoking is not good for my health, but I feel that stopping at the moment would be difficult, as I find smoking relaxes me, and my pain seems to be worse when I am under stress.

Candidate: I can understand … everyone has a misconception that smoking is relaxing them or helping them get rid of stress, but actually, it will put you in even greater danger in the future.

I know how difficult it is for anyone to stop it, but I want to reassure you that many people have successfully stopped smoking by participating in the smoking cessation clinic. Does it make sense for you, Mrs Murphy?

Patient: Yes doctor! I understand and will take the necessary steps for this.

Candidate: Thanks for your understanding. Another thing is you are taking two glasses of wine every evening. If we count that in terms of as a unit, it is around 28 units per week that are over the recommended amount suitable for a man. This is actually very alarming for you because you have already some problems with your liver. Your liver test result is abnormal on your last checkup; alcohol, obesity, and your medication (methotrexate) may be the reason for this. Have you ever thought that way?

Patient: No doctor … I am scared now. So, what should I do?

Candidate: It would be better to cut down your amount of alcohol intake to a safer limit and do regular exercise to lose weight, and this will help you normalize the liver function.

Moreover, exercise regularly can help relieve stress, help keep your joints mobile and flexible, and strengthen the muscles supporting your joints.

Patient: Yes doctor! I used to cycle to work which kept me fit, and I regret not cycling since I developed joint pain and stiffness. My weight has increased due to a lack of exercise. I want to know, is it possible for me to do such types of exercise?

Candidate: I am delighted to know that you were used to cycling, and you realize that exercise helps you keep fit. I would like to advise you to do exercise regularly and start cycling again. There will be a little trouble initially, and it is usually best to gradually increase the amount of exercise you do. Try low-impact activities that put less strain on your joints, such as swimming, cycling, walking, and aqua aerobics. If you need more guidance, a physiotherapist is an excellent person to advise you on suitable exercise types. Is that okay with you?

Patient: Doctor … I would like to be doing more exercise as I know the lack of exercise makes me unfit and puts weight on. However, I feel that more exercise will increase my pain and might damage my joints. Will exercise damage my joints?

Candidate: It is highly appreciable that you would like to do exercise, and you are right, excess weight puts extra strain on your joints, and it causes more pain. I know it's difficult for anyone to exercise with pain, but I want to tell you that your arthritis is a different type of arthritis, not like old-age arthritis. Please try to keep active as much as possible. The muscles around the joints will become weak if they are not used. Regular exercise may also help to reduce pain and improve joint function.

You can also just modify your daily habits to simplify your activity like if you use public transport, you can get off one to two stops before reaching home and walk instead. If you drive, please walk when you are going to buy something from your local shop. If you live in a flat, you can climb the stairs instead of using the lift. Am I clear so far?

Patient: Doctor, should I worry about the abnormal liver function tests?

Candidate: That is really a good question. As I mentioned earlier, your overweight, alcohol intake, and RA medication can cause it. However, be sure that if you maintain a healthy lifestyle by reducing your weight and alcohol consumption, it will return to an average level; if not, then we need to think about the side effects of the methotrexate, and we will change methotrexate and use other drugs.

We will follow-up with you every 4–6 weeks and check your liver enzyme levels to see if it raises further or not, and we will refer you to a joint doctor (rheumatologist) who can make a proper decision about your medications. Do you have any other concerns?

Patient: Doctor ... Please tell me, can any diet help with my arthritis?

Candidate: There is no substantial evidence to suggest that specific dietary changes can improve RA. However, it is vital to ensure your overall diet is still healthy and balanced. Having a sensible diet will help in controlling your weight and reduce the risk of further complications. Try to avoid salty, fatty, and oily food, avoid eating out, and cook at home as much as possible. Please try to have plenty of fruits and vegetables in your diet. Is that clear?

Patient: I understand, but it's really tough to cook for me. I have an extremely busy schedule, Doctor.

Candidate: Eating out is not healthy as they use a lot of salt, sugar, and fat to make it tastier. I understand it may be challenging to cook every day, but you can cook once or twice per week, store it in the refrigerator, and use it for the whole week. So, you don't have to eat outside every day.

Social History

Candidate: Mrs Murphy, as you said before, you are a software engineer, and this disease is affecting your job; therefore, I can refer you to an occupational health worker as your job is affected. An occupational therapist can provide training and advice that will help you to protect your joints, both while you are at home and work.

Patient: Thank you so much, doctor! It will be a great favor for me.

Candidate: Now tell me, with whom you are living? Are they doing well? Who is supporting you at home? Are you financially supported?

Patient: I am living with my husband and my children; they are all in good health. I am self-independent, and my husband also helps me a lot.

Make a Management Plan

Candidate: That's all right. So, we will now refer you to the MDT involving a joint doctor, specialist dietician, physiotherapist, occupational therapist, and social worker; they can give you proper advice regarding your lifestyle and disease. Mrs Murphy, is there anything that I haven't explained to you properly?

Patient: No. you have explained everything very well.

Make Summary

Recheck Understanding: May I know how much did you get from our discussion today?

Help
Candidate: I will give you some leaflets, brochures, and the National Rheumatoid Arthritis Society website address to read more about the disease. I will give you my contact details and contact me if you have any worries or queries.

Thank you so much for spending time with me.

Patient: Thank you.

Shake hands!

Rheumatoid Arthritis

Your role: You are the doctor in the rheumatology OPD clinic.

Problem: New diagnosis of rheumatoid arthritis.

Patient's name: Mrs Shayla Rahman, a 30-year-old lady.

Scenario: Mrs Shayla Rahman was referred to the Rheumatology Clinic last month with multiple joint pain and swelling of the hands. She was seen by your consultant, and he advised some blood tests and X-rays of both hands. The results came back with a strongly positive rheumatoid factor (RF), and anti-CCP and the X-rays showed ulnar deviation with abnormal left metacarpophalangeal (MCP) joints, which favor the diagnosis of rheumatoid arthritis (RA). Her FBC, CRP, and U&E were done and showing normocytic normochromic anemia with high erythrocyte sedimentation rate (ESR) and CRP with normal renal function test. Unfortunately, your consultant is busy doing his post-take round, and he asked you to see the patient.

Your task: You have to explain the diagnosis and management plan and address her concerns.

Introduction, Permission, and Confirmation of the Agenda

Candidate: Hello, Mrs Rahman. I am Mohammad Ali, one of the working doctors here today. I am sorry to tell you that my consultant is busy right now, so I have come here to talk to you about your blood test results. Is that okay with you?

Patient: Hello, Doctor, it's all right.

Candidate: Do you want to invite anyone else to our discussion today?

Patient: No.

Check Understanding

Candidate: Do you have any idea what has been happening to you so far? Do you know why we did the blood tests and what we were looking for? Did your consultant explain the prescribed diagnosis at your last appointment?

Patient: I don't have any idea, actually. I was fit and well, but I have had pain, swelling, and stiffness in my hand joints for the last few months, which is worse in the early morning. So, I met my consultant, he did some blood tests on me, and now I am here for the results.

Candidate: Mrs Rahman, the results of blood investigations as well as X-rays have been released, and it's not as we expect ... (Stop for a while ...).

It reveals that you have a disease called rheumatoid arthritis (RA) (stop for a while ... let the patient express her feelings and thoughts) ... Do you have any idea about this disease?

Patient: No, Doctor, I don't have any idea about it. What is it, Doctor? Is it a serious condition, Doctor?

Candidate: I appreciate your concern; actually, it can be serious if left untreated, but we are going to do our best to control your disease. I am here to discuss the disease. Do you want me to explain to you more about it?

Patient: Yes, sure.

Explain the Disease Simply without Jargon

Candidate: It is a disease due to disturbance in our defensive system, which is supposed to attack bugs and germs. Sometimes our defense system, instead of attacking germs and bugs, go crazy for an unknown reason, and it starts attacking our own tissues; in your case, it is attacking the joints, and the tissues (capsule) surround it.

Symptoms of Rheumatoid Arthritis

The main symptoms of the disease are pain and stiffness of multiple joints, particularly the joints of hands, which are commonly affected. The stiffness is usually worse in the morning or after taking some rest. Sometimes inflammation causes swelling around the affected joints. Over time, the inflammation can damage the joints, cartilage and part of the bone near to the joint.

Complications and Prognosis

In a few cases, inflammation may damage other organs such as the lungs, eyes, heart, or blood vessels. However, modern treatments can often limit or even stop the progression of the disease and limit joint damage. Moreover, our role as a medical team is to do a regular follow-up to ensure that your main symptom is managed and to detect any complications early if they tend to occur. Am I clear so far, Mrs Rahman?

Patient: Yes, it's a lot of information, and I am not actually expecting this RA. I am feeling hopeless.

Candidate: I am absolutely agreed with you; I am giving you much information, but don't worry, we'll talk to you again later, and since it's a long-term illness, we'll tell you everything through a series of conversations.

Treatment

Patient: Is it curable, Doctor? How could you treat me? Can you tell me some about the treatment options of RA?

Rheumatoid arthritis is not curable, but it is controllable. Treatment can make a big difference to reduce symptoms and improve the outcome, and there are many available treatment options here that actually depend on whether and how severely RA affects you.

During the acute attack, we usually start treatment with simple painkillers and a steroid for short periods to manage your symptoms. However, most importantly, we have to give more potent medications such as immunosuppressive drugs (DMARDs) that may suppress the crazy defense system in your body. These immunosuppressive medications are vital to reduce further complications such as joint deformity or damage and other extra-articular manifestations such as lung and eye problems. Are you following me, Mrs Rahman?

Patient: Yes.

Side Effects of Immunosuppressants

Candidate: However, these types of medications have their own risks (increased chance of infections) at the same time have their own benefits, and if you think about the benefits versus the side effects, the benefits will outweigh the issues of side effects. Is that okay, Mrs Rahman?

Patient: Yes.

Candidate: Well ... nonpharmacological interventions are also essential, such as exercises to increase muscle strength, which supports the joints, relaxation techniques, the use of splints for inflamed or deformed joints, etc.

Patient: Doctor, you want to give me a steroid? I don't want to take it. I have heard steroids have many side effects.

Candidate: I would like to assure you that the use of steroids in your case would hopefully be for a short course while you are established on more long-term medication and treat any acute flare-ups. The frequency of side-effects (e.g., bone loss, hyperglycemia, weight gain, and thinning/bruising of the skin) is relatively low if you are on a low dose of steroids for a short duration and most importantly that side-effects are generally reversible.

You will be monitored closely in the clinic for side effects of steroids and any other medications you are started on. Moreover, I want to mention that you will not be forced to go on any medication you are not keen on.

Address the Patient's Concerns

Candidate: Do you have any concerns, Mrs Rahman?

Patient: Doctor, actually, I am terrified about being dismissed from work if my boss feels that arthritis will affect my job. May I need to let my office know about it?

Candidate: Before moving on, may I know what are you doing for a living? And how much does your illness impact your job and usual daily activity?

Patient: I am an architect, and I have to work with my hands for making designs and many other things, it's quite difficult for me to work because of pain.

Candidate: I appreciate your concern ... However, I assure you that you are not bound by statutory law to tell your employers about your diagnosis, and the doctors will also maintain your confidentiality.

I would like to inform you that RA is usually well controlled with appropriate medication, and you should be able to carry out your job without restriction.

However, if you face any difficulty performing your job, you should speak to the occupational health department in your workplace. In addition, the National Rheumatoid Arthritis Society (NARS) can be an excellent source to support patients with RA.

Patient: If I want to be pregnant, what will I do?

Candidate: If you want to be pregnant, then we have to ensure that your disease is well controlled with safe drugs. In that case, you can become pregnant without complications. Furthermore, most importantly, when you want to become pregnant, it will be better to inform your obstetrician and the joint doctor to make an MDT give you full care during your pregnancy. Do you have any other questions?

Social History

Candidate: Would you mind if I ask you some questions about your lifestyle, Mrs Rahman?

Patient: Yes.

Candidate: Do you smoke? If yes, then how many sticks per day? How long?

Patient: Yes, I have been smoking 15 sticks in a day for the last 10 years.

Candidate: I want to inform you that smoking may cause your RA symptoms to worsen and other complications such as heart disease, lung cancer, stroke, etc. I strongly advise you to stop smoking. Have you ever tried to stop? If you want, then I can refer you to a smoking cessation clinic where you will meet people who have successfully stopped smoking.

Do you drink? If yes, for how many years? What is the amount?

Patient: I have been drinking 2/3 glasses of wine every evening for many years.

Candidate: Alcohol also has some harmful impacts on RA patients; I recommend you reduce your amount of alcohol intake to a safer limit.

With whom you are living? Are they doing well? Who is supporting you at home?

Patient: I live with my husband.

Make Summary

Recheck Understanding: May I know how much did you get from our discussion today?

Help

Candidate: I have given you a large amount of information to take in ... I completely understand that it's impossible to remember everything that we have discussed. I will give you some written information that you can take away with you and read this in your leisure time. I will give my contact details as well to contact me if you have any worries or concerns anytime. Thank you so much for spending time with me.

Patient: Thank you.

Shake hands!

Transient Ischemic Attack

Your role: You are the doctor in a neurology clinic.

Problem: A new diagnosis of transient ischemic attack (TIA).

Patient: Mr Kelvin, a 50-year-old man.

Scenario: The patient has hypertension (HTN), and type 2 diabetes mellitus (T2DM) was seen yesterday as an emergency with a TIA. He developed left-sided weakness and speech disturbance during his work. All of the symptoms were improved on the way to the hospital, and he had fully recovered by the time he was seen. His blood glucose level was normal. The patient has diabetes and HTN, which are controlled with metformin and ramipril. He smokes 10–15 cigarettes/day. His usual medication comprises metformine, ramipril, and rosuvastatin. Aspirin was started following the event. The patient has been referred to the neurology clinic for further assessment. On examination, his pulse was 84 beats/min and regular, and his blood pressure was 135/80 mm Hg. There were no carotid bruits or cardiac murmurs. Fundoscopy was normal, and urinalysis showed glucose 1+. His most recent glycated hemoglobin (HbA1c) was 7%.

You have already discussed the situation with your consultant, who has advised further investigations by CT scan of the head and carotid Doppler scan. Treatment with aspirin should continue, and advise the patient to stop smoking.

Your task: You have to explain the plan of management to the patient and address the patient's concerns.

Introduction, Permission, and Confirmation of the Agenda

Candidate: Hello, Mr Kelvin. I am Mohammad Ali, one of the working doctors here today. I have been asked to talk to you about your condition. Is that okay with you?

Patient: Hello, Doctor, it's all right.

Candidate: Do you want to add anyone else to our discussion today?

Patient: No.

Check Understanding

Candidate: Okay, Mr Kelvin, would you please tell me how much you know about your condition? What is your expectation?

Patient: I have been under my family doctor's care for several years as I have diabetes, high blood pressure, and high cholesterol controlled by medications. Yesterday I was seen for the first time as an emergency because I had a weakness affecting my left arm and some speech disturbance. However, my symptoms had resolved spontaneously by the time when I reached. The doctor told me that I had a mini-stroke or TIA; he gave me aspirin to take and let me go home with an appointment for review in the brain clinic today. Now I am scared as the doctor told me that I am lucky not to have suffered a permanently disabling stroke, but there is a possibility in future. Will I get another one, Doctor?

Candidate: I am sorry, but it is possible that you may have it again! I will talk through all of this in detail. Before that, as you know, you had a condition called TIA. Do you have any idea about TIA?

Patient: Not at all. I just know it is a mini-stroke.

Candidate: May I explain to you more about your condition?

Patient: Yes.

Explain the Mechanism of Transient Ischemic Attack

Candidate: Okay. Please don't hesitate to interrupt me at any time for any query.

A transient ischemic attack or TIA is a temporary stroke. Here transient or temporary means symptoms start suddenly and usually goes within an hour in most cases. However, in some cases, it can last up to 24 hours. This is because different parts of our brain control different parts of our body, and the symptoms will depend on which area of the brain is affected. Therefore, it can present with weakness of a hand, arm, or leg; difficulties with speech or swallowing; tingling, and numbness of a part of the body; loss of vision, or double vision.

Transient ischemic attack is mainly caused by a tiny blood clot that becomes stuck in small blood vessels in the brain, causing a lack of blood supply to the part of the brain. The clot usually breaks up quickly; therefore, the affected part of the brain is without oxygen for just a few minutes and soon recovers.

A fatty lump (atheroma) inside the lining of the main artery in the neck is the common site for this clot formation, and sometimes a tiny clot forms in a heart chamber. These are then carried in the bloodstream, toward the brain, and the clot travels in it until it becomes stuck; when it becomes stuck and blocks the artery that stops the blood supply to the part of the brain. Am I clear so far? Do you have any questions till now?

Patient: No.

Explain to the Patient What Investigations are Required to Evaluate the Symptoms and Determine Future Treatment Recommendations

Candidate: I have discussed the situation with your consultant, who has advised further investigation by carotid Doppler scan and CT scan of the head. Would you like to know more about it?

Patient: Yes please.

Candidate: Actually, a magnetic resonance imaging (MRI) scan/CT scan can show which part of the brain is affected or whether there was a small bleed into your brain or other problem such as a brain tumor that cause the similar symptoms.

Ultrasound scan of your carotid artery (carotid Doppler) can help to see a severe narrowing of one of these arteries. If one or both of the carotid arteries are >50% furred up, you may be referred urgently for surgery (carotid endarterectomy) to unblock them.

Tell about the Treatment Options

We have already started aspirin, which is an anti-clot forming medicine that helps to prevent a future stroke. So, I strongly recommend that your treatment with aspirin should continue along with other lifestyle modifications. May I ask you some questions about your lifestyle?

Patient: Yeah, sure.

Candidate: Do you smoke or drink alcohol? How many sticks and for how long?

Patient: I don't drink alcohol, but I have been smoking 10–15 cigarettes a day for the last 10 years.

Emphasize the Importance of Risk Factors and Lifestyle Modification

Candidate: It's a lot. I strongly advise you to stop smoking. It really brings a good impact on your health. Have you ever tried to do it?

Patient: My GP told me to stop, and I tried to stop, but I failed.

Candidate: Okay, then I can help you in that matter. I can refer you to the NHS's stop smoking clinic, and I assure you that many people successfully stop smoking in this way.

Not only stopping smoking, maintaining a healthy lifestyle with regular exercise, a healthy diet, and weight reduction are also important.

Patient: Why has this happened to me at such a young age?

Candidate: That's a really good question … I also want to talk about the risk factors. Some common risk factors can be changed and some cannot … such as high blood pressure, high blood sugar, high cholesterol, having some diseases that are more prone to form blood clots, and importantly smoking, alcohol consumption, and so on ... I am afraid that you have most of the risk factors. Therefore, I want to inform you that it is important to reduce risk factors, which will reduce the chances of having a stroke or TIA.

Please Provide Appropriate Information about the Risk of Further Stroke

In terms of your query about having a future permanent disabling stroke, I want to mention that a TIA itself does no harm or permanent damage to the brain, and the symptoms go soon. However, a TIA indicates that you tend to form blood clots in your blood vessels or heart. Therefore, if you have a TIA, you have a higher-than-average risk of developing a larger blood clot, which may cause a stroke or heart attack in the future.

But I want to tell you that early initiation of existing treatments after TIA was associated with an 80% reduction in the future stroke risk. Does it make sense for you?

Patient: Yes, it is. Do I need better medicines than my doctor has given me so far?

Candidate: I appreciate your concern. Be sure that your GP gives you the proper medicines, particularly aspirin, to prevent the clot. However, the main treatment of this mini-stroke is controlling the risk factors by tight control of your blood pressure, blood sugars, cholesterol, stopping smoking, and other lifestyle modifications, as I said.

Meanwhile, we will assess you further by a scoring system often used to assess your risk of a future stroke earlier after having a TIA, and if you need it, we will add some other medications too (in paroxysmal AF-anticoagulation).

Address the Patient's Concern

Candidate: So, Mr Kelvin, do you have any other concerns?

Patient: What is the evidence that stopping smoking will help?

Candidate: I know stopping smoking is really a tough decision for anyone, but the chemicals in tobacco are carried in your bloodstream that can damage your arteries. Much research has been done on it and proves that stopping smoking can greatly reduce your risk of stroke and many other diseases such as heart attacks and lung cancer.

Okay, Mr Kelvin, may I ask you some questions? Do you drive? Do you drive for your living?

Patient: Yes, I drive to go to my office.

Candidate: Mr Kelvin, I am sorry to tell you that you have to stop driving for a month. As it is your first TIA, you may not need to inform the DVLA. However, if, you have several TIAs over a short period of time, you must inform DVLA and stop driving until at least 3 months after your last TIA.

Candidate: So, Mr Kelvin, is there anything that I haven't explained to you properly?

Patient: No. You have explained everything very well.

Social History

Take relevant social history to manage your patient.

Make Summary

Recheck Understanding

May I know how much did you get from our discussion today?

Help

Candidate: I will give you some written information and website address to read more about stroke and TIA; I will give you my contact details as well to contact me if you have any worries or queries ... Thank you so much for spending time with me.

Patient: Thank you.

Shake hands!

Addison's Disease

Your role: You are the doctor in the endocrine OPD clinic.

Problem: New diagnosis of Addison's disease.

Patient's name: Mrs Sarah Kaur, a 27-year-old lady.

Scenario: Mrs Sarah Kaur was referred to the endocrine clinic with unexplained fatigue and has undergone some blood tests that revealed Addison's disease. The patient has returned to the clinic for her test results.

Your task: You have to explain the diagnosis and management plan and counsel the patient for management in some special circumstances.

Introduction, Permission, and Confirmation of the Agenda

Candidate: Hello, Mrs Sara Kaur. I am Mohammad Ali, one of the working doctors here today. I have come here to talk to you about your test results. Is that okay?

Patient: Hello, Doctor, it's all right.

Candidate: Do you want to add anyone else to our discussion today?

Patient: No.

Check Understanding

Candidate: So, Mrs Kaur, how are you feeling now? Do you have any idea what has been happening to you so far? Do you know why we did the blood tests and what we were looking for?

Patient: I don't have any idea, actually. I was completely fine 3 months back, after that I have been feeling too tired. I can't do my household works even I am failing to take care of my 3-year-old child. That is really frustrating. Sometimes I feel dizzy especially while I stand from a sitting position. So, I met my GP, and he referred me to the consultant who did some blood tests, and now I am here for the results …

Candidate: Okay, Mrs Kaur, I can understand. The results of blood investigations have been released and reveal that you have a disease called Addison disease (stop for a while—let the patient express her feelings and thoughts). Have you heard it before?

Patient: No, Doctor, I haven't. What is it? Is it serious, Doctor?

Candidate: I appreciate your concern; actually, it can be serious if left untreated, but we will do our best to control your disease. I am here to discuss the disease. Would you want me to explain more about it?

Patient: Okay.

Candidate: Basically, we have two small adrenal glands that lie just above each kidney. Cells in the adrenal glands make various proteins called hormone, which acts on different parts of the body. It is a condition in which your adrenal glands are not working as well as they should. So, they cannot produce as much steroid hormone as they normally do. Steroid hormone is vital for health, regulating blood pressure, the immune system, and responding to stress.

Causes

Most commonly (80% cases), it is caused by an autoimmune disease means disturbance in our defensive system, which is supposed to attack bugs and germs. Sometimes our defense system, instead of attacking germs and bugs, goes crazy for an unknown reason, and it starts attacking our own tissues. In your case, it is attacking your adrenal gland cells, which make steroids.

Other causes are infections such as TB or other viral and bacterial infections, drugs or hereditary, etc.

For deficiency of this hormone, you may have generalized weakness, become easily tired, lose weight, decreased BP, dizziness, decreased glucose level, tanned skin, feeling and getting sick, and electrolyte disturbance.

Patient: But doctor, I don't have any other symptoms besides tiredness. So why do I have this disease?

Candidate: In some cases, it may present with vague symptoms initially.

Addison's Crisis

One thing I would like to inform you is that the most serious consequence of this disease is the Addisonian crisis, where the level of steroid falls to become very low, and you can become very ill within a short time. At that time, you may develop severe vomiting and diarrhea, low blood pressure, dehydration, tummy pain, or even may develop collapse; therefore, you have to seek immediate medical help.

It is a medical emergency; you may become severely ill and even die if the cause of the symptoms is not diagnosed properly and treated quickly. It is often triggered by another illness such as infection or stress such as surgery. During this time, you will need extra steroids, if you have Addison's disease, you cannot make extra steroids, and you may quickly develop Addison's crisis.

But let me assure you that we will guide you regarding all of the bad symptoms and follow-up you regularly to prevent any unwanted situations.

Patient: Doctor, it's such a scary thing! I didn't expect this today! I haven't imagined that I have such a dangerous disease! This is really a bad day for me!

Candidate: I am really sorry for this bad information today. But be sure that we will do our best for you.

Patient: How will you treat me now? Is there any treatment for this? Any medicine or anything?

Treatment

Candidate: Yes, definitely, there are available treatment options for you, and the main treatment is the replacement of this steroid hormone you no longer make. You can take it as an oral tablet and you should never miss taking your steroid as it is vital for your well-being. You will need regular follow-ups at the outpatient clinic to make sure your hormone levels are well maintained.

Drug Interaction with Steroids

Candidate: Well, in terms of using the steroid, we need to keep in mind that some medicines used to treat other conditions can interfere with the steroid used to treat Addison's disease. Therefore, the dose may need to be adjusted. Always inform your doctor that you are being treated for Addison's disease if you are prescribed any other medicine. Okay, Mrs Kaur?

Patient: Okay.

Special Circumstances

Candidate: Now, I would like to discuss some special situations with Addison's disease, if that's okay with you ...

Patient: Okay please.

Candidate: It is vital for anyone having Addison's disease that he/she takes the right amount of steroid replacement every day. Without this replacement medicine, you can become very ill. Therefore, you must be strictly adherent to this. If you are sick or have an illness such as fever, vomiting or diarrhea, you will need to take a double dose of steroids until it is settled.

If you need an operation, dental procedure or any medical procedures, you must make sure that the doctor knows you have Addison's disease because you will need an extra dose of steroids in such situations.

When you go on a holiday, take ample supplies steroid along with you as emergency support.

If you take part in heavy exercise or sport, you will need extra steroids and fluids, so it is advisable to take advice from your doctor on how to adjust the dose to suit you.

If you are planning for pregnancy, you have to inform your obstetrician and gland doctor to make MDT, give you full care, and avoid complications during pregnancy.

Patient: It's quite a lot, Doctor! How could I remember so many things?

Candidate: I know I'm giving you a lot of information, it's very difficult to remember everything but don't be panicked, it's not just a single conversation. We will arrange a series of conversations to further discuss all the issues again with you.

Patient: Okay ... Thank you. But there are lots of restrictions ... How will I maintain so many things?

Candidate: Yes, it's really tough to maintain. I can understand ... But, I can make things easier for you by advising you some general "sick day rules" where you can know what to do in different situations involving stress, trauma, or illness, and you can handle such unusual situations or avoid an adrenal crisis.

Medic Alert Bracelet and Carrying a Letter

I strongly recommend that you wear a Medic Alert bracelet to let others know about your condition and carry an ample of steroids with you in case of emergency. Does that make sense, Mrs Kaur?

Patient: Yes. Okay.

Address the Patient's Concern

Candidate: So, Mrs Kaur, do you have any other concerns?

Patient: Is it a curable condition, Doctor?

Candidate: I am sorry to tell you that it is not curable, but it can be controlled on medication, and if you are completely compliant with your medications and following regular follow-up, you can live near-normal life and enjoy your life... Any other concerns?

Patient: What about complications of steroid therapy, Doctor?

Candidate: Steroids will be given for you as replacement therapy to reach the normal level so that there is no risk of developing complications of the long-term use of steroids. Am I clear so far?

Patient: Yes.

Social History

Take relevant social history to manage your patient.

Candidate: So, Mrs Kaur, is there anything that I haven't explained to you properly?

Patient: No. You have explained everything very well.

Make Summary

Recheck Understanding

May I know how much did you get from our discussion today?

Help

I am giving you some written information and the Addison's Disease Self-help Group website address where you can get a wealth of information about handling difficult situations with Addison's disease. Moreover, I will give you my contact details, if you have any worries or queries you can contact me. Thank you so much for spending time with me.

Shake hands!

Ulcerative Colitis with the Refusal to Admit Hospital

Your role: You are a doctor in the Acute Medicine Department.

Problem: Exacerbation of ulcerative colitis (UC).

Patient's name: Mrs Angela Murphy, a 32-year-old lady.

Scenario: The emergency department has referred Mrs Murphy to the medical team because of worsening diarrhea and abdominal pain in the background of UC. The consultant has received the patient and advised hospital admission for IV therapy. The nurse has informed you that the patient does not want to be admitted. Your consultant has asked you to talk to the patient.

Your task: You have to explain to the patient her diagnosis and management plan and determine if she is competent to refuse admission to the hospital.

Introduction, Permission, and Confirmation of the Agenda

Candidate: Hello, Mrs Murphy. I am Mohammad Ali ..., one of the working doctors here today. I have been asked to talk to you about your condition. Is that ok with you?

Patient: Hello, Doctor, it's all right.

Candidate: Do you want to add anyone else to our discussion today?

Patient: No.

Check Understanding

Candidate: Ok, Mrs Murphy, how are you feeling now? How much do you know about your condition?

Patient: I am not feeling good, Doctor. I have had UC for the last 4 years, which was well-controlled on medication. But over the last 7 days, I have developed increased motion. I am taking mesalazine tablet and mesalazine enema.

Candidate: Hmm ... I can understand. Before proceeding further, I would like to ask you some questions; it will help me get a clear picture of your condition if that's ok.

Patient: Yes.

Candidate: You have mentioned increased bowel motion recently, so how many times per day? What about the amount? Is it mixed with blood or mucous? Any fever and abdominal pain? And what about your waterworks?

Patient: I am passing loose stool mixed with mucous and blood several times per day, even at night. I am taking fluid more and more to get ease ... I have no tummy pain, actually, but there is slight discomfort present right now. No problem with my waterworks and I have no fever.

Candidate: It's ok, thank you ... May I explain to you more about your condition?

Patient: Sure ...

Candidate: Please don't hesitate to interrupt me at any time for any query. We have done some blood tests and stool tests to assess you more ... as you are passing frequent loose stool several times per day, even at night, and you are taking more and more fluid to get ease, all this together suggest you have an acute flare of UC ...

You are taking orally as well as per rectal mesalazine regularly ... But it's not improving. It suggests this drug is not working at this moment. Does it make sense for you, Mrs Murphy ...?

Patient: Oh ... yes, it makes sense a lot, Doctor, even I can understand that it is actually not working this time.

Candidate: At this moment, we think you need immediate hospital admission for intravenous steroids and intravenous fluid as well as monitoring regularly ... And we decided to admit you immediately to control your flare of UC as early as possible. Is that ok with you, Mrs Murphy?

Patient: But I don't want to admit to the hospital. I don't like to stay here!

Candidate: I can understand. Actually, no one wants to stay in the hospital, it's not a pleasant place to be, but here it's a matter of your health and life. May I ask you why you don't want to admit? Is there any particular reason here?

Patient: Because it is very difficult for me at this moment ... My sister is a doctor. She agreed to give me support at home. It will be more comfortable to remain at home than in the hospital.

Candidate: Ok, but may I explain to you more why we are thinking about your hospital admission at this moment?

Patient: Ok ... you can tell me, but I will not change my decision.

Candidate: Since you are competent, I will not impose any decision on you. But as a doctor, it is my duty to give you all the information so that you can make the right decision.

Sometimes if the flare-up gets out of control, then the colon can be very inflamed and swollen and can burst if left untreated ... in the technical fancy term, it is called toxic megacolon. This would be a serious problem and would need an emergency operation. On the other hand, as you are passing frequent loose stool, you may become dehydrated, and your kidney may fail if it is not corrected adequately ...

However, the good thing is ... the I/V steroid is very good at controlling flare up and preventing this more serious problem. With steroid treatment, we find that patient tends to improve quite quickly. So, Mrs Murphy, do you understand my point? (Is she aware of the seriousness of her condition?)

Patient: Yes, I can. You are right in your place, I know. Still, Doctor, I don't want to stay here, it's not possible for me, it is very important to stay at my home. I have to take care of my son; his final exam is near. And besides, the whole family is dependent on me. So please, Doctor, give me some tablets that I can take home.

Candidate: I understand your situation, but right now, we need to prioritize your health, and only when you are healthy you can take care of others. Moreover, regarding tablets, I can give you the steroid in a tablet, but I am afraid it will not be as effective as injections because you need more powerful doses, which can only be given by injections. Therefore, I strongly recommend you to admit to the hospital at least for a short period so that we can give you the proper treatment.

Patient: Doctor, I will rest at home, drink fluids and do whatever it needs, but I will not be admitted. Please give me the tablet. I believe it will be enough for me, and my sister is a doctor. I talked to her, and she will take care of me.

Candidate: Well, Mrs Murphy, you have the capacity to take the decision (legal issue: competent) as you understand your condition and the possible outcome of not being admitted. You are legally allowed to refuse treatment (ethical issue: patient autonomy). Therefore, I can't enforce you for your admission.

I will give you oral steroids, but you should regularly be monitored by your sister and take adequate fluid to prevent dehydration. Does your sister live with you?

Patient: No, but she will visit me regularly.

Candidate: Please tell her to visit you once or twice a day, and if you feel very unwell, you must try to reach the hospital as early as possible. And I will discuss your case with my consultant as well as. Is that ok with you?

Patient: Ok.

Candidate: I am sorry to tell you that it's a legal issue, so that you need to sign a form as you insist on not being admitted against the medical decision.

Patient: No problem. I will do it.

Address the Patient's Concern

Candidate: So, Mrs Murphy, do you have any other concerns?

Patient: No. Thank you.

Social History

Take relevant social history to manage your patient.

Candidate: So, Mrs Murphy, is there anything that I haven't explained to you properly?

Patient: No. You have explained everything very well.

Make Summary

Ok, Mrs Murphy, I am going to summarize the important things from our discussion today ... you have been a known case of UC for the last 4 years. You were well-controlled with oral medication. But over the last 7 days, you have developed worsening diarrhea mixed with blood. The investigation report suggests it is a flare of UC. So, we advised you to get admission for intravenous therapy for early recovery as well as to prevent complications ... but you don't want to admit to the hospital at this moment because of some personal problems. Legally I can't enforce you for your admission. So, I am giving you oral steroids at this moment and advice for supportive care. Is that ok, Mrs Murphy?

Recheck Understanding

May I know how much did you get from our discussion today?

Help

Finally, I would like to say ... you must share the information with your other family members ... If you change your mind, then I will ask you to admit the hospital for the best care of management.

I will give you my contact details and the contact details of a specialist nurse ... If you have any worries or queries, please don't hesitate to contact me ...

Thank you ...

Shake hand!

Celiac Disease

Your role: You are the doctor in the gastrointestinal tract (GIT) OPD clinic.

Problem: New diagnosis of celiac disease.

Patient's name: Mrs Jasmine Gupta, a 27-year-old lady.

Scenario: Mrs Jasmine Gupta was referred to the GIT clinic with unexplained anemia and has undergone an oesophago-gastro-duodenoscopy (OGD) and colonoscopy. The OGD and colonoscopy were negative, but the biopsy was taken from the D2 of the duodenum, which along with relevant blood tests [positive anti-tissue transglutaminase antibody (anti-TTG-Ab), iron deficiency anemia, low folic acid] has come back positive for celiac disease. The patient has returned to the clinic for her investigation reports.

Your task: You have to explain the diagnosis and management plan and counsel the patient on appropriate modification that needs to be made to her diet.

Introduction, Permission, and Confirmation of the Agenda

Candidate: Hello, Mrs Gupta. I am Mohammad Ali, one of the working doctors here today. I have come here to talk to you about your blood and camera tests result. Is that, ok?

Patient: Hello, Doctor, it's all right.

Candidate: Do you want to add anyone else to our discussion today?

Patient: No.

Check Understanding

Candidate: Do you have any idea what has been happening to you so far? Do you know why we did the camera test and blood test and what we were looking for?

Patient: I have had weakness and diarrhea for the last 3 months. I have lost weight also. I went to my GP, and he did some blood tests and told me I had anemia. After that, he referred me to the hospital. The doctors then did some blood tests and camera tests, and I am waiting for the result.

Candidate: Well ... I have your test results with me and unfortunately, they revealed that you have a condition called UC ...

Patient: Oh! I see ... Celiac!

Candidate: Do you have any idea about celiac disease?

Patient: No. Not at all.

Candidate: It's all right. Let me explain to you more about the disease. Please don't hesitate to interrupt me at any time for any queries.

Celiac disease is an autoimmune disease; our immune system makes white blood cells and antibodies to protect against foreign objects such as viruses, bacteria, and other germs. Sometimes our immune system, instead of attacking germs and bugs, go crazy for an unknown reason, and it starts attacking our own tissues. In your condition, it attacks the lining of part of the gut, causing inflammation. Are you following me, Mrs Gupta?

Patient: Yes.

Candidate: The most important issue here is that the inflammation is triggered by food containing gluten, which is part of certain foods—mainly foods made from wheat, barley, and rye. People with celiac disease make antibodies against gluten, so here, the gut mistakes gluten as a harmful one and reacts against it as if it were fighting off a germ. These antibodies cause inflammation in the lining of a part of your gut called the small intestine.

Our small intestine lining contains millions of tiny tube structures called villi. These help digestion and absorption of food and nutrients. As a result of inflammation, the villi become flattened; digestion and absorption of food become affected which may cause a deficiency of vitamins, iron, and other nutrients and may make you feel tired and weak.

Your anemia is due to poor absorption of iron and weight loss due to poor absorption of food. As the fat part of the food is poorly absorbed, the stool becomes loose, pale, smelly, and difficult to flush away. Does that make sense, Mrs Gupta?

Patient: Yes, it is, but how will you treat me now?

Candidate: Fortunately, the symptoms can be kept away by having a diet completely free from gluten. Once you stop eating any food that contains gluten, the symptoms go within a few weeks. The main foods to stop are any that contain wheat, rye or barley. Many common foods contain this ingredient: bread, cake, pasta, pastry, and many kinds of cereal. To avoid symptoms and complications, I strongly recommend you avoid all foods that contain gluten.

Patient: Complications? What complications, Doctor?

Candidate: Actually, the untreated and inadequately treated celiac disease may develop many complications such as developing thinning of the bones (osteoporosis) as a result of nutritional deficiency, having a baby that has a low birth weight or born prematurely. Although it is rare, in the long run, it may lead to certain cancer in the gut called lymphoma. Fortunately, all of these complications can be avoided if you completely avoid any type of food containing gluten. So, the main step of treatment is to avoid a gluten-free diet. Am I clear so far, Mrs Gupta?

Patient: Yeah. It seems very serious, but I don't have much more symptoms other than this tiredness and diarrhea.

Candidate: Well, actually, initially, the symptoms may be vague as yours. In most cases, this is not so bad, especially if you avoid gluten-containing foods.

Patient: Doctor ... I don't want to go on a special diet because I think it may be unpalatable and unhealthy ...

Candidate: I can understand your feelings, but we will involve an experienced dietician who can guide you regarding your diet, be sure that most people can follow a gluten-free diet without any difficulties, and they will have a major beneficial effect on their symptoms. In fact, fish, meat, vegetables, potatoes, fruits, rice, corn, maize, and dairy products are fine. You can also buy or order special gluten-free flour, pasta, bread, and other available foods from health food shops.

We will manage you under an MDT involving your gut physician, dietician, and specialist nurse. We will regularly follow-up you, and any problem will be dealt accordingly.

Address the Patient's Concern

Candidate: So, Mrs Gupta, do you have any concerns or expectations?

Patient: Is it curable, Doctor?

Candidate: I am sorry to tell you that it is not curable, but it is treatable. The single treatment for celiac disease is a lifelong, strictly gluten-free diet. If you can avoid foods containing gluten, your condition will be completely controlled, and you can live a near-normal life.

Social History

Take relevant social history to manage your patient.

Candidate: So, Mrs Gupta, is there anything that I haven't explained to you properly?

Patient: No. You have explained everything very well.

Make Summary

Candidate: Thank you. Now I am going to summarize the important things from our discussion today.

Your blood and camera tests reveal that you have celiac disease. In this disease, your bowel cannot tolerate the gluten-containing diet. So our main step of management is to avoid all diets containing gluten. We will refer you to MDT involving a gut physician, dietitian, and a specialist nurse. Is that ok, Mrs Gupta?

Recheck Understanding
May I know how much did you get from our discussion today?

Help
I will give you some written information and the website address of the celiac disease society of UK to read more about the disease; I will give you my contact details as well to contact me any time if you have any worries or queries ...

Shake hands!

Patient with the First Fit

Your role: You are the doctor in the acute medical ward.

Problem: Patient with the first fit.

Patient's name: Mr Albert Soames, a 33-year-old man.

Scenario: Albert Soames, admitted the day before, was found unconscious while shopping. An electroencephalogram (EEG) and CT scan of the brain were done and they were normal. The diagnosis is a first fit/seizure, and the patient is now ready for discharge; your consultant has asked you to explain to the patient about the diagnosis, management plan, and any restrictions resulting from having had a seizure.

Your task: You have to explain to the patient his diagnosis, management plan, and any restrictions they need to place upon their activities.

Introduction, Permission, and Confirmation of the Agenda

Candidate: Hello, my name is Mohammad Ali. I am one of the working doctors here today. I understand you were found unconscious while shopping and got admitted yesterday. I have been asked to talk about your condition, is that okay with you?

Patient: Ok.

Candidate: May I start by taking your full name, age, and where are you from, please?

Patient: Mr Soames, 35 years old, I am from Dublin.

Candidate: Do you want to invite anyone else to our discussion today?

Patient: No.

Check Understanding

Candidate: Would you please tell me exactly what happened to you?

Patient: I collapsed suddenly while shopping. I remember walking into the supermarket and smelling something strange, but then I woke up in the ambulance. The passers-by told the paramedics I collapsed to the floor next to the freezer cabinet ... started shaking, and they could not rouse me for about 4–5 minutes. They told the paramedics that after the shaking stopped, I was drowsy and confused for half an hour. I improved when I was in the ambulance on the way to the hospital. This has happened for the first time in my life ... There are no previous episodes.

Candidate: Ok ... How are you feeling now?

Patient: Fine ...

Candidate: That's good. I am glad to hear that you are completely fine now. Do you have any idea what has happened to you?

Patient: No doctor.

Candidate: It's ok, no problem. Let me tell you about your condition. We did a special test called EEG and a CT scan of your brain. Fortunately, they are normal. However, your symptoms are consistent with a seizure, and the nerve doctor is suspecting this may be a first epileptic fit.
(Stop for a while, let the patient express his feeling and thought) ...

Patient: Oh! ... That was a seizure!

Empathy and Sympathy

Candidate: I can understand this is not something you expected. Be sure that we are going to give you the full care and support we can.

Do you have any idea about epilepsy? May I explain to you more about epilepsy?

Patient: I don't know much about it; I just heard about it. Please explain it to me, Doctor.

Candidate: Ok ... Please don't feel hesitate to interrupt me any time for any query.

Explain the Disease

The brain contains millions of nerve cells that constantly send tiny electrical messages down the nerve to all parts of the body. Different parts of the brain control different functions of the body, so symptoms depend on which part of the brain is affected. However, epilepsy is an active focus in the brain, sending an abnormal electrical impulse to the body, causing shaking of the body due to uncontrollable muscle contractions.

In many cases, no cause for the seizure can be found, but sometimes it may be familial (idiopathic epilepsy), in some cases underlying brain damage (such as a patch of scar tissue in the part of the brain, stroke, growth or tumor, infection) causes epilepsy that may irritate the surrounding brain cells and trigger seizure. However, your brain scan and blood tests exclude these possibilities as all are normal.

It can come in the form of unpredictable shaking of the body with loss of consciousness, tongue biting, frothing from the mouth, and maybe uncontrolled waterworks. It can be precipitated by high fever, strong flashes such as strobe lighting or video games, stress or anxiety, and lack of sleep ... so you have to avoid these factors. Does it make any sense for you ... Mr. Soames?

Patient: Yes, but doctor, will it happen again?

Candidate: I wish I could tell you that it won't happen again. Unfortunately, it can be possible that you will get another attack of seizure in future.

Patient: Is there any way to prevent this from happening or any treatment for me?

Candidate: As it is the first seizure and has no specific etiology, EEG, and CT scans are normal, we will not start antiepileptic drugs at this moment to prevent a further attack. If another episode occurs (recurrent seizures confirm epilepsy), then we have to start the medications. The treatment of the condition is oral medication will be prescribed by the nerve doctor. And you have to be completely compliant with these medications to control your condition and decrease the chance of any further attacks.

So, we are going to refer you to an MDT involving a nerve doctor, social worker, occupational health worker to give you the proper care and management plan ... is that ok, Mr Soames?

Patient: Ok, Doctor.

Driving History

Candidate: Do you drive? Do you drive for a living?

Patient: Yes, I do, and driving is my job.

Candidate: I am sorry to tell you, but you have a legal obligation to inform the DVLA to explain the situation, and they will assess when you can drive. Does it make any sense for you, Mr Soames?

[If the patient intends to drive ...]

Patient: Doctor, I have to drive. It's my job. I've been doing this for the last 10 years, my family is dependent on me, and I'm the only earner in the family. It's not possible to stop. How could you tell me that there is a legal obligation? I'm absolutely fine now.

Candidate: I appreciate your feelings .... I know stopping driving is very difficult for you as your living depends upon it, but your condition is risky for yourself and the others during driving.... I am afraid that you could get this attack while driving, which could be very serious for you and put your life at risk.

If you are driving, imagine yourself driving your child home and you got this fit which would stop you from thinking and even hitting the brakes, you will get an accident with your beloved son, which I am afraid might end your life. So for your health and public health, it is your legal obligation to inform the DVLA.

Patient: Ok, I understand what you are trying to say. Will you inform DVLA, if I don't?

Candidate: If you do not do so, I am obliged to inform DVLA (break his confidentiality). If you have been driving and caused a car accident after the doctor advised you not to do, you will be fully accountable for that, your insurance may not redeem, and sometimes the police may charge you.

Patient: Oh! I feel anxious, doctor, I don't know how I manage everything now!

Candidate: I completely understand, it can be difficult. You can contact the epilepsy society as they deal with managing epilepsy with work or driving. It would be useful for you to connect with them and also you can inform your occupational health team, they could do you a replacement with another suitable job for the duration of the bar in the same company. Do you like us to write to them?

Patient: Ok. That will be better.

Candidate: I would like to inform you that to avoid potentially serious injury during seizure—do not use open fire—a microwave oven is much safer than a conventional oven, kettle, or hot plate. Showers are safer than a bath. If you are having a bath, tell someone not to leave you alone. And leave the door unlocked. Make sure there are sufficient guards or rails in any high situations. Use electrical tools with power breakers and avoid using sharp furniture or tools during day-to-day activities. However, it is sensible to tell people (such as friends, relatives, and work colleagues) about your epilepsy so that they might wish to learn about the recovery position when you are unconscious during an epileptic attack. Mr Soames, are you comfortable with my advice?

Patient: Yes, thanks, Doctor.

Candidate: Well, do you have anyone with you right now whom we can tell about your recovery position and what should do if you have a seizure in future?

Patient: No.

Candidate: Please bring any of your family members or friend next time.

Social History

Take relevant social history to manage your patient.

Candidate: Is there anything else that we have not explained? Do you have any other concerns or any expectations from me?

Make Summary
Check Understanding

May I know, please, how much did you get from our discussion today?

Help

Candidate: I will give you some written information and the website address regarding epilepsy to learn more about it. I will give my contact details as well to call me if you have any worries or concerns anytime. Mr Soams, since you are not permitted to drive, is there anyone to drive you home?

Patient: No problem, I will call my wife to drive me home.

Candidate: Thank you for spending time with me.

Patient: Thank you.

Shake hands!

Emphysema with Smoking Cessation

Your role: You are the doctor in the lung clinic.

Problem: Smoking cessation advice in an active smoker with new emphysema.

Patient's name: Mrs Christina Bunch, a 50-year-old woman.

Scenario: Mrs Christina Bunch was admitted 4 days ago with worsening shortness of breath on exertion, which then came on at rest with wheezing and purulent productive cough and treated appropriately with antibiotics, steroids, and nebulizer. Spirometry revealed moderate chronic obstructive pulmonary disease (COPD), she is now ready for discharge, and the consultant on the ward has asked you to discuss with her smoking cessation, given that she has a diagnosis of COPD.

Your task: You have to explain to the patient about the condition and discuss the cessation of smoking.

Introduction, Permission, and Confirmation of the Agenda

Candidate: Hello, Mrs Christina Bunch, I am Mohammad Ali, one of the working doctors here today. I have been asked to talk to you about your condition ... Is that ok with you?

Patient: Hello, Doctor. It's all right.

Candidate: Do you want to invite anyone else to our discussion today?

Patient: No.

Check Understanding

Candidate: Ok, Mrs Christina, how are you feeling now?

Patient: Well, I'm definitely improving, but I don't feel as well as I should. My cough is a lot better, but still, I am facing breathing difficulty.

Candidate: I know it's tough for you, but would you please tell me how much you know about your condition?

Patient: I have had a chronic cough and sputum with increasing breathlessness for several years. I just feel more breathless when I walk too long or up the stairs, and also exercise tends to make the breathing problem worse. 4 days ago, I was hospitalized with my shortness of breath and a bad cough. The doctor told me that I have emphysema.

Candidate: Ok, you already know about emphysema. Is this something that has ever been discussed with you? Or how much do you know about it?

Patient: I know this is a condition where I may have some lung damage, and sometimes also I may get some infections like this time.

Candidate: Ok, would it be ok if we talked a bit about your disease process, its causes, and a few recommendations that might relate to the disease?

Patient: Yes, please

Candidate: Please don't hesitate to interrupt me any time for any query ...

Emphysema is a chronic lung problem. It is mainly due to the damage to the airway lining causing obstruction. It is slowly progressive that's why you are feeling progressive breathlessness on exertion for several years and on-off cough with phlegm. 4 days ago you had a flare-up of emphysema due to an infection in your lung. You needed oxygen and some powerful antibiotics to treat it.

Patient: That's a real concern; when I was admitted to the hospital, the doctors gave me oxygen, and I never thought I would be the person who would need oxygen like that; that was too scary. I'm terrified of needing an oxygen tank, carrying it around with me, and having the tubes in my nose.

Candidate: I know, it seems scary, and we have a spirometry today, which is a breathing test that you did, and we compared it with the test 6 months ago you had; it is quite a bit worse now.

Patient: Oh! It's another shocking news!

Candidate: It must be. However, let me discuss how can we help you and what type of lifestyle changes can help with your condition. In particular, I want to talk about smoking. I understand that you do smoke.

Patient: Yes, I do.

Candidate: Is it ok if we have a chat about your smoking habit?

Patient: It's all right.

Candidate: How many cigarettes a day do you smoke? And how long have you been smoking?

Patient: It's been around 25 sticks per day for the last 20 years.

Candidate: It's quite a lot of smoking. Unfortunately, smoking causes damage to the lungs. I am sorry to say that if you have emphysema and continue to smoke in such a way, the severity of emphysema will worsen rapidly. When you carry on smoking, you will feel more breathless. You may not be able to do day-to-day activities. Even with carry-on smoking, you may find simple things start to make you breathless, for example, just walking on the flat for a small distance or sometimes even room-to-room can make you shorter of breath and even turn into a point where you may need home oxygen. As you already mentioned, you are scared about oxygen, so I highly recommend you stop smoking because if you stop smoking, it will help slow down the rate at which emphysema will deteriorate.

Not only this lung problem, but smoking also causes premature death by increasing the risk of lung cancer and heart diseases such as heart attack, brain stroke, etc.

Patient: Does that happen really, Doctor?

Candidate: Yes, unfortunately, it really does. However, the good news is that by giving up smoking, the risk will reduce significantly. Moreover, you will notice a difference in breathing soon after stopping, you have your smell better, your taste better, and you will be financially better off. In addition, your risk of developing lung cancer will start to fall, and you can set a good example to others like your children ... Moreover, I think it's a good opportunity to discuss if you have any thoughts about stop smoking?

Patient: Well, but I think it's tough.

Candidate: I know that smoking is habit-forming and challenging to stop ... but have you ever tried to stop before, and have you been successful?

Patient: I tried, but I failed.

Candidate: What challenges have you faced when you tried to quit? Do you have any fears of stopping smoking (nicotine withdrawal syndrome)?

Patient: I found it difficult. It was awful, I had headaches, irritability, and palpitation that's why I never tried again.

Candidate: I agree ... it may not be easy, but I am sure that you can do it. And what about your other family members? Are they smoke?

Patient: My father is also a smoker. He has been smoking 40 cigarettes for the last 60 years, and he hasn't got any health problems.

Candidate: This is not always the case. It is good that your father is fine.

Patient: If smoking is bad. Why do all the doctors smoke?

Candidate: What doctors do is not always the right thing to do.

Patient: You know, it's my hobby; I like to smoke even with my work, it just relaxes me, I feel good.

Candidate: Many claim that it relaxes them and relieves their stress. Nicotine withdrawal can increase stress as the stress of withdrawal feels the same as other stresses. It seems like smoking is reducing other stresses, but this is not the case. Even many researches show stress levels are lower after they have stopped smoking. You can find many ways to relieve your stress; for example, you can go for yoga or meditation.

Would it be ok to explain some things that we can do to help you give up smoking? Because we know smoking is a very addictive habit and tough to stop, people can still find it difficult even if they are determined.

Patient: Ok.

Candidate: There are different types of approaches to quitting smoking. First, we can refer you to a smoking cessation clinic where smoking advisors help people stop smoking; they will chat with you, set targets, talk about some things that can help you, for example, behavioral modification techniques. It is a 12-week program. Initially, you will be in 1 to 1 session then will add to group sessions.

Another method we can call prescription tablets—bupropion and varenicline. These will actually help you by reducing the urge to smoke and withdrawal symptoms and, therefore, reducing craving.

The main reason that people smoke is—they are addicted to nicotine, so nicotine replacement therapy (NRT) is another option. NRT is a medication that gives you a low level of nicotine without the tar, carbon monoxide, and other poisonous chemicals present in tobacco smoke. These can be given in the form of a patch, spray, or chewing gum. In addition, it can help reduce unpleasant withdrawal effects such as bad mood, irritability, and craving, which may happen when you stop smoking.

It would always be better for anyone who wants to quit smoking should try a combination of all the above measures. How do you feel about everything we discussed today?

Patient: Nicotine? Isn't it smoking?

Candidate: Not actually; even nicotine getting from NRT is much safer than from cigarettes. Besides causing addiction, nicotine is not thought to cause disease when taken for a few weeks. The health problems from cigarettes, such as heart and lung diseases, are due to the tar and other harmful chemicals in cigarettes; also, the nicotine from smoking is absorbed rapidly and has a quicker effect than NRT. The dose of nicotine in NRT is not as high as in cigarettes. So, taking NRT in place of smoking is one step toward a healthier life.

Patient: I see ... that's good. It is good for me, but I am very much habituated to smoking; I smoke while working and walking in the evening. It's become a part of my life; how can I avoid it?

Candidate: In that case, to avoid temptation, you can change your routine in the difficult first few days in situations where you would like usually smoked ... I know it's difficult, but if you once achieve it, you will feel much better in your future life.

Patient: What should I do if I fail?

Candidate: If you fail to quit, we won't judge or nag you or take it personally. We are a friendly face that understands how difficult it is to quit, and we will help you get back on track to becoming a non-smoker.

You can find much online support, such as the NHS Smoke-Free Website, which can boost your chance of success in stopping smoking. In addition, you can call the Smokefree National Helpline.

Address the Patient's Concerns

Candidate: Ok, Mrs Christina ..Is there anything else that we have not explained properly? Do you have any concerns or questions?

Patient: Is it worth stopping smoking now? Isn't it just too late?

Candidate: Lung damage due to smoking is irreversible, so you won't regain lost functions if you give up now. Your lung function will continue to decline the same as anyone else's. If you keep on smoking, it will get worse much faster. So, it is never too late to stop smoking ... It is worth stopping as it reduces the ongoing damage to your lung.

Patient: Doctor, if I fail again to do it?

Candidate: Please don't be hopeless if you fail. After that, we will find the reasons why you felt it difficult this time and we will try to make you stronger next time. I want to assure you that, on average, people who eventually stop smoking have made three or four previous attempts. So, Mrs Cristina, would you like to do that?

Patient: I will definitely try to stop it.

Candidate: That's appreciating, and I highly encourage you to stop smoking. So I will give you a prescription, and also I will arrange another appointment just after 2 weeks to reinforce the issue discussed.

Social History

Candidate: Well, just some more questions about your lifestyle …
- Do you drink alcohol? If yes, how many drinks would you have been in a week?
- Are you working now? What are you doing for a living?
- Are you married? With whom you are living? Are they doing well? Who is supporting you now? Are you independent in activities of daily living?

Patient: I work as a manager in a private company. I don't drink at all, Doctor.

Make Summary

Recheck Understanding

May I know how much did you get out discussion today?

Help

Candidate: I have given you a large amount of information to take in … I completely understand it's impossible to remember everything that we have discussed. I will give you a leaflet, and "quit smoking helpline" website address. I will give my contact details and contact me if you have any worries or concerns anytime.

Thank you so much for spending time with me.

Patient: Thank you.

Shake hands!

Counseling of an Alcohol Drinker

Your role: You are the doctor in the general medical clinic.

Problem: Counseling for reducing alcohol consumption.

Patient's name: Mrs Lara Taylor, a 56-year-old lady.

Scenario: Mrs Taylor was referred to the outpatient clinic with uncontrolled hypertension, and during the assessment, it was found that she is drinking over and above the recommended weekly limit of alcohol. The consultant has asked you to counsel the patient on reducing alcohol consumption.

Your task: You have to explain the effects of continued excess alcohol consumption and counsel the patient to reduce alcohol consumption.

Introduction, Permission, and Confirmation of the Agenda

Candidate: Hello, Mrs Taylor. I am Mohammad Ali, one of the working doctors here today. I have come here to talk to you about your blood pressure. Is that, ok?

Patient: Hello, Doctor, it's all right.

Candidate: Do you want to add anyone else to our discussion today?

Patient: No.

Check Understanding

Candidate: Mrs Taylor, I understand your GP has sent you to the clinic because of your blood pressure. Could you please tell me more about what has been going on?

Patient: Three months ago, I went to my GP for a checkup, and at that time, my blood pressure was high. I have been taking regular medication since then, but it was not controlling. I went to my GP again 1 month ago, and he changed my medication. Today he sent me to the hospital because I have had high blood pressure till now.

Tell Her about Uncontrolled Blood Pressure

Candidate: I understand your blood pressure is not being under control, and you are taking medication for it. Have you been taking the medication regularly?

Patient: Yes. I am taking it every day.

Candidate: Well, ... you are taking your medication regularly, but your blood pressure is still high, which means it does not really control your blood pressure.

Patient: Yes, but why it is not working, Doctor?

Figure Out the Causes of Uncontrolled Blood Pressure

Candidate: I want to talk to you about some of the reasons why your blood pressure is not controlled. There are different kinds of things we have to look at, particularly caffeine and alcohol.

Do you drink lots of coffee or tea at all? As we know that tea and coffee contain caffeine, which can raise blood pressure. So it would be helpful to reduce it.

Patient: Not so much, Doctor. I take coffee only two times a day.

Take a Brief History of Alcohol Intake

Candidate: Well, that's absolutely fine. May I ask do you drink alcohol?

Patient: Yes.

Candidate: Regularly? For how many years? Every day or once a week? What types of it?

Patient: I usually drink two and a half glasses of wine in the evening for 15 years.

Candidate: Ok ... So, every day you drink two and half glasses of wine. Do you drink more than this?

Patient: Very rarely.

Candidate: Ok, very rarely you drink >2.5 glasses ... When is it?

Patient: When I go out with my friends, most probably it's Saturday night or on holiday.

Candidate: Ok, how often does that happen?

Patient: It's normally once a week.

Candidate: Regularly?

Patient: Yeah.

Candidate: What is the maximum amount when you go out? Have you drunk more than that?

Patient: It's a little more.

Candidate: Ok. When you are at home and have these 2.5 glasses, is that a pub measure or a home measure? (Remember, a pub measure of spirits that equals 1 unit. A home measure is often a double).

Patient: It's a pub. Just the little one.

Measure the Drinking Amount

Candidate: So, you are taking a medium glass of wine, and it's around two and a half glasses. If we count that as a unit—a medium glass of wine would be about two units of alcohol. If you are drinking two and half glasses at night—you are taking five units, and if you take it for 7 days, you are taking around 35 units per week. Moreover, if you take more on Saturday night or go out, it is even higher than that.

Tell the Recommended Safe Limits of Alcohol

The recommended amount for anyone, both men and women, no >14 units of alcohol in a week, no more than three units in any 1 day, and have at least two alcohol-free days in a week.

Patient: But Doctor ... are you sure? I think it is different for men and women.

Candidate: Well, previously, it was 21 units for men and 14 units for women. However, after much research, it is proved that alcohol causes harmful effects on the human body, especially later. Therefore, it was found that even 21 units is much higher, so it is cut down to 14 units as women.

Moreover, as I mentioned earlier, you can't drink a maximum of 14 units at all once; binge drinking can be harmful even though the weekly total may not seem too high.

Cut Down, Annoyed, Guilty, and Eye-opener–Tolerance Withdrawal—Questionnaire

Do you mind if I ask you some questions about your daily life?

Patient: It's ok.

Candidate: Well ... Have anyone in your family asked you to cut down on your drinking?

Patient: Yes, my husband always says to me to reduce it, but I don't listen to him.

Candidate: And also, some other quick questions, [Cut Down, Annoyed, Guilty, and Eye-opener–Tolerance Withdrawal (CAGE-TW)]
- Have you ever felt you should cut down on your drinking?
- Have people annoyed you by criticizing your drinking?
- Have you ever felt bad or guilty about your drinking?
- Have you ever had a drink first thing in the morning to steady your nerves or get rid of a hangover (eye-opener)?
- Do you feel that you have to increase the amount of alcohol you drink to achieve the same effect? (Tolerance)
- What happens if you do not drink for a day or two? (Withdrawal)

Patient: Why are you asking all these questions to me? It annoys me, Doctor.

Candidate: I am sorry. I did not mean to offend you. I just wanted to see if we can help you. Are you ok to continue?

Patient: Ok.

Candidate: I asked you some questions, and it sounds that you haven't any alcohol dependency, but drinking this sustained and excess amount of alcohol can cause dependency later in your life, and I think it already started the problem with your blood pressure. Your blood pressure is not well controlled. I believe the amount of alcohol you consume may be the cause.

My recommendation would be to reduce to the recommended level. I am not telling you to stop drinking altogether; it is just about to cut down to a safer limit. It will have some positive impact on your blood pressure and your whole health. Does it make sense for you?

Patient: Ok. But how much should I reduce it?

Candidate: You can reduce it in one glass directly in the evening, or you can measure out how much you are drinking in a week and remain within a safer limit.

We can give you some support about how much you should drink and figure out the correct amount by making a drinking diary for a couple of weeks or so; or using smartphone apps to monitor how much you are drinking.

We have different ways to help—we can refer to the Alcohol Anonymous (AA) team if you feel that you need the motivation to stop. AA group is a support group for people who are alcoholics or with drinking problems. The only requirement for someone to go there is the desire to quit drinking. What usually happens there is that people usually sit in a group and share their experience about what type of things have helped them cut down or quit alcohol. How does that sound to you?

Patient: Ok, it would help me, I think.

Candidate: Talking therapy (cognitive behavioral therapy) is another option. It helps identify thoughts or beliefs that may contribute to alcohol dependence. Even your family members can help you. For example, if your husband is supportive, he can accompany you to AA.

You may not need all of this; it is just to know what help is available. Are you interested in any of these?

Patient: I will think about it, and I will let you know. Actually, this is really tough for me right now, but I will definitely try it.

Candidate: Ok. At any point, if you require any help to cut down your drinking amount, please come back to us. We are always here to help you.

Address the Patient's Concern

Candidate: Do you have any other concerns?

Patient: Why should I have to cut it down? I am completely fine, and I don't have any symptoms at all.

Candidate: The long-term effects of alcohol are more dangerous, and in your case, it is already creating a problem with your blood pressure. If you are not aware of this now, it could lead to even greater danger in the future as it increases the risk of developing serious problems such as stroke, heart attack, and many complications with the liver.

Social History

Take relevant social history to manage your patient.

Candidate: Is there anything that I haven't explained to you properly?

Patient: No. You have explained everything very well.

Make Summary
Recheck Understanding
May I know how much did you get from our discussion today?

Help

Candidate: I will give some leaflets or web addresses to read more about alcohol-related health problems. I will give you my contact number and contact me at any time if you have any worries or queries.

Thank you so much for spending time with me.

Patient: Thank you.

Shake hands!

Discussion on Breaking Bad News

Breaking Bad News

Bad news is any news that seriously and adversely changes patient's view of his/her future. Therefore, the gap between the patient's expectations and the reality of the patient's medical condition widen. You can't tell how any bad news is (and how badly it may affect the patient) unless you have some ideas of what the patient's perceptions and expectations of the situation are first when giving bad news (or actually any important medical information) it is important that: before you tell ... ask the patient what he/she already knows and continues with the Setting-Perception-Invitation-Knowledge-Exploring Emotions-Strategy and Summary (SPIKES) protocol. Doing well can help the patient come to terms with his/her illness and minimize psychological stress. There is no hard and fast rule, but a patient-centered approach often helps.

SPIKES

S—setting: Make sure to review the records and be ready for questions. Start by minimizing distractions so that you will be totally attentive to the family. Then, sitting down in a place when possible, use a quiet, comfortable room to discuss. Remember being seated is more comfortable and calming. Open questions to start with, active listening, not interrupting, and facilitation techniques are also key parts of the setting.

P—perception of the patient: Ask the patient or family what they know or suspect about the disease/symptoms and how they view the condition's seriousness. Questions help to clarify what the family already knows about the illness. *"Would you please tell me how much do you know about your condition? Do you know why we did the CT scan and what we were looking for?"* As the patient replies—listen to the level of comprehension and vocabulary the patient is using, accept or denial by the patient (but don't confront it at this stage).

I—invitation from the patient to give information: Asking permission, and respect the patient and the family's right to know about the disease. *"Would you like me to explain what happened with you?"* Now break the bad news— *"The results are not as we hoped ... I am afraid I have got some bad news (warning shot)."*

K—knowledge: Giving medical facts, some useful rules are: Aligning—using language intelligible to a patient, starting at the level he or she finished. Give the information in a palatable way and with small chunks; check the reception—confirm that they understand and respond to their reactions. As you talk, you listen—as you listen, you acknowledge and respond.

E—explore emotions with "EVE" protocol: Identify the cause or source of emotion and respond appropriately.

Explore the emotions: *"I can see that came as a shock for you/I can see that this has come as unexpected/I can see that this is very distressing for you."*

Validate the emotions: *"I can only imagine what you are going through/I can understand why you are distressed."*

Empathetic response: *"I am sorry for what has happened/I am sorry for what you are going through."*

In case the patient is crying, offer tissue or water and ask if there is any help she needs, e.g., call someone for her ... *"Would you like me to call someone for you?"*

S—strategy and summary: At the end of the interview, you have to propose a strategy; close the interview with summarizing and clarifying what you have discussed; offer to the patient to raise any other major important issues that need to be addressed even if you can't discuss them at the moment at least you can set the agenda for the next meeting.

Pancreatic Carcinoma

Your role: You are the doctor in the GIT outpatient clinic.

Problem: New diagnosis of pancreatic carcinoma (advanced).

Patient's name: Mr Ahammed, a 60-year-old man.

Scenario: Mr Ahammed was referred to the clinic with pale stool, weight loss, and painless jaundice. A CT scan of the abdomen and pelvis reveals a mass in the head of the pancreas with metastasis to the liver and spleen. The patient has come into the clinic for the result of the CT scan.

Your task: You have to explain to the patient his diagnosis and management plan and address his concerns.

Setting

Candidate: Hello, Mr Ahammed. I am Mohammad Ali, one of the working doctors here today. I understand you are here for your scan result, and I have been asked to talk with you regarding this. Is that okay?

Patient: Hello, Doctor, it's all right.

Candidate: Well, how are you feeling now?

Patient: Fine.

Candidate: I am glad to know that. Have you come to the hospital on your own today?

Patient: Yes.

Candidate: Is there anyone you would like to be in this discussion today? Or, before we go into details, would you like to call someone?

Patient: No.

Perception

Candidate: Okay, Mr Ahammed, would you please tell me how much you know about your condition? Do you know why we did the CT scan and what we were looking for?

Patient: I was completely fine 6 months back. After that, I lost 6 kg weight and I have tummy pain, particularly after having a meal. Over the last 2–3 weeks, my skin and eyes get yellowish, and my stool gets pale. My GP did some blood tests; after that, he referred me to the hospital for a CT scan, and I am waiting for my result.

Invitation

Candidate: Obviously I have the test results with me, is this the right time to discuss your test results?

Patient: Yes, please.

Knowledge

Candidate: As you have significant weight loss, yellowish skin, which we called jaundice, feeling unwell, tummy pain, we are concerned about your symptoms and we have done some blood tests as well as a CT scan of your tummy.
　　Unfortunately, I am sorry to say, I don't have any good news for you …
　　(warning shot) (… Stop for a while) …

Patient: What?

Candidate: I am afraid your condition is more serious than we thought (stop for a while … you must use facial expression and nonverbal cues here, it is mandatory). Unfortunately, they reveal that you have cancer in your pancreas.

Patient: Oh! ...
(Stop for a while and let the patient express his feelings. Hence, it is advisable to ensure the patient listens to what is being told by asking him a question)

Explore the Emotion

Patient: Cancer! ...
(Acknowledge his distress and be prepared to deal with anger and derail. Facilitate expression of emotion)

Candidate: I can see that this has come as a shock to you.

Patient: How is it possible! Are you sure?

Candidate: The scan looks very suspicious for cancer of the pancreas, and I am afraid ... the appearances are very typical for cancer!

Patient: I just feel a little unwell. Otherwise, I am well. My pain is also very mild. Just after taking some food, I think it's only due to my erratic lifestyle!

Candidate: I am really sorry for what has happened. I can't even imagine what you are going through. Actually, your symptoms are highly suspicious. Unfortunately, the blood tests and image tests are done for you revealed that you have advanced cancer in the pancreas spread to the other organs such as the liver and spleen.

I am sorry to say that your cancer seems to be in a very advanced stage.

Patient: I can't believe that! (May be the patient is starting to cry)

Candidate: I completely understand this has come as unexpected ... it's really hard to take in ... I am really sorry for this bad information today. Mr Ahammed, would you like to have some tissue?
(The patient might still be crying ... Offer water) ... Would you like to have some water?

Candidate: Mr Ahammad, are you okay?

Patient: You know... I have had regular checkups with my GP; I check my blood pressure, diabetes, liver, and kidneys. I have no other problems at all ... I don't know how I could get cancer! Even no one in my family has ever had cancer.

Candidate: Unfortunately, despite routine checkups, cancer can occur in anyone.

Patient: Doctor, how long have I had it?

Candidate: It's very hard to tell, but you probably have had this for several months as you have had symptoms for the last 6 months!

Patient: Oh! ... 6 months!.....(patient may turn down his head ... acknowledge this again with empathy and offer help)

Candidate: Are you okay, Mr Ahammed? Would you like me to call someone for you?

Patient: I feel so bad, Doctor. I don't know what I will do, I haven't imagined that!

Strategy and Summary

Candidate: I can sense how challenging to cope up the situation for you. Are you in a state to hear me more? I just want to talk with you regarding our next step.

Patient: Yes, please tell me what is next? What will you do for me?

Candidate: When we receive a scan report like this, we refer the patient to the expert team called MDT. I will refer you to an MDT straight away. It will be an urgent referral within 2 weeks. In an MDT, the cancer specialist, scanning specialist, surgeon, Macmillan nurse, and so on will all together to decide your treatment. Does that make sense so far, Mr Ahammed?

Patient: Will they operate on me?

Candidate: This will actually depend on the decision of the cancer specialist and the surgeon. The next step is to confirm the histological diagnosis of your cancer by doing a snip test or biopsy. Most likely, they will recommend chemotherapy or combined chemo and radiotherapy as you have advanced cancer with spreading to the liver and spleen. Unfortunately, surgery may not be effective enough here, but the decision will depend on the MDT's opinion.

Patient: Doctor, will I get well?

Candidate: I wish I could tell you would be fine, or nothing will happen to you! But I can't…. We are here to support you in any way we can, and we will provide the best medical care for you.

Patient: My neighbor had colon cancer, and I saw him in a horrible state. Doctor, I don't want to be in pain like he was!

Candidate: We will address your pain and all the symptoms you're having, and we're going to be available for you every time whenever you need us.

Address the Patient's Concern

Candidate: So, Mr Ahammed, is there anything else I can do for you now?

Patient: I am going to die, Doctor! There is no hope, Doctor!

Candidate: Unfortunately, I am sorry to tell you that cancer seems to be very advanced. However, we are going to do our best to give you full care and proper management.

Patient: For how long I am going to live, Doctor?

Candidate: I am afraid … not for a long time as your condition is very advanced, but be sure that we will do our best and give you full care and keep you pain-free for the rest of your life. We will also support you socially and psychologically.

Social History

Take relevant social history to manage your patient.

Candidate: Mr Ahammed, is there anything that I haven't explained to you properly?

Patient: No. You have explained everything very well.

Make Summary

Help

Candidate: Here are my contact details for you. It has my number, and I will write down the referral letter for you also to an MDT. Would you like for me to explain any of this to your family?

Patient: Yeah. Okay. I'll bring my wife.

Candidate: Okay, all right … I will come again after a while and talk to your wife. Again, I'm hoping for the best for you, and no matter what happens, we are here for you.

Patient: Okay. Thank you.

Shake hands!

Multiple Sclerosis

Your role: You are the doctor in the neurology clinic.

Problem: A new diagnosis of multiple sclerosis.

Patient: Mrs Mark, a 32-year-old lady.

Scenario: The young lady presented to the clinic 3 weeks ago because of a 4-day history of blurred vision in the left eye. Twelve months ago, she had an episode of unsteady gait and slurred speech with complete recovery within a few days, and the consultant did suggest the possibility of multiple sclerosis. An MRI scan performed 3 weeks ago is shown multiple demyelinating plaques in the brainstem and periventricular regions; visual evoked potential reveals delayed response, and the cerebrospinal fluid (CSF) study reveals oligoclonal bands—all are consistent with multiple sclerosis. Mrs Mark is now at the clinic and waiting for the result.

Your task: You have to explain to the patient about the condition and address the patient's concerns.

Introduction, Permission, and Confirmation of the Agenda

Candidate: Hello, Mrs Mark, nice to meet you, I am Mohammad Ali, one of the working doctors here today. I have been asked to talk to you, is that okay with you?

Patient: Nice to meet you, Doctor, it's all right.

Candidate: Is there anyone you would like to be in our discussion today? Or, before we go into details, would you like to call someone?

Patient: No.

Check Understanding

Candidate: I know that you were in the hospital 3 weeks ago with a visual problem. How are you feeling now? Has there been any improvement?

Patient: Yes, I am well now, Doctor.

Candidate: As you know, we did the MRI and some other tests 3 weeks ago. Do you have any idea what has been happening to you so far? Do you know why we did the MRI scan and what we were looking for?

Patient: There were lots of tests they did on me, but I don't have any ideas. The symptoms have gone away, and I feel fine now, but I don't know why it happened.

Candidate: Well … We have got all the test results back, and we have got the diagnosis for you. So, is this the right time to discuss your test results?

Patient: Yes, please.

Candidate: Unfortunately, I am sorry to say I don't have any good news for you. I'm afraid it is a serious diagnosis.
(warning shot) (… Stop for a while) …

Patient: What do you mean by serious, Doctor? What is it?

Candidate: I am sorry to say, but the test results and the symptoms that you've had all suggest that you have got multiple sclerosis. Have you heard it before? (Take a pause …) I can see that it was a big shock for you.

Patient: I can't believe … it's MS!

Candidate: You look upset. I can understand this has come as unexpected.

Patient: I have heard of it. But I can't believe that I would have the disease. I have seen people around in wheelchairs and using sticks with this disease, and it's really horrible. Even I feel fine now, I mean everything has gone away! Are you sure, Doctor, these are my results?

Candidate: I do appreciate your concern, anyone in your position would feel the same. We have checked all that, and these are definitely your results. Let me just explain the test results if that's okay with you.

Patient: Yes, please. How could you be sure I have got MS?

Candidate: The symptoms you have had with walking and now with the vision coupled with the test results—the scans, the vision tests, and the lumbar puncture all point to MS. The MRI of your brain and spine shows the areas of inflammation and scarring, which we call plaques, resulting from multiple sclerosis. Another test we did on your eye called the visual evoked potential that shows slowing, and abnormal pattern in the nerve's electrical impulse in your eyes suggests inflammation, which is another indicator of MS.

Patient: But, last time, why I was told the lumbar puncture test result was normal, and the doctor sent me home from the hospital?

Candidate: I agree, but when we tested the fluid by a lumbar puncture that we took out from your spine, it looked normal and found no evidence of infection could cause such nerve damage in the brain. However, we found a protein (oligoclonal band) in it that you tend to get in multiple sclerosis. We only find that protein after running it through the analyzer and the result comes back a couple of days later. So that's why last time, they told you the lumbar puncture test was normal.

Patient: I don't understand why am I being told after so long that I have had MS?

Candidate: Actually, MS is such a big diagnosis, and it is very difficult to make a confirmed diagnosis initially because almost all symptoms that can occur with MS can also occur with other diseases. It is often difficult to be sure if the first episode of symptoms is due to MS, such as you may have an episode of blurring of vision or numbness in your leg for a few weeks, which then goes, it may be the first relapse of MS or may be due to other causes. A confirmed diagnosis of MS is often not made until two or more relapses have occurred. So, we don't like to tell people that in case it's not. At first, we like to get all the test results together. There is no single test that can ever prove the diagnosis of MS, all the tests together and your symptoms make us sure that it is multiple sclerosis.

Patient: But doctor, I am only in my early thirty! How could I get this?

Candidate: In Europe, this is about the age that MS does begin to affect people. Unfortunately, it can be a bit younger, but generally, this is the age.

So, you said that you had seen people in wheelchairs and with sticks. May I ask how much you know about the disease multiple sclerosis?

Patient: No, not in detail.

Candidate: Let me explain to you what multiple sclerosis actually is. It is a disease due to disturbance in our defensive system, which is supposed to attack bugs and germs normally. However, sometimes our cells of the immune system, instead of attacking germs and bugs, go crazy for an unknown reason, and it starts attacking our own tissues ... in your condition, it attacks the myelin sheath, which surrounds your nerve fibers in the brain and spinal cord that leads to small patches of inflammation. The inflammation around the myelin sheath stops the affected nerve fibers from working properly, and symptoms develop. The symptoms during a relapse depend on which parts of your brain or spinal cord are affected.

The most important thing about MS is, nearly 9 in 10 people with MS have the common relapse remitting form of the disease. So, you have a flare (relapse) where the nerves are inflamed like in your eyes and legs, over days or weeks that will tend to recover (remit). However, each time the nerves recover, they don't always recover to a full extent. So, as I said, we can't predict exactly how it will affect you in the future.

Patient: You mean my leg problem and my vision problem both were for MS? Will it affect me again?

Candidate: I am afraid MS is a very variable disease, some people are very well with it, but some may progress more quickly. The pattern generally depends on time, but with multiple sclerosis, it's very difficult to say how it will affect anyone in future.

Patient: What about my job? How is that going to affect my career?

Candidate: Most people with MS will continue to walk and function at their work for many years after their diagnosis. Some people with MS do become disabled over time, and a minority becomes severely disabled. However, multiple sclerosis is a very variable disease which means that we can't predict how it will affect you in the future, and we can't predict which one of those you will be. Unfortunately, it may affect your job, or you may not be able to do your job in future. Right now, you have no restrictions to work as you have no symptoms.

Patient: You mean as time goes on, and if I have other episodes, it will just deteriorate me even more?

Candidate: Unfortunately, that is how it tends to happen each time the nerve is damaged, it will recover but may not full extent. I am sorry, but it might be possible.

Patient: It's really frustrating! I didn't expect it today, Doctor! What about my driving? Am I able to drive?

Candidate: In the point of view of driving, at this moment, there's no restriction in your driving because your vision and your legs are quite normal now, but in future, you might not be able to drive if your symptoms get worsen.

Patient: I've recently got married. We are planning for pregnancy shortly! I mean, what about my children? Will they get it from me?

Candidate: Multiple sclerosis doesn't affect your fertility, and there's no reason that you can't have children. I suppose the only concern for yourself, and your husband is that MS is a chronic disease, and you don't know how well you are going to be in the future, so looking after children might be more difficult, but there's no reason you can't have children. You can become pregnant without complication, but if you are planning for pregnancy, inform your obstetrician and the nerve doctor to make an MDT to give you the full care.

Multiple sclerosis is not purely genetic, so your children won't definitely have MS, but there is a slightly higher risk that they might develop it in the future.

Patient: Why I have got the MS? What is the reason behind this?

Candidate: We don't really know what causes MS, and there is a lot of research being done that is trying to establish what factors can increase the risk of developing the condition. Many factors such as genetic, stress, or environmental factors influence it, but we can't predict how and who will get it.

Patient: So, how will you treat me now? There must be an available treatment for it that might stop any further episodes with me. What are those?

Candidate: I am afraid ... There is nothing really that will stop any more episodes from happening. Unfortunately, there isn't any treatment that has a magical effect on MS, but some treatments (I/V natalizumab, oral fingolimod) can possibly help reduce the number of relapses in some cases, and they are not suitable for everyone with MS. Whenever you get an episode, we can give you a high dose of steroids for a few days to reduce inflammation that shortens relapse duration.

Patient: Steroids? Why will you give it to me, isn't it dangerous?

Candidate: There are different kinds of steroids that will help to dampen down all the inflammation in your nerves, and they reduce the length of time that the flare lasts for in each episode of MS. Obviously, there are some side effects from the steroids, but the benefits outweigh the risks (whatever your level of risk, the benefits greatly exceed any of those hazards). Is that clear so far?

Patient: So there's nothing for me that may treat my MS? Can't you just tell me how could I be able to prevent this from happening in future?

Candidate: As I said, we still don't really know what causes multiple sclerosis or what causes flares. It's very difficult for us to tell you what to avoid and how to make it better.

Moreover, I'm not an expert on this, but I will make an appointment for you to see someone from the MS specialist service so that they can discuss things with you.

Patient: Will I be dependent on a wheelchair in future?

Candidate: I am not hiding anything. As I said, it tends to be the ones with severe disease, but hopefully, you will stay as good as now, and we will make sure to follow-up you regularly so that you will be able to report any changes in your condition to us.

Patient: If it could have been diagnosed when I had the problem a year ago, would my treatment have made a difference?

Candidate: Multiple sclerosis is a quite difficult disease to diagnose because, as I said, it's very variable; some people will develop one episode like your leg problem but never come back with another episode. So generally, we don't make the diagnosis until someone's had two episodes. As there is no treatment you haven't missed anything because of this delay.

Patient: But I'm still unable to believe that actually what I have got? I mean, is there any way I can get a second opinion?

Candidate: That's absolutely fine. I will arrange another appointment with my consultant or anyone MS specialist in the next week for you.

Patient: I don't know how I could face all of this: how could I tell my husband! What should I do now? I feel my life is finished!

Candidate: I know it's quite unpleasant to take in it. It will be better to be open with your husband and say—what is MS and what's likely to happen in the future. I can make another appointment with either myself or my consultant in the next week for you to come back with your husband and chat with us about all the test results and go over what we have found. How does it sound?

Address the Patient's Concern

Candidate: So, Mrs Mark, do you have any other concerns?

Patient: What should I do if I get new symptoms shortly?

Candidate: Still, you can see your GP as the first port of call if you are worried about any new symptoms. You can always contact the MS specialist nurse to discuss new symptoms or problems with medication. Moreover, I suggest you keep a diary of symptoms so that you can report any changes when you come to the clinic.

Social History

Take relevant social history to manage your patient.

Candidate: So, Mrs Mark, is there anything that I haven't explained to you properly?

Patient: No. You have explained everything very well.

Make Summary

Recheck Understanding

May I know how much did you get from our discussion today?

Help

Candidate: I will give you some leaflets, brochures, and website addresses to read more about MS; I will give you my contact details as well to contact me if you have any worries or queries.

Thank you so much for spending time with me.

Patient: Thank you.

Shake hands!

Delayed Diagnosis of Cancer

Problem: Dealing with a concern about a delayed diagnosis of cancer.

Patient's name: Mr Jacob Barlow, a 71-year-old man.

Relative's name: Mr Gareth Barlow, the patient's son.

Scenario: Mr Jacob Barlow presented to the hospital with an acute MI and was advised for a coronary angiogram 6 months ago. At that time, his routine blood tests showed microcytic, hypochromic anemia with a hemoglobin concentration of 88 g/L. It was felt that endoscopy/colonoscopy was risky at that point due to his MI and thought that this anemia was likely due to his chronic NSAIDs use for his rheumatoid arthritis. The plan was made for regular follow-up the patient. The patient received two units of blood and then had coronary angiography, which revealed the three-vessels disease. After that, he had coronary artery bypass grafting, which was uneventful, and he made a good recovery. Low-dose aspirin was continued, as his hemoglobin appeared stable at that time. He stopped all NSAIDs and continued only paracetamol. The patient returned to his GP 4 weeks ago because he was feeling progressively weak. Repeat blood testing showed a recurrence of iron deficiency anemia. Further investigation by colonoscopy and biopsy revealed the presence of cecal carcinoma. Now the patient has been admitted to the ward for staging and definitive therapy. Mr Gareth Barlow, the patient's son, asked to see you, and he believes that the delay in the diagnosis of malignancy has reduced Mr Jacob Barlow's chances of survival and that your hospital has poorly served him.

Your task: You have to discuss the issue with the patient's son and manage his concerns.

Introduction, Permission, and Confirmation of the Agenda

Candidate: Hello, Mr Barlow, I am Mohammad Ali, one of the working doctors here today. I am here to talk to you about Mr Jacob Barlow, can I just confirm your relationship with him first?

Relative: He is my father.

Candidate: Are you the next of kin?

Relative: Yes.

Candidate: Ok. Are you on your own today? Do you want to call anyone from the family in our discussion today?

Relative: No.

Check Understanding

Candidate: Mr Barlow, I am currently looking after your father. It would be helpful if you just could tell me what has been happening so far? How do you expect it to be?

Relative: My father had a heart attack 6 months ago. At that time, he had anemia also. The doctors told me this had probably occurred because of my father's painkillers for his arthritis. Now my father has developed anemia again, and doctors say he has cancer in his bowel. I am very upset and want to know why the delay in diagnosis occurred. I believe that there was a delay in diagnosing my father's cancer and I feel that the hospital has badly served him.

Explain the Situation to the Patient

Candidate: I am really sorry to hear about your father's condition. I can see you are really upset; it is reasonable to be upset. We will look into things and check where things went wrong. But before we move on, may I explain to you what exactly happened to him?

Relative: Yes, please.

Candidate: Six months ago, your father presented to the hospital with a heart attack (myocardial infarction), which means insufficient blood supply to the heart, causing chest pain. At that time, a coronary angiogram, a relatively minor procedure to allow visualization of the blood vessels that supply the heart, was advised.

However, routine blood tests showed that he was anemic, which means his blood had a reduced ability to transfer oxygen. At that time, we thought this had probably occurred because of the painkillers your father was taking for his rheumatoid arthritis. As a result, your father received two units of blood for the correction of his anemia.

After that, he had a coronary angiogram that showed severe heart disease, and he had heart bypass surgery. He has no further chest pain and makes a good recovery. His blood level appeared to be stable, and he was treated with low-dose aspirin. All painkillers are stopped other than paracetamol.

Four weeks ago, your father returned to his GP because he felt weak and repeat blood tests showed a recurrence of anemia.

I am sorry to tell you, but he had further tests, including a telescope examination of the bowel (colonoscopy) and snip test (biopsy); unfortunately, colon cancer was confirmed. He has now been admitted to the ward to determine whether cancer has spread (staging) and for definitive treatment.

Relative: Well ... I heard you all ... But why was this not picked up during his first admission? He had anemia 6 months back. Now you are saying he has cancer. Why was my father's anemia not investigated any further?

Candidate: I can see this has really affected you, anyone in your position would feel the same. Basically, at first, we thought the cause of your father's anemia was due to bleeding from the stomach, which may have been due to his painkiller or from the bowel with a possibility of cancer too. Therefore, we planned to keep the situation under review.

Moreover, your father had a big heart attack, and it was felt that a telescope investigation that could confirm the cause of his anemia was not appropriate at that time. So, we planned to do your father's test after 6 weeks which was appropriate in such a situation.

Relative: What are my father's chances of survival now?

Candidate: I am sorry to tell you that right now it's really difficult to say, and the outcome will depend on whether the tumor has spread or not so our next step would be staging cancer by doing some further investigations.

Relative: Doctor, would that not be considered negligence and malpractice?

Candidate: All the steps were taken according to our protocol in the best interest of your father's health. At that time, a heart attack was a medical emergency, and we gave the best treatment, and it is dangerous for any heart attack patient to undergo such an invasive test such as a telescope immediately. Moreover, after giving two units of blood, your father felt better, and his anemia was corrected. That's why we decided to follow-up with him after 6 weeks with the telescope test. I am sorry to tell you that sometimes patient symptoms are not clinically obvious, and diagnosis becomes delayed.

Relative: What could have been done if his malignancy had been discovered before his bypass?

Candidate: It completely depends on the patient's health status. The bypass is major surgery; we usually avoid it in a cancer patient who is critically ill. In your father's case, he was apparently healthy other than this anemia, and the cancer was not known to us. So, according to the treatment protocol, we treated him with the surgery.

Relative: Is the cancer related to my father's rheumatoid arthritis or the treatment he took to control the pain?

Candidate: It can be possible; however, I am not sure about it at this moment. I will read more about it from my textbook, talk to my consultant, and let you know about it.

Address the Patient's Concern

Candidate: Do you have any other concerns?

Social History

Take relevant social history to manage your patient.

Candidate: Is there anything that I haven't explained to you properly?

Patient: No. You have explained everything very well.

Make Summary

Recheck Understanding

May I know how much did you get from our discussion today?

Help

Candidate: I am really sorry about what has happened to him. I hope the best for your father. I will give you my contact details as well to contact me if you have any worries or queries …

Thank you so much for spending time with me.

Relative: Thank you.

Shake hands!

Dementia

Your role: You are the doctor in the general medicine ward.

Problem: Palliative care of a patient with severe dementia.

Patient's name: Mrs Jenny Walker, an 82-year-old lady.

Relative's name: Mr Jack Walker, the patient's son.

Scenario: Mrs Jenny Walker has had severe dementia for the last 5 years and got admitted to the ward 3 days ago because of progressive weight loss. She has been on treatment for dementia to improve her memory, but she has continued to deteriorate, and now she is in a very advanced stage, and despite the help of others, she neither knows how to eat nor shows any interest in eating. She is very weak and only tolerates taking a sip of water. All the investigations, including blood tests, X-ray, ECG, US, and CT scans of the abdomen and brain, are normal. She is not in distress, and the weight loss is only because of dementia. Your consultant decided that further aggressive therapy and investigation are not appropriate, and palliative care is the best approach for her.

Your task: You have to speak to the patient's son, explain his mother's present health status, and discuss any issues he raises.

Introduction, Permission, and Confirmation of the Agenda

Candidate: Hello, Mr Walker, I am Mohammad Ali, one of the working doctors here today. I am here to talk to you about Mrs Jenny Walker, can I just confirm your relationship with her first?

Relative: She is my mother.

Candidate: Are you the next of kin?

Relative: Yes.

Candidate: Ok. Are you on your own today? Do you want to call anyone from the family in our discussion today?

Relative: No.

Check Understanding

Candidate: I know that your mother has been in hospital for the last couple of days because she has not been well. Can you tell me how much you know about what has been happening to your mom or how much have you been informed?

Relative: My mom has had dementia for the last 5 years. My mother is not taking any food for the last 3 weeks and losing weight. She does not talk to me anymore, sometimes she yells at me and does not recognize me. Last Monday, she vomited several times and got admitted to the hospital. Doctors did lots of tests, and they said everything was normal. I don't know what has been happening to her or why she is losing weight. I am really worried about her condition.

Candidate: I can understand your worriedness. As you know that the blood tests and other tests were done, and all came back normal. The medical team looked for all other possible causes of weight loss, and we have found nothing else after lots of investigations and examinations. Actually, she has been losing weight due to a lack of eating, and that lack of eating is because of her dementia.

Relative: Dementia? But I thought it was causing the problem with memory ...

Candidate: Unfortunately, in the advanced stage of dementia, the patient is not aware of eating and can cause weight loss. May I explain to you more about dementia and what we can do for your mother in the future?

Relative: Yes.

Candidate: Dementia is a chronic and progressive condition. Normally dementia affects one's memory and behavior. However, with time it can affect people to stop eating and drinking, leading to weight loss like your mother. Mrs Walker has been reviewed and assessed by our medical team, and unfortunately, dementia in your mom's situation has now progressed to advanced or end-stage. I am sorry to tell you that there is a very limited treatment option. As dementia is an irreversible condition, any aggressive treatment such as assisted feeding or I/V fluids or feed will no longer help her.

Relative: Doctor, as you say that my mother is not aware of eating for dementia and losing weight, why not feed her differently? You have decided that aggressive treatment would not help my mom, it's not fair! You must try to give her food. Can't you give her food through the nose tube or something else? I am really worried that not eating will kill her quickly!

Candidate: I can understand how difficult this is for you, but unfortunately, things are unlikely to get better, as the condition will likely continue progressing. Nose tubes or tubes into the stomach are unlikely to help. With NG tube patients usually feel uncomfortable and they try to pull out the tube which can lead further injuries, and this also increases the risk of choking.

At this stage, we can make a referral for palliative care for your mom. Do you have any idea what palliative therapy is?

Relative: No. What is this?

Candidate: Palliative therapy is offered by a team of doctors, nurses, social, and healthcare professionals just to make sure that the patient is comfortable. It focuses on managing pain and any other symptoms, such as nausea or any distress. They can provide you with specialist advice on managing the symptoms and how to provide basic care. They can also provide emotional support to patients and relatives in coping with the illness. Does it make sense, Mr Walker?

Relative: Oh, yes.

Candidate: May I ask you a few questions about how your mom is normally at home? Like, what about her mobility? Is she bed-bound or does she need help in getting into and out of bed? Who else at home? Who is taking care of your mom? Can she communicate with you?

Relative: I live with my mom, and I have been a full-time carer for my mom. She is totally bed-bound. I love my mom so much, and I have been caring for my mom for the last 5 years on my own.

Candidate: I appreciate it. Mr Walker, are you financially supported, or do you need any help in looking after your mom?

Relative: Yes, I am. I have no financial problem.

Candidate: Okay, that's fine. We can offer you some help looking after your mom in terms of day-to-day care and someone to support you emotionally.

Relative: Thank you, Doctor. Can I take her home?

Candidate: You can take your mom home before that we just need to make sure you have all the necessary help to look after your mom. Does your mom have any advance directive or living that will help us to know her wishes for her care?

Relative: No ... nothing like this.

Candidate: Okay, then I need to speak to my consultant just to make sure how we can make that possible and appropriate.

Address the Patient's Concern

Candidate: So, Mr Walker, do you have any other concerns?

Relative: Doctor, how long will my mom live?

Candidate: I am sorry to say she is at the end stage of life. At the moment, it is difficult to predict, maybe a few more days only!

Relative: Doctor, my mom doesn't talk to me, even sometimes she can't recognize me! She doesn't even recall my name most of the time!

Candidate: As the disease progresses, it becomes difficult for someone with dementia to express themselves verbally. As dementia mainly affects memory, it would be difficult for her to remember your name most of the time. People with dementia have got good days and bad days. Some days they can have a good memory and be able to recognize and unfortunately some days their memory can be bad. She can actually hear you, but it is difficult for her to reply to you. You can try to remind her of your name, and continue to talk to her.

Relative: Sometimes, she shouts and yells at me. It's really frustrating for me.

Candidate: I am sorry to hear about what you and your mom are going through. Unfortunately, this usually happens with dementia if it has reached an advanced stage. Sometimes with dementia, you can lose the ability to communicate and shouting or yelling can be a form of communication, so if she is shouting or yelling, you need to check she is comfortable that she is not in pain or any form of discomfort. Also, as she is bed-bound, you need to check that her beddings are not wet and lying comfortably.

Relative: Doctor, is there any hope? Will my mom get better?

Candidate: Unfortunately, your mom is unlikely to improve from this condition. As the condition progresses, your mom may get more and more sleepy and will talk or communicate less. She may spend most of her time sleeping and opening her eyes very less. Eating and drinking may become more and more difficult.

Relative: What should I do for my mom at the moment? I want to take care of her, and I love her a lot. I will do everything for her. How can help her to feed?

Candidate: It really sounds good that you care about your mom a lot. You can give her plenty of time to eat and remind her to chew and swallow carefully. Give her a small and frequent meal, serve it in liquid or puree form so that she can easily take it. When eating, keep the drink in her hand so she can take it if she has trouble swallowing. Always try to take care of her oral health, moisten her mouth with a straw and help her feed or give her a drink as much as she tolerates.

You can help her stay in a quiet environment. Try to being around her, and try to talk to her, sometimes you can hold her hand thus making her feel supported.

Social History

Take relevant social history to manage your patient.

Make Summary

Recheck Understanding

May I know how much did you get from our discussion today?

Help

Candidate: We can also give you support so that you do not become exhausted. We can refer you to social services, which can help provide some carers who can come to your home and help you look after your mom. There is another type of care called hospice which you might find very helpful. Hospice care is just like palliative therapy, but it can be offered at home, as a daycare or in an inpatient unit. It can allow you to be seen by doctors, nurses, social, and healthcare professionals without being admitted to the hospital. Is this something that you would be interested in?

Relative: Yes, it must be helpful for me.

Candidate: Okay, I will arrange for you. I will also give you some written information and my contact details to contact me for any queries. So, Mr Walker, is there anything that I haven't explained to you properly?

Relative: No. You have explained everything very well.

Candidate: Thank you.

Shake hands!

Renal Biopsy

Your role: You are the registrar in the kidney disease clinic.

Patient's name: Mrs Karen Thomson, a 35-year-old lady.

Scenario: Mrs Karen Thomson was diagnosed with a case of SLE 1 year ago. She was on regular follow-up and treatment, but recently she presented with hematuria, proteinuria, oliguria, and biochemical evidence of AKI due to lupus nephritis. The consultant decided to do a renal biopsy to know the staging of her kidney involvement to start proper treatment.

Your task: You have to counsel her about the renal biopsy and manage her concerns.

Introduction, Permission, and Confirmation of the Agenda

Candidate: Hello, Mrs Thomson. I am Mohammad Ali, one of the working doctors here today. I have come here to talk to you. Is that okay?

Patient: Hello, Doctor, it's all right.

Candidate: Do you want to invite anyone else to our discussion today?

Patient: No.

Check Understanding

Candidate: Mrs Thompson, I understand that you are coming today for a kidney snip test, and I am here to answer your questions and concerns about the procedure. However, before that, can you please tell me how much do you know about the condition and how far you were told about the procedure?

Patient: Doctor ... I got SLE 1 year ago. It was well controlled with some drugs. I have never been hospitalized before. I became unwell 3 days ago with bloody urine. My consultant did some blood and urine tests, but now he is asking me to do a kidney snip test. I don't have any idea about this.

Explain about SLE

Candidate: I am here to discuss everything with you and will address your all concerns. Let me explain your disease first. It is a disease due to disturbance in our defensive system, which is supposed to attack bugs and germs. Sometimes our immune system goes crazy for an unknown reason, instead of attacking germs and bugs, it starts attacking our own tissues. As SLE is a multi-system disease that may attack the joints, skin, and the lining of the heart and lungs, as you used to have.

But unfortunately, this time, it hits your kidney. You know ... SLE has a variable way of presentation, and also it can affect the kidneys in different ways. Sometimes, painkillers can cause kidney disease, therefore, another possibility for your kidney problem can be because of your painkillers.

As you are passing less urine than normal, so that blood and urine tests are done for you; unfortunately, it revealed that you have blood and protein in the urine, and kidney function tests revealed your kidney is not working well. And the kidney consultant decided that a kidney snip is definitely needed to assess your kidney condition and accurately diagnose the cause of your kidney damage. Do you have any idea about the procedure of kidney snip?

Patient: No. I don't know, what is this?

Candidate: Would you like me to tell you more about this procedure?

Patient: Yes. Definitely, Doctor.

Explaining the Procedure

Candidate: It is a procedure that we do on the renal ward on a daily basis, and almost always, it passes uneventfully....

Your kidneys lie toward the side and back of your upper tummy, just under the ribcage. So, you will usually be needed to lie on your front on a bed. Then, the skin over a kidney is appropriately cleaned with an antiseptic solution. A local anesthetic is then injected into a small area of skin and tissues just over the kidney to be sampled (biopsied). This stings a little at first for a couple of seconds but then makes the skin numb, and you will not feel anything. How does that sound, Mrs Thompson?

Patient: Hmm ...

Candidate: During the snip test, an ultrasound scanner is often used to help the doctor visualize and localize the kidney, so the biopsy needle is inserted in the right place. After that, a special hollow needle is then pushed through the skin and muscle into the kidney tissue to obtain a small snip. Because of the local anesthetic, again, you would not feel any pain. However, you may feel some pressure in your back as the doctor pushes on the needle. Finally, the needle is inserted and withdrawn quickly, carrying out a small snip of kidney tissues.

After the procedure, you will need to lie on a bed and be observed for 6-7 hours to check that you have no complications or bleeding. Am I clear so far?

Patient: Yes.

Indications and Benefits

Candidate: This procedure is very important as it will give us an idea about the cause of your kidney problem, how much your kidney is affected, and the stage of your kidney disease. According to that, you will receive the proper treatment. Let me assure you if we can treat lupus nephritis appropriately by getting the biopsy report, the outcome is excellent. Without this procedure, we can't find out the stage of your kidney disease and we can't give you the proper treatment. Your kidney function may deteriorate, and I am sorry to tell you even you may have kidney failure and may need renal replacement therapy in future. Do you understand, Mrs Thompson?

Patient: Yes.

Explain Disadvantage

Candidate: Like every procedure, it also has complications such as bleeding, infection, injury to an internal organ, and having inappropriate snip. However, such complications are extremely rare, and benefits outweigh the risks (whatever your level of risk the benefits greatly exceed any of those hazards).

Preparation is Needed before a Kidney Biopsy

I would like to ask you ... Are you on any blood-thinning medications?

Patient: I am not sure about it. It would be better if you checked my medication list.

Candidate: Okay, then I will check your medication list. Shortly before the snip test, you will usually have a blood test, and this will check how well your blood will clot—to make sure that you will not be likely to bleed following the test. You may be advised not to take any blood-thinning medicines such as aspirin and warfarin 1 week before the biopsy. Moreover, it is better to discuss with your doctor if you take such medicines for other conditions. Is that okay with you, Mrs Thompson?

Are you hypertensive? (Blood pressure should be well controlled before the procedure)

Patient: No doctor ...

Candidate: So .... Mrs Thomson ... What do you think? Are you prepared to have it done?

Patient: I am scared to do such a procedure, doctor ... I have a needle phobia, and I am also thinking about pain ...

Candidate: Yeah ... I know it is painful, but we are going to give you local anesthesia to numb the area of insertion so that you will feel very little pain. Furthermore, if you feel any pain, just let us know, we could always put more local anesthetics.

Patient: Doctor …. I am also scared about infection, as you mentioned …. I don't want such a procedure where there are so many complications ….

Candidate: I really appreciate your feelings …. But be sure that we usually do excellent skin cleaning, and the possibility of getting any infections from the procedure is extremely unlikely….Also, I want to inform you that this procedure is done by an expert doctor who did such procedure hundreds of times before, so chances of complications are much lower here……

Does it make sense for you, Mrs Thomson?.......

Patient: Yes.

Address the Patient's Concerns

Candidate: Do you have any other concerns?

Patient: Doctor… Is there any way to catch the diagnosis other than this invasive procedure?

Candidate: It is the best way to diagnose the cause of your kidney disease to have a snip from your kidney, which allows us not only for diagnosis but also for staging your kidney disease….we can go alternatively for some scanning of kidneys, but this will not be as much as accurate as of the snip…….

Patient: Doctor…. Do you need to perform biopsy both kidneys?

Candidate: No…. we will just take it from one of your kidneys….

Patient: When do I get my result back?

Candidate: The result of the biopsy may take a week or so to come back.

Patient: Doctor…. If I refuse to snip, won't you give me any treatment?

Candidate: We will give you the treatments, and we will manage you as much as we can, but as I told you that to give you the correct treatment, we need to check at which stage it is affecting.

Patient: Doctor…. When do I need to do this test? Can I delay it for a while?

Candidate: If you agree, then we should go for the test as soon as possible….because as long as we leave it without proper treatment, it will continue to damage your kidney…

So…. Mrs Thomson, are you feeling about going ahead with kidney biopsy?

Patient: Actually doctor…. I need some time, and I want to think about it more…..

Candidate: Okay, Mrs Thomson, I will give you some time to think about it, and maybe share the opinion with one of your family members. I will involve my consultant as well to convince you more about the procedure.

Consent

Meanwhile….if you accept to do the procedure, you have to sign a consent form agreement containing all the pieces of information, and you can withdraw any time if you change your mind.

Furthermore, I want to advise you … not to take part in any contact sports such as rugby for a certain period of time after the procedure. This is to make sure the kidney has a chance to heal properly. Is that clear, Mrs Thompson?

Social History

Take relevant social history to manage your patient.

Candidate: So, Mrs Thompson, is there anything that I haven't explained to you properly?

Patient: No. You have explained everything very well. I will think about it and inform you of my decision.

Make Summary
Recheck Understanding
May I know how much did you get out discussion today?

Help
Candidate: I will give you some leaflets, brochures, website addresses to read more about the procedure; I will give you my office contact number

as well to contact me if you have any worries or queries …

Anyone to drive you home?

Patient: Yes, my husband is with me.

Candidate: Thank you so much for spending time with me.

Patient: Thank you.

Shake hands!

Percutaneous Endoscopic Gastrostomy Tube Insertion

Your role: You are the registrar in the GIT clinic.

Patient's name: Mr John Harvey, a 72-year-old man.

Relative's name: Mrs Polin Harvey

Scenario: Mr John Harvey is a hypertensive patient. He was admitted 2 weeks ago with a stroke that has left him with marked left-sided weakness and poor swallowing. Over this period, there have been no signs of improvement in his swallowing which was assessed by speech and language therapists. He is receiving nutrition through an NG tube, but he has not tolerated it well and the tube has become dislodged on several occasions. The multidisciplinary team has considered that a percutaneous endoscopic gastrostomy (PEG) would be appropriate for his long-term feeding care. The medical team assessed Mr Harvey's mental health status, and he was able to consent to the procedure. Mrs Harvey has come to discuss the long-term feeding issues of her husband.

Your task: You have to explain to Mrs Harvey what options are available for feeding her husband and the MDT recommends that a PEG is an option for his feeding care.

Introduction, Permission, and Confirmation of the Agenda

Candidate: Hello, Mrs Harvey, I am Mohammad Ali, one of the working doctors here today. I am here to talk to you about Mr John Harvey, can I just confirm your relationship with him first?

Relative: He is my husband.

Candidate: Do you want to invite anyone else to our discussion today?

Relative: No.

Check Understanding

Candidate: I understand that you have come here today to discuss the long-term feeding issues of your husband, but before that, can you please tell me how much you know about his condition?

Relative: My husband has had high blood pressure for a long time, for which he was taking medicine. But 2 weeks ago, he had a stroke and was admitted to the hospital. Since then, he could not swallow food, for which he is being fed through a nasal tube. Doctors told me they would assess his swallowing by the specialist, and I am here to know about my husband's long-term feeding care. Feeding through the nose tube is big trouble for him, he doesn't like it at all and opened it 2/3 times. It's very difficult for me to see him this way. I am expecting now that the doctor will arrange to feed him by mouth.

Explain about His Condition

Candidate: I can understand your feelings that it's a very difficult time for both of you, but let me tell you more about his condition. Mr Harvey was admitted 2 weeks ago with a stroke that has left him with marked left-sided weakness and poor swallowing.

I am really sorry to say that, over the past week, there have been no signs of improvement in his swallowing when assessed by the speech and language therapists. He has been receiving nutrition via a nasogastric tube, but he has not tolerated it well. As you know, the tube has become dislodged on several occasions.

It is very important to maintain his nourishment as he is unable to take his food by his mouth normally. So, we discussed with the multidisciplinary team plans for his feeding, and they have considered that a PEG would be appropriate.

Meanwhile, we assess his mental status, and the medical team thinks that Mr Harvey is able to consent to the procedure.

Do you have any idea about this PEG tube feeding?

Relative: What is it, Doctor? I don't know ... How will it work? Is it another form of the nasal tube?

Explaining the Procedure

Candidate: It's not the nasal tube. It is a tube used to give food, fluids, and medicines directly into the tummy by passing a long thin tube through the skin to the stomach. May I explain to you more about this? How it will work, or how will it be put on?

Relative: Yes, please.

Procedure/How it is put in?

Candidate: PEG means percutaneous endoscopic gastrostomy. Here percutaneous means through the skin, endoscopic means a small, long, thin, and flexible tube with a light and camera at the tip of the tube called an endoscope is used to position the PEG feeding tube into the stomach; and gastrostomy means making an opening into the stomach. This feeding tube has a small plastic disc inside your stomach and another small disc on the top of your skin where the tube is inserted. Here, these discs prevent the tube from coming out or the whole tube ending up in your stomach. During the procedure, a sedative injection is usually given to the patient to make him/her sleepy and relaxed, and we use a local anesthetic in the throat and tummy wall to numb the area of skin where the PEG tube is to be inserted. Am I clear so far, Mrs Harvey?

Relative: Yes, doctor, but why it is necessary to take this tube?

Indications and Benefits

Candidate: This is the best approach for tube feeding over a long period. PEG feeding tubes are easier to use and more comfortable than nasal tubes. This feeding tube can also be hidden under his/her clothes so that no one will know he/she has got one.

Explain Disadvantage

Candidate: Apart from some discomfort for the first few hours after the insertion, people having a PEG tube inserted usually don't have any problems; however, minor problems can occur, such as infection at the site of insertion or some leakage from the site of the tube.

Major complications are very rare, including bleeding, breathing problems during or after the tube is inserted, the tube causing a hole in the bowel (perforation), infection within your tummy, and minimal risk of death.

However, I want to assure you that the procedure is done by an expert doctor who has done such a procedure hundreds of times before, so the chances of having these complications rates are very, very low ....

So .... Mrs Harvey ... how does that sound?

Address the Patient's Concerns and Questions

Do you have any concerns or questions?

Relative: Yes, Doctor, why aren't you feeding him normally?

Candidate: We always prefer patients to drink and eat normally if they can, but I'm afraid that the stroke has damaged the nerves that control their swallowing. So, if they try to eat or drink normally, that causes a risk of swallowed food going into their lungs rather than in their stomachs, which can cause serious infection or pneumonia that can endanger their lives.

Relative: Doctor, a PEG tube in the stomach sounds horrible. Are there any alternatives?

Candidate: Well, I understand what you're saying. A PEG tube does sound horrible, but it's not as scary as it sounds. We've already tried feeding him with a nasogastric tube—but, as you know, he has not tolerated it well, and the tube has been dislodged on several occasions. A PEG tube obviously doesn't go through the nose but straight through the abdominal wall and into the stomach, so patients find it much less irritating.

Relative: How can you be sure that he understands what having a PEG tube means?

Candidate: I agree that it's difficult to know exactly what a patient understands sometimes. However, we have talked to your husband about the reasons for recommending a PEG to maintain his nutrition. We discussed the issues, and he understands that he needs to have food and drink, that he can't eat and drink normally. He feels that the tube through the nose is uncomfortable and keeps falling out several times. We've explained to him how a PEG tube is put in and its possible complications. We think he understood everything well and wanted to take some time to consent to the procedure. We will arrange another chat with him to discuss and to take his consent soon.

Relative: Doctor, will he need this PEG for the rest of his life?

Candidate: It is difficult to say at this moment, but he may need it. Some patients with swallowing difficulties caused by a stroke can improve as time goes on. Sometimes they improve to the point of not needing the PEG anymore, in that case, it can be removed very simply by pulling it out.

Relative: Will he be able to do everything if he is attached to a PEG?

Candidate: Yes, we try to do all the feeding overnight so that day is free for other things such as physiotherapy.

Relative: Will the PEG be obvious?

Candidate: No, it will not be visible when it is not being used. When your husband is not attached to the feeding bag and tube, the PEG tube lies close to the skin and is not usually visible under clothes.

Relative: Doctor ... what would happen if we choose not to put in a PEG?

Candidate: If we cannot give him adequate nourishment and hydration, he will deteriorate and would find activities such as physiotherapy more difficult. We think other methods of giving him food and drink will be less effective and have more problems than a PEG.

Social History

Take relevant social history to manage your patient.

Candidate: So, Mrs Harvey, is there anything that I haven't explained to you properly?

Relative: No. You have explained everything very well.

Make Summary

Recheck Understanding

May I know how much you get from our discussion today?

Help

Candidate: I will give you some leaflets, brochures, website addresses to read more about the procedure; I will give you my contact details as well to contact me if you have any worries or queries.

Thank you so much for spending time with me.

Relative: Thank you.

Shake hands!

Intercostal Chest Drain

Your role: You are the doctor in the respiratory ward.

Problem: Patient with empyema requiring intercostal drain

Patient's name: Mrs Lara Smith, a 42-year-old lady.

Scenario: Mrs Smith presented with pneumonia confirmed by chest X-ray (CXR), which has not improved with intravenous broad-spectrum antibiotics. A chest CT revealed an empyema, and the consultant advised the patient of an intercostal drain. You have been asked to get informed consent for the intercostal drain.

Your task: You have to explain the diagnosis and management plan and obtain informed consent for the intercostal drain.

Introduction, Permission, and Confirmation of the Agenda

Candidate: Hello, my name is Mohammad Ali, one of the working doctors here today. I have come to talk to you about your test results. Is that okay with you?

Patient: Hello, Doctor, it's all right.

Candidate: Do you want to invite anyone else to our discussion today?

Patient: No.

Check Understanding

Candidate: Okay, Mrs Smith. How are you feeling today? May I know how much do you know about your condition? Do you know why we did the CT scan and what we were looking for?

Patient: Not so good... I have been taking injection antibiotics for a couple of days for my chest infection, but it's not working. Still, I have chest pain, cough, and breathlessness, along with fever.

Candidate: I am sorry to hear about that. May I explain more about your condition, like why it's not improving and what should we do next?

Patient: Yes, sure.

Candidate: Basically, you have pneumonia. When we see the infection in a chest X-ray, it is called pneumonia, and I am sorry to say it is a serious infection. We have started injectable antibiotics for a couple of days. The majority of people usually improve with antibiotics.

But unfortunately, you are not improving. So, we did the CT scan to see the chest more details. Unfortunately, it shows there is pneumonia, which is complicated by a bowl of pus in your chest wall cavity that means around your lung. The condition is called empyema.

Patient: Oh! Is it serious?

Candidate: I am sorry, but yes, it is serious if it is not treated adequately. May I explain more about this condition and what will be the best treatment for you?

Patient: Yes.

Candidate: Please don't feel hesitate to interrupt me any time for any query.

In empyema, the bowl of pus is covered by a thick layer, and antibiotics can't penetrate the layer, so it does not act properly. That's why you are not improving. The best way to treat the condition is to drain the pus by inserting a tube into the chest cavity called intercostal tube drainage, and after that, antibiotics will act properly. In that case the treatment outcome is good. Do you have any idea about intercostal tube drainage?

Patient: Chest tube? How it would be done? I don't know.

Candidate: May I explain to you more about this procedure?

Patient: Yes.

Candidate: It's a minor procedure, and we do the procedure in the ward on a daily basis, and almost always, it passes uneventfully. As it is a minor procedure, no anesthesia or deep sedation is required. We will use the local anesthetic to numb the area before inserting the tube. Once the area is completely numb, we will give a small incision (2–3 cm) between the 4th and 5th rib space. Then we will introduce the chest tube through the incision site. If fluid begins to drain through the tube, then it is in the right place. Another end of the tube will be attached by a chamber containing water. Then we will suture the tube to fix into the chest wall and cover the insertion site with a gauze piece. Does it make sense for you?

Patient: I am scared, Doctor! It sounds horrible! How can you get it in? Will it hit my lung?

Candidate: I want to assure you that it will be done by an expert doctor who has done such a procedure hundreds of times before, and the procedure will be done by USG-guided imaging. So we can see the structure properly; therefore, the chance of complications will be low.

Patient: Okay .... But why do you want to do such a complicated thing?

Candidate: This procedure is very important for you; otherwise, the infection will not be controlled, and if I give you the antibiotic without draining out this pus, it will not act actually, and your condition will worsen further. Am I clear, Mrs Smith?

Patient: I understand. But is there any risk of having this tube?

Candidate: That's a good question, even I want to discuss this with you. Like any invasive procedure, there are some risks, such as bleeding, infection, pain, and injury to the lung. However, such complications are extremely rare, and benefits outweigh the risks (whatever your level of risk the benefits greatly exceed any of those hazards).

So .... Mrs Smith ... What do you think? Are you prepared to have it done?

Patient: I need some time to discuss it with my husband.

Candidate: Okay, that's fine. I appreciate your decision; you can take your time, but please don't be so late because it's very important; the sooner we start treatment, the better for you.

If you accept to do the procedure, you have to sign a consent form (legal issue) containing all the information of the procedure and you can withdraw anytime if you change your mind ... Is that okay with you?

Patient: Yes. I will contact you as early as possible.

Address the Patient's Concerns

Candidate: Do you have any other concerns?

Patient: Is there any other option, Doctor?

Candidate: I am sorry to tell you that it is the only way to solve your problem at this moment. The procedure is prescribed to you by the chest specialist who is an expert in such a case.

Social History

Take relevant social history to manage your patient.

Candidate: So, Mrs Smith, is there anything that I haven't explained to you properly?

Patient: No. You have explained everything very well. I will think about it and inform you of my decision.

Make Summary

It's okay, and now I am going to summarize the important things from our discussion today. So you have pneumonia, and you are getting IV antibiotics for a couple of days to control the infection. But you are not improving as your pneumonia is complicated by a collection of pus in your chest wall cavity called empyema. At this moment, the best way of treatment would be intercostal tube drainage. It will help to confirm our diagnosis as well as for appropriate treatment. I have explained the advantages and disadvantages of the procedure as well as the steps of the procedure, but at this moment, you are not going to give consent to do the procedure. So, I am giving you some time to think. And in our next meeting, I will involve our chest consultant to convince you more about the procedure. Is that okay, Mrs Smith?

Patient: Yes, thank you, Doctor.

Recheck Understanding

May I know how much did you get from our discussion today?

Help

Candidate: I will give you some written information and website address to read more about the procedure; I will give you my office contact number as well to contact me if you have any worries or queries.

Shake hands!

Hickman Line

Your role: You are the registrar in the renal clinic.

Patient's name: Mr Tom Watson, a 45-year-old man.

Scenario: Mr Tom Watson has complained of high fever with night sweats, weight loss, and lymphadenopathy for the last 2 months. Positron emission tomography-computed tomography (PET-CT) scan was done, and a diagnosis of Hodgkin lymphoma (grade 2b) is confirmed. He needs chemotherapy, and the oncologist decided to insert the Hickman line for a regimen of chemotherapy.

Your task: You have to break the news, counsel him about the Hickman line and manage his concerns.

Introduction, Permission, and Confirmation of the Agenda

Candidate: Hello, Mr Tom Watson. I am Mohammad Ali, one of the working doctors here today. I have come here to talk to you. Is that okay?

Patient: Hello, Doctor, it's all right.

Candidate: Do you want to invite anyone else to our discussion today?

Patient: No.

Check Understanding

Candidate: Mr Watson, how are you feeling now?

Patient: I am fine, Doctor.

Candidate: Do you have any idea what has happened to you so far? Do you know why we did the CT scan and what we were looking for? Did your consultant explain the possible diagnosis at your last visit?

Patient: I don't know anything, and I just hope my test reports come back normal.

Breaking the News

Candidate: The results of blood investigation and imaging (PET-CT) have been released, and unfortunately, I don't have good news for you at the moment....

Pause...

It reveals that you have a disease called Hodgkin lymphoma. Unfortunately, this is a type of cancer of lymph glands.

Pause... (let the patient express his feelings and thoughts)....

I am really sorry for this bad information today; I know how hard this news is for you, but be sure that we will do our best for you.

Explaining the Disease

Candidate: Are you comfortable to talk now? Would it be fine to explain more about the disease?

Patient: Yes.

Candidate: It is a nasty growth in your lymph glands that has some symptoms in the form of loss of weight, fever, night sweat, anemia, and infection.
However, the good news is that this is a treatable as well as curable cancer; in many cases, patients become wholly cured after adequate treatment. Would you like me to talk more about it?

Patient: Yes, please tell me about that.

Explaining the Treatment Plan

Candidate: Our oncologist has reviewed your case and decided that you need chemotherapy to treat your cancer. Chemotherapy is the combination of some specific medications that can destroy cancer cells and may cure cancer completely. However, it needs a specific pathway to put in your body; I want to talk about it with you. Is that okay?

Patient: Okay.

Hickman Line Explanation

Candidate: Chemotherapy has to be given through a wide-bore needle called the Hickman line.

The wide-bore needle will be inserted in a large blood channel under aseptic precautions and under local anesthesia to numb the insertion area. It will be done by an expert doctor who did such a procedure hundreds of times before.

The advantages of this line are in the form of providing easy access for giving chemotherapy. However, like every procedure, it has some complications in the form of bleeding, infection, injury to the surrounding tissues, or maybe blockage of the line, but all of these complications are infrequent.

Are you comfortable with my advice, Mr Watson?/Do you understand what I have said about the procedure?

Patient: Yes. Doctor.

Address the Patient's Concerns

Candidate: Do you have any concerns?

Patient: Is it curable?

Candidate: As I told you before, this is curable cancer, but in some cases, it may fail, or some may have a recurrence. However, we should think positively and hope for the full cure.

Patient: Do I have to decide right now about this? Can I take some time to think, Doctor?

Candidate: You don't have to make a decision right now, but we can't wait too long, because without treatment the disease will get worse and I'm sorry to say it can be very dangerous for you. It would be better if you think things over, and I will arrange another chat later to discuss your decision. Also, I will ask one of the specialist nurses to come and talk to you and give you more information about how the treatments will be given; and the available support.

Patient: But, Doctor, someone in my family received chemotherapy and developed infertility. Does chemotherapy cause infertility?

Candidate: Unfortunately, infertility is one of the complications of chemotherapy which sometimes may not be reversible. However, we can overcome this problem alternatively by saving some of your sperm in a sperm bank to use in the future; you can bring your wife next time to discuss the issue with both of you.

Consent

Candidate: After knowing all the information, you need to read and sign a consent form to continue the procedure. One thing I would like to add is that if you change your mind, you can withdraw it anytime.

Patient: I will go for the treatment and all the necessary procedures.

Candidate: That's really appreciable. I will admit you and arrange another meeting along with the consent form for you shortly.

Social History

Take relevant social history.

Candidate: So, Mr Watson, is there anything that I haven't explained to you properly?

Patient: No. You have explained everything very well.

Make Summary

Recheck Understanding

May I know how much did you get out discussion today?

Help

Candidate: I will give you some leaflets, brochures, and website addresses to read more about the procedure; I will give you my office contact number as well to contact me if you have any worries or queries.

Shake hands!

Lumbar Puncture

Your role: You are the registrar in the neurology clinic.

Patient's name: Mrs Stela Johnson, a 31-year-old lady.

Scenario: Mrs Johnson was admitted with a blurring of vision. On examination, she had evidence of bilateral papilledema. Then an MRI and magnetic resonance venography (MRV) of the brain were done, which excluded any mass lesion and/or cerebral venous sinus thrombosis. A diagnosis of idiopathic intracranial hypertension is made, and the consultant neurologist has asked for a lumbar puncture to measure the CSF pressure and therapeutic aspiration if needed.

Your task: You have to explain idiopathic intracranial hypertension and encourage her to consent for a lumbar puncture.

Introduction, Permission, and Confirmation of the Agenda

Candidate: Good morning, Mrs Johnson. I am Mohammad Ali, one of the working doctors here today. I have come here to talk to you. Is that okay?

Patient: Good morning, doctor, it's all right.

Candidate: Do you want to invite anyone else to our discussion today?

Patient: No.

Check Understanding

Candidate: Mrs Johnson, how are you feeling now? Can you please tell me how much do you know about your condition?

Patient: I have had blurred vision for the past 3 weeks. After that, I went to my GP, and he detected some problems in the back of the eyes. I had a scan of my brain, and I am waiting for the result. I am worried that I may go blind. I was told that I needed another test involving a needle in my back.

Explain about the Disease

Candidate: Well, I have the test result back ... And the good thing is, there is no evidence of a tumor. The most likely diagnosis for your visual problem is a condition called idiopathic intracranial hypertension. Have you ever heard about that?

Patient: No. I don't know what it is ....

Candidate: Okay, may I explain to you more about the condition?

Patient: Yes, please.

Candidate: Idiopathic intracranial hypertension is a benign condition, and there is increased fluid around the brain and spinal canal, which is putting increased pressure on the back of the eyes, causing blurred vision. Idiopathic means that the cause is unknown. The main symptoms are loss of sight and headache. Women of childbearing age who are overweight or obese are commonly affected by this condition.

The best way to diagnose and treat the condition is to have a lumbar puncture, which allows the spinal fluid pressure to be measured through a needle in the back. If this is found to be raised, it will be treated by taking away some of the spinal fluid.

So, our consultant decided to do a lumbar puncture to confirm your diagnosis as well as treat you .... How do you feel about it? Do you have any idea about this procedure of spinal tap? May I explain to you more about this procedure?

Patient: Not so much ... I have heard only that this will involve inserting a needle on my back and I am so much worried about it. Doctor, please explain it to me.

Explaining the Procedure

Candidate: I can understand your feelings. Inserting a needle in the back is really scary for anyone, but actually, it's not as scary as it sounds. Let me explain to you more about the procedure; for this test, you will lie on your left side with your knees pulled up against your chest or sit up and lean forward on some pillows. Your lower back area will be adequately cleaned with antiseptic. Then the doctor will numb the area of skin between two lower spinal bones by injecting some local anesthetics. This sting a little at first, but later you will not feel anything.

The doctor then pushes a needle through the skin and tissues into the space around the spinal cord between two vertebrae filled with cerebrospinal fluids (CSFs); as because the skin is numbed with a local anesthetic so you do not feel pain.

A certain amount of CSF is removed, and the needle is then taken out. Then you will lie on your back for 4-6 hours to minimize any risk of a headache. Am I clear so far?

Patient: Yes, but why it is necessary to do such a complicated procedure?

Indications and Benefits

Candidate: Actually, this is the best way to confirm your diagnosis, as I mentioned earlier.... Unfortunately, if your CSF pressure is found to be raised then you will need the procedure repeating every few days until the CSF pressure is back to normal.

Explain Disadvantage

Although it is rare but like every procedure, it has some complications—you may develop a headache after the test that usually goes after a few hours. It is best to lie down for a few hours after the test, as this makes a headache less likely to develop. Rare possibilities are, for example, bleeding or infection at the site of needle insertion. Any damage to the spinal cord as a result of the procedure is very rare. So .... Mrs Johnson ... What do you think? Are you prepared to have it done?

Address the Patient's Concerns

Do you have any concerns?

Patient: I am afraid doctor.... I don't want a needle in my back; what else can you do? ...

Candidate: I can understand your point.... As you have a visual problem, the most effective treatment for your condition would be the repeated spinal tap, but as you do not want to have serial lumbar punctures to drain it, other options are available. This includes weight loss and drugs that lower CSF production, but these measures are less effective alone.

Patient: Doctor ... am I going blind?

Candidate: Well... I appreciate your concern but be sure that the outcome is good with proper treatment, and it is important to have regular eye checkups and spinal fluid pressure checks to minimize the risk of visual loss. Does it make sense for you, Mrs Johnson?...

Patient: Doctor, I am very scared about the procedure ... I think it must be very painful ... Will I be conscious throughout this period?

Candidate: I can assure you that the only pain is just like a stinging similar to a bee sting that you may experience initially when anesthetizing the area. You will be conscious throughout the period, and we will assess you for any discomfort.

Patient: Doctor .... What would happen if I decided not to have the lumbar puncture?

Candidate: In that case, we have to manage you blindly with some medications, but this may cause great harm to you ... It doesn't always work well with medicines; I am sorry to say but, if the CSF pressure continues to rise, then at some point, you may go blind.

Patient: Doctor .... Could I end up paralyzed if you make a mistake?

Candidate: I want to assure you that this procedure is done by an expert doctor who has done such procedures hundreds of times before .... so the chances of any mistakes are very low ....

So, Mrs Johnson …. Are you feel about going ahead with lumbar puncture (LP)?

Patient: Actually doctor …. I need some time, and I want to think about it more …..

Candidate: Okay, Mrs Johnson, I will give you some time to think about it, and I suggest discussing the issue with one of your family members. Meanwhile, I will involve my consultant as well to convince you more about the procedure.

Consent

Mrs Johnson, after knowing all the information, you need to read and sign a consent form to continue the procedure. One thing I would like to add is that if you change your mind, you can withdraw it anytime.

Social History

Take relevant social history to manage your patient.

Candidate: So, Mrs Johnson, is there anything that I haven't explained to you properly?

Patient: No. You have explained everything very well. I will think about it and inform you of my decision.

Make Summary

Recheck Understanding

May I know how much did you get from our discussion today?

Help

Candidate: I will give you some written information and website address to read more about the procedure; I will give you my contact details; if you have any worries or queries, please contact me.

Thank you so much for spending time with me.

Patient: Thank you.

Shake hands!

Oesophago-gastro-duodenoscopy Procedure

Your role: You are the registrar in the GIT disease clinic.

Patient's name: Mrs Angela Markel, a 65-year-old lady.

Scenario: Mrs Markel has had a history of hematemesis and melena for the last 2 weeks and was admitted to the hospital 3 days back. She has had some "alarm" symptoms such as anorexia, weight loss, with altered bowel habits. She has hypertension and takes amlodipine. She is hemodynamically stable now, and her blood tests are unremarkable except for a hemoglobin count of 8.5 g/dL and mean corpuscular volume (MCV) 72 fL. Two units of blood transfusion were given in the last 24 hours, and she is awaiting an oesophago-gastro-duodenoscopy (OGD), which is scheduled for tomorrow morning.

Your task: You have to explain to Mrs Markel the likely cause for her symptoms and obtain informed consent for the OGD.

Introduction, Permission, and Confirmation of the Agenda

Candidate: Hello, Mrs Markel. I am Mohammad Ali, one of the working doctors here today. I have come here to talk to you. Is that okay?

Patient: Hello, Doctor, it's all right.

Candidate: Do you want to invite anyone else to our discussion today?

Patient: No.

Check Understanding

Candidate: Mrs Markel ... How are you feeling today? Have you had any more episodes of passing black stools or blood from the back passage? Do you vomit anymore? (with or without blood)

Patient: No, now I am fine ...

Candidate: Do you have any idea? What has been happening to you so far? Did your consultant explain further investigations or treatment before?

Patient: I don't know, Doctor, why all of these happened! I got admitted 3 days back with some black tarry loose stool and also bloody vomitus. Doctors gave me blood through the needle, but honestly speaking, I don't know anything. Can you please tell me about my condition?

Explain about Symptoms

Candidate: Oh, sure ..., I am here today to answer your questions and concerns.

Mrs Markel, you have passed blood mixed stool and also throwing up some blood, which is unusual and implies severe bleeding in the tummy or bowel.

Meanwhile, the blood loss was confirmed by the blood tests carried out. We did some blood tests on admission and confirmed that you were anemic because of the blood loss, which then needed to be corrected first with the blood transfusion.

I am really sorry to tell you that the causes of your symptoms might be something serious ... we are not sure about it, but possibly there is a bad growth in your tummy or bowel.

Patient: What do you mean, Doctor? Is it cancer? Please explain it to me the Doctor ... What is it? I want to know ....

Candidate: I know this is really hard for you, but as I have said, it is certainly a possibility that we need to look for. I am not hiding anything when I say that we do not know what causes the problem at the moment. It could turn out to be cancer, or it could turn out to be something much more straightforward. So we must try to confirm this as early as possible, and the best way to check any bad growth in your bowels or tummy is OGD. Do you have any idea about this?

Patient: No. I don't know what it is!

Candidate: Would you like me to tell you more about this procedure?

Patient: Yes. It will be better.

Explaining the Procedure

Candidate: It is a procedure called an OGD that we do on the GIT ward on a daily basis, and almost always, it passes uneventfully ....

So in this procedure .... we will help you swallow a long thin, flexible tube (telescope) called an endoscope that passes into your upper gut. The tube is less than the thickness of a pen and has a light and camera at the tip of the endoscope to see inside and to take images of the gullet (esophagus), stomach, and upper part of your gut, known as the duodenum. Then, images are transmitted to a viewing screen and most importantly, any source of bleeding if found that can be treated at the same time.

Indications and Benefits

This procedure is essential as it is the best way to know what has caused the blood loss and to find out any bad growth in your tummy or bowels.

If any bleeding area is seen, it might be possible to inject medications or by doing other procedures such as ligation, cautery, or banding to stop further bleeding. Alternatively, we may take a small snip if there is any bad growth and send it to the lab for a test and look under a microscope; this will help us to confirm our diagnosis. Does it make sense for you?

Patient: Doctor, I am very scared about the procedure ... I think it must be very painful ... Will I be conscious throughout this period?

Candidate: It is a routine test that is commonly done. The doctor may numb the back of your throat by spraying on some local anesthetics or give you an anesthetic lozenge to suck. You may be given a sedative to help you relax, which is given by an injection into a vein in the back of your hand. The sedative can make you drowsy; however, it does not put you to sleep completely as it is not a general anesthetic. How does that sound, Mrs Markel?

Patient: Thank you, Doctor. It will be fine.

Explain Disadvantage

Candidate: The procedure has some complications such as other procedures, but these are rare. In this case, that would include bleeding from any trauma by the telescope that may require a blood transfusion; perforation that may require surgery; and reaction to the sedative medication. However, such complications are extremely rare, and benefits outweigh the risks (whatever your level of risk the benefits greatly exceed any of those hazards). Is that clear so far?

Patient: Yes.

Preparation is Needed before an Oesophago-gastro-duodenoscopy

Candidate: If you decide to go for the test, you will need some preparations before your test. Commonly, the stomach needs to be empty so that you should not eat for 4-6 hours before the test. However, small sips of water may be allowed up to 2 hours before the test. Importantly, some medications may need to be stopped before the test.

Address the Patient's Concern

Is that okay, Mrs Markel? Do you have any concerns?

Patient: Doctor .... Is it a major surgery?

Candidate: It is a very simple test that we do on the GIT ward on a daily basis, and almost always, it passes uneventfully ....

Patient: Why can't you do an X-ray or a scan?

Candidate: It is not possible to make an accurate diagnosis by an X-ray or other scans. This is the best way because it can directly visualize the inside of your stomach and small bowel. So .... Mrs Markel, are you feeling about going ahead with OGD?

Patient: Actually, Doctor .... I need some time, and I want to think about it more ...

Candidate: Okay, Mrs Markel, I will give you some time to think about it, and maybe share the opinion with one of your family members. I will involve my consultant as well to convince you more about the procedure.

Consent

And .... if you accept to do the procedure, you have to sign a consent form agreement containing all the information and you can withdraw at any time if you change your mind.

Social History

Take relevant social history.

Candidate: So, Mrs Markel, is there anything that I haven't explained to you properly?

Patient: No. You have explained everything very well. I will think about it and inform you of my decision.

Make Summary

Recheck Understanding

May I know how much did you get from our discussion today?

Help

Candidate: I will give you some leaflets, brochures, website addresses to read more about the procedure; I will give you my contact details as well to contact me if you have any worries or queries.

Thank you so much for spending time with me.

Patient: Thank you.

Shake hands!

Offer a Blood Transfusion

Your role: You are the registrar in the hematology clinic.

Patient's name: Mr Jack Lorimer, a 79-year-old man.

Scenario: Mr Jack Lorimer has been referred to the hospital because of tiredness and normocytic normochromic anemia. His hemoglobin count is 7.2 g/dL. Investigations have included a normal upper gastrointestinal (GI) endoscopy and a barium enema which only revealed mild diverticulosis in the large bowel. The consultant wonders whether the anemia may be due to myelodysplasia in the presence of normal hematinics and no obvious GI pathology. He suggests offering a blood transfusion of two units.

Your task: You have to explain the results of the tests and offer Mr Lorimer a blood transfusion.

Introduction, Permission, and Confirmation of the Agenda

Candidate: Hello, Mr Lorimer. I am Mohammad Ali, one of the working doctors here today. I have come here to talk to you. Is that okay?

Patient: Hello, Doctor, it's all right.

Candidate: Are you comfortable?

Patient: Yes, doctor.

Candidate: Do you want to invite anyone else to our discussion today?

Patient: No.

Check Understanding

Candidate: I understand that you come today for your camera test and barium enema reports. I have your test results with me. Before discussing the results, can you please tell me how much you know about the condition?

Patient: Apart from tiredness, I was reasonably well 3 weeks back. Then the doctor told me that I have anemia, and referred me to the clinic for investigations. Today I am here for my reports and want to know the cause of my tiredness.

Candidate: I have the test result with me and fortunately, your upper GIT camera test is normal. You have mild diverticulosis on the other test.

Patient: Are you sure it is not cancer? My doctor said that was a possibility, and that's why he wanted to investigate my bowels.

Candidate: Yes, Mr Lorimer, you don't have any cancer or bad growth, and we did the barium enema test of your bowels, which showed only small diverticula.

A diverticulum is a small pouch with a narrow neck that sticks out from the gut wall. When it causes no symptoms, we can call it diverticulosis. It is unlikely that the diverticulosis itself would have caused the anemia, and we are suspecting that the bone marrow is not as active as previously, therefore, fewer blood cells are being produced, contributing to the anemia.

A normal blood count is 12–14 g/dL for an adult, but your count is 7.2 g/dL. As a result of your anemia, you have been getting symptoms of tiredness.

The best way to treat this is to give blood through a transfusion. So how do you feel about having a blood transfusion?

Patient: Doctor, are there any alternatives?

Candidate: Okay, Mr Lorimer .... I assure you that the blood is being offered in your health's best interests. The advantage of having blood is that it will improve your blood count and help to improve tiredness.

And I am really sorry to tell you that actually there is no suitable alternative in terms of tablets to reverse the anemia because this is due to dysfunction of your bone marrow. Tablets or other medications will not work here.

Patient: Doctor, I am afraid about the risks of blood transfusion.

Candidate: I appreciate your concerns, but I would like to tell you that in the UK, a blood transfusion is safe, and some strict regulations are now in place to ensure safety.

Before giving blood, certain things we do to prevent errors such as we will check that the correct blood type by cross-matched and check patient identification labels with the labels on the blood bag to ensure wrong blood is not given, so that the chances of mistakes are very low.

Other risks with a blood transfusion include allergic reactions to the blood, which presents with an itch and wheals within minutes of commencing the transfusion. However, if this happens, treatment is available to counter it.

Patient: Doctor .... I've heard of people getting nasty infections from blood transfusions—is that going to happen to me?

Candidate: In the UK, all donated blood is checked for viruses such as human immunodeficiency virus (HIV), hepatitis B and C and the risk of contracting an infection is extremely low.

Address the Patient's Concerns

Candidate: Do you have any other concerns, Mr Lorimer?

Patient: Okay, doctor, but will this blood transfusion will correct my anemia completely?

Candidate: As your bone marrow is not working properly, unfortunately, there is a chance that you will become anemic again, and you may need blood transfusions several times a year. We have to regularly follow-up you in the blood clinic to check your level; if it gets low, we must correct it again.

So .... Mr Lorimer, what do you think? Are you prepared to have it done?

Patient: Yes, doctor. I think I should proceed.

Candidate: Thank you for your understanding. I assure you that a blood transfusion is safe, and we can arrange a date for this to be done, and you can go home the same day after a post-transfusion blood test. You will then be seen again in the clinic to have the blood count checked. We will follow-up on your blood levels from time to time after that.

Consent

As you are ready for the transfusion, you have to sign a consent form. Mr Lorimer, is there anything that I haven't explained to you properly?

Patient: No.

Social History

Take relevant social history to manage your patient.

Make Summary

Recheck Understanding

May I know how much did you get out discussion today?

Help

Candidate: I will give you some leaflets, brochures, website addresses to read more about the blood transfusion; I will give you my contact details as well to contact me if you have any worries or queries ...

Candidate: Thank you so much for spending time with me.

Patient: Thank you.

Shake hands!

Needle Stick Injury

Your role: You are the registrar in the general medical clinic.

Patient's name: Mrs Bridgel Harvey, a 27-year-old lady.

Scenario: Mrs Bridgel Harvey, 27 years old, a nurse in your medical unit had a needle stick injury when trying to have a blood sample from one patient who is a known case of HIV. She has been very anxious since that event and wants to discuss with you the issue.

Your task: You have to counsel her about needle stick injury and address her all concerns.

Introduction, Permission, and Confirmation of the Agenda

Candidate: Hello, Mrs Harvey; I am Mohammad Ali, one of the working doctors here today. I have been asked to talk to you. Is that ok with you?

Patient: Hello, Doctor, it's all right.

Candidate: Do you want to invite anyone else to our discussion today?

Patient: No.

Check Understanding

Candidate: Ok, Mrs Harvey, would you please tell me what happened exactly?

Patient: I have been asked to see an HIV-positive patient who is already on numerous therapies including zidovudine, didanosine, indinavir, and septrin. The patient has been admitted for unexplained dyspnea, and it's possibly due to *Pneumocystis jiroveci* pneumonia. I wore two pairs of gloves, but after taking the blood and with the syringe full, I have had a needle stick injury with the green needle entering about 0.5 cm into the pulp of my right index finger. I panicked and disposed of the whole syringe and needle into the sharp bin. I washed the contaminated area with water and soap and allowed the injured side to bleed freely.

If the history couldn't make it complete, then the important questions to be asked—

Candidate:
- Were you gloved? Did you take universal precautions (gloves, mask, and gown)?
- Was it a wide or narrow bore needle?
- Was it superficial or deep injury?
- Any visible blood on the needle?
- Did you dispose of the needle into the sharps bin?
- What happened after the injury?
- Did you squeeze the sight of injury, and did you wash your hands with soap and alcohol?
- Did you tell someone else to take the blood from the patient?
- Tell me about your patient. Moreover, how is he now?

Reassurance

Candidate: I am really sorry for what has happened to you today. Needlestick injury may carry a risk of HIV, HCV, and HBV infection as well. But I want to assure you that the chance of HIV infection after needle stick injury is only 0.3%, for HCV is 3%, but HBV is almost 30%. A large number of medical staff had a history of needle stick injury with a minimal case of infection.

However, as you told me that you were gloved and the injury was superficial, you washed your finger with soap, which was great, so you should not worry.

Did you receive immunization for HBV before? You told your patient is HIV positive and taking therapies for that, but do you know that patient's HBV and HCV status?

Patient: No! I don't know … ! What will happen now?

Make a Plan and Reassure

Candidate: I can see you are worried and it's reasonable to be worried. Anyone in your position would feel the same but be sure that we will give you the full care and support we can. May I explain what are we going to do now? Please don't feel hesitate to interrupt me any time for any queries.

At first, we will write down an incident report.

We will give you the prophylaxis treatment as early as possible, which is anti-HIV triple therapy that includes zidovudine, lamivudine, and indinavir and should be taken for 28 days. These medications should be prescribed up to 72 hours after exposure, but the golden time is within 1 hour after the exposure. Before starting medication, we need to know about your general health, and we may do some blood tests, including your liver and kidney function tests. Would that be okay with you?

Patient: Ok, Doctor.

Candidate: We would like to do some blood tests, particularly for HCV, HBV, and HIV infection now, and we will repeat the test after 3 months as well. There is no point in testing this sample for blood-borne viruses at this stage. We just do this for medico-legal purposes.

Before doing the HIV test, signed consent will be required first. The result will be released after 24–48 hours and will be completely confidential, and it will be released only to you but not by e-mail or phone. Does it make sense for you?

Patient: Yes. Please do it as early as possible, Doctor.

Candidate: I can understand your situation, we will do it without any delay, and we will refer you to an infectious disease doctor and an occupational health worker to give you the proper plan of care and follow-up.

Moreover, I want to inform you that if you have a fever, skin rash, malaise, or any abnormal swelling in the neck, armpit, or groin, you have to seek medical care immediately (seroconversion syndrome). Is that ok, Mrs Harvey?

Patient: Ok. And if the test result comes negative, I have no more tension, right, Doctor?

Candidate: This is not for all time. May I explain more about the tests Mrs Harvey?

Patient: Yes.

Candidate: The test may have a false positive and false-negative result. If the test is positive, it means you have an HIV infection. You may have anxiety and mood changes. You may lose your future insurance, but prior insurance will be preserved, but the advantage is that we will start early treatment to avoid complications (AIDS). You have to change some lifestyle and job modification.

If the test is negative, you may have some relief, but it must be repeated after 3 months to be sure you are completely free from the virus. This is because in the early stage of infection, it may be falsely negative. Is that clear so far, Mrs Harvey?

Patient: What types of modification, Doctor?

Modification of Lifestyle

Candidate: Until confirming that you are completely free from the virus (for at least 3 months), you have to make some lifestyle modifications:
- Most importantly, you have to have safe sex until confirming that you are free from the virus completely …. so you have to use a condom during sex.
- At work, you have to avoid the procedures and direct contact with the patient. I am going to involve an occupational health team to provide office work for you.
- You have to avoid blood transfusion during that time.
- You have to keep your personal instruments such as a razor, mouth brush for your personal use.

Mrs Harvey, are you comfortable with my advice? Do you have any queries?

Patient: Yes, Doctor.

Candidate: Do you have any stable partner? Are you pregnant? Or planning pregnancy soon?

Patient: I am 4 months pregnant, doctor … What will I do?

Candidate: That's a valid concern. I will confirm to my seniors whether we can give you anti-HIV triple therapy just now; in fact, zidovudine and lamivudine are not contraindicated in pregnancy, but experience with other therapies like indinavir is limited; however, the advantage outweighs the risk and most importantly, it is known to reduce the risk of viral transmission to your baby (vertical transmission).

Patient: I am in shock, doctor! I don't know how it happened to me! I have always been careful at work. I still can't believe I made such a mistake. I had to be a little more careful.
[Showing empathy and sympathy reassure again]

Candidate: I understand it was an unexpected event and it is so unfortunate that it has happened to you. We are going to give you the best care and I want to reassure you again that chance of catching the infection of HIV is extremely low (0.3%) after a needle stick injury.

Social History

Take relevant social history to manage your patient.

Address the Patient's Concerns

Candidate: Is there anything else that we have not explained properly before I go on, do you have any concerns?

Patient: I don't want to inform the hospital occupational health team, doctor.

Candidate: May I know why you don't want to inform them?

Patient: Because I am afraid to lose my job.

Candidate: I know it is tough for you to cope up the situation. But it is better to inform them and stop dealing with blood, they might arrange for another job not dealing with blood, and you know that this carries a risk to your patient. I am afraid that if you don't inform them, I will have to take advice from a senior colleague in a very confidential way, but I am afraid it might reach to the General Medical Council (GMC).

Make Summary

Recheck Understanding

May I know how much did you get out discussion today?

Help

Candidate: I am sorry again for what happened to you today. I am going to arrange necessary investigations and I will refer you to the infectious disease clinic for post-exposure prophylaxis (PEP) therapy.

I will give you some leaflets and website addresses regarding HIV. You can read to know more about the disease. I will give you my contact details and call me if you have any worries or concerns anytime.

Shake hands!

Newly Diagnosed Human Immunodeficiency Virus

Your role: You are the registrar in the infectious disease clinic.

Patient's name: Mrs Bridgel Harvey, a 27-year-old lady.

Scenario: Mrs Bridgel Harvey, a 27-year-old hospital staff member who had a needle stick injury when withdrawing blood from an HIV patient. She met your colleague at that time, who advised her to inform the Occupational Health Department and refer her to an infectious diseases consultant who started PEP. Her first HIV test done 1 hour after the injury was negative, but according to the protocol, she needs to repeat it in a 3-month duration. Her repeated test turned to be positive, unfortunately. The patient has returned to the clinic for the result of her investigation.

Your task: You have to discuss her positive test and to start her on GENVOYA. GENVOYA is a single tab combination of four antiretroviral drugs. Most common side effects—dark urine, nausea and vomiting, headache, insomnia, and jaundice.

Introduction, Permission, and Confirmation of the Agenda

Candidate: Hello, Mrs Harvey. I am Mohammad Ali, one of the working doctors here today. I have come here to talk to you about your test result. Is that, ok?

Patient: Hello, Doctor. It's all right.

Candidate: Do you want anyone to be with you in our today's discussion?

Patient: No.

Check Understanding

Candidate: Do you have any idea what has been happening to you so far? Do you know why we did the blood tests and what we were looking for?

Patient: Yes, Doctor, I know that ... I had a needle stick injury 3 months back, and I was very anxious; then, I met one of your colleagues in the hospital who started PEP. They did the test for HIV at that time, and fortunately, it was negative. But according to the protocol, they told me that I would have to do the test again after 3 months.

Check Expectation

Candidate: So, we did the test again as per protocol; what is your expectation regarding this test result?

Patient: Yeah, Doctor, as I had a negative test result during the injury, so I believe it may turn to be negative.

Candidate: The result of the test has been released. Would you like to know about it?

Patient: Yes, sure, Doctor ...

Start Breaking Bad News Gradually with Some Tragedy

Candidate: Mrs Harvey, I am really sorry to tell you that the test results are not as you expect .... (stop for a while) ... Unfortunately, they came back positive for HIV .... (stop for a while and let the patient express the feelings)

Patient: Do I have HIV? What do you mean, doctor? Are you sure, doctor? Could it be falsely positive?

Candidate: I am extremely sorry that I am giving this information to you, but unfortunately, we have double checked it and it has confirmed that you have HIV.
(Acknowledge her distress and be prepared to deal with anger or denial)

Patient: Doctor, the first time, it was negative, and I had received the PEP. How is it possible?

Candidate: I do appreciate your question and I know how much this news is hard for you.... Actually, blood tests are the most accurate test for HIV. However, it takes 1–3 months (modern tests will pick up the infection in a month after first being infected as opposed to 3 months with the older tests) after infection to give a reliable result, this period we called window period, viral markers may not appear in blood by this time, and a false negative result is not so uncommon at an early stage.

Give some time to absorb the news ... Mrs Harvey, would you like to have some water?

I know this is really shocking news for you ... But I want to assure you that, although there is currently no cure for HIV, with early diagnosis and effective treatments, most people with HIV will not develop any AIDS-related illnesses and can expect to lead a near-normal lifespan.

Patient: What do you mean, Doctor? Do you think am I going to lead a healthy life with HIV?

Candidate: Certainly, there are very effective drug treatments. With proper treatment and regular follow-up, we can control the disease and also prevent possible complications. We will give you the full support and care that enable you with the virus to live a long and healthy life.

Check Idea

Candidate: Do you have any idea about HIV? I know it's really a stressful moment for you; however, if you are able to hear me, I can tell you more about the disease.

Patient: Yes, Doctor.
(Explain the disease simply without jargon)

Candidate: Please don't hesitate to interrupt me at any time for any queries. HIV is a virus that damages the cells in your defense system and weakens your ability to fight everyday infections and diseases.

Symptoms of HIV

When you first become infected with that HIV, it is called the primary infection. The most common symptoms are sore throat, high temperature, and skin rash (sometimes known as the classic triad).

About 80% of people with HIV develop symptoms at this time. Other symptoms may include feeling sick, diarrhea, swollen glands, tiredness, headache, and generalized body aches.

In advanced stages of HIV infection (AIDS), it can cause multiple symptoms, including fever, cough, breathlessness, diarrhea, weight loss, oral ulcers, lumps, and bumps in your body, mainly due to opportunistic infections in your body.

However, I want to assure you that people treated early in an HIV infection do not develop this stage.

Further Investigations

As you are confirmed to have HIV, we will do another two important blood tests are:
1. *HIV viral load test:* A blood test that monitors the amount of HIV in your blood.
2. *Cluster of differentiation 4 (CD4) lymphocyte cell count:* It measures how HIV has affected your immune system.

And according to this, we may manage you with either only virus killing drugs alone or add other medications for prophylaxis to prevent opportunistic infections ...

For example, if you have a CD4 count <200, you should receive the Pneumocystis pneumonia (PCP) prophylaxis; if it is <100, there is a special protocol; if it is <50, there is also a special protocol.

These tests will be done from time-to-time to assess how far the disease has progressed and the response to treatment.

Patient: What you are going to do for me now?

Treatment

Candidate: At this moment, we are planning to treat you with GYNOVA, a tablet containing four medicines. They work in different ways, but all medicines stop HIV from copying (viral replication) itself. This method of treatment is called highly active antiretroviral therapy (HART). However, it is essential to take medications regularly and exactly as prescribed to maintain success and prevent the virus from becoming resistant to the drugs.

Side Effects of Medicine

Like other medicines, antiretroviral medicines can cause side effects in some cases. Unfortunately, GYNOVA also has some of these, such as dark urine, nausea and vomiting, headache, insomnia, jaundice, etc.

However, the side effects of HIV medicines are usually mild and go away after a few weeks. To avoid these side effects, we advise you to be in a regular follow-up with our OPD clinic.

Drug Interaction

Besides, some of these medicines can react with other commonly used medications. Therefore, always check with your HIV clinic staff or your GP before taking any other medicines to see if these medications are suitable with ZYNOVA or not.

Are you getting me, Mrs Harvey ...? Do you have any concerns?

Patient: Yes, doctor, I want to know when my treatment will be started?

Candidate: The British HIV Association recommends that anyone with HIV ready to carry out the treatment should start taking it as soon as possible regardless of CD4 count.

Patient: May I know, doctor, what is the usual length of treatment/how long do I have to take this medication?

Candidate: Once you have started treatment, you will need to take these medicines for the rest of your life to keep your immune system competent and prevent you from getting other infections.

Follow-up

In addition to that, you need to do regular blood tests to monitor how well these drugs are working. Before starting treatment, you will usually have a CD4 T-cell count and a viral load blood test as a baseline measurement. After starting treatment, these tests will be repeated after 1 month and then about every 3 months thereafter. If your treatment is effective, your CD4 count will increase, and your viral load will decrease.

When a patient with HIV takes effective treatment, it reduces his/her viral load to undetectable levels. This means that HIV in the blood is so low that it can't be detected by a test. Having an undetectable viral load for 6 months or more means the virus will not pass during sex.

You may need other blood tests if you feel sick or develop symptoms due to an infection.

Patient: What happens if I do not take HIV medicines?

Candidate: If you have HIV and do not take medicines, eventually, your viral load increases and the number of CD4 T cells decreases significantly over several years. Your immune system becomes very weak, which means you are open to getting infections, and your body cannot fight against infection. These infections can become serious and enormous for your body, and you are likely to die.

Patient: What to do if I miss a dose?

Candidate: If you forget to take a dose, take your medicines as soon as you remember. However, do not take two doses at the same time to make up for the missed dose. If in doubt, speak with your doctor or pharmacist.

Patient: Doctor ... am I having AIDS?

Candidate: At this moment, you don't have any symptoms of AIDS. AIDS is the name used to describe some potentially life-threatening infections and illnesses that happen when HIV has severely damaged your defense system. And I want to assure you that we can prevent developing AIDS by proper treatment and regular follow-up in most cases.

Social Circumstances

Besides the treatment, certain precautions have to be taken by yourself, which I want to discuss with you. But, before that I would like to ask you some personal questions, is that ok?
- Are you sexually active?
- Do you have a stable partner? How many partners have you had in the last 6 months?

I believe that the last time when you had a needle stick injury, you were advised to have a safe sex/intimate relationship with your partner. Are you complying with it?

It would be advisable to talk to your partner about your test result so that she can support you.

It is also advisable to tell your GP about your results because if you have any problems with your health, he will be the 1st point of contact, and he should know.

You have to avoid blood transfusion; you have to keep your personal instruments such as razors, mouth brushers for only your personal use.

Seeking Compensation

Mrs Harvey …. Before finishing, I have some good news for you. Do you know that you have the right to seek compensation?

Patient: What do you mean that, Doctor?

Candidate: Yes, Mrs Harvey … because you got the virus due to the needle stick injury while doing your job, and your HIV status was negative before that. So, it is an occupational or industrial related disease. Have you ever heard about this?

Patient: No … please explain to me …

Candidate: You have the right to seek compensation, and there is a special form; you can get this from the local social security office. I advise you to bring that, fill it properly, and resubmit this form again as soon as possible because any delay in submitting the paper is going to result in a loss of your right. I will help you at every point, and after that, they will visit you to assess you, and according to the degree of this ability, you will get your compensation. So, I will arrange another meeting with you to tell you the next step.

Do you have any other concerns?

Social History

Take relevant social history to manage your patient.

Clarification

Summary

Leaflets, contact numbers ….

Hospital Superbug-1

Your role: You are the doctor in the general medical ward.

Problem: Patient with *Clostridium difficile (C. difficile)* infection.

Patient's name: Mrs Colin Andrew, a 68-year-old lady.

Relative's name: Mr John Andrew, patient's son.

Scenario: Mrs Colin Andrew has been admitted to the hospital with sepsis due to pneumonia and treated with broad-spectrum antibiotics for the last 10 days. Yesterday, she developed a few episodes of diarrhea and stool cultures have been sent off for *C. difficile* toxin, and the result is awaited. She is otherwise well, and the plan is to discharge her once her diarrhea resolves. Her son, Mr John Andrew, has come to the ward to see her and finds that she has been moved into a side room because of diarrhea. The nurse-in-charge of the shift has already explained the situation to him, but he wants to speak to a doctor. After talking to relatives of other patients on the ward, he was already aware that there has been an outbreak of diarrhea in the hospital recently.

Your task: You have to address the son's concerns about his mother's infection and isolation.

Introduction, Permission, and Confirmation of the Agenda

Candidate: Hello, Mr John Andrew. I am Mohammad Ali, one of the working doctors here today. Are you the son of Mrs Colin Andrew?

Relative: Yes, I am.

Candidate: Thank you for coming. I have been asked to talk to you about your mother's condition. Is that, ok?

Relative: Yes, sure.

Candidate: Do you want to invite anyone else to our discussion today?

Relative: No.

Check Understanding

Candidate: Ok. Mr Andrew, how much do you know about your mother's condition?

Relative's reply: My mother was admitted to this hospital with pneumonia and has been receiving treatment with antibiotics for several days. She seemed to be doing well, and I was expecting to take her home soon. However, when I came to see her today, the nurse-in-charge told me that she has developed diarrhea since yesterday and moved to a side room. I have been chatting to the relatives of another patient on the same ward who mentioned "an outbreak of diarrhea in the hospital". I am anxious about my mother's condition … Can you explain to me, please? What's happening with her?

Candidate: I am sorry about your mother's condition. I can see you are really anxious, and I can understand why you are anxious. I am here to explain everything to you.

As you know, she was initially admitted with pneumonia which is a serious infection in the lung. It can be fatal in an elderly patient, so we have to treat that with I/V antibiotics according to her culture and sensitivity report.

Relative: Yes, even she was improving, Doctor.

Candidate: Yes, she was really doing well, and her chest infection seems to start improving. However, unfortunately, since yesterday, she has developed a few episodes of diarrhea, and a stool sample has been sent to establish the cause of it, mainly looking for a bug called *C. difficile*, and the results are not back yet.

Relative: What is it? Doctor, I am afraid, what you say about the bug? *C. difficile*? I have read about a "hospital superbug" that can be serious and can even cause death. Is it the same?

Candidate: I appreciate your concern, and actually, our medical team is also concerned about this. Therefore, her stool has been sent to the lab to investigate the bug called *C. difficile*.

We take all the necessary steps to give her better treatment and expect an early recovery. Even if Mrs Andrew's diarrhea is confirmed to be due to *C. difficile*, she will be given the proper treatment and monitored closely for any complications with daily examinations, X-rays, or blood tests if needed, and you will always be kept informed of her progress.

Relative: But why does my mother get this bug and how?

Candidate: I know you are concerned about your mother. Let me explain more about this bug and the disease process so that things become clear for you.

Relative: Yes, please.

Candidate: In our bowels, there are millions of bacteria, some are good, and some are bad, but normally, bad bacteria such as *Clostridium* in our gut remain in tiny numbers and are not active. They don't cause any infection as good ones have the upper hand over bad ones, the good one's help digest our food and they protect against invading bad bacteria to our bowel. The body's defense system gets disturbed whenever one's getting such a serious infection, particularly in elderly patients like your mother's pneumonia. Antibiotics which are used to treat bad bacteria causing pneumonia also kill the good bacteria of the gut because they can't recognize good or bad ones, so the bad bacteria such as *C. difficile* in the bowel wall are taking the upper hand over the good one and multiply their numbers and produce toxins causing diarrhea.

However, I want to assure you that it is completely treatable with specific antibiotics in most people but very rarely can lead to complications such as severe bowel inflammation and obstruction.

Relative: What doctor?... The antibiotic for pneumonia causes the diarrhea ... Why did you give it, as you know this is harmful?

Candidate: I am really sorry for what has happened to her, but these antibiotics were given in the best interest of your mother's health. We can't predict it initially as it does not happen in all cases. However, the elderly, hospitalized patients, especially those with other comorbidities, are particularly susceptible to getting this infection.

Relative: Who gave my mother this bad antibiotic? I want to know; I want to complain about him ... tell me who is responsible for all of this?

Candidate: Ok ... Mr Andrew, I can understand your feelings that you can't rely on us right now, but I would like to tell you, all the treatments are given according to the protocols, and the treatment was not given by a single doctor. It was a team decision that we called a multidisciplinary team approach. However, if you want to complain, I can give you the contact details of the Patient Advisory Liaison Service (PALS) or the complaints department of the hospital.

Relative: Doctor ... Why have you moved my mother to a side room? ... I have also been asked to wear an apron and gloves when going in to see my mother. But why?

Candidate: I would like to tell you that regardless of the stool culture result, the hospital takes all cases of diarrhea seriously in case it is due to an infectious agent, and precautions have to be taken to avoid the spread of infection. That's why she has been moved to a side room to reduce the chances of picking up the bug or transmitting it to others. It is a specialized ward, and there are trained staff, equipment, procedure, and protocol to treat this type of patient.

Precautions are required for all staff and visitors: namely to wear an apron and gloves when going into her room to reduce the chances of picking up the bug or transmitting it to others.

Relative: Doctor ... is it true that there has been an outbreak of diarrhea in the hospital?

Candidate: Several patients in the hospital may have diarrhea or other infections for a variety of reasons. However, if there is any suspicion of an outbreak, the infection control team will advise on the containment of infectious diseases in the wards. This team is responsible for carrying out a thorough investigation, reporting it to higher authorities, and prescribing measures to reduce the risk of spreading by closing off certain wards or bays.

Relative: Doctor ... I think the staff is not taking adequate hygiene measures in this hospital and that may be the reason for my mother's diarrhea ....

Candidate: I am sorry for your bad experience, but may I know why do you think so? Have you ever noticed anything like this? If so, then I can assure you I will note down any specific examples, and I will also speak to the ward manager about it and take every possible step to overcome any unusual acts or events.

Relative: How will you treat this bad bug now?

Candidate: If the culture test confirmed this superbug infection, then we will treat this infection with some other specific antibiotics that are very specific for this kind of bug infection. At the same time, we have to change her present antibiotics to treat pneumonia which is causing *C. difficile* infection; also, we need to keep a close eye on her and will need a regular blood test.

Relative: What do you mean, doctor? You are telling me that antibiotics may have caused this, yet you plan to give her more ....

Candidate: Yes .... actually, this is the treatment protocol; some specific antibiotics are used in *C. difficile* infection. But before that, we have to wait for the reports. Am I clear, Mr Andrew?

Relative: So, how long this diarrhea will continue? It's really awful for my mother, and I think she is so weak and lethargic.

Candidate: Well, actually, this varies from patient to patient, some people get recovery soon, and some are not. I completely understand your concern; we are giving her fluids through the I/V route to prevent dehydration, and also we will start antibiotics soon after getting the reports.

Address the Patient's Concerns

So, Mr Andrew, are there any other concerns?

Relative: Not actually. I feel pretty relieved now. But, Doctor, how long my mother has to remain in the hospital?

Candidate: It's quite difficult to say, and she is definitely not ready to leave the hospital right now. The minimum treatment for this infection is 10 days. However, if her condition gets improved, we can treat her on an outdoor basis.

Social History

Would you mind if I ask some questions about your mother's lifestyle?
- With whom your mother is living?
- Are they doing well?
- Are they financially supported?

So, Mr Andrew, is there anything that I haven't explained to you properly?

Patient: No. You have explained everything very well. Thank you.

Make Summary

Recheck Understanding

May I know how much did you get out discussion today?

Help

Candidate: I will give you some leaflets, brochures, website addresses to read more about the bug; I will give you my contact details as well to contact me if you have any worries or queries ...

Thank you so much for spending time with me.

Relative: Thank you.

Shake hands!

Hospital Superbug-2

Your role: You are the doctor in the general medical ward.

Problem: Patient with Methicillin-resistant Staphylococcus aureus (MRSA) carrier.

Patient's name: Mr Daniel, a 60-year-old man.

Relative's name: Mrs Daniel, patient's wife.

Scenario: Mr Daniel was admitted to the hospital 5 days ago due to infective exacerbation of COPD. His condition improved after getting usual antibiotics (amoxicillin) and supportive care (oxygenation and nebulization). A nasal swab has been taken. The result shows MRSA. But he has no evidence of MRSA infection with negative blood culture and sputum culture for MRSA. The patient has been isolated, and all necessary precautions have been taken.

Your task: You have to talk to the wife and address her concern. Consent from the husband has been taken.

Introduction, Permission, and Confirmation of the Agenda

Candidate: Hello, I am Mohammad Ali, one of the working doctors here today. May I confirm you, Mrs Daniel, the wife of Mr Daniel?

Relative: Yes, I am.

Candidate: Thank you for coming. I have been asked to talk to you about your husband's condition. Is that, ok?

Relative: Yes, sure.

Candidate: Do you want anyone to be with you during our today's discussion?

Relative: No.

Check Understanding

Candidate: Ok. Mrs Daniel, how much do you know about your husband's condition?

Relative's reply: My husband has a smoker's cough, and suddenly his condition got worse, and he couldn't take a breath properly; then I called an ambulance and took him to the hospital. He was then admitted to the hospital, and doctors were treating him well. My husband was doing well, but I don't know why he was shifted to a separate room, and doctors are wearing different clothes and masks. I'm not being allowed to go inside. I am so worried about him; please tell me what's happening?

Candidate: I am glad that he is doing well. However, I can see you are worried about your husband and not so happy about shifting him to a separate room; let me explain everything so that things become clear for you.

I understand from his case notes that he has COPD and was admitted because of a chest infection. We have been treating him according to our hospital's protocol, and fortunately, he is responding well. We investigated him to look for infection in his blood, sputum and took some swabs from his nose. Has anyone told you about the results?

Relative: No.

Candidate: The result of the nasal swab shows he has MRSA. Do you know what MRSA is?

Relative: I heard about it. It is a superbug with no treatment, and it is very dangerous.

Candidate: MRSA stands for Methicillin-resistant *Staphylococcus aureus*. It is a type of bug that doesn't respond to usual antibiotics. However, we have many powerful antibiotics that can fight against this bug. This bug is not more aggressive or infectious than other subtypes of *Staphylococcus aureus*.

Relative: Doctor, does it spread from dirty hands because people don't wash hands properly?

Candidate: MRSA spreads from person-to-person, usually through direct skin-to-skin contact. That's why we shifted him to a separate room, and we are continuing his treatment according to his infection status. This is for the best interest of his health and other patient's health in the hospital. However, as he is weak, we need to be more cautious, and we don't want your husband to catch any other bugs, which can be dangerous for him, and we don't want this bug to spread in the hospital. Does that make sense, Mrs Daniel?

Relative: Yes. But I am so scared! My husband gets a superbug infection! What will happen now, Doctor?

Candidate: I am really sorry. I should have been clearer. At the moment, he doesn't have any infection, and he is just carrying this bug on his nose.

If a person is healthy, MRSA usually won't cause infection. We call this person MRSA carrier, but this bug can be infective when someone has a poor defense system. Fortunately, he has no evidence of MRSA infection; he is only an MRSA carrier.

Relative: So, how will you treat him?

Candidate: When a person is an MRSA carrier, we will consider decolonization, which involves using antibacterial (chlorhexidine) body wash or powder and shampoo to remove MRSA from the skin and scalp. This must be used daily for 5 days. It must be used as a shower gel to the whole body, including the groin and armpit.

An antibacterial cream (mupirocin nasal ointment 2%) can be used to remove MRSA from inside his nose and should be used three times daily for 5 days.

He should wash every day during the decolonization process, ideally using a fresh towel to dry himself each time. He should wear a clean set of clothes each day. The bedding will also be changed daily.

He will be rescreened 48 hours after completion of 5 days course. If he still has MRSA positive, then decolonization should be completed up to two times after the course.

Address the Patient's Concerns

So, Mrs Daniel, is there anything else that we have not appropriately explained before I go on ... Do you have any questions or concerns?

Relative: I heard people can die from this bug? Will my husband die?

Candidate: As we discussed, your husband hasn't developed any MRSA infection. He is only the MRSA carrier, and hopefully, we can clear the bug from his body with the help of the medication I already mentioned. However, as your husband has a low immune system, we may find it difficult to treat him if this becomes an infection. This can become a bit serious. However, even if he develops MRSA infection, we have many good antibiotics that can fight against MRSA and most patients respond to these antibiotics. These antibiotics are usually given through blood vessels as a drip.

Relative: Can I visit him?

Candidate: You should be able to visit him, but you need to wear protective equipment such as an apron, gloves, and mask.

Relative: Can I get this from him?

Candidate: You may get this from him as you live with him. In that case, you can get screened for MRSA. However, you need to speak to your GP to have screened for MRSA.

Relative: Can I take him home?

Candidate: MRSA on the skin can be treated at home as well, but as we have started treating him, let him finish his treatment. We will do another screening. After that, if he cleans the MRSA, he will be able to go home.

Social History
Take relevant social history to manage your patient.

Make Summary
Recheck Understanding
May I know how much did you get out discussion today?

Help
Candidate: I will give you some leaflets, brochures, website addresses to read more about the bug; I will give you my contact details and contact me if you have any worries or queries …

Thank you so much for spending time with me.

Relative: Thank you.

Shake hands!

Genetic Counseling

Your role: You are the specialty registrar in the genetic clinic.

Problem: Counseling a patient's daughter for Huntington's disease (HD).

Patient's name: Mr Albert Fred, a 50-year-old man.

Relative's name: Mrs Lucy Smith, daughter.

Scenario: Mr Fred was admitted a few days ago with progressive confusion, memory loss, and a movement disorder. Investigations were done for progressive memory loss and dementia, and the genetic test confirmed a diagnosis of Huntington's disease.

Your task: You have to explain to the patient's daughter about the condition, provide details of her own potential testing and outline a management plan.

Introduction, Permission, and Confirmation of the Agenda

Candidate: Hello, are you Mrs Smith? Daughter of Mr Fred?

Relative: Yes, I am.

Candidate: I am Mohammad Ali, one of the working doctors here today. I have been asked to talk to you. Is that ok with you?

Relative: Ok.

Candidate: Do you want to invite anyone else to our discussion today?

Relative: No.

Check Understanding

Candidate: Ok, Mrs Smith, would you please tell me what brings you here today?

Relative: My father was admitted a few days ago with progressive confusion, memory loss, and movement disorder. His genetic test came positive for Huntington's chorea. I have come here today to be tested for HD because of my father's recent diagnosis.

Candidate: I am sorry to hear about your father's recent diagnosis. Do you have any idea about Huntington's disease and the genetic test?

Relative: No, Doctor.
(Try to obtain a family tree …)

Candidate: Before we move on, tell me about your family members. How many brothers or sisters, aunts, uncles, and cousins do you have? Do other members of your family have the same problem?

Relative: I have two brothers, they are well, but my uncle has a similar illness.

Candidate: I see … How is your uncle doing?

Relative: He has also movement disorder and dementia and is now housebound.

Candidate: May I explain to you more about Huntington's disease?

Relative: Yes, please.

Candidate: Please don't feel hesitate to interrupt me any time for any queries. Huntington's disease is an illness that predominately affects the brain. It is a slowly progressive condition that interferes with the movement of the body. The most common movement problem is chorea—sudden, jerky, involuntary movements that tend to affect your hands, face, arms, and legs. It can also affect your awareness, thinking, and judgment, and can lead to change in your behavior. In an advanced case, it can cause dementia, as in your father's case.

It is a genetic disorder. Here genetic means the condition is passed on through families by special codes called a gene. Each cell of your body contains chromosomes, which are made up of many genes. A defective gene causes HD in chromosome 4. If one of your parents has a defective *HD* gene, there is a 50–50 chance that you will also have HD (autosomal dominant disorder).

The disease in the next generation usually comes at an earlier age and with more severe symptoms (anticipation and expansion). However, this is unpredictable when the symptoms will appear exactly and how severely they will be affected. So, it varies from one to another.

Unfortunately, there is no cure for HD; no treatment is found to delay the onset of the symptoms or progression of symptoms. Therefore, treatment aims to control symptoms as much as possible when they develop (such as tetrabenazine for chorea). Is that ok, Mrs Smith?

Relative: Ok. I understand. But I want to test for it. How could I do it, Doctor?

Candidate: Ok, I want to give you some sorts of information like what the options for you in terms of testing are, what that means for you and what you need to know about the test and so on. If there are any queries, then I can answer before you decide… So, may I explain to you more about the test?

Relative: Yes, Doctor.

Candidate: The genetic test is a blood test; it involves taking a blood sample from a vein. After the sample has been taken, it is sent to the laboratory for testing. It may take 2-4 weeks for the result to come back. Importantly, the result will not be released by email or telephone. You will be the only one to receive the result (legal issue: confidentiality).

The purpose of the screening is to establish the presence or absence of a specific gene mutation (defective gene) causing HD inherits from your parents.

But this test has a small possibility of false positivity (that means the test may be positive without having the disease) and false negativity (that means the test may be negative, but the patient has the disease). However, the chance of false positivity and false negativity is very low. Does it make any sense to you?

Relative: Ok, but if I become test positive, then what will you do?

Candidate: If the test is positive, the advantage will be, we will refer you early to MDT for regular follow-up and management (for candidate: As HD is untreatable and the patient is asymptomatic at the time of consultation, you need to explore the reason for the test and warn the patient if the test turns to be positive). It may affect your mood and may have a bad psychological impact, and you may lose your future insurance, but prior insurance will be preserved.

If the test is negative, in that case, the advantage is—you will be relaxed, and you can continue your life without having HD. But the disadvantage is that it may be rarely false-negative, and in that case, we will repeat the test to confirm our future diagnosis. Do you want to do the test now or want to take time?

Relative: I want to think about it.

Consent

Candidate: Well, take your time, and if you agree to do this test, you must sign a consent form in which all the information about the test is mentioned. If you want to withdraw anytime, you have the complete right to that (patient autonomy).

Relative: I think it would be better for me to discuss with my husband first.

Candidate: Ok, in that case, you can bring your husband next time to share the information and decision with you. Postponing the test will not alter the outcome of the disease. Does that make sense so far?

Relative: Yes.

Social History

Take relevant social history to manage your patient.

Address the Patient's Concern

Candidate: So, Mrs Smith, do you have any other concerns?

Relative: If I have the disease, when will the symptoms appear?

Candidate: I appreciate your concern. Unfortunately, it is unpredictable when and how severe the symptoms will appear exactly. It varies from one to another.

Relative: What about my children, doctor? May they have the disease?

Candidate: If you are confirmed to have the disease, I am sorry to tell you that every one of your children has a chance of 50% to have the disease.

Relative: What if I plan to be pregnant, doctor?

Candidate: There are several options for you if you test positive and wish to have children in the future, such as prenatal testing by chorionic villus sampling or amniocentesis. This can show whether your baby has the defective gene and, therefore, whether they will develop HD. However, the test is not always 100% accurate. Preimplantation genetic testing (PGD) is also available if one parent carries the defective gene. It involves the couple undergoing IVF treatment so that embryo can be tested for HD before implanting in the woman's womb, and the only embryos without the defective *HD* gene are implanted.

Meanwhile, we will refer you to MDT involving the genetic counseling team to help you in this issue to make a test of your interest.

Candidate: Is there anything else that we have not explained? Do you have any other concerns or expectations from me?

Relative: No.

Make Summary
Check Understanding
May I know, please, how much did you get from our discussion today?

Help
Candidate: I will give you some written information and the website address regarding HD and a genetic test to learn more about it. I will give you my contact details and call me if you have any worries or concerns anytime. Thank you for spending time with me.

Patient: Thank you.

Shake hands!

Counseling for Anticoagulation

Your role: You are the doctor in the hematology clinic.

Problem: Young woman requiring anticoagulation

Patient's name: Mrs Angela, a 25-year-old lady.

Scenario: You are a medical doctor in the hematology clinic, and Mrs Angela is a 25-year-old young lady recently diagnosed with atrial fibrillation during her cardiology follow-up. She has a history of tissue aortic valve replacement 1-year back. The cardiologist decided to give her an anticoagulant.

Your task: You have to explain about different types of anticoagulation medications and advice the most suitable one for the patient.

Introduction, Permission, and Confirmation of the Agenda

Candidate: Hello, Mrs Angela. I am Mohammad Ali, one of the working doctors here today. I have been asked to talk to you about your condition. Is that ok with you?

Patient: Hello, Doctor, it's all right.

Candidate: Do you want to add anyone else to our discussion today?

Patient: No.

Check Understanding

Candidate: Would you please tell me how much do you know about your condition?

Patient: I had an aortic valve replacement 1 year ago. I came to the heart clinic for a follow-up. They found irregular heartbeats, and then they referred me to you for further management. I have diabetes and have been taking insulin for the last 2 years.

Candidate: Ok, Mrs Angela ... I understand from your case note that you have atrial fibrillation and tissue aortic valve replacement. Do you have any idea about your atrial fibrillation?

Patient: I don't know much more ...

Candidate: Well .... May I explain to you more about the condition?

Patient: Ok.

Candidate: Please don't feel hesitate to interrupt me any time for any query....

Firstly, think about the heart. It is a physical and electrical pump. The upper chamber collects the blood from the periphery as well as from the lung then it passes to the lower chamber. Then lower chamber passes blood all over the body. In fact, these things are done by effective contraction and relaxation of the heart chambers.

Atrial fibrillation can interfere with the blood flow in the heart chamber, which sometimes leads to a small blood clot formation in a heart chamber. A clot can travel in the blood vessels until it becomes stuck in a smaller blood vessel in the brain or sometimes in other parts of your body. As a result, part of the blood supply to the brain may then be cut off by a clot suddenly and permanently, which causes a stroke. So our main concern is—atrial fibrillation increases the risk of having a stroke.

On the other hand, as you have diabetes, it also potentially increases the risk of stroke. To reduce the risk of stroke, we have to use blood thinner medications called anticoagulants. However, it does not actually thin the blood but alters certain chemicals in the blood to stop clot-forming so easily. Blood thinner medications come in two forms—daily injections (heparin, enoxaparin) and tablets—either warfarin (traditional options) or one of the newer agents called NOAC (novel oral anticoagulants) such as rivaroxaban, dabigatran, and apixaban.

Each drug has different advantages and disadvantages. May I explain more about these three drugs? So that you can decide which one will you prefer.

Patient: That would be fine.

Candidate: In terms of daily injections (heparin/enoxaparin), you have to take the medication just like insulin therapy daily. This is weight-based with a predictable response. Although it increases the risk of bleeding in the puncture site and other sites, but this injection is the best drug for those planning for pregnancy or during the pregnancy period as it has no harmful effect on your baby like other oral drugs.

May I ask if you have a partner? Or are you planning for pregnancy?

Patient: Not right now, but I will think in future.

Candidate: Well … now, in case of warfarin, it is a widely tested and trusted drug as an anticoagulant … It is a very strong drug as a blood thinner medication and the chance of bleeding (major/minor) is more common than other drugs. This is a very tricky drug and does not have fixed dose like other drugs. Even the same drug dose shows variable response (increased/decreased) from person-to-person. Therefore, it is very important to monitor drug response by doing a regular blood test (PT with INR).

The increased response causes an increased risk of bleeding; on the other hand, decreased response can cause the drug's failure; therefore, we have to do a regular blood test to get an adequate response. However, if we keep the range of blood-thinning within INR-2-3, the chance of bleeding will be extremely rare.

Another disadvantage of the drug is drug-drug interaction. It can interact with many drugs that may increase or decrease the effectiveness of the drug. So, if you are going to receive any new medication, you have to inform your physician.

Unfortunately, some types of food may alter warfarin effect as well … So if you take the drug, we will refer you to a dietician who can guide you regarding the type of food you have to avoid. Are you following me, Mrs Angela?

Patient: Yes …

Candidate: The good thing is—it has a reversal agent that means we can use the antidote (Vitamin K) to revert the effect of warfarin if required.

In terms of newer drugs (NOAC: Rivaroxaban)—these drugs have a predictable response to our body. The main advantage of this drug is—it has a fixed-dose. No drug monitoring is required. In contrast to warfarin, it has a lower risk of bleeding, but the main disadvantage is, it has no reversal agent. Does it make sense for you, Mrs Angela?

Patient: Yes.

Address the Patient's Concern

Candidate: Ok…Mrs Angela … Is there anything else that we have not explained properly before I go on … Do you have any questions or concerns?

Patient: No … Thank you for explaining everything to me.

Candidate: It's my pleasure. May I know which one will you prefer?

Patient: I think the newer one would be better. I want this one as it's easy to handle.

Candidate: It's all right.

Social History

Take relevant social history to manage your patient.

Make Summary

Recheck Understanding

May I know how much did you get from our discussion today?

Help

So, I will prescribe rivaroxaban, the newer one for you, and I will give you some written information about this drug, which you can read in your leisure time at home and if any questions arise, please note it and inform me in your next visit.

Thank you

Shake hands!

Patient with Poor Compliance

Your role: You are the specialist registrar in the general medical unit.

Problem: Dealing with a poor compliant patient.

Patient details: Mr Robert, a 47-year-old man.

Scenario: Mr Robert is a known case of DM taking insulin, and his HbA1c in the last visit was 11.2%. The diabetic nurse mentioned his uncontrolled DM is most probably due to noncompliant with medication.

Your task: You have to discuss this issue with him.

Introduction, Permission, and Confirmation of the Agenda

Candidate: Hello, I am Mohammad Ali, one of the working doctors here today; I have been asked to talk about your condition. Is that, ok?

Patient: Yes.

Assess the Patient's Current Health

Candidate: Ok, thank you for coming back to see us. I understand from your case notes that you have had diabetes for the last 10 years. Mr Robert, how have things been going in your point of view?

Patient: Recently, I have been feeling tired and thirsty. I have lost almost 3 kg weight over the last 2 months.

Approach the Issue of Compliance in a Nonconfrontational Manner

Candidate: Well, you had some blood tests that showed your HbA1c is 11.2%. HbA1c is the test to measure DM control in the last 3 months. Unfortunately, in your case, it is very high and means your diabetes is not controlled.

Patient: Oh! I see …

Candidate: Mr Robert, I am concerned about your uncontrolled blood sugar. I just wanted to talk and explain why that might happen and figure out what we can do to look after you. Would it be all right if I asked you some questions first?

Patient: Yes.

Candidate: Mr Robert, has there anything changed recently in your lifestyle, such as your eating habits or your workload or exercise?

Patient: No … not at all. I am eating as usual and maintaining a diet as my dietician said, and also, I am doing regular exercise.

Candidate: I appreciate it. Moreover, in terms of your medications, what are the medications are you taking?

Patient: My GP changed my oral antidiabetic medications to insulin for the last 3 months. Now I am taking insulin only.

Candidate: Ok … generally, insulin in most cases achieves quite good control of blood sugar. By this point, would you think you take your insulin regularly? Or have you missed your doses sometimes?

Patient: Actually, yes, I do. Sometimes I missed my doses.

Candidate: Just be sure that we are here not to judge you … we are here to offer you the full care and help. Would you think you missed it quite often?

Patient: Yah, maybe.

Candidate: Is there any particular reason for that?

Patient: It's really hard for me to remember it every time before the meal. By the time I remember insulin, it's too late.

Candidate: I can understand. In that case, we can help you by giving you a reminder aid device to remind you every time for your injection.

Patient: I don't want to take injections. Why don't you give me insulin in tablet form instead of injection?

Doctor: I am sorry to say, but the insulin does not come in tablet form and therefore, it must be given as a small injection just underneath the skin. And it's crucial to take insulin properly because, in diabetes, your body can no longer control sugar properly without insulin; your pancreas is not producing insulin as much as required, so we need to give you insulin to maintain a normal blood sugar level.

Patient: Don't you think it's a really tough piercing needle on your own body? Even I told my GP not to give insulin. I have a needle phobia.

Candidate: I know it seems tough and scary for anyone initially, but it will actually not be an issue whenever you are habituated with it. Our diabetic nurse can teach you or one of your family members how to inject you perfectly.

I want to inform you that there are many different advanced devices and equipment for treating DM; one of them is an insulin pump to avoid repeated injections. I will refer you to a diabetic nurse to explain different devices, and you can choose the most suitable one for you. Is that ok with you, Mr Robert?

Patient: Ok. It's sound good. But why do you want to put me on insulin forcefully? I don't want it. Please give me back my oral medications. I was perfectly ok with that. Can I get some strong tablets instead of insulin?

Explain the Importance of Compliance to Control DM and Prevent Complications

Candidate: I am insisting on you about insulin because I am concerned about your poor sugar control. Oral medications are no longer working for you, your sugar levels are high, and right now, insulin is the best way for you to control sugar level.

Moreover, diabetes can cause many serious complications silently, such as kidney problems, vision problems, increasing the risk of brain stroke, heart attack as well.

But if you are completely compliant with insulin, your glucose level will be well controlled, and you can avoid all these complications. Does it make sense for you, Mr Robert?

Patient: Ok, I can understand.

Address the Patient's Concerns

Candidate: Do you have any other concerns?

Patient: Well. But what about hypoglycemia? I heard people with insulin have more risk of it.

Candidate: That's really a good question, and I also want to discuss it with you. To be honest, keeping tight control of your blood glucose with insulin increases the risk of hypos. However, if you are a little conscious, there are lots of steps you can take to reduce the risk of hypos such as regular checking of your blood sugar level, learning about the correct dose of insulin you need, not skipping or delaying snacks or meals, adjusting your insulin if you're exercising heavily and avoiding alcohol as well.

We will guide you about the typical symptoms of hypoglycemia and how to avoid it; even if you ever have it, you will be taught how to overcome and deal with it. It is simply can avoid by keeping a supply of sugary drinks, fruit juice, or glucose tablets to hand always so that you can treat symptoms early.

Patient: But it's really tough, Doctor. I can understand your point, but you know, it's tough for me.

Candidate: I understand your reluctance, and many people would think the same. But it would be best if you prioritized your health. Given the risk associated with nonadherence, I strongly advise you to consider my advice.

Patient: Ok, doctor. But I am thinking about the other advanced equipment that you said ....

insulin pump. Maybe it will be a better option for me, what do you think?

Candidate: Certainly… I will give you the contact details of a specialist nurse, you can choose the device, and you can also learn the techniques of giving insulin.

Patient: Ok. Thank you.

Candidate: I would like to add that besides drug compliance, you must make some lifestyle modifications to control your DM, particularly regular walking or exercise and dietary modification is very important as well.

Social History

Candidate: May I ask you some questions at this moment?
- Are you working now? What are you doing for a living? Are you married? With whom you are living? Are they doing well? Who is supporting you now? Are you independent in activities of daily living?
- Do you smoke? If not, then ask, have you ever smoked? If yes, then ask, how many years are you smoking? How many sticks per day?
- Do you drink alcohol? If yes, how many drinks would you have been in a week?

Patient: I am a shopkeeper, lives independently. Do not smoke or drink alcohol.

Candidate: So, Mr Robert, is there anything that I haven't explained to you properly? Do you have any other questions or concerns or expectations from me?

Patient: No. You have explained everything very well.

Make Summary

Recheck Understanding
May I know how much did you get out discussion today?

Help
Candidate: Ok, Mr Robert, we can go through your prescription and modify the insulin dose for you. And I am giving you some leaflets, which you can read after you go home and my contact details if you have any questions, you can contact me.

Thank you for spending time with me.

Shake hands!

Nonorganic Disease

Your role: You are the doctor in the general medical ward.

Problem: Explain nonorganic disease.

Patient's name: Mrs Elsa Maria, a 35-year-old woman.

Scenario: Maria has been admitted with an acute exacerbation of her chronic pain, for which she has undergone multiple investigations, including blood tests, CT chest and abdomen, MRI spine and numerous gynecological investigations as well. All the test results have come back normal. She will be discharged today. The patient wants to talk to a doctor about her condition.

Your task: You have to explain the diagnosis and management plan and answer any questions that she may have.

Introduction, Permission, and Confirmation of the Agenda

Candidate: Hello, Mrs Maria, nice to meet you. I am Mohammad Ali, one of the working doctors here today.

Patient: Nice to meet you, Doctor

Candidate: I understand you wanted to talk to a doctor about your condition and I have been asked to talk to you. Is that ok with you?

Patient: Yes, Doctor, it's all right.

Candidate: Do you want to invite anyone else from the family to our discussion today?

Patient: No.

Check Understanding

Candidate: May I know how much do you know about your condition?

Patient: I have pain everywhere, I always feel pain in the different parts of the body, not so severe pain, but there is always some pain. I am taking different medications, but no medication is working at all. I have seen many doctors and done different tests, but no one can tell me what is causing my pain ....!

Candidate: Can you tell me more about how it's affecting your life, and is there anything else that particularly increases or decreases your symptoms?

Patient: What should I say, doctor? I'm always in pain. There is pain somewhere. When I go to sleep, I feel pain; when I wake up, I feel pain. I can't work properly, sleep properly! My performance in the office is getting worse day by day.

Candidate: I can understand you are suffering a lot. It is affecting your all-daily activities as well as your job. I understand from your case note that many investigations were done, and you are seen by different physicians several times, but all the test reports are normal. What do you think about that?

Patient: Should I think about it, or should you?

Candidate: I can see that you are very angry ... can you tell me what thoughts are going through your mind?

Patient: What do you mean, doctor? The tests are normal ... I am medically fit! Do you think I am acting? Do you want me to go back to my husband and tell him that all the blood tests, CT scans, and MRIs are normal, and he thinks I'm such a big liar? I've been suffering for so long, so many tests are being done, but no one can say what happened to me!

Candidate: I really appreciate your feelings ... I can understand that you are suffering a lot. It's affecting all activities of your life. I did not say you lie, or you are acting at all. I admit your suffering, and you have something that we have to manage. We are here to give you the full help and care. May I explain to you more about your condition?

Patient: Ok.

Candidate: Please don't hesitate to interrupt me at any time for any query. I can understand that you have pain all the time with you ... you are seen by different doctors, and they have done different tests to identify the cause of your pain. You have taken the different forms of medications, but no medication is working well ... you still have pain with no improvement, and all the test reports are normal repeatedly.

Patient: Yes, and if you need more tests, do it, but tell me what happened to me?

Candidate: I think no test is required at this moment to identify the cause as all the relevant tests have already been done.

I think you are suffering from a condition called "medically unexplained syndrome".

Patient: What do you mean by unexplained?

Candidate: It is termed when no known physical cause can be found for a physical symptom. It is mostly due to stress, and when someone is under mental stress, he/she may express physical symptoms such as headache, neck pain, back pain, joint pain, and so on. Does it make sense to you, Mrs Maria?

Patient: I don't understand how stress causes my symptoms! Doctors ask me about the stress. Yes, I am under stress. But I am under stress due to my pain, nothing else. How could this be the cause of my pain?

Candidate: The relationship between the mind and body is complex and not fully understood. Mental stress can cause such physical symptoms, and often the symptoms go when mental and emotional factors ease. We don't realize the physical symptoms are due to a mental factor; we just think that we have a physical disease and see a doctor about it.

Make a Management Plan

However, I want to reassure you that we must help you as much as possible and do our best to manage your condition. We will refer you to an MDT involving a social worker and psychiatrist to give you the proper care and support. Is that ok with you?

Patient: Psychiatrist!!! Why? Do you think I am mad, doctor?

Candidate: I am sorry that we have given you such impressions. The psychiatrist is not for mad people only. Many people seek medical care from a psychiatrist for their mental support and relief when they are under a lot of stress. He may help you by talking therapy, such as cognitive behavior therapy (CBT), which may help you understand your symptoms and may prescribe some medications (such as low dose SSRI), which improve your mood and relieve your stress.

Address the Patient's Concerns

Candidate: Ok, Mrs Maria ... Is there anything else that we have not explained properly before I go on ... Do you have any concerns?

Patient: I have a long-standing headache ... I want to do imaging for my head.

Candidate: Actually, your headache is one of the symptoms secondary to stress. We don't have any indication to do imaging for the brain at this moment.

Patient: Well .... but I want to be sure that my brain is ok, and I don't have anything serious.

Candidate: In fact, our consultant has decided that there is no need for further investigation. Imaging has some side effects such as exposure to radiation and you do not need to be exposed to radiation without a clear indication.

Patient: Please, doctor, I want to do it. I think it is really very important to me.

Candidate: Well, I will inform my consultant regarding this issue ... ok, Mrs Maria?

Social History
Take relevant social history to manage your patient.

Make Summary
Recheck Understanding
May I know how much did you get from our discussion today?

Help
I am giving you some written information about the disease; you can take it and read it in your leisure time. I will give you my contact details if you have any worries or queries you can contact me. Thank you so much for spending time with me.

Shake hands!

Medical Error-1

Your role: You are the doctor in the general medical ward.

Problem: Medical negligence.

Patient's name: Mrs Yali Watkins, a 55-year-old lady.

Relative's name: Mrs Baegi Kathey (next of kin).

Scenario: Mrs Watkins was admitted this morning with a history of fever and cough. A CXR revealed left lower lobe pneumonia. Her daughter relayed a message to the casualty triage nurse that Mrs Watkins is allergic to penicillin. Unfortunately, this message was not passed on to you because of the various breakdowns in the communication pathway. The GP letter had no mention of the allergy, and the patient has dementia; therefore, she was unable to give a proper history. Unintentionally, IV amoxicillin was prescribed and given by yourself. As a result, she developed rash and vomiting, treated with IV chlorpheniramine, hydrocortisone, and metoclopramide. Mrs Watkins is stable now, and the vomiting was settled. Mrs Watkins's daughter is upset about this incident and wants to make complaints.

Your task: You have to talk to her and address her concerns.
(How to approach a medical error:
- Patient safety—a patient safety incident occurs.
- Document the incident in the patient's record.
- Being honest by informing the patient/his/her family/carers what error happened and apologize.
- Report the incident by your local reporting system.
- Learning—how will my report inform local and national learning.
- Complaint—what if the patient wants to make a complaint, involve the PALS service if needed)

Introduction, Permission, and Confirmation of the Agenda

Candidate: Hello, I am Mohammad Ali, one of the working doctors here today. May I confirm that you are Mrs Baegi Kathey ... Daughter of Mrs Watkins? And are you next kin of Mrs Watkins? (Confirm who is speaking to you and make sure she is her next of kin).

Relative: Hello, Doctor. Yes, I am.

Candidate: I have been asked to talk with you to about your mother's condition, Is that ok?

Relative: It's all right.

Candidate: Do you want to add anyone else to our discussion today?

Relative: No. Who did this mistake, Doctor? I want to know! I will complain against him. How is this possible in such a big hospital! How did such a mistake happen?

Check Understanding

Candidate: I can see that you are very angry ... (Explore the situation; the daughter's ideas and expectations and concerns; acknowledge she is angry and try to explore why, let the daughter express her feelings and anger without interruption, listen attentively, resist the temptation to interrupt, keep calm, and don't raise your voice.)

Relative: Who did this mistake, Doctor? I want to know! I will complain against him. How is this possible in such a big hospital! How did such a mistake happen?

Candidate: I understand that this event has really affected you. We will look into things and see where things went wrong, before that can you please tell me how much do you know about your mother's condition?

Relative: My mom has been admitted today with a fever and cough. After doing CXR, the doctor said that she has pneumonia. I told the casualty nurse that my mom is allergic to penicillin, but the doctor prescribed her intravenous amoxicillin. Unfortunately, just after giving the injection, she became unwell, started vomiting and developed a rash. I am really upset about this incident, and I want to make a complaint.

Candidate: It is completely understandable why you feel that way; I am really sorry for what happened to your mother. On behalf of the medical team, I apologize for this mistake. (In this clinical scenario, a true break in the communication system, so I apologize for what happened to the mother, be honest and transparent and explain the incident).

Relative: Last year, she was given penicillin for something, and it was awful …. she became unwell at that time and was in the hospital for about 2 weeks! She had severe vomiting, fever, rashes, and so on … and doctors told me the penicillin had been the thing that made her so ill. Now I bring her into the hospital, and she has been given penicillin again! I don't know how the doctors made this. You are a doctor … you must be aware of allergies and appropriately respond to the allergies.

Apologize again …

Candidate: I am really sorry again for what has happened to your mother. It should not have happened. I know how much your mother is precious to you. Your feelings are highly appreciated. It is mainly due to the breaking of communication or missed information, and we will investigate what happened seriously. May I explain to you more what happened exactly?

Relative: Yes …, please.

Explain the incident:

Candidate: Your mother was admitted due to pneumonia, but there was a breakdown in communication, which should not have happened.

I really did not know she is allergic to penicillin. The antibiotic was given in good faith in the best interest of your mother. In fact, it was the best treatment and was given when I did not know she is allergic to penicillin. Unfortunately, she developed an allergy to penicillin with some skin rashes and vomiting. The antibiotic was stopped immediately, then she was given anti-allergic treatment, and her condition was stabilized. Now she is under close monitoring.

Relative: How could you say that you don't know? I said to the nurse that my mom has a penicillin allergy! Something bad could have happened to my mother. She could even die! I heard the allergies were nasty, and last time my mother was in a horrible situation.

Candidate: I do appreciate your concern as a caring daughter, sometimes allergies can become serious, however, fortunately your mom is stable now …. As your mother has dementia, she could not give us the proper history, and the GP's letter had no mention of the penicillin allergy.

I want to assure you that we are here to help your mother as much as we can, and any harm to your mother was not intended at all, and this matter will handle very seriously. Let me explain things that we will do next ….

Explain how you wish to resolve the situation and the actions you intended to make to ensure that similarly does not occur.

I will check further your mother's file to know whether penicillin allergy is mentioned or not and what happened in detail. After that, I will write in clear, obvious notes in your mother's file that she is allergic to penicillin and not be given to her in the future.

I will write down the incident report for what has happened, and I will fill out an "incident form /datix" and investigate the error. Meanwhile, I will inform my consultant and nurse-in-charge.

I will discuss this issue in the next morbidity and mortality meeting to avoid this in the future.

In addition, I will refer this issue to the risk management team to investigate what happened. Is that ok with you?

Relative: Ok. Please do it.

Address the Patient's Concern

Candidate: So, Mrs Kathey? Do you have any concerns or expectations?

Relative: I never expect this from such a big hospital. It's really disgusting, and I want to make a complaint, doctor.

Candidate: Definitely, this is your right .... As your mother is not competent so you can make a complaint on behalf of her. I can get you in touch with PALS (the Patient Advice and Liaison Service) service, and it is a service where you can make formal complaints if you strongly feel that your care is compromised. We will follow-up on the result of your complaint and be sure that your mother's management plan will not be affected at all. Do you have any other concerns?
[Where a patient is not satisfied with a verbal apology, it is important to appreciate the complaints procedure. It is good practice to ensure a dated response within three working days of receiving a written complaint.

Legal issue: Only the patient can make complaints if he/she is competent, but in this scenario, the patient has dementia (lack of capacity), so the relative can make the complaints here; if the patient is competent, then we have to say ... we will have to discuss this first with Mrs Watkins as she is competent if she wants to make a complaint, I will help her to fill the form and send it to the Trust Legal Department.]

Relative: I want the sister's name who forgets to inform the information of penicillin allergy of my mother to the doctor?

Candidate: I am not defending my colleague, but we are working here as one team; all team members are responsible for your mother's condition. However, I need to reassure you that this event raises our concern as a medical team, and it will be a matter of investigation. The aim of investigating the event is to improve the medical services and keep the patient's safety rather than pointing to someone, as mistakes happen, but we need to address how to avoid them. (Never point to any one of your colleagues but reassure the patient that this will be a matter of investigation)

Social History

Take relevant social history to manage your patient.

Candidate: So, Mrs Kathey, is there anything that I haven't explained to you properly?

Patient: No. You have explained everything very well.

Make Summary
Recheck Understanding
May I know how much did you get from our discussion today?

Help
I will give you my contact details if you have any questions; please don't hesitate to contact me any time ... you can visit the Trust Website and know what the policy of the trust is and how you could raise your concerns and complaints online. It is always nice to give feedback that may help to improve the services.

Thank you.

Shake hands!

Medical Error-2

Your role: You are the doctor in the general medical ward.

Problem: Medical error

Patient's name: Mr Jane, a 50-year-old gentleman.

Scenario: Mr Jane presented to the hospital 2 days ago with central chest pain and sweating and has been admitted to the hospital. Three days before his admission, he attended the accident and emergency (A&E) department complaining of chest pain. ECG was done at that time, but the diagnosis was not picked up. He was sent home with the diagnosis of musculoskeletal pain before getting the troponin results. After discharging him, the troponin result came back positive. Now this time, your consultant reviewed his ECG, which was done during his first attendance at the hospital. T-wave inversion has been found, and a diagnosis of nonST-elevation myocardial infarction (NSTEMI) has been made. The patient was medically managed in the CCU and has shifted to the medical ward.

Your task: You have to talk to the patient, assess his condition, explain the medical error, and address his concerns.

Introduction, Permission, and Confirmation of the Agenda

Candidate: Hello, I am Mohammad Ali, one of the working doctors here today. May I confirm your name and date of birth, please?

Relative: Hello, Doctor. I am Jane; my DOB is 12/5/1972.

Candidate: I have been asked to talk with you, is that ok?

Patient: It's all right.

Candidate: Do you want to add anyone else to our discussion today?

Patient: No.

Check Understanding

Candidate: I understand that you came to the hospital 2 days ago. Am I right?

Patient: Yes, Doctor.

Candidate: Have you been told about the reason why you are in the hospital?

Patient: Yes, I came to the hospital with chest pain, and they did some investigations. I was told that I had a heart attack.

Candidate: Yes, you are right; you came to the hospital and were diagnosed with a heart attack. How are you feeling now?

Patient: I am feeling fine now.

Candidate: Do you have any symptoms such as chest pain/breathlessness/heart racing/swelling in the legs/cough?

Patient: No.

Candidate: I am glad to know that you are fine now and have shifted to the ward. If I am not wrong, you came to the hospital a few days ago as well. May I know why?

Patient: Yes. I had this chest pain 5 days ago. I came to the hospital, doctors did some tests and told me that it was just muscle pain. So they gave me some painkillers and sent me home.

Candidate: Well, Jane, I am here to talk to you about an error that has happened in your treatment. Has anyone mentioned it to you already?

Patient: No. What do you mean?

Candidate: It is important that, being a doctor, we are open and be honest in these things if any error happens. It is your right to know everything. Let me explain it to you. Unfortunately, the first time when you came to the A&E, you actually had a heart attack and somehow, which was missed at that time. Our colleagues in the A&E could not pick the abnormality in your ECG, and before the blood results came back, they sent you home; unfortunately, your blood result was positive for heart attack.

Patient: How can this be possible?

Candidate: This really should not have happened, and I am really sorry for what has happened. Please accept my apology on behalf of our team. We will look at everything that went wrong regarding not waiting for the blood results and not reading your ECG correctly. I am glad that you are fine now, and we are taking proper care of you in the hospital.

Patient: How could it happen? How could anyone miss a diagnosis? You are a doctor; you shouldn't miss it. Don't you think it's a big mistake? I can't take it, Doctor!

Candidate: It's quite understandable how much this frustrates you. I agree with you this is really a big mistake; I apologize again, and we will make sure that it won't happen in the future.

Patient: How will you make sure?

Candidate: In such situations, we have a system in our hospital. I will write down this incident in your notes, inform my consultant, and fill an incident form to let the hospital authorities know about the incident. In this way, the hospital authorities can promptly reduce the risk of further events and improve the service we provide in the hospital. Even these incidents are reported nationally as well in order to prevent them from happening elsewhere.

Patient: I never expect this from such a big hospital. It's really disgusting, and I want to make a complaint, Doctor.

Candidate: Definitely, this is your right. You can make a complaint. I can get you in touch with PALS (the Patient Advice and Liaison Service), and it is a service where you can make formal complaints if you strongly feel that your care is compromised. We will follow-up on the result of your complaint and be sure that your management plan will not be affected at all. Do you have any other concerns?

Patient: No. But I am really upset, Doctor.

Candidate: I am sorry that you feel that way. I will make sure you get the best possible treatment and nothing like this happen in the future. I will tell my consultant to come and speak to you. We are going to have a closer look at you. We will take all necessary actions to prevent any further incidents.

Patient: Ok, Doctor.

Social History

Take relevant social history to manage your patient.

Candidate: So, Mr Jane, is there anything that I haven't explained to you properly?

Patient: No. you have explained everything very well.

Make Summary
Recheck Understanding
May I know how much did you get from our discussion today?

Help
I will give you my contact details if you have any questions; please don't hesitate to contact me any time ... you can visit the Trust Website and know what the policy of the trust is and how you could raise your concerns and complaints online. It is always nice to give feedback that may help to improve the services.

Thank you.

Shake hands!

Medical Trial

Your role: You are the doctor in the ward.

Problem: New clinical trial.

Patient's name: Stephan, a 45-year-old man.

Scenario: Mr Stephan is attending the clinic for routine follow-up of asthma, this is usually well-controlled, but last year he had a couple of hospital admissions due to exacerbation of asthma symptoms. Mr Stephan is leading a normal life now but given he has recently struggled with recurrent hospital admissions. Your consultant has suggested a new drug that is undergoing testing might be suitable to trial for Stephan as he is eligible to see whether it works.

Your task: You have to explain to the patient about a new clinical trial, assessing the efficacy of new medicine in controlling asthma symptoms, and preventing further hospital admission.

Introduction, Permission, and Confirmation of the Agenda

Candidate: Hello, Mr Stephan, I am Mohammad Ali, one of the working doctors here today, I have been asked to talk to you about your condition. Is that ok with you?

Patient: Hello, Doctor. It's all right.

Candidate: Do you want to add anyone else to our discussion today?

Patient: No.

Check Understanding

Candidate: I understand from your case note that you have come here for an asthma assessment. Do you have any idea what's has been happening to you so far?

Patient: I was reasonably well-controlled, but I had a couple of hospital admissions last year due to acute exacerbation. As a result, my GP sent me to the clinic for regular follow-ups.

Candidate: Thank you …, we have done some blood tests for your asthma assessment. Here we see one of the cells (eosinophil) in your blood is very high, and you have recurrent hospital admission due to exacerbation in the last year …. My consultant thinks that a new drug undergoing testing might be suitable for trial for you as you are eligible for the trial to see whether it works. May I explain more about the trial if you don't mind?

Patient: It's ok.

Candidate: I want to assure you that I am just sharing the information about the trial, and you have no obligation to participate in the trial. I would like just to invite you to take part in the research study. We will add the new drug with your present treatment, just to see the benefit of the drugs in terms of reducing hospital admission and symptoms.

The advantage of taking part in the study is that some doctors will monitor your condition more closely than usual. It is possible that your condition may improve, although there is no guarantee, and it may help develop a new therapy for others with a similar condition.

Address the Patient's Concern

Candidate: Is that ok, Mr Stephan? Do you have any concerns at this time?

Patient: Is there any side effect of the drug, Doctor?

Candidate: This is definitely a good question; in fact, there is no drug clearly without side effects; this is a phase 2 study for the drug.

Initially, the drug was tested in the labs on the animal. It did not show any major side effects. Then it was tested on the healthy volunteer men without asthma to see any side effects of the drug to a healthy person. This is called the phase-I trial. In this trial, it showed that the side effects are very rare. There is no evidence of major side effects at this moment. So, now the drug is in the phase II trial will be given to the asthmatic patient, particularly those with high eosinophil count and recurrent hospitalization despite adequate existing treatment.

If something goes wrong or any side effect occurs, they would be treated appropriately by the team. I would like to add that your identity in this study would be treated as strictly confidential. Records identifying you would not be made publicly available, and if the trial result is published, your identity will remain confidential. I want to add that there are many patients in our center who have participated in the study. Do you have any other questions or any concerns?

Patient: May I withdraw anytime from the study?

Candidate: This participation is totally voluntary. If you don't want to take part, then your management by the team would not be altered in any way. You would be treated in the usual way. If you decide to take part, you can still withdraw at any time, which would not affect your treatment's future conduct.

You don't need to decide everything right now. I will give you some leaflets or written information as well as a website address to know more about the study. You can share the information with your family members as well.

Finally, I would like to say that if you decide to participate in the study, you have to sign a consent form attached to the information sheet.

Social History

Take relevant social history to manage your patient.

Candidate: Is there anything that I haven't explained to you properly?

Patient: No. You have explained everything very well.

Make Summary
Recheck Understanding

May I know how much did you get from our discussion today?

Help

Candidate: I will give you my contact details as well to contact me if you have any worries or queries.

Thank you so much for spending time with me.

Patient: Thank you.

Shake hands!

Cancer Withhold

Your role: You are the registrar in the General Medical Clinic.

Patient's name: Mrs Mona Parker, a 72-year-old lady.

Relative's name: Mr John Parker, the patient's son.

Scenario: Mrs Mona Parker, aged 72, presented to the hospital with confusion due to UTI. Further investigations, including a CT scan, have been done, and the diagnosis of bowel cancer has been made. Your consultant decided to talk to her daughter instead as the patient was confused. Now her confusional status has improved, and she is stable. The patient has been assessed and has the full mental capacity now. Her son, Mr John Parker, was not present at that time. He has come to the hospital to talk to the consultant urgently. The consultant is not available. He told the nurse that he didn't want anyone to talk to his mother about her cancer.

Your task: Please talk to Mr John Parker and address his concerns. Consent has been taken from Mrs Mona to talk to her son. Diagnosis hasn't been disclosed to the patient yet.

Introduction, Permission, and Confirmation of the Agenda

Candidate: Hello, I am Mohammad Ali, one of the working doctors here today. May I confirm, are you Mr Parker? And how are you related to Mrs Mona Parker?

Relative: Hello, yes, I am. She is my mother.

Candidate: I understand you wanted to talk to the consultant. I would like to apologize that he is very busy now, and I am here to address all of your concerns. Is that, ok?

Relative: It's all right.

Candidate: Do you want anyone to be with you in our discussion today?

Relative: No.

Check Understanding

Candidate: Well .... Mr Parker, how may I help you?

Relative: My mom has got cancer, your consultant spoke to my sister, and I was not present there at that time. Doctor, please don't tell her that she has cancer.

Candidate: I am really sorry to hear about the diagnosis of your mother. I know it is a very tough time for you and your family, but may I know why don't you want us to tell her?

Relative: I am afraid it will affect her deadly if she comes to know about her condition.

Candidate: I understand your care for your mother; this is really big news for anyone. However, let me explain some of the challenges that we may face if we don't explain the situation to your mom:

At the moment, your mom is capable of understanding everything and making decisions for herself. Legally, it's your mom's right to know about her condition.

She might ask us directly "What has happened to me?", in that case, we cannot hide anything from her. As a doctor, we have to tell everything to your mom, and we cannot lie to our patients.

She has cancer, so we need to do further investigations to make a proper management plan for her and review her condition. Sometimes investigations and treatments come with some invasive procedures, and we won't be able to provide any of these without her consent. She will ask us why we are doing all these tests then we have to explain it to her otherwise she might not allow us to do these.

Relative: Doctor, my mom is old and weak. It will be really hard for her; she won't digest the news that she has cancer.

Candidate: I can hardly imagine what you are going through. We will handle this conversation sensitively. We will break the news into layers. At first, we will check her ideas about her condition; then we will ask her whether she wants to know about her condition. If she wants to know, then we will give her the diagnosis in an empathetic manner. We will give her some time so that she can absorb the news.

Relative: Doctor, please don't tell her. I'm her son; I am the head of the family and take all her decisions.

Candidate: Mr Parker, is there any particular reason you don't want us to tell her about her condition?

Relative: My dad had cancer, and he died because of cancer, my mom was the one looking after him. She saw my father's suffering very closely, and she lost my father only 2 years ago, now she has cancer. It will be very difficult for her to accept, that's why I am telling you please don't tell her about her condition.

Candidate: I am deeply saddened by the loss that you and your family have encountered. My deepest condolences to you! Now I can fully understand why you don't want to tell her about cancer.

As you told me that your dad had cancer and she was the one looking after him. Don't you think sooner or later she will come to know about her illness? At that time, she will not trust anyone. She will not trust you. She will not trust us, and no treatment will be effective for her.

Relative: Doctor. She is a very simple lady; tell her that she has an infection and treat her for cancer.

Candidate: Mr Parker, the treatment for cancer and infections are different. Soon she will come to know that she has cancer as she knows about cancer symptoms because she was taking care of your father.

Relative: Ok, Doctor. Just don't use the word cancer in front of her as I mentioned she knows about this word.

Candidate: What we can use instead of cancer. There are words such as tumor or growth, but these are medical words, and she may not understand these words. She has got full mental capacity; we have to tell her that she has got cancer to discuss the further plan of management with her.

Relative: Doctor. She doesn't understand English.

Candidate: Don't worry, we will arrange an interpreter for your mom. So that is not an issue.

Relative: Can I be an interpreter?

Candidate: Mr Parker, we have a specialist in this field who knows how to give information to our patients. I am so sorry you cannot be our interpreter.

Relative: Can I be there while you are talking to my mom?

Candidate: Yes, of course, you can be with us when talking to your mom if she wants. As long as she is happy, we don't have any problem having you on her side.

Relative: Doctor. Can I interrupt you while you are talking to my mom about her condition?

Candidate: May I know why do you want to interrupt us?

Relative: Because I know my mom. Maybe you tell her something that will hurt her sentiments.

Candidate: I know you know your mom better than anyone, and I would say it would be helpful to talk to us now regarding anything that might be helpful for us. However, I don't think it would be appropriate to interrupt us while talking to your mom and discussing her condition.

Address the Patient's Concerns and Questions

Do you have any concerns or questions?

Social History

Take relevant social history to manage your patient.

Candidate: So, Mr Parker, is there anything that I haven't explained to you properly?

Relative: No.

Make Summary

Recheck Understanding

May I know how much did you get from our discussion today?

Thank you so much for spending time with me.

Relative: Thank you.

Shake hands!

Live Organ Donation

Your role: You are the registrar working in the renal unit.

Patient's name: Miss Jayeta Hasan, a 30-year-old lady.

Relative's name: Mrs Urmi Hasan, patient's mother.

Scenario: Mrs Jayeta is a 30-year-old lady who has been suffering from lupus nephritis and has started hemodialysis for 2 years. She is on the waiting list for a cadaveric transplant; it has been mentioned to the patient and her family that it will take a long time and there will be no guarantee that she will get a kidney. Mrs Urmi (mother of Jayeta Hasan) has been wondering whether to donate one of her kidneys and requested a meeting with the team. Your consultant is busy in the clinic, and he asked you to meet Mrs Urmi.

Your task: You have to give Mrs Urmi an overview, including the pros and cons of acting as a living donor and to answer all concerns.

Introduction, Permission, and Confirmation of the Agenda

Candidate: Hello, Mrs Urmi. I am Mohammad Ali, one of the working doctors here today. Are you the mother of Miss Jayeta?

Patient: Yes, Doctor.

Candidate: Thank you for coming. We are here today to discuss some issues that you have requested to discuss with my consultant; I would like to apologize that he is very busy at this moment, and I am here to address all your concerns. Is that ok, Mrs Urmi?

Patient: Yes, it's ok.

Candidate: Do you want to add anyone else to our discussion today?

Patient: No.

Check Understanding

Candidate: Ok. Mrs Urmi, how much do you know about your daughter's condition?

Relative: Actually, doctor, my daughter struggles with lupus nephritis. Unfortunately, her kidney function has switched off, and they initiated for her some sort of renal replacement therapy that may be called hemodialysis. For the last 2 years, she has been regular for these hemodialysis sessions. Doctors put her name on the waiting list for a cadaveric transplant, but she has not had any calls yet. We have been informed it will take a long time, so for my daughter's sake, I want to donate one kidney to her.

(Doctor's actions in case of organ donation: Explore the negativity, explore the positivity, and explore the procedure)

Explore the Negativity

Candidate: I am really sorry hear about your daughter's condition. However, as you have been informed, there is no guarantee for how long your daughter will wait until we have a suitable organ for her. For the last 2 years, she has been on the waiting list, and till now, we don't know exactly when a suitable kidney will be available for her.

Patient: Yes, that's why I am thinking to donate one kidney to my daughter.

Explore Positivity

Candidate: I really appreciate your decision to donate one kidney to your daughter. It will be the most precious gift ever for your daughter. I want to inform you that live organ donation has a better outcome than cadaveric donation. A kidney from living donors does not need to be transported from one place to another, so the organ is in a better condition when it is transplanted. Mrs Urmi, you will give your daughter almost and nearly a normal life if you do such a step.

Do you have any idea about kidney donation/how much you know about kidney donation?

Patient: Not at all.

Explore the Procedure

Candidate: Ok, Mrs Urmi, I want to tell you that kidney donation is one of the most common types of donations worldwide, but it is actually a long process. It needs around 3-6 months to finalize all the issues. So we can proceed with kidney donation as early as possible because this needs a lot of preparation for you and your daughter.

The Issue of Assessment

Do you have any ongoing medical conditions such as HTN, DM or any family history of kidney disease?

Patient: No. I don't have any.

Candidate: That's good news for both of you. Because having these illnesses is one of the important barriers to donation.

At the same time, there are lots of medical and psychological assessments because not everyone is ready to do such a step, and sometimes one can decide to donate the kidney emotionally, and finally, when it comes to donation, they don't want to donate anymore. So, there should be a psychological assessment of the donor and the recipient as well. The mood doctor is going to involve later on for the assessment of both donor and recipient. Are you following me, Mrs Urmi?

Patient: Yes, Doctor.

Candidate: Moreover, regarding medical assessment, both of you will undergo several tests such as crossmatching, tissue typing as well as checking for HIV, HBV, HCV infections, and scan test to make sure that you don't have any hidden renal disease and the donation would be safe for you in the first place.

During the assessment, it may reveal an illness that may also have psychological and medical implications, such as you may have positive blood samples for hepatitis B or any other disease.

So, retaining back to our conversation ... It's a long process, and it takes around 3-6 months to finalize all issues because there should be medical and psychological issues for both of you.

Patient: Ok, so it will take much more time.

Candidate: Yes, it is.

The Issue of Surgical Complications and Rejections

I am sorry to tell you, but honestly, the surgery itself has some complications. Although the chances are very low, it has its own risks, such as anesthetic risks, risks of infections, risks of rejection, and so on.

At the same time, Mrs Urmi, I would like to tell you that, even after doing all of the procedures, the most important fact is that transplant may fail what we called as transplant rejection, where her immune system suddenly begins to attack the donated kidney because it recognizes it as a foreign tissue; however, if it does occur, it can often be successfully treated with a short course of more powerful immunosuppressant medications. As I mentioned earlier that the living donor has a better outcome and there are fewer chances of rejections in contrast to the cadaveric donor. The percentage of successful transplantation with a living donor is around 95%.

Patient: Doctor, can I live a normal life having only one kidney left?

Candidate: People can live a normal life with one kidney. Fortunately, you don't have any long-term disease which could affect your kidneys so that you can lead a nearly normal life after transplantation. Only a minority of people may develop HTN later on.

Patient: How long will I have to stay in the hospital, and how long it will take for complete recovery?

Candidate: I appreciate your concern. The surgery is usually a laparoscopic operation. It has a low risk of complications. Our donors usually leave the hospital in 2-3 days and resume their normal life with limited activity in 2-6 weeks. And after 6 weeks, life as it was before donating.

The Issue of Checking Implications
Mrs Urmi, I strongly advise you that you need to check with your insurance company before getting into this step. So, you should check the implications of an organ donation. Some insurance companies have a particular chapter concerning organ donation; you should revise this chapter with your insurance company. Also, the insurance company may not cover some expenses, so you should check it first to go and donate safely. Is that ok, Mrs Urmi …?

Patient: Ok.

The Issue of Immunosuppressants
Candidate: Your daughter will have to be on life-long medications (immunosuppressive) to prevent or decrease the issues of rejection after kidney transplantation. Furthermore, these types of medications have their own risks (infection) at the same time have their own benefits and whatever your level of risk, the benefits greatly exceed any of those hazards.

Concerning this issue, if you agree, we can arrange another meeting with the transplant team, who will give you full detail about the transplant, and your daughter will be a part of our next meeting with the transplant team. Is that ok with you, Mrs Urmi?

Patient: Yes, doctor, I will think about it. Thank you …

Address the Patient's Concerns
Candidate: Do you have any other concerns?

Patient: No.

Social History
Take relevant social history to manage your patient.

Candidate: Is there anything else that we have not explained? Do you have any other concerns or expectations from me?

Summarize
Check Understanding
May I know, please, how much did you get from our discussion today?

Help
I will give you some written information and the details of the kidney donation society to know more about the renal transplant; I will give you my contact details. If you have any worries or queries, please don't hesitate to contact me.

Thank you

Shake hands!

Advance Care Decision

Your role: You are the doctor in the respiratory ward.

Problem: Advance care decision.

Patient's name: Mrs Watkins, a 65-year-old lady.

Relative's name: Miss Collins, Daughter.

Scenario: You are the doctor in the respiratory ward, and the patient Mrs Watkins presented with a chest infection on a background of severe pulmonary fibrosis. This is the patient's 3rd admission in the last 6 months, and she has deteriorated significantly over that period. She is dependent on care for all activities of daily living and housebound and is having long-term oxygen at home. She also has a history of dementia. Your consultant has asked you to talk to the patient's daughter about future admission to the hospital and advanced care planning.

Your task: You have to explain the situation and discuss the issue of advance care planning for the patient with a relative.

Introduction, Permission, and Confirmation of the Agenda

Candidate: Hello, Miss Collins. I am Mohammad Ali, one of the working doctors here today. I am here to talk to you about Mrs Watkins, can I just confirm your relationship with Mrs Watkins first?

Relative: Hello, Doctor, she is my mother.

Candidate: Well, thank you for coming. Are you the next of kin?

Relative: Yes.

Candidate: Ok. Do you want to add anyone else to our discussion today?

Relative: No.

Check Understanding

Candidate: Ok ... Miss Collins ... How much do you know about your mother's condition/do you have any idea what has been happening to your mother so far?

Relative: My mom has been admitted to this hospital with breathlessness, and the doctor told me she gets a chest infection. She has had a lung problem for the last 2 years, may be called lung fibrosis, and her condition is getting worse day-by-day. This is her 3rd admission in the last 6 months. Over that period, she has become housebound and is having long-term oxygen therapy at home.

Candidate: Yes, and I understand from her case note that she has forgetfulness and dementia as well. Is that right?

Relative: Yes, she has dementia and needs a full-time caregiver.

Candidate: I know it's difficult to handle independently at this stage. I am sorry to tell you that your mother is very ill and we need to make sure that we make the right decision for her. May I explain more to you about your mother's present condition?

Relative: Yes.

Candidate: This time, she is admitted due to a chest infection, and we have had started IV fluids and antibiotics as well as oxygen. The good thing is she is improving gradually.

However, this is her 3rd admission in the last 6 months, and she has deteriorated significantly over that period and become housebound. She is having long-term oxygen therapy and has a preexisting lung problem in technical fancy term this is called lung fibrosis. She also has dementia.

So, she cannot understand what's going on with her. Unfortunately, both of the conditions are deteriorating gradually. Even with quite a minor infection in the chest, she gets very unwell and comes to the hospital for antibiotics.

One of the reasons, I want to talk with you that ... what would be her decision in her future admission, as we have seen each time in her admission she is deteriorating.

Relative: Yes, but she is improving.

Candidate: Yes ... But each time, she is getting more and more deteriorated. I think she is at high risk for a further chest infection, and she will again require hospitalization. In case of severe infection such as pneumonia, I am sorry to say she may require ICU admission for intensive care [intensive therapy unit (ITU)].

Relative: Oh! I see ... But she is well now, Doctor. Why will she get it?

Candidate: I know she is well now, but I am talking about her future condition as she is deteriorating than earlier. Do you have any idea about ITU care, Miss Collins?

Relative: No ...

Candidate: Here, a tube passed into the windpipe connected to a breathing machine (ventilator), which helps to rest her lungs. There may be other tubes in the arms and neck to give antibiotics, fluids, and other treatments. It will be done under sedation to overcome the distress of the tube.

But the risks of ventilation and ITU admission are further infection, difficulty in weaning off the ventilator, psychosis and unfortunately in the worst case—sometimes death.

Miss Collins, does your mother have a living will or Power of Attorney? Do you have any idea about her wishes about ITU admission and ventilation when she was all right? And how does the rest of the family feel about ventilation or ITU admission?

Relative: No. Nothing, she never expressed anything about this! Regarding families, I am the one who takes care of my mom, and I think my mom should get all kinds of medical services if needed.

Candidate: I appreciate your feelings. However, as you know that your mother has poor general health, this will not be a good decision to put her in ITU in the future.

Relative: Why? How could you tell this?

Candidate: I have discussed with my consultant and the medical team, and we believe that she would not be an appropriate candidate for ventilation because of the high morbidity and mortality risk plus high chance of difficulty in coming off the ventilator; therefore, a decision not to ventilate was taken in the best of your mother's condition. Are you following me, Miss Collins?

Relative: You mean, like, if my mom's condition is getting worse, you can't treat her! My mother will die, and you won't do anything for her?

Candidate: I understand how you feel .... I would think the same if I were in your place. This decision only relates to a ventilator or ITU admission, but this is not an "all or none" decision about her care. I want to assure you that her basic medical and nursing care will not be affected.

Relative: But I have heard that people come back healthy through ventilators. Then why don't you do it for my mother?

Candidate: We decide everything based on risk and benefit ratios. In terms of your mother's condition, she may worsen with a ventilator, and the chances of regaining from the ventilator are very low for her. It will do more harm and will prolong her suffering. So, the risks of using a ventilator for your mother will outweigh the benefits.

Relative: Well, I can understand, but I can't let my mother die like this. I want to give all the treatment for whatever the risk is.

Candidate: Ok ... I know this is really very stressful for you, and I am not telling you to make the decision right now, it's an ongoing process, and we will talk about it again, and if you want a second opinion, I can arrange for a second opinion for you, is that ok with you?

Relative: Yeah, yeah, that will be fine. I need one, I think ...

Candidate: Well. I will arrange another meeting for you with my consultant and ITU specialist; you will know all the details from them and ask any questions you may have.

Address the Patient's Concern

Candidate: So, Miss Collins, do you have any other concerns?

Relative: Can I take my mother home? If the infection happens again in the future, what should I do?

Candidate: Your mother is improving, but this is not the right moment to take her home. She needs some more time to stay here and complete her treatment. And next time, if she again develops chest injection, I think the best approach will be for her that you must ask your GP to come to your home. She may need to start oral antibiotics as early as possible .... However, if she feels very ill, she will need to be readmitted.

Relative: Is there any powerful medicine that can prevent her from getting worse? Can't you tell me the best option for her? You know, I have no one in this world but my mother.

Candidate: I know how precious your mother is to you. I am sorry to tell you, but watchful waiting will be the best option for her .... Unfortunately, there is nothing that can prevent her deterioration!

Relative: Oh!

Candidate: I know how hard this news is for you, and I want to reassure you that the decision was taken in the best interest of your mother's condition ...

Is there anything else that we have not explained properly? Do you have any questions or concerns, or expectations to me?

Relative: No. Thank you.

Social History

Take relevant social history to manage your patient.

Candidate: Miss Collins, as you mentioned, your mother is housebound and needs support from others for her daily living. I can help you in that case; I can arrange the social health worker support for her if that's ok with you.

Relative: Yes, please. It will be a great favor.

Recheck Understanding

May I know how much did you get from our discussion today?

Help

Candidate: I will arrange our next meeting, and I will arrange the social worker team to meet your mother and give her appropriate support. I will give you some written information about what I have said about the end of life decision, and I will give you my contact details as well to contact me if you have any worries or queries.

Is there anything that I haven't explained to you properly? Do you have any other questions or concerns?

Relative: No.

Candidate: Thank you so much for spending time with me. I am hoping best for Mrs Watkins.

Relative: Thank you.

Make Summary

Now I am going to summarize the important things from our discussion today.

So, this is your mother's 3rd admission for the confirmed chest infection in the last 6 months on a background of severe pulmonary fibrosis. She also has a history of dementia and requires full-time care. She has deteriorated significantly over that period of time. So, we have discussed her future admission to the hospital as well as advance care planning.

I have discussed with some of my colleagues, and we think she would not be an appropriate candidate for ventilation because of the high morbidity or mortality risk. Is that ok, Miss Collins?

Shake hands!

Decision about Do-not-resuscitate

Your role: You are the doctor in the ICU.

Problem: Consent to do not attempt cardiopulmonary resuscitation (DNACPR).

Patient's name: Mrs Stella Newsman, an 82-year-old lady.

Relative's name: Mr Eric, son of the patient.

Scenario: Mrs Stella Newsman was admitted to the hospital with sepsis secondary to pneumonia and dementia with a background history of Alzheimer's disease, type 2 diabetes mellitus, and HTN. Despite IV fluids and IV antibiotics, she has deteriorated on the ward and developed multiorgan failure. She is dependent on care for all activities of daily living and living in nursing care. Your consultant has asked you to talk to Mr Eric, her son, and discuss a DNACPR.

Your task: You have to explain the deteriorating clinical situation and discuss the issue of not attempting cardiopulmonary resuscitation.

Introduction, Permission, and Confirmation of the Agenda

Candidate: Hello, Mr Eric. I am Mohammad Ali, one of the working doctors here today. I am here to talk to you about Mrs Stella Newsman, can I just confirm your relationship with her first?

Relative: Hello, Doctor, she is my mother.

Candidate: Well, thank you for coming. Do you want to add anyone else to our discussion today?

Relative: No.

Check Understanding

Candidate: Ok. Mr Eric, how much do you know about your mother's condition?

Relative: My mom was admitted to this hospital for a chest infection. I am really worried that despite getting intravenous antibiotics and intravenous fluid treatment, she is deteriorating. She has some other problems such as diabetes and HTN, and also, she has had dementia for last 2 years.

Candidate: Unfortunately, she is very ill and we need to make sure that we make the right decision for her. May I explain more to you about your mother's present condition?

Relative: Yes.

Candidate: Your mother was admitted to the hospital due to pneumonia. Now the infection has spread to the bloodstream. In fancy technical terms, this is called sepsis. She has a background history of uncontrolled DM and HTN. We were started with intravenous fluid and broad-spectrum antibiotics to clear up infections. Since she had developed severe breathlessness, and she couldn't take a breath by herself; therefore, we put her into a breathing machine (ventilator) to take breaths. Despite treatment, she is not improving, and unfortunately, she has developed multiorgan failure, which means her heart, lungs, kidney, and brain are not working well. Does that make sense so far, Mr Eric?

Relative: Oh! But she is on ongoing treatment. She might get better. I hope so.
(Use the pause to tell the message to sink in)

Candidate: I am sorry to tell you that my consultant reviewed your mother this morning during the ward round and felt that there is a possibility that she may deteriorate further and die shortly.

Relative: Oh! I know her condition is not good, but why don't you do the best treatment for her?

Candidate: I can sense how difficult this news is for you. I want to assure you that we are giving your mother the best treatment as much as possible.

And there is one thing I should discuss with you that relates to what we might do in the event of things going very wrong with her health. I am sorry and not that I'm expecting it to happen …. But there is always the possibility, as, with any unwell patient, things could go very wrong and get worse despite everything we have tried—that the heart could stop and we may need to re-start the heart with CPR or heart-starting machines (DC shock).

Did your mother express her wishes before about CPR when she was all right? How do you and the rest of the family feel about the CPR?

Relative: No. My mother never expresses anything about it. And we also never think like that way.

Candidate: Ok, it's all right. I am sorry to say, as your mother is very frail with multiple comorbidities, and from the medical point of view, it would be futile to resuscitate her if her heart stops. Therefore, the treating medical team decides in the best interest of your mother's condition not to be resuscitated if she had cardiac (heart) arrest.
(Use the pause to let the message sink in)

Relative: How it is possible! I can't even imagine all such things! The CPR! Heart-stopping! I can't take this!

Candidate: I can understand how stressful all of this is for you …

Relative: Yes, it is … It is …, Doctor!

Candidate: Although this is a difficult subject to talk about. Do you have any ideas about what resuscitation or CPR is?

Relative: No, not at all.
(Explain resuscitation to the son)

Candidate: When a patient's heart stops beating, we start to do resuscitation by jumping on the chest to do forceful compression, sometimes using the heart starting machine (DC shock) to start the heart and give some medications through a needle to stimulate the heart to work again. I am sorry to say, in your mother's case, ultimately, it would be futile.
(Explain complication of resuscitation)

Unfortunately, resuscitation has its own complications, like your mother may have a fractured rib, bleeding, or deformity in the chest. Do you understand my point?

Relative: Yes, I can.

Candidate: Well. Mr Eric, does your mother have a living will or lasting Power of Attorney?

Relative: What does it mean?

Candidate: It's something where one can make a decision about your mother's health when she is incompetent. Do you know anything about this?

Relative: No. There is no such thing.

Candidate: Well. As your mother has poor general health, the chance to revive her again is extremely low and resuscitation attempts may do more harm than good by prolonging the dying process. Therefore, a decision not to resuscitate is taken in the best interest of your mother's condition.
(Showing empathy and sympathy again) (If he starts crying … Allow him to express his emotion and sadness. Comfort him and offer him a box of tissues if handy)

How do you feel now, Mr Eric? Would you like to save some water?

Relative: I feel so hopeless. My mother is going to die! Oh! How could I bear all this! Even you won't give her the treatment! Doctor, my mother will die shortly, and you even won't give her the treatment!

Candidate: I know how much this news is hard for you, and be sure that this decision was taken in the best interest of your mother's condition.

I want to make sure that this decision relates to CPR only, and this is not an "all or none" decision about her care. She will continue to receive conventional treatment appropriate for her, such as I/V fluids and antibiotics.

[Manage the dilemma of rejection of her son to (DNR: do-not-resuscitate)]

Relative: Doctor, please do anything to keep my mother alive.

Candidate: I appreciate your feelings; I know how much your mother is precious to you, and be sure that she is precious for us too. As your mother does not have an advanced directive, living will or Power of Attorney, so that the medical team has the right to make a decision in the best interest of the patient's condition.

Relative: It's really hard for me …. I can't accept your decision at all.

Candidate: I know it must be, but we can arrange another meeting involving anyone else of your family members whom you can trust. We can involve our consultants-in-charge of patient's care to reply to any worries or queries you still have.

Address the Patient's Concern

Candidate: So, Mr Eric, do you have any other concerns?

Relative: There is nothing to do, Doctor?

Candidate: I am sorry, but to be honest, there is nothing to do actually, but we can assure you that we will give your mother all the supports except CPR or other advanced treatment, which she can't tolerate at all.

Social History
Take relevant social history to manage your patient.

Make Summary
Recheck Understanding
May I know how much did you get from our discussion today?

Help
Candidate: I will give you some written information and the website address of CPR and the address of "The Human Rights Act, 1998" to know more about the end-of-life decision. I will arrange our next meeting, and I will give you my contact details, if you have any worries or queries, please don't hesitate to contact me.

Is there anything that I haven't explained to you properly? Do you have any other questions or concerns?

Relative: No.

Candidate: Thank you so much for spending time with me.

Relative: Thank you.

Shake hands!

End of Life Decision

Your role: You are SHO in the medical ward.

Problem: End-of-life decision.

Patient: Mr Mirza Abbas, an 80-year-old man.

Scenario: Mr Abbas was readmitted yesterday with breathlessness and responded to initial noninvasive ventilation from which he has been successfully weaned. He has a severe chronic obstructive pulmonary disease with long-term oxygen therapy and a background history of ischemic heart disease with heart failure. He is dependent on care for all activities of daily living and has been confined to his house. Shortness of breath is his main limitation, and over the last year, he has been admitted to the hospital four times with increasing frequency and exacerbations of breathlessness, sometimes precipitated by infection. However, his resuscitation status has not been documented yet.

Your task: Discuss his resuscitation status and make decisions about "do not resuscitate" and "do not intubate" orders as part of the advance directive. You may assume that you were involved in his care during this and his previous admissions, and he knows who you are.

Introduction, Permission, and Confirmation of the Agenda

(Introduction, setting, and rapport-discussion about resuscitation should be between a patient and ideally a doctor who has already created a rapport with that patient, even if brief. The setting should ideally be quiet and without distractions).

Candidate: Hello, Mr Abbas; I am Mohammad Ali, one of the working doctors here today. I have come here to talk to you about your care and particularly plans for the future. Is that, ok?

Patient: Hello, Doctor, it's all right.

Candidate: Would you like anyone to be with you in our discussion today?

Patient: No.

Check Understanding

Candidate: How are you feeling now, Mr Abbas? What do you know about your current condition?

Patient: Well, I am feeling quite a bit fine now. But I know my heart and lung condition are not good at all. I feel more and more breathless nowadays, and even I have difficulty breathing when doing normal things like getting out of bed. I realize that day-by-day, my condition is getting worse. I can feel it. You know, the worst part is? ... I have to depend on others, which I don't like at all.

Candidate: I'm so sorry to see you like this. You have been in hospital rather a lot over the last year, and now you're back in hospital sooner than you and your doctors had hoped.

Patient: Yes, I am ... you are right.

Candidate: Well, as you know about your illnesses; so, what are you expecting or how do you expect your condition?

Patient: Oh! Nothing much! I know I don't have lots of time. Doctors told me that things like my illnesses are going to be worse and significantly shorten my life. I can feel the changes in my body; I have no energy at all. I am not expecting anything, actually.

Candidate: Well, at the moment, you can understand what is happening, and you can make decisions. I would like to have a conversation about how we will take care of you in future and make some important decisions and sign your papers. Can I go ahead?

Patient: Ok.

Candidate: Mr Abbas, do you have any living will or lasting power of attorney?

Patient: No, what do you mean by the lasting power of attorney?

Candidate: To appoint someone as your lasting power of attorney means, in the future, you might not be able to make decisions by yourself; this person will decide for you. You can appoint someone on behalf of you to make decisions for you; this can be anyone you trust and can also take decisions similar to what you think. It is a legal issue, and if you want to appoint anyone, you can speak to your GP, who can make arrangements for signing the document.

Patient: Ok, I will think about it.

Tell Him about His Condition and Resuscitation

Candidate: Ok. Unfortunately, someone with a heart and lung condition as bad as yours may suddenly take a turn for the worse. I am sorry and not that I'm expecting it to happen .... However, there is always the possibility, as, with an unwell patient, things could go very wrong and get worse despite everything we have tried—if your condition gets worse, your heart may stop beating. You may develop cardiac arrest, and we would usually do chest compression to bring it back, called CPR (cardiopulmonary resuscitation).

Similarly, your lungs may also fail to breathe; usually, we will put tubes in your lungs, and the machine will do the breathing for you.

Have you ever thought about what your wishes might be in that situation? Or would you wish us to try to restart things with CPR (cardiopulmonary resuscitation) or heart-starting machines (DC shock) or breathing tubes, and so forth?

Patient: Doctor, No ... I don't really want to suffer so much anymore. I really don't want to be a burden to my family. Not that my kids or wife don't love me, but I don't want to be their burden. But I'm asking out of curiosity, how would you restart my heart again or what you called CPR is?

Explain CPR Briefly

Candidate: Ok, sure, I can make it clear for you. Actually ... if things go horribly wrong, and your heart or breathing stops, we start to do resuscitation and try to reback it by jumping on the chest to do forceful compression, and in that case, you may have fractured ribs. Putting a big tube in the throat, and giving some medications through a needle to stimulate the heart to work again, all together is called CPR. The best outcomes are for previously fit patients with no heart or lung problems. However, the outcome is doubtful if there is a background of many comorbidities and chronic medical diseases. Does it make sense?

Patient: Oh, yes .... I saw that on TV, such a horrible thing! I understand.

Candidate: Yes, it is ... I am sorry to say; ultimately, it would likely be futile.

Patient: Oh! I got it.

Candidate: I can see that you find this difficult. We could talk about it later if you prefer, or, if you wish, with members of your family here (if you know there are family members), or some patients simply prefer that we do what we think is the very best for them.

Patient: No.. it's all right, doctor.

Candidate: So, what is your thought about resuscitation?

Be Prepared to Deal with Emotions with Empathy and Sympathy

Patient: No ... No Doctor, I can't hurt my body so much; it must feel so bad that you said to put a pipe in the throat, to fix the heart by pressing on the chest! Everything feels so bad and painful. I don't want to suffer anymore!
(Sometimes, the patient may want to leave it on medical's decision, and he/she may say, "I would leave it in your hands, doctor. Do as you think best?")

Candidate: I appreciate your decision, and I spoke to my consultant and the medical team; we believe that in terms of your current severe illness and presence of your multiple comorbidities,

CPR at this stage will have poor outcomes, may do more harm than good and even if it works it will just be prolonging your days of suffering and would lead to very poor quality of life. We think that it's in your best interest to be declared not for resuscitation. How does it sound?

Patient: Yes. Right.

Reassure the Patient about the Rest of His Care

Candidate: I want to make sure that this decision relates to CPR only, and your basic medical and nursing care such as I/V fluids, antibiotics, oxygen therapy as well as NIV support will not be affected at all. However, if it gets worse, no escalating to ITU for ventilator support or CPR.

Patient: Yes, I think I should share everything with my family, they love me dearly and may be depressed by my decision, but to be honest, I don't want to be a burden to anyone.

Candidate: Well, I will arrange another chat for you and your family on a later day. So, Mr Abbas, if you go with nonattempting resuscitation, we will fill out the Red form or DNAR form, and it will be placed into your medical notes; however, you may change your mind any time as long as you are competent. Ok, Mr Abbas?

Patient: Yes.

Address the Patient's Concern

Candidate: So, Mr Abbas, do you have any other concerns?

Patient: No, not actually.

Social History

Take relevant social history to manage your patient.

Candidate: Mr Abbas, as you are concerned about not bothering anyone for your daily needs, may I arrange social worker support for you? I think it would help you with your current and future status.

Relative: Yes, please. It will be a great favor.

Make Summary
Recheck Understanding

May I know how much did you get from our discussion today?

Help

Candidate: I will give you some written information and the website address of CPR and the address of "The Human Rights Act, 1998" to know more about end-of-life decisions. I will arrange our next meeting and arrange for the social worker to meet you and fulfill your daily needs more comfortably. I will give you my contact details, if you have any worries or queries, please don't hesitate to contact me.

Is there anything that I haven't explained to you properly? Do you have any other questions or concerns?

Patient: No.

Thank you so much for spending time with me.

Patient: Thank you.

Shake hands!

Brainstem Death Testing

Your role: You are the doctor in the ICU.

Problem: Patient in ICU suitable for brainstem death testing.

Patient's name: Mrs Lee Chaung, a 55-year-old lady.

Relative's name: Mr Taan Chaung, patient's son.

Scenario: You look after Mrs Lee Chaung in the intensive care unit (ICU), who presented with a sudden collapse at home. The patient was brought to A/E by ambulance and found a catastrophic subarachnoid hemorrhage after a CT scan of the brain. The patient was intubated before the diagnosis and has been in ICU for the last 3 days without any sedation and has made no signs of life. The MDT involving neurology consultants and the intensive care specialists have decided the next appropriate action is to carry out brainstem death testing to confirm that the patient has suffered a complete neurological failure.

Your task: You have to explain the relative reason for brainstem death testing, how it is done, and finally, what it means.

Introduction, Permission, and Confirmation of the Agenda

Candidate: Hello, Mr Taan Chaung, I am Mohammad Ali, one of the working doctors here today. I am here to talk to you about Mrs Lee Chaung, can I just confirm your relationship with her first?

Relative: She is my mother.

Candidate: Are you the next of kin?

Relative: Yes.

Candidate: Ok. Are you on your own today? Do you want to call anyone from the family in our discussion today?

Relative: No.

Check Understanding

Candidate: Mr Chaung, I am looking after your mother in ICU at this time. It would be helpful if you just could tell me what's been happening so far?

Relative: My mother suddenly collapsed at home, and we immediately called the ambulance. The doctor told me that my mother's condition was not so good, she had bleeding in her brain, and they put her on a ventilator and did lots of tests, but I don't know why my mother was given a ventilator. Now I'm waiting for my mother's recovery and hoping for the best.

Tell Him about Her Condition

Candidate: I'm sorry for what has happened to your mother. Mr Chaung, let me give you a bit more information about the tests, what we have done and what we have found out, is that ok?

Relative: Yes.

Candidate: Exactly as you said, your mother was found unconscious, and the paramedics brought her to the hospital, and she has been in ICU on life support since then. One of the 1st tests we did at that moment was the CT scan of the brain; this is a scan of the head.

As we need to explain why she gets unconscious …. The scans show that she has had something called "subarachnoid hemorrhage", which means that she has had bleeding inside the scalp.

Unfortunately, there is a large amount of bleeding that affecting her brain and causing damage to it. Bleeding tends to result from a blood vessel that was burst and the blood escaping from the blood channel, ultimately damaging the brain.

Moreover, this is the reason for her unconsciousness, and it is actually similar to a stroke because it also causes damage to the brain. Are you following me, Mr Chaung?

Relative: Yeah, yes...

Candidate: Unfortunately, your mother has had very extensive bleeding on the scan, so there is a very significant amount of blood damaging the brain. (Take a pause ... to absorb the information)

Relative: Oh! I see ... bleeding in the brain! That's must be very serious ...

Candidate: I am afraid it is really serious. Obviously, that is more serious than a little or tiny leakage of blood vessels causing minimal damage.

We give her the maximum treatment she could have; we give her medications to support her heart and increase its performance, and put her on a breathing machine (ventilator) to help her breathing. But unfortunately, I am sorry to say, she is not responding at all and our medical team believes she will not regain her consciousness because the brain's maestro is not working anymore; the maestro of the brain is the vital part of our brain that handles our breathing and controls our heart beating. Therefore, it is unwise to keep her suffering anymore.
(Again, take a pause, give some time to react and respond empathically according to the relative's reaction)

Relative: Doctor ... Is there any operation that you can do for her?

Candidate: It is a valid question. There are some types of subarachnoid hemorrhages where an operation can be effective. But I am sorry to tell you, unfortunately, in your mother's case the bleeding is so extensive that it won't bring good results or any benefit in having an operation. We have already discussed her case with a specialist doctor who operates the brain called a neurosurgeon, he/she thoroughly checked the scans, but unfortunately, his/her advice is that actually, he/she has nothing to do to improve your mother's condition.

I appreciated that this is the last thing you wanted to know ... but I really have to be honest with you and explain the situation as we have discovered it yet. (Take a pause again ... To absorb it, and answer any question sensitively)

Relative: Oh! There is nothing to do! So, you are doing nothing for my mother!

Candidate: I can sense what you are going through and where the question is coming from. We have been assessing her every day, looking after her and making various observations on your mother, and one thing that we know from her scan is when the damage to the brain is extensive, it is something irreversible ... the brain cells cannot be replaced once damaged and will not recover...

Relative: But my mom is breathing now ...

Candidate: Unfortunately, the only thing that is currently keeping her alive is the ventilator that she is attached to.. and this would instantly cease to function if the machine is stopped, and her heart would stop soon after.
(Retake a pause ...) I am really sorry to give you such horrible news in such terms ...

Relative: So, doctor, what will you do next?

Candidate: Yes, the situation now arises about what we should do next to look after your mother ... actually, as your mother's heart and lungs are being artificially maintained, and her brain has irreversible damage, so we will go for something called brainstem death testing .... It is going to make a serious assessment of the brain to see if there is any chance that the patient has a survivable illness or not ... (Take another pause ... offer some water or tissue or other support if needed)

I would like to discuss with you briefly about the test if that's ok.

Relative: Yeah... please.

Candidate: We will involve two senior doctors; one of them is a consultant to assess the patient separately; we will stop all the medications, including anesthetics and will do tests involving:

A torch is shone into both eyes to see if she reacts to the light (absent pupillary light reflex); or pressure is applied to the forehead (supraorbital pressure) to see if there's any movement of the limbs in response (absent motor stimulation); and finally, we will stop the ventilator for a short period to see if she attempts to breathe on her own (assess response to apnea testing).

Two different doctors conduct all the tests at different times, not in front of each other and if both have the same results, unfortunately, the patient is unlikely to recover. (Again, give another moment to take in all the bad news …)

Relative: My mother was completely healthy. I can't believe it! Just 3 days ago, my mother was fine, was at home!

Candidate: I can understand this has come as a shock to you and I know this is a really really hard time for you. Do you want to call anyone from your family?

If your other family members, would like to talk to me or one of my colleagues or if you would like a further chat later in the day, that's absolutely fine … Is there anything that I haven't explained to you properly? Do you have any other questions or concerns?

Relative: No. Thank you ….

Brainstem Death and Organ Donation

Your role: You are the registrar in the ICU.

Problem: Brainstem death and organ donation.

Patient's name: Mr Pitter Watson, an 80-year-old man.

Relative's name: Miss Jenny Watson, daughter.

Scenario: Mr Watson was admitted to the ICU 2 days back with a large intracerebral hemorrhage. The CT scan has shown extensive hemorrhage with midline shift. He was intubated on arrival in the A/E, started on intravenous propofol, and transferred to the intensive care unit. Sedation was stopped 36 hours ago. The neurosurgeons, intensivists, and your consultant reviewed the patient and felt that the prognosis was extremely poor and that neurosurgical intervention would be inappropriate. Since stopping sedation, the patient has shown no neurological response, and now he has been confirmed brainstem dead by two consultants. Now, he is in sinus rhythm, is normotensive, and a ventilator supports his respiration. The daughter has been informed of the poor prognosis and has been told that special "brain testing" is being performed. She is now waiting for an update.

Your task: You don't need to discuss the brainstem testing details but sensitively approach the idea of organ donation.

Introduction, Permission, and Confirmation of the Agenda

Candidate: Hello, Jenny, I am Mohammad Ali, one of the working doctors here today. I am here to talk to you about Mr Pitter Watson, can I just confirm your relationship with him first?

Relative: He is my father.

Candidate: Ok. Are you on your own today? Do you want to call anyone from the family in our discussion today?

Relative: No.

Check Understanding

Candidate: Jenny, I am at this time looking after your father in the ICU. It would be helpful if you just could tell me what's happening so far?

Relative: I was not at home at that time. My father fell down the stairs and then somehow the neighbors noticed and brought him to the hospital. After calling me, I went straight to the hospital. The doctors said that my father had a brain hemorrhage. His condition is also very critical. I'm so worried about my dad; I just think if I hadn't left him alone at home, this accident wouldn't happen.

Breaking the Bad News

Candidate: I know how difficult time it is for you, but I am afraid, I don't have any good news for you.

Relative: What do you mean, Doctor?

Candidate: Unfortunately, Mr Watson has shown no signs of improvement, and there have been no indications at all that he will recover consciousness.

As a result of the brain hemorrhage, Mr Watson has suffered irreversible brain damage. The brain cells cannot be replaced once damaged, so these cells will not recover; thus, your father will never wake up.

I am sorry to say that he is now brainstem dead, as confirmed by two experienced consultants. This means that he is technically or legally dead.

Relative: Doctor .... How is it possible? Surely he can't be dead—his heart is still beating, and he is breathing, right?

Candidate: I am sorry to tell you that your father depends on the machine to do the breathing for him, and this would instantly cease to function if the machine is stopped, and his heart would stop soon after. Thus, your father's heart and lungs are being artificially maintained, and that brainstem death equates with the death of an individual.

Therefore, the next appropriate step is to stop the artificial ventilation. I must say that this is not to cause your father to die, but he is already technically dead, so continuing ventilation will not bring him back.
(Take a pause, give some time to react and respond empathically according to the relative's reaction)

One thing I would like to discuss with you, I know it's a difficult topic to talk about, and it's really awful, but we are obliged to talk to relatives about the possibility of organ donation. Do you think that you can talk about this at the moment?

Relative: Oh! It's really hard for me! ....

Candidate: Jenny, I am really sorry to give you such horrible news, I can hardly imagine what you are going through, as your father has died and there has been no damage to the other organs, it is common in such situations for the family to be approached about the concept of organ donation. Would that be okay if I ask you some questions about your father?

Was your father a kind person? Did he love to help other people? Did he mention anything about organ donation before?

Relative: Yes, he was a very kind person. But he didn't mention anything like that before!

Candidate: I know this is very difficult for you to talk about at the moment. I just want to tell you that your father's kidney can help another person to have a near-normal life. Many people having kidney damage are dependent on a dialysis machine, and they are not leading a normal life, they are struggling, and there is a very long waiting list for organ donation. (If he is holding an organ donation card—"This was the wish of your father, he was looking behind life to helping other sick people. Do you want to fulfill the last wish of your beloved father?")

What do you think about it? Do the family members have any strong feelings? Are there any religious obstacles?

Relative: Doctor, I can't understand anything right now. This news comes as a real shock for me!

Candidate: I can understand your situation ...

Relative: How long will he have after you turn off the breathing machine?

Candidate: I am afraid ... He may die within minutes ...

Relative: If we agree to go ahead with the transplantation, will that delay his funeral? Will his body become disfigured?

Candidate: If you and your family agree to organ transplantation, the ventilation will continue until the organs are retrieved. Once done, ventilation would be withdrawn after that you can take him for funeral .... Moreover, I want to assure you that he will not suffer any distress or pain as your father is brainstem dead.

Our experienced organ transplantation team will make a small clean cut and take the organs, and the wound will be closed cleanly, and he will be dressed carefully, his dignity will be respected throughout the procedure.

So, Miss Watson .... What do you think? Do you agree with this donation?

Relative: I need some time to sink in all the things. Please give me some time and also, I need to inform my family.

Candidate: Definitely, please take your time and inform your family. I will speak to the transplant team, who then may/will talk to you.

For donation, there will be routine microbiological screening tests, e.g., for hepatitis B and C, and I would like to ask you about his past medical health to make sure there are no contraindications.

So, had he any history of cancer? Or any history of long-term diseases?

Relative: No ....

Candidate: I know this is a hard time for you ... you can take your time to think about this donation, but if you have other family members who would like to talk to me or one of my colleagues or if you would like a further chat later in the day, that's absolutely fine ...

Is there anything that I haven't explained to you properly? Do you have any other questions or concerns?

Relative: No.

Thank you ....

Hospital Postmortem

Your role: You are the doctor in the neurology ward.

Problem: Request for hospital postmortem.

Patient's name: Mr Tan Palmer, a 65-year-old man.

Relative's name: Mrs Angela Bowman, patient's daughter.

Scenario: The patient was admitted with an infective COPD exacerbation with type-2 respiratory failure 7 days ago. He was known case of chronic kidney disease (CKD) and old MI, and he was a heavy smoker and used to smoke 30 cigarettes a day. He was treated with IV antibiotics and NIV. He was improving but still poorly. Last evening, he suddenly collapsed in the toilet and, unfortunately, died despite attempts of resuscitation. After that, you review his X-rays, and you have a suspicion that he may have a left lung carcinoma behind the heart, which was somehow missed by the team. You informed your consultant, and he suggests asking for the next of kin's permission for a hospital postmortem to decide if the patient died from a pulmonary embolism and whether he had a lung carcinoma. If the patient's family refuses the postmortem, you or your consultant will be happy to issue a death certificate.

Your task: You have to ask the next of kin, Mrs Bowman, for permission to arrange a hospital postmortem.

Introduction, Permission, and Confirmation of the Agenda

Candidate: Hello, Mrs Bowman. I am Mohammad Ali, one of the working doctors here today. I am here to talk to you about Mr Palmer, can I just confirm your relationship with him first?

Relative: He is my father.

Candidate: And are you the next of kin of Mr Palmer?

Relative: Yes, I am.

Candidate: Would you like anyone to be with you in our discussion today?

Relative: No.

Check Understanding

Candidate: Mrs Bowman .... I am really sorry to hear about the sudden death of your father.

(Pause ...)

It is a huge loss, and the news saddens all the staff looking after him and me.

(Pause to allow Mrs Bowman to express her emotions)

Tell Her about his Condition

He was very sick when he came in with a lung infection, and despite the appropriate management, he continued to remain poorly. We were all beside him, we were taking care of him, but suddenly something strange happened, he had another chest pain, we gave him medications, and we did life-saving manoeuvers for him, but unfortunately, he didn't respond to our manoeuvers.

Relative: My dad was improving, I met him, and he talked to me last afternoon ... after that, all of this happened; I was really in shock when I was told that my father suddenly collapsed and he is no more. It is really shocking, surprising! Why did it happen?

Explain Your Suspicions and Request the Postmortem

Candidate: The suddenness of his death surprised us also. He may have had a clot in his lung, but I am also concerned he may have had lung cancer–although we are not sure on either point.

Relative: Doctor ... Everyone has told me my father had something like a bad infection in his lung and died because of it—why are you suddenly thinking of something else now?

Candidate: We reviewed his X-rays, and have a suspicion that he may have a left lung cancer behind the heart, which was somehow missed by the team. Actually, this does not always obvious on the chest X-ray, especially when it is behind the heart shadow. Maybe that's the reason we missed it. The only way of knowing exactly what may have caused the sudden deterioration is a postmortem.

How do you feel about this? Have you heard about a postmortem?

Relative: Postmortem? How will you do it?

Explain the Procedure

Candidate: An experienced pathologist with the help of a technician will do it in an examination room that looks similar to an operation theatre. The examination room is licensed and inspected by the Human Tissue Authority (HTA).

There are two parts—the external and the internal examination. Externally, they will look at the body more closely. They may do some imaging such as an X-ray, CT scan or MRI. In an internal examination, the person's body is opened, and the organs are removed for examination.

A diagnosis can sometimes be made by looking at the organs. However, some organs may need to be examined in close detail while a postmortem and these investigations can take several weeks to complete.

After the postmortem has been completed, the pathologist will return the organs to the body and stitch the body. Sometimes, they need to keep the organ in the laboratory for examination. In this case, we will close the cut so you can take the body for the funeral. Then, of course, the organs can be given to you later, but I assure you no organ will be missing if you deny that.

Sometimes additional tests such as genetic testing may also be done.

Relative: Doctor, it's a really complicated procedure and even will take a longer time. Why do you want to do this?

Benefits of a Postmortem

Candidate: That's a valid question. Let me explain why this is important—it could be something that may run in the family, a disease or a condition that the family doesn't know about; we don't want any family member to suffer the same situation. It is important to be sure that he has withheld no treatment could have saved him, and this will give the team further experience, which will help them in any similar situations. It also helps the families deal better with bereavement when they know the cause of death.

Relative: What will happen to my father's body if you do the postmortem? This is already a tough time for the family—I just want to get on with the funeral arrangements without any delay.

Candidate: I assure you his dignity will be maintained throughout the procedure, and after the procedure, he will be dressed cleanly with no wounds visible on the day of the funeral, there will be no delay in the funeral, and I will sign the death certificate for you. So ... Mrs Bowman, what do you think about it?

Relative: I am feeling so uneasy about this procedure, doctor .... It sounds horrible ...! My father's whole body will be cut off !!! It would be tough for me ....

Candidate: I appreciate your feelings, Mrs Bowman .... If you feel uneasy about a full postmortem and if you prefer, then we can go for a limited postmortem of the chest only; that will also be helpful.

I also want to inform you that if they find anything suspicious, like lung cancer, unless there is a specific objection, this organ may be kept to confirm the diagnosis and possibly be used for educational or research purposes. If you have any objection, another option is for the tissue of interest to be fixed, examined, and returned to the body before release. I can assure you again that organs would not be kept.

Moreover, if you wish, you can get the postmortem results as they are sent to the consultant looking after your father, and I can arrange an appointment with him to explain the findings.

(If she refuses the whole thing; thank her and assure her that the procedure is not going to be carried on) Ok, Mrs Bowman …. I respect this decision wholeheartedly and will issue a death certificate straight away, and I am going to write on the certificate about cause of death, i.e.,

A. Lung failure (respiratory failure)
B. Lung infection
C. Chronic lung disease (chronic obstructive pulmonary disease)
D. Kidney failure
E. Disease was due to blocking of the heart vessels (myocardial infarction).

(If she agrees, sign the agreement form and arrange an appointment for her with the consultant to discuss the results of the postmortem) Ok, then I am going to arrange the necessary documents, which need to be signed. I will inform my consultant, and arrange a meeting with you to discuss the postmortem report.

Do you have any other concerns?

Thank you …

Coroner's Postmortem

Your role: You are the doctor in the neurology ward.

Problem: Request for Coroner's postmortem.

Patient's name: Mr Park Waller, a 41-year-old man.

Relative's name: Mrs Jenny Waller, patient's wife.

Scenario: Mr Park Waller was a married 41-year-old young businessman in reported good health previously. He was developed severe abdominal pain, profuse bloody diarrhea, nausea, and vomiting since he attributed it to "food poisoning" from the "bad" potato salad he had eaten the day before. He was admitted to the ward this morning, and after evaluation, it was suspected as a case of homicidal unknown poisoning. He was treated with IV fluids and antibiotics, and the necessary investigations were sent, but the patient became profoundly short of breath and had a generalized seizure, followed by cardiopulmonary arrest and unfortunately died. Since it is suspected as a homicidal poisoning and not knowing how or why Mr Waller died or by whom he was given poison, it is now a police case and an inquest and a coroner's postmortem need to be carried out.

Your task: You have to explain to Mrs Waller with empathy and talk about the need for a coroner's postmortem and what it will mean for the family.

Introduction, Permission, and Confirmation of the Agenda

Candidate: Hello, Mrs Jenny Waller. I am Mohammad Ali, one of the working doctors here today. I am here to talk to you about Mr Park Waller, can I just confirm your relationship with him first?

Relative: He is my husband.

Candidate: Ok. Are you on your own today? Do you want to call anyone from the family in our discussion today?

Relative: No.

Check Understanding

Candidate: Mrs Waller ... I am really sorry to hear about the sudden death of your husband ...

Pause ...

Relative: Hm ...

Candidate: The news saddened all the staff and me looking after him.
(Pause to allow Mrs Waller to express her emotions)
   Mrs Waller, may I ask, what actually happened to Mr Waller? Do you have any thoughts in your mind about his sudden death?

Relative: My husband was completely healthy. Yesterday, he came home from work, drank tea with me and talked for a while. Then he suddenly got a call from his friend and requested him to leave. Around 7.30, he returned to the house and said that he was feeling unwell, then he vomited several times and got very sick. I called the hospital and took him to the hospital by ambulance. The doctor's interrogation revealed that he had eaten something poisonous. My husband died within a few hours! I am really in shock.

Candidate: I am really sorry to hear all about him. We are also in shock. Mr Waller came to us with severe abdominal pain, vomiting, and bloody stool, we immediately started the treatment, but he collapsed and lost consciousness straight away.
   We tried to save his life by doing some life-saving measures, but he didn't respond to our maneuverers and unfortunately, he died.

Explain Your Suspicions and Inform Her about the Decision Taken for Postmortem

(Be prepared to give her enough time to express her grief as the loss of her husband in such a tragic way may not necessarily have sunk in. You should be prepared for anything in such a situation, as no particular reaction can be predicted. None of us knows how we would react in such an awful situation, so do not take it personally and accept the fact. The patient's relative might say, "My husband died due to this nasty procedure in your hospital. You killed my husband. What have you done! I want to make a complaint; I will sue you!" Prepare yourself to deal this with patience.

Relative: I know, the doctors did everything.

Candidate: Actually, we are not sure about what happened, and we need to talk to you before you can have the funeral for your husband. I want to ask you if you have already been spoken to the police or other hospital staff concerning the procedure of dealing with your husband's death?

Take a pause ... and give some time to express her feelings ...

Relative: I can't believe now that my husband is dead! I did not speak to the police or anyone else.

Candidate: I know this is a tough time for you, but I am sorry to tell you that Mr Park's case is now being considered as homicidal poisoning, and it will be referred to the police and the criminal justice system for further inquiry.

Relative: No doctor ... We just want to bury my husband, and you can't stop us.

Candidate: I realize that what I say now is likely to be upsetting, but it is important because it is not clear at this stage exactly what happened to Mr Park. Therefore, a coroner's postmortem (PM) examination of the body will need to be carried out.

Unfortunately, this is the only way to get a death certificate, and only the coroner will sign the death certificate to take him for the funeral.

I want to inform you how and what is involved in a postmortem. Have you ever heard about it?

Relative: I heard, not know much actually, but why do you want to do this? My husband is dead already, isn't it enough thing for us?

Explain the Procedure of the Coroner Postmortem

Candidate: Mrs Waller, I can hardly imagine what you are going through and right now you are not in a state of thinking anything. However, it will help the police investigation and enable justice to be sought for your husband's death.

An independent officer responsible for the legal investigation of death with the help of an experienced pathologist and a technician will make a small clean cut in your husband's body and examine the organs of suspicion. After the procedure, he will be dressed cleanly. No scar will be visible on a funeral day. After the procedure is done, a representative from the coroner's office will contact you to discuss the outcomes and sign for you the death certificate.

Relative: We don't want anything like this for my husband's body. We have the right to say "NO."

Candidate: I can understand your situation. If I were in your place, I would do the same. As because there is criminal activity here, the case has to go to the coroner, and a coroner's postmortem will have to be carried out. Therefore, the family has no right to object.

Take a pause ...

Relative: Doctor ... I won't let you steal my husband's organs.

Candidate: I know you are hurt now, but unfortunately, the pathologist may need to retain some of Mr Park's organs or tissues for further tests or until the criminal investigation is complete. Once the retained organs or tissues are no longer required, these may be returned to the family if requested or disposed of by burial or cremation.

Relative: Doctor ... give us his death certificate, and I just want to get on with the funeral arrangements without any delay.

Candidate: I am sorry it's out of my hands. I can't sign the death certificate, and only the coroner can sign it.

I assure you the coroner's postmortem examination usually takes place without delay, and after the procedure, he will be dressed cleanly with no wounds visible on the day of the funeral.

A coroner's officer and a police family liaison officer will inform you about the situation and offer advice.

Thank you for your patience (even if you don't think she has been patience), and are there anything else you would like to talk about or do you have any questions about the matters discussed?

Relative: No.

Candidate: Mrs Waller, I can understand that you may want to talk about this with your other family members and that I can give you some time to do it.

Please let us know if you need any help to inform your family. Moreover, I can arrange another meeting later on.

Thank you.

Index

Page numbers followed by '*f*' figure.

A

ABCDE manner 331
Abdomen 157
  examination of 77
  inspect 195
Abdominal bloating 183
  analyze 183
Abdominal malignancy 266
Abdominal scar 30*f*
Abduct thumb 312
Abstinence 274
Acanthosis nigricans 265
Accessory nerve, XI 320
Accident and emergency
   department 467
Accommodation reflex 318
Acetylcholine receptor 139
Achilles tendinitis 62
Acid-fast bacilli 172, 284
Acknowledgment technique 373
Acquired immunodeficiency
   syndrome, related illnesses 444
Acromegaly 15, 16*f*, 47
  analyze complaint 47
  discussion with examiner 50
  etiology 48
  focused examination 49
Adalimumab 306
Addison's crisis 388
Addison's disease 4, 52, 55, 387
  analyze symptoms 52
  causes 387
  drug interaction with steroids
     388
  focused history 52
  important targeted histories 53
  medic alert bracelet and
     carrying a letter 389
  self-help group website 389
  social history 389

special circumstances 388
treatment 388
Adenocarcinoma, case of 254
Adrenal insufficiency 55
  acute 55
Airway obstructions, large 251
Alcohol
  consumption, chronic 274
  drinker, counseling of 403
  excess 334
  free period 274
  intake, reducing 378
Alcoholic
  anonymous 274
  hepatitis 273
  liver disease 272, 277, 278
Alkaline phosphatase 278, 281
  raised 253
Allergic bronchopulmonary
   aspergillosis 172
Alopecia areata 4, 4*f*
Alpha-1 antitrypsin deficiency 269,
   280
Alzheimer's disease 24, 480
Ameobiasis 296
Amifampridine 139
Amiodarone 36, 52, 328
  facies 10, 10*f*
  pigmentation 231
Amlodipine 189
Amoxicillin 249
Amylase 304
Amyloidosis 85, 265
Analgesics 73
Anaplastic large 255
Anemia 155, 217, 394
  risk of 37
Angela 160
Angioedema 14, 14*f*
Angiotensin II receptor blockers
   105

Angiotensin-converting enzyme
   inhibitors 105
Angular stomatitis 266
Ankle clonus 315
Ankylosing spondylitis 60
Antibacterial cream 451
Anticancer drugs 328
Anticoagulation
  counseling for 456
  long-term 219
Anti-double stranded
   deoxyribonucleic acid 73
Antimuscarinic 353
Anti-muscle-specific kinase 362
Anti-myelin-associated
   glycoprotein 335
Antineuronal-Ab 330
Antinuclear antibodies 73, 236
Antiparkinsonism drugs 321
Antiretroviral medicines 445
  highly active 444
Antiseptic liquid 194, 264, 314
Antitachycardia pacing 226
Antithyroid drugs 36
Antithyroid peroxidase antibody
   36
Antiviral therapy 270
Aorta, coarctation of 194
Aortic area 211
Aortic coarctation 222
Aortic dissection 149
Aortic regurgitation 61, 194, 200
  evidence of 150
Aortic stenosis 198
Aortic valve replacement 149, 194,
   456
Apex loudest in expiration 207
APLA syndrome 147
Appetite, loss of 284
Argyll-Robertson pupil 201
Arm's length away 323

Arnold–Chiari malformation 323, 325
Arrhythmias 211, 279
Arsenicosis 25, 25f
Arterial blood gas 172
   sampling 244
Arterial dorsalis pedis 58
Arthralgia 278
Arthrodesis 80
Ascites 283
Aspergillus serology 172
Aspergillus species 241
Assess soft palate and uvula 320
Asthma, follow-up of 469
Ataxic gait 321
   broad-based 365
Ataxic nystagmus 325
Athlete's foot 18
Atrial fibrillation 127
   analyze symptoms 127
   differential diagnoses of 127
   evidence of 341
   focused examination 128
   increases risk of stroke 456
Atrial flutter 221
Atrial septal defect 220
Atrioventricular node re-entrant tachycardia 127
Autoantibody 55
Autoimmune arthritis 78
Autoimmune cause 36
Autoimmune disease 164, 240, 269
Autoimmune disorders 4
Autoimmune hemolytic 290
Autoimmune hepatitis 265, 269, 270, 272, 277
Autoimmune screening 306
Autonomy 374
Autosomal dominant disorder 55, 360, 454
Autosomal dominant polycystic kidney disease 292
Axilla, examine 265
Azathioprine 73, 155, 306

B

Baby hippopotamus 347
Back pain 65
   focused history 65
Bacteria, millions of 448

Bacterial peritonitis, secondary 284
Balanitis 161
Basal honeycombing 238
Becker's muscular dystrophy 8, 9f, 9
Beclomethasone 247
Bedside clues 264, 310, 314
Belimumab 73
Benedikt syndrome 324
Benzodiazepine 274
Benzylpenicillin 151
Beta agonists, short-acting 252
Beta-blockers 130, 135, 206, 363
Beta-interferon 353
Bibasal crepitations 204
Bicuspid aortic valve 201
Biliary cholangitis, primary 280
Biliary cirrhosis, primary 272, 277
Blood escaping 487
Blood loss (chronic), evidence of 7f
Blood pressure 346
   causes of uncontrolled 403
Blood sugar 50
   control of 458
   random 172
Blood transfusion, offer 438
Blue sclera 18, 210
   and dentinogenesis imperfecta 18f
Body language 373
Body mass index 264
Bone marrow suppression 155
Boutonniere's deformity 82, 231
Bowel cancer 185
Bowel, colonoscopy 415
Bradykinesia 364
Bradykinin-mediated angioedema 14
Brain injury 307
Brain's maestro 487
Brainstem
   dead 489, 490
   testing 486
   demyelination 324
   infarction 324
   sign 324
   stroke 97
Breaking bad news 406
Breaking confidentiality 374

Breath, shortness of 53
Breathing machine 478, 480, 487
Breathing test 400
Breathlessness 276
Bronchial asthma 251
Bronchial obstruction 240
Bronchiectasis 231, 239
   bilateral 250
   causes of 240
Bronchiolitis obliterans 85, 237
Bronchiolitis obliterans syndrome 260
Bronchogenic carcinoma 231
Brown–Séquard syndrome 352
Budd–Chiari syndrome 269, 283
Bulbar palsy 356
Bulbar, presence of 344
Bullectomy 248
Bullous pemphigoid 7, 7f
Burkholderia cepacia 241

C

Cachexia 231
Café-au-lait spots 6
Caffeine 145
Calcium channel blockers 363
Calgary Cambridge framework 2
Cancer, delayed diagnosis of 414
Cancer withhold 471
   check understanding 471
Capacity, lack of 466
Capillary dilatation 71
Caplan's syndrome 237
Capsule endoscopy 166
Carcinoid syndrome 276
Card test 312
Cardiac
   catheterization 221, 224
   cause 38
   examination 81
   failure 269
   resynchronization therapy 226
   surgery 191
Cardiology case presentation 197
Cardiomyopathy 278, 279
Cardiopulmonary resuscitation 480, 484
   explain 484
Cardiorespiratory examination 150

Cardiovascular disease 310
Cardiovascular system 207
  examination 194, 198, 210, 212, 214, 216, 278
Carotid bruit 146
Carotid dissection 144
Carpal tunnel scar 265
Carpal tunnel syndrome 8, 32, 48, 50
CD4 T-cell count 445
Coeliac disease 164, 266, 393
  diagnosis of 393
Cell carcinoma, large 254
Cell lymphoma kinase 255
Central chest pain 467
Central nervous system 71, 347
Central scotoma 326
Cerebellar ataxia 350
Cerebellar disorder 310, 314, 322, 349
Cerebellar lesion 319
Cerebellar nystagmus 325
Cerebellar sign 280, 365
Cerebellar syndrome 350
Cerebellum 311
Cerebral aneurysms 292
Cerebral artery, middle 347
Cerebral autosomal dominant arteriopathy 144
Cerebral palsy 307, 335, 347
Cerebral vascular accident 326
Cerebrospinal fluid 331
Cerebrovascular disease 346
Cervical lymphadenopathy 266
Cervical myelopathy 341, 344
Cervical rib 338
  bilateral 338
Cervical spondyloradiculopathy 338
Charcot–Marie–Tooth 336, 337
  disease 311, 336, 338
  genetic studies 336
  phenotype 337
Chest
  asymmetry 232
  auscultation of 233
  drains 230
  examination 81
  pain 214
  percussion of 232

scars 30, 31*f*
wall deformities 196
Chlamydia 162
Chlamydia pneumoniae 250
Chlamydia spp. 245
Chlordiazepoxide 274
Chlorhexidine 451
Chloroquine 328
Chlorpromazine 365
Cholinergic crisis 363
Cholinesterase inhibitor, role of 139
Chorea 368, 453
Choreoathetosis 311
Chronic obstructive pulmonary disease 118, 246
  analyze symptoms 118
  focused history 118
  moderate 399
Churg–Strauss syndrome 335
Chylous ascites, case of 285
Cirrhosis 279
Clarithromycin 249
Claw hand 338
Clinical consultation station 2
Clinical examination skills, practical assessment of 2
Closing session 3
Clostridium 448
Clostridium difficile 447
Clostridium difficile toxin 166
Clubbing 20, 21*f*
Cognitive behavior therapy 274, 462
Cognitive function 364
Cold exposure 77
Collapsing pulse 246
Color Doppler echocardiography 218
Combined ulnar and median nerve lesion 338
Comfortable versus tachypnea 230
Communication and ethics 372
Complete blood count 172
Complex ophthalmoplegia 324
  left-sided 324
Compound muscle action potential 329
Compressive lesion 324
Computed tomography pulmonary angiography 73

Computed tomography, high-resolution 171, 236
Concomitant coronary artery disease 216
Confidentiality 374
Congestive cardiac failure 131, 276
  analyze complaint 131
  focused examination 133
  focused history 131
Congruous homonymous hemianopia 326
Connective tissue disease 74, 231, 324, 328
  evidence of 201
Consciousness, level of 271
Consensual pupillary reflex 318
Consent form, signing 374
Consolidation 253
Constrictive pericarditis 269
  chronic 276
Continuous positive airway pressure 230
Conventional bradycardia pacemaker 226
Copious respiratory secretion 250
Cord compression 342
Corneal arcus 195
Coronary angiogram 207, 415
Coronary artery bypass graft 135, 194
  coexistent 216
Coronavirus 245
Coroner's postmortem 495
  explain procedure of 496
Cor-pulmonale 249, 250
Corrigan sign 195
Corticospinal tract 311
Corticosteroids 73
Coxiella spp. 245
Cranial nerve 96, 319
  examination of 317
Craniopharyngioma 325
Creatine phosphokinase 139
Crigler–Najjar syndrome 272
Crockery 368
Crohn's disease 163, 164, 266
  analyze symptom 163
  diagnosis 165
  differential diagnoses 163
  focused history 163

Cullen's sign 267
Cushing syndrome 32, 43
   analyze symptoms 43
   focused examination 45
   focused history 43
Cushingoid face 15*f*
Cushingoid feature 157
Cyclophosphamide 73
Cyclosporin 155
Cystic fibrosis 231, 242, 243
   related diabetes 243
Cytomegalovirus 245, 340
   retinitis 29*f*

D

Damaging airways 171
Deep vein thrombosis 24, 24*f*, 25, 348
   differential diagnosis 24
   sign of 233
Deep-seated infections 190
Deformity polyarthritis 281
Degenerative disorders 356
Delirium tremens 274
Dementia 417, 419
   cause 453
   social history 419
Demyelination 341
Deoxyribonucleic acid, double-stranded 369
Dermal-epidermal junction 73
Dermatitis herpetiformis 164, 184
Dermatomyositis 9*f*
   associated 77
Des-gamma-carboxy prothrombin 281
Diabetes mellitus 324
   control and prevent 459
   sign of 240
Diabetic foot 17, 17*f*, 56
   focused examination 58
   focused history 56
   quick systemic review 57
Diabetic maculopathy 105
Diabetic retinopathy 26, 26*f*
Diarrhea in hospital, outbreak of 447
Diffuse cutaneous systemic sclerosis 15
Diffuse parenchymal lung disease 8

Digoxin 135, 206
Dilated cardiomyopathy 279
Dilated pulmonary arteries 215
Dilated vein 267
Diplopia 94
   analyze symptoms 94
   focused history 94
Direct light reflex 318
Direct skin-to-skin contact 451
Disease-modifying antirheumatic drugs 83, 376
Disequilibrium, examination for 321
Distal myopathy 332
Dive-bomber potentials 359
Dorsal column 352
Dorsal column sign 341
   evidence of 341
Dorsiflexion 315
Dorsum of hands, examine 265
Down syndrome 24, 24*f*, 194, 210, 220, 294
Doxycycline 249
Driving issue 375
Drug-induced side-effect 155
Duloxetine 329
Dupuytren's contracture 22*f*, 265, 278, 280
Dysdiadochokinesia 312
Dysesthesia 329
Dyslipidemia 146
Dystonia 311

E

Ecchymosis 195
Ectopic adrenocorticotropic hormone 253
Educate patient 372
Edward syndrome 294
Ehlers–Danlos syndrome 19, 19*f*, 201, 210
Eisenmenger syndrome 221
Ejection systolic murmur 211, 220
Electrical impulse, abnormal 397
Electroencephalogram 396
Embolic phenomenon 211
Emotion
   explore 406, 408
   validate 406
Empathetic response 406

Empathy 372
   and sympathy 396
Emphysema 277
   with smoking cessation 399
Empyema 230
Encephalitis lethargica 365
End of life decision 483
Endocrine cause 52
Endocrine neoplasia, multiple 49
Endothelin receptor antagonist 78
End-stage liver disease 271
Enophthalmos 324
Enoxaparin 456, 457
Epidermal growth factor receptor 255
Epididymitis 161
Erythema 232
Erythrocyte sedimentation rate 328
Ethical issues, principles of 374
   autonomy 374
   beneficence 374
   justice 374
Excoriations 265
Exercising regularly 378
Explanation and planning 3
Extra-articular manifestations, detect 80
Extractable nuclear antigens 73
Eye
   contact 373
   examination of 40, 92, 323
   movement 40, 319, 323
Eye-opener-tolerance withdrawal 404

F

Fabry's disease 205
Facial nerve 320
Facial nerve palsy 16, 17*f*, 310
Facilitation technique 373
Fasciculation 310, 311
Fatigability 332
   test 138
Fat-soluble vitamin 282, 303
Felty's syndrome 83, 265, 288, 289
Fibrosis 241
   score 277
Fine needle aspiration cytology
   guided 172
   test 36

Firdapse 139
Flame-shaped hemorrhage 26
Flapping tremor 246
Fluticasone 247
Folate deficiency 266
Foot, vascular examination of 58
Foreign body 251
Foster–Kennedy syndrome 27, 27f, 93
Friedreich's ataxia 93, 311, 341, 345
Fundoscopy 26, 40, 92, 319
Furosemide 151, 206

G

Gabapentin for neuropathic pain 353
Gait, examine 321
Gamma-aminobutyric acid 274
Gamma-glutamyl transferase 281
Gastrointestinal tract 5, 14
  examination 264
Gathering information 2
Genetic counseling 453
Genetic disorder 453
Genetic test 278, 454
Geniculate ganglion 326
Genitalia, external 161
Gentamicin 363
Gilbert's syndrome 272
Glatiramer acetate 353
Glaucoma 27, 28f
Glossitis 266
Glycopyrronium 247
Golden minutes 376
Gonorrhea 162
Gout 86
  analyze symptoms 90
  examination 88
  focused examination 92
  focused history 86, 90
Gram staining 172
Granulomatous disease 325
Graves ophthalmopathy 325
Graves' disease 38, 40
  focused examination 40
  focused history 38
  quick systemic review 39
Graves' ophthalmopathy 39, 102
Grey turner sign 267

Gridiran incision 29
Gross hearing testing 320
Guillain–Barré syndrome 327
Gum hypertrophy 266
Gynecomastia 266

H

Haemophilus influenzae 291
Hamman-Rich syndrome 236
Hand 77, 195
  and nail 71
  close inspection of 231
  pain, differential diagnosis of 32
Headache 103, 173, 445, 462
  analyze complaint 173
  relevant family history 175
  social history 175
  treatment history 175
Heart attack 415
Heart block 362
Heart disease 274
Heart failure 77
  management of 209
  treatment of 151, 198, 206
Heart sound 196
  first 204, 207
  second 204, 207
Heart-starting machines 481
Heel-Shin test 315, 334
Heliotrope rash 77
Hematological malignancy, features of 266
Hemiplegic migraine 144, 146
Hemochromatosis 269, 270
  features of 273
Hemolytic anemia 272, 290
  chronic 266
  secondary 290
Hemophilus influenzae 241
Hemoptysis 25, 168
  analyze complaint 168
  detailed history 168
  past medical and surgical history 170
  treatment history 170
Heparin 456, 457
Hepatic arteriovenous malformations 273
Hepatic bruit 273
Hepatic carcinoma 273

Hepatic encephalopathy 271
  signs of 273
Hepatic hemangioma 273
Hepatocellular 272
  carcinoma 270, 272
Hepatocyte injury 272
Hepatojugular reflux 196
Hepatomegaly 22f
Hepatorenal syndrome 272
Hepatosplenomegaly 265, 286
Hereditary hemochromatosis 272, 278
Hereditary hemorrhagic telangiectasia 6, 7f
Hereditary neuropathy 329
Hereditary spastic paraparesis 341
  case of 341
Hereditary spherocytosis 290, 291
Herpes zoster rash 16
  in-ears 317
Hickman line 430
  explaining disease 430
  social history 431
High steeping gait 321
Histamine-mediated angioedema 14
Hoffman's sign 312
Holter-monitoring 129
Homonymous hemianopia 326
Horner's syndrome 23, 23f, 120, 231, 323, 324
Hospital postmortem 492
  benefits of 493
  explain procedure 493
Hospital superbug-1 447
Hospital superbug-2 450
  social history 452
Hot joint, acute 17, 18f
Human immunodeficiency virus 53, 172, 340
  drug interaction 445
  early diagnosis 444
  effective treatments 444
  investigations 444
  newly diagnosed 443
  related illnesses 444
  side effects of medicine 445
  social circumstances 445
  symptoms of 444
Human T-lymphotropic virus type 1 340

Huntington's disease 367, 453
　case of 369
　cure for 454
Hydralazine 135
Hydrocortisone 249, 252
Hydronephrosis 294
Hydroxychloroquine 80
Hypercholesterolemia 36
Hyperglycemia 368
Hypertension 292
　control of 130
Hypertensive retinopathy 26, 26f
Hyperthyroidism 4
Hypertonia 315
Hypertonic saline 243
Hypertrophic cardiomyopathy 214
Hypertrophic obstructive
　　cardiomyopathy 198
Hyperuricemia-induced gout 288
Hypoglossal nerves, XII 320
Hypomimia 364
Hypophonia 364
Hypoproteinemia 279
Hypothyroidism 32, 37, 334
　focus history 33
　focused examination 35
　referral 32
　relevant family history 34
　treatment history 34
Hypotonia 311, 315
Hypoventilation disorder 250

I

Ice pack test 362
Idiopathic epilepsy 397
Idiopathic Parkinson's disease,
　diagnosis of 364
Idiopathic pulmonary fibrosis 236
Idiopathic thrombocytopenic
　purpura 265
Ileostom 267
Iliac fossa, left 267
Illegal drugs 375
Immotile cilia syndrome 240
Immune deficiency 266
Immune suppression,
　complications of 261
Immune-mediated neuropathies
　335
Immunoglobulin level 240

Immunosuppressant medications
　475
Immunosuppressants 73
　issue of 476
　side effects of 382
　social history 383
Impaired sensation, evidence of
　351
Implantable cardioverter
　defibrillator 135, 194
Implantable device treatment
　options 227
Indomethacin 80
Infection, chronic 52
Infective endocarditis 190, 290
　confirming 190
　signs of 212
　stigmata of 216
Inflammatory bowel disease 106
Inflammatory demyelinating
　polyneuropathy, chronic 327,
　332
Inflammatory marker 147
Infliximab 306
Infraclavicular scar 196
Inhaled corticosteroid 247
Inhaler machine 230
Inherited neuropathy 327
Insomnia 445
Insulin 459
　injection site 327
Intensive care unit 486
Intensive therapy unit 478
Intercostal chest drain 427
　social history 428
Interferon therapy 36
Internal carotid artery aneurysm
　96, 324
Internuclear ophthalmoplegia 319
Interstitial lung disease 85, 230,
　235
Intestinal arteriovenous
　malformations 273
Intra-abdominal hemorrhage 307
Intracardiac device 226
Intracranial pressure, raised 48
Intravalvular hemolysis 217
Intravenous immune globulin 139,
　331
Involuntary movement 311, 368
Iron 266

Iron deficiency anemia, signs of
　7f, 7
Irritable bowel syndrome 76
Ischemic heart disease 114, 127
Isolated splenomegaly 288
Ivabradine 135

J

Janeway lesion 195, 216, 265
Jaundice 22f, 22, 217, 290
　classification of 272
　indicates malignancy 232
Jaw jerk 320
Jendrassik maneuver 312
Jerky 453
　pulse 198
Jock itch 18
Joint hypermobility 19, 210
Joint pain 178
　analyze complaint 178
　detailed history 178
　differential diagnoses 181
　treatment history 180
Joint position sense 313, 316
Jugular venous pressure 71

K

Kayser–Fleischer ring 280, 365
Kennedy's disease 354
　signs for 354
Keratoconjunctival sicca 80, 368
Kidney biopsy, preparation
　needed 421
Kidney disease, chronic 266
Kidney donation society 476
Kidney transplantation 476
Kissing ulcer 308
Klebsiella pneumoniae 241
Kocher incision 28
Koilonychia 7, 7f, 265
Kulchitsky cells 254
Kyphoscoliosis 250

L

Labial gland biopsy 335
Lambert–Eaton myasthenic
　syndrome 76, 136, 254
　analyze symptoms 136

focused examination 138
treatment history 137, 138
Laminectomy 80
Laryngeal nerve palsy, recurrent 254
Laurence-Moon-Bardet-Biedl syndrome 294
Leber's hereditary optic atrophy 90, 326
Leber's optic atrophy 93
Leflunomide 80
Leg, inspect 195
Leg lift 315
Leg roll 315
Legal issue 374, 466
Legionella 244
Legionella antigen 244
Legionella spp. 245
Lethargy, differential diagnosis of 32
Leukoencephalopathy 144
Leukoplakia 55
Lewis-Sumner syndrome 335
Lewy body dementia 365
Lichen planus 4, 5f
Lid lag 40
Lifestyle change, importance of 377
Life-threatening hypoxemia 250
Limbs 138
Limited cutaneous systemic sclerosis 15
Lip hyperplasia 266
Lipase 304
Listening skills 373
Lithium 36, 363
Live organ donation 474
  explore negativity 474
  explore procedure 475
  issue of
    assessment 475
    surgical complications and rejections 475
Livedo reticularis 147
Liver cirrhosis 279
Liver disease
  chronic 269, 271, 276
    stigmata of 327
  common cause of 278
Liver function tests 36, 172

Liver transplantation 282, 298
Lobectomy 256, 257
Loin pain 12, 293
Loop-diuretics 272
Lower limb
  examination of 314
  neurologically 336
Lower motor neuron
  lesions 311
  signs 355
Lumbar puncture 432, 434
  explain about disease 432
  explaining procedure 433
Lung biopsy scars 266
Lung cancer 253, 254
  different treatment options for 255
  histological diagnosis 254
  treatment of 254
Lung collapse 241
Lung for carbon monoxide 236, 247
Lung function test 171, 356
Lung transplant 260
  criteria 261
  indications for 260
Lung volume reduction surgery 248
Lymph node biopsy, scars of 265
Lymphadenopathy 265
Lymphadenopathy, evidence of 239
Lymphoma 108
Lymphoproliferative disorder 288, 290

M

Macrolides 363
Macular edema 105
Magnetic resonance angiography 97
Maintenance and reliever therapy 252
Malar flush 194
Malignant cell 172
Malignant hypertension 78
Malignant pleural effusion 230
Marfan syndrome 148, 194, 201, 210
  differential diagnoses 148

evidence of 150
eye examination 150
focused examination 149
McBurney's point 29
Meckel-Gruber syndrome 294
Medical error-1 464
Medical error-2 467
  make summary 468
Medical jargon 3
Medical negligence 464
Medical trial 469
  social history 470
Medic-alert bracelet 264
Medically unexplained syndrome 462
Melanocyte-stimulating hormone 55
Meningioma 96, 324
Mental state examination, mini 364
Metabolic complication 155
Metabolic syndrome 277
Metallic valve replacement 194
Methicillin-resistant *Staphylococcus aureus* 250, 450
Methotrexate 80, 379
Methyldopa 365
Meticulously 314
Metoclopramide 365
Metronidazole 306
Microstomia 77
Mid sternotomy scar 194, 196
Migraine
  headache 175
  type of 146
Miller Fisher syndrome 325, 330
Miller Fisher variant 331
Minocycline 52
Mitochondrial myopathy 325
Mitral facies 11, 11f
Mitral regurgitation 62, 207
Mitral stenosis 204
  causes of 205
Mitral valve prolapse 210
Mitral valve replacement 194
Mixed aortic valve disease 202
Mixed mitral valve disease 212
Monoclonal antibody therapies 73
Monoclonal gammopathy 329

Mononeuritis multiplex 324
Moraxella catarrhalis 250
Morquio syndrome 210
Motor 320
Motor axonal neuropathy, acute 331
Motor neuron disease 338, 354, 356
Motor sensory axonal neuropathy, acute 330
Motor sensory neuropathy 329
Motor stimulation, absent 488
Motor system examination 330
Mucopolysaccharidoses 205
Multidisciplinary team 172, 377
Multifocal acquired demyelinating sensory 335
Multifocal motor neuropathy 329, 333
Multi-system disorder 304
Mupirocin nasal ointment 451
Murmur 196
  diastolic 62
  mid-diastolic 212
  systolic 134
Muscarinic antagonist, long-acting 247
Muscle state, examine 314
Musculoskeletal system 243
Myasthenia gravis 281, 314, 332, 357
  complication of 363
  ocular 361
  thymectomy for 311
Myasthenia, worsening of 363
Mycobacterium abscessus 241
Mycobacterium tuberculosis 241
Mycophenolate mofetil 73
Mycoplasma 244
Mycoplasma pneumoniae 245
Myeloproliferative disorder 108, 288
Myocardial infarction 415
Myopathic face 317
Myotonia 310
Myotonic discharge 359
Myotonic dystrophy 323, 358
Myxedema 283
Myxedematous face 10, 10*f*
Myxedematous facies 283

N

Nail-fold capillaroscopy 78
Nails, spooning of 265
Naproxen 64
Nasal speech 361
Natalizumab 353
National Institute for Health and Care Excellence 274
  guideline 203
Nebulized salbutamol 252
Nebulizers machine 230
Neck and chest 157
Neck, examine 40
Neck for thyroid gland, examination of 35
Neck pain 462
Necrobiosis lipoidica 5, 5*f*, 327
Needle stick injury 440
  modification of lifestyle 441
  reassurance 440
Neisseria meningitis 291
Nelson syndrome 52
Nephrotic syndrome 266
Neurofibroma 338
Neurofibromatosis type-1 6, 6*f*
Neurological disorders 307, 335
Neurological examination 111, 129, 138, 146, 338, 346, 368
Neurological manifestation 280
Neurological signs 350
Neuromuscular disorders 250
Neutropenia 155
New York Heart Association 205
Nicotine replacement therapy 401
Night sweats 187
  analyze complaint 187
  detailed history 187
  quick systemic review 188
  referral 187
  treatment history 189
Nitrates, long-acting 135
Nonalcoholic fatty liver disease 273
non-Hodgkin's lymphoma 85
Nonorganic disease 461
  explain 461
  management plan 462
  social history 463
Nonsteroidal anti-inflammatory drugs 7, 64, 376

Nonverbal communication skills 373
Noonan's syndrome 194, 214
Norfloxacin 275
Nose tubes 418
Nystagmus 310, 317
  approach 325

O

Oat cell carcinoma 254
Obstructive sleep apnea 231
Oesophago-gastro-duodenoscopy procedure 435
  consent 437
  explain about symptoms 435
  indications and benefits 436
  preparation needed before 436
Ophthalmoplegia 324
  approach to 324
Optic atrophy 27, 27*f*, 90, 102, 327
Optic chiasma 325
Optic neuropathy, evidence of 353
Oral anticoagulation, evidence of 216, 218
Oral antidiabetic medications 458
Oral glucose tolerance test 50
Oral ulcer 13, 13*f*
Organ donation 489
Organ transplantation team 490
Organizing pneumonia 237
Organomegaly 329
Osler's node 195, 216
Osler–Weber–Rendu syndrome 266
Osteogenesis imperfecta 152, 201, 210
Oxybutynin 353
Oxygen therapy 485
  long-term 172

P

Painful red eye 60
Painless jaundice 407
Palmar erythema 40, 265, 327, 246
Palpate aortic area 196
Palpate pulmonary 196
Pancoast syndrome, evidence of 120
Pancoast tumor 231, 338
Pancreatic ascites 284

Pancreatic carcinoma 407
  diagnosis of 407
  social history 409
Pancreatic tumor 49
Pancreatitis, chronic 303
  examination 303
Pansystolic murmur 207, 212
Papillary muscle dysfunction 208
Papilledema 26, 26f
Paracetamol-induced acute liver failure 300
Paradoxical embolism 144
Paramedian scar 266
Paramyotonia congenita 360
Paraneoplastic 330
  neuropathy 328
  syndrome 330
Parasellar tumor 96
Parathyroid hormone-related protein 253
Parkinson plus syndromes 365
Parkinson's disease 307, 364, 365, 367
Parkinsonian 321
Parotid enlargement 278, 317
Patau syndrome 294
Patent ductus arteriosus 224
Patient Advisory Liaison Service 448
Patient with first fit 396
Peak expiratory flow monitoring 251
Pectus carinatum 231
Pectus excavatum 196
Peek sign 362
Penicillamine 363
Penicillin-allergic 151
Penis 160, 161
Percutaneous endoscopic gastrostomy 307, 374
  tube, insertion 267
    explaining procedure 425
    social history 426
Perioral puckering 77
Peripheral edema 207, 276
Peripheral motor neuropathy 338
Peripheral neuropathy 80, 327
  atypical features of 330, 334
  evidence of 58
Peripheral signs 120, 165

Peritoneal dialysis 266
Pernicious anemia 4
Peutz–Jegher's syndrome 55, 266
Phalen's sign 81
Phenothiazine 52
Phenytoin 363
Photosensitive rash 11, 11f
Physical examination 3
Physical space 372
Pink-blue mottling 71
Pinprick sensation 316
Pituitary tumor 325
Plantar extensors 365
Plantar fasciitis 62
Plasma exchange 139
Plethoric face 13f
  differential diagnosis 13
Pleural effusion 114, 253, 254
  analyze symptoms 114
  differential diagnosis 114
  focused history 114
Pneumococcal antigen 244
Pneumonectomy 256, 258
  complications of 259
Pneumonia 244
Pneumothorax, recurrent 241, 294
Polyarteritis nodosa 71
Polycystic kidney disease 201, 293, 294
Polycythemia 292
Polymyalgia rheumatica 141
Polyneuropathy 327, 329
Porphyria cutanea tarda 7, 8f
Portal hypertension, cirrhosis with 273
Positron emission tomography 254
Postencephalitis 365
Posterior cerebral artery aneurysm 324
Post-transplant lymphoproliferative disease 158, 261
Post-transplant lymphoproliferative disorder 155
  analyze symptoms 156
  focused examination 157
Pramipexole 365
Prednisolone 139, 249
Pregnancy, toxemia of 37

Preimplantation genetic testing 455
Pretibial myxedema 10, 10f
Procainamide 363
Prochlorperazine 365
Progressive back pain, differential diagnosis of 60
Progressive supranuclear palsy 364
Prolonged prothrombin time 270
Pronator drift 311
Propafenone 363
Prophylactic antibiotics 275
Prosthetic aortic valve 216, 218
Proteinuria and hematuria 244
Proximal muscle weakness 330
Pseudoathetosis 311, 351
Pseudobulbar dysarthria 344
Pseudogout 279
Pseudomonas aeruginosa 241
Pseudoxanthoma elasticum 201
Psoriasis 13, 13f, 110
  focused history 110
Ptosis
  approach to 323
  bilateral 22, 23f
    differential diagnosis 22
    improvement of 362
Pulmonary adenoma 256
Pulmonary complications 259
Pulmonary edema 251, 259
Pulmonary embolism 25, 73, 122
  analyze complaints 122
  differential diagnosis 122
  focused history 122
Pulmonary fibrosis 10, 239
Pulmonary flow, quantification of 215
Pulmonary function test 236
Pulmonary hypertension 196
  signs of 71
Pulmonary nodule 237
Pulmonary rehabilitation 121
Pulmonary stenosis 214
Pulse rate 32
Pupil 96
Pupillary light
  reflex 488
  response 92
Pupillary reflex 318

Pursuit movement 319
Pyoderma gangrenosum 106
   analyze symptoms 106
   causes of 106
   focused history 106
Pyramidal lesion 311
Pyramidal signs 364, 365

Q

Quincke's sign 195
Quinidine 363
Quinolones 363
Quit smoking helpline 402

R

Radial pulse 195
Radiation burn 231
Radiation therapy, using 288
Ramipril 138
Ramsay Hunt syndrome 16, 320
Raynaud's disease 281
Raynaud's phenomenon 71
Reactive arthritis, principal management of 182
Recombinant deoxyribonuclease 243
Red blood cells 272
Reflux pancreatitis 302
Refsum's syndrome 99
Relapsing-remitting multiple sclerosis 353
Renal biopsy 420
   explaining procedure 421
   indications and benefits 421
Renal cysts, bilateral 294
Renal function test 172
Renal replacement therapy 265
   evidence of 155, 157
Renal transplant 295, 476
   causes of 155
Renal-pancreas transplant 301
Respiratory physician 240
Respiratory system 77, 218
   examination 230, 239, 246
Respiratory ward 477
Resuscitation 484
Retinal vein occlusion 27, 28f
Retinitis pigmentosa 27, 98
   and polydactyly 29f

differential diagnosis 98
   focused history 98
Rheumatic heart disease 127, 201
Rheumatoid arthritis 32, 79, 231, 265, 381
   complications and prognosis 382
   diagnosis of 381
   lifestyle modification of 376
   related lung disease 237
   symptoms of 382
   treatment 382
Rheumatoid feet 8f, 8
Rheumatoid hand 8f, 8
Rheumatoid lung 237
Rhonchi, added sound 121, 233
Rinne's test 320
Rituximab 73
Rivaroxaban 457
Romberg test 322
Rose Bengal test 335
Rutherford Morrison's scar 266
Ruzurgi 139

S

Saccadic eye movement 319
Sacral edema, check for 197
Sarcoidosis 12, 12f, 108, 231, 325
   differential diagnosis 12
Scalp 18
Scars 29f
Schirmer's test 335
   positive 63
Sclerodactyly 265
Scleroderma 281
Scleromalacia 80
Sclerosing cholangitis, primary 277
Sclerosis, multiple 341, 349, 352, 410, 412
   diagnosis of 353, 410
Scrambled egg 28
Seeking compensation 375
Seizures confirm epilepsy, recurrent 397
Semi-conscious 374
Sensation
   assessment of four modalities of 58
   examine for 312, 316
   loss of 319

Sensory 319
   ataxia 334, 351
   nerve action potential 329
   sign 352
      absence of 355
   symptoms 350
Sepsis secondary 480
Serological testing 84, 244, 270
Serotonin-noradrenaline reuptake inhibitor 329
Serum albumin 281
Serum angiotensin converting enzyme 328
Serum ascitic albumin gradient 285
Serum bilirubin 278
Serum ferritin 270, 281
Serum glutamic oxaloacetic transaminase 281
Serum glutamic pyruvic transaminase 281, 376
Serum phytanic acid level 351
Severe systemic disease 73
Sexually transmitted infection 159, 161
   analyze symptoms 159
Sigmoiditis 183
Simple cysts, multiple 294
Single palpable kidney 294
Sjögren's syndrome 80, 264, 281, 324, 330, 335, 368
Skin biopsy 73
Slurred speech 310
Small cell carcinoma 52, 254
Smoking, stopping 378
Snip test (biopsy) 415
Sodium valproate 365
Spastic paraparesis 340
Speech 314
Spider nevi 266
Spinal cord compression 342
Spine, examination in 165
Spirometry with reversibility test 251
Spironolactone 135, 151, 206
Splenomegaly 290
   mild 288
   moderate 288
Splinter hemorrhage 150, 195, 212, 216, 265

Spontaneous bacterial peritonitis, in case of 284
Sporadic myxomatous degeneration 211
Spot diagnosis 4
Sputum pots 249
Squamous cell carcinoma 254
Staccato speech 310
Staphylococcus aureus 241, 451
Starvation 145
Steatohepatitis 273
Steroid 139
   sparing agent 73
   therapy 264
Stigmata 150
Stomas 267
Stone formation, recurrent 294
Streptococcus pneumoniae 241
Striae 267
Stroke 211, 346, 307
   mini 146
Sturge-Weber syndrome 5, 5*f*
Subcortical infarcts 144
Subpleural reticulation 238
Sudden death 211
Sulfasalazine 80
Superior venacaval obstruction 21, 21*f*
Supraclavicular lymphadenopathy 21
Suprasellar meningioma 325
Supraventricular tachycardia 127, 359
Swan neck deformity 82
Swanson's arthroplasty 81
Swinging light test 318
Sydenham's chorea 368
Syndrome of inappropriate antidiuretic hormone secretion 253
Syringobulbia 323
Syringomyelia 338
System atrophy, multiple 349
Systemic embolic risk 130
Systemic inflammatory response syndrome 164
Systemic lupus erythematosus 7, 69, 231, 324
   focused history 69
   important targeted histories 70
Systemic sclerosis 15, 15*f*, 75

T

Taboparesis 345
Tacrolimus 155
Takayasu's arteritis 201
Tar staining 195
Tardive dyskinesia 367
Telangiectasia 77, 266
Telephone receiver 368
Tenckhoff catheter 266
Tender hepatomegaly 283
Testis 161
   examine 161
Tetracyclines 363
Tetranucleotide 359
Thalassemic face 23, 23*f*
Thrombocytopenia 155, 265
Thumb
   abduction 311
   and wrist signs 151
   Z-deformity of 8, 82, 108
Thyroid acropachy 40
Thyroid disease 108
Thyroid faces 129
Thyroid gland enlargement 129
Thyroid status 40
Thyrotoxic face 11, 11*f*
Thyrotoxicosis 38, 128, 184
Tinea corporis 18, 18*f*
Tinel's signs 81
Tiotropium 247
Todd's paresis 144, 145, 347
Tone, examine 311, 314
Tongue 266
   muscles 361
Total lung capacity 247
Tourette's syndrome 367
Toxic dilatation 166
Tracheal position 232
Tracheostomy 327
Traction bronchiectasis 238
Transbronchial lung biopsy 254
Transient ischemic attack 140, 384
   analyze symptoms 140
   clinical problem 140
   focused history 140
   importance of risk factors 385
   in young female 144
      analyze symptoms 144
      differential diagnosis 144
      focused history 144
   lifestyle modification 385
   mechanism of 385
Transjugular intrahepatic portosystemic shunt 272
Transplant rejection 475
Tremor 310
Trichomonas vaginalis 162
Tricuspid regurgitation 196
Trigeminal nerve 319
Trinucleotide repeat expansion 359
Trisomies 13 294
Trust legal department 466
Tubercular ascites 284
Tuberculosis 324, 325
Tuberous sclerosis 19, 20*f*, 294
Turner syndrome 19, 194

U

Ulcer, examination of 58
Ulcerative colitis 166
   exacerbation of 390
   with refusal to admit hospital 390
Ulnar styloidectomy 80
Upper limb 349
   examination of 310
   flexion of 311
Urea and electrolyte 36
Urinary tract infection 67
Urine dipstick 77
Ursodeoxycholic acid 281, 282
Urticaria 14*f*

V

Valsalva maneuver 211
Valve leakage 217
Valve replacement 151, 203
Valve thrombosis 217, 219
Vancomycin 151
Varicella zoster virus 245, 340
Varicose vein 25, 25*f*
Vasculitic lesion 71
Vasculitis 78, 330
Vein harvesting scars 195
Ventilation-perfusion 73
Ventricular failure, right 196
Ventricular hypertrophy, left 50
Ventricular septal defect 222
Ventricular tachycardia 359
Vertebrobasilar infarction 323

Vestibulocochlear nerve 320
Vibration sense 313, 316
Viral hepatitis 272, 277
Viral screening 277
Virchow's node 266
Visceral perforation 307
Visible choroidal pigment 18
Visible peristalsis 165
Visual acuity 40, 92, 96, 142, 317
Visual-evoked potentials 93
Visual field 318
　defect, approach to 325
　testing 93
Vitamin
　B12 266, 341, 349
　　deficiency 93, 326, 334
　D 154
　E 349
　　deficiency 350
　K deficiency 304

Vitiligo 4, 4*f*
Vitreous hemorrhage 102
　analyze symptoms 102
　focused examination 104
Vivid hallucinations and delusions 274
Voltage-gated calcium channel 139
von Hippel–Lindau syndrome 294

W

Waddling gait 321
Warfarin 141, 206
　therapy, signs of 212
Warm periphery 246
Weber's test 320
Weight gain, differential diagnosis of 32
Wernicke's dysphasia 347

Wernicke's encephalopathy 275, 325
Whipple's disease 274
　evidence of 280
Wilson's disease 269, 365, 270
　serum ceruloplasmin for 270
Worms, bag of 6

X

Xanthelasma 23, 23*f*, 194, 195, 266
Xiphisternum-T6 316
X-linked recessive inherited disorder 9

Y

Yellow nail syndrome 239
Yersinia spp. 296

EU GSPR Authorised Reprsentative
Logos Europe, 9 rue Nicolas Poussin
1700, La Rochelle, France
Phone: +33 (0) 6 67 93 73 78
E-mail: contact@logoseurope.eu

www.ingramcontent.com/pod-product-compliance
Ingram Content Group UK Ltd.
Pitfield, Milton Keynes, MK11 3LW, UK
UKHW050430150426
5217IPUK00019B/1320